Anatomy and Physiology of
Domestic Animals

Anatomy and Physiology of Domestic Animals

R. Michael Akers and D. Michael Denbow

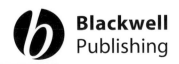

Blackwell
Publishing

R. Michael Akers, Ph.D. completed his B.S. (Biology) and M.S. (Dairy Science) at Virginia Tech and his Ph.D. at Michigan State University in 1980. He is currently the Horace E. and Elizabeth F. Alphin Professor of Dairy Science at Virginia Tech and Department Head of Dairy Science. He and his colleagues and students have co-authored more than 160 original research articles, reviews, and book chapters in the areas of lactation biology and endocrinology. He also authored the book *Lactation and the Mammary Gland,* which was published by Iowa State Press in 2002. He has received numerous university and professional society awards for research excellence, including the Young Scientist, Borden, and Pharmacia and Upjohn Physiology Awards from the American Dairy Science Association and the Animal Growth and Development Award from the American Society of Animal Science. In 2006 he was named a Fellow of the American Dairy Science Association.

D. Michael Denbow, Ph.D. is a professor of Animal Science at Virginia Tech. He completed his B.S. and M.S. in Animal Science at the University of Maryland and his Ph.D. in physiology from North Carolina State University in 1980. He enjoys a reputation as an excellent teacher and researcher. He has received numerous awards for outstanding teaching, including Purina Mills Award for Teaching Excellence, Teaching Award of Merit, National Association of Colleges and Teachers of Agriculture, and the W. E. Wine Award for Excellence in Teaching from Virginia Tech. He has authored or co-authored over 165 papers in the areas of neurophysiology and, especially, control of feed intake in birds.

Blackwell Publishing Professional
2121 State Avenue, Ames, Iowa 50014, USA

Orders: 1-800-862-6657
Office: 1-515-292-0140
Fax: 1-515-292-3348
Web site: www.blackwellprofessional.com

Blackwell Publishing Ltd
9600 Garsington Road, Oxford OX4 2DQ, UK
Tel.: +44 (0)1865 776868

Blackwell Publishing Asia
550 Swanston Street, Carlton, Victoria 3053, Australia
Tel.: +61 (0)3 8359 1011

Authorization to photocopy items for internal or personal use, or the internal or personal use of specific clients, is granted by Blackwell Publishing, provided that the base fee is paid directly to the Copyright Clearance Center, 222 Rosewood Drive, Danvers, MA 01923. For those organizations that have been granted a photocopy license by CCC, a separate system of payments has been arranged. The fee codes for users of the Transactional Reporting Service are ISBN-13: 978-0-8138-0329-6/2008.

First edition, 2008

Library of Congress Cataloging-in-Publication Data
Akers, R. Michael.
   Anatomy and physiology of domestic animals / R. Michael Akers and D. Michael Denbow.
     p. cm.
   Includes bibliographical references and index.
   ISBN-13: 978-0-8138-0329-6 (alk. paper)
   ISBN-10: 0-8138-0329-2 (alk. paper)
 1. Veterinary anatomy. 2. Veterinary physiology. I. Denbow, D. Michael. II. Title.

   SF761.A55 2008
   636.089'2–dc22

2007043408

The last digit is the print number: 9 8 7 6 5 4 3 2

Table of Contents

Preface

In our view, it is virtually impossible to adequately understand or study physiology without consideration of anatomy. Although the fundamental focus of this text is physiology, we strived to include sufficient system, organ, tissue, and cellular anatomy to enable students to better appreciate the integration of both topics—in short, to appreciate that structure and function are intimately interconnected.

The goal of this book is to provide a foundation so that undergraduate students in agricultural and biological sciences will be successful in upper-level specialty courses, such as nutrition, reproduction, lactation, growth biology, biotechnology, and the like. We also anticipate that this text will provide new graduate students with a readily understandable source for review of basic principles.

We thank our wives (Cathy Akers, 37 years and counting; Dr. Cindy Denbow) for their love, support, and understanding through these long hours of figure making, writing, and editing. We also thank our graduate students, colleagues, and students in our classes for inspiration, a helping hand, and lots of questions. We especially thank Ms. Sara Robinson and Dr. Rebecca Splan for preparing several drawings and Drs. Ray Nebel, Frank Robinson, and Frank Gwazdauskas for photographs used in the reproduction chapter.

R. Michael Akers
D. Michael Denbow

Anatomy and Physiology of
Domestic Animals

1 Introduction to anatomy and physiology

Contents

Although there are many good anatomy and physiology texts that focus on humans, there is a paucity of such options for animals. Since animals have physiological and anatomical differences relative to humans, a human text does not do the study of animals justice. Animals walk on four legs, whereas humans walk on two. Ruminant animals have adaptations to their digestive system that make them unique from humans. The respiratory system of birds differs from that of humans, thus making birds able to fly at high altitudes. The focus of this text will be to emphasize the anatomy and physiology of animals in order to appreciate their unique systems.

Anatomy and physiology

Anatomy (derived from the Greek words meaning "to cut open") is the study of the morphology, or structure, of organisms. Therefore, anatomy deals with form rather than function. It can be divided into macroscopic (gross) or microscopic anatomy. Macroscopic anatomy deals with structure that can be seen with the naked eye, whereas microscopic anatomy deals with structure that can be seen only with the aid of a microscope.

Macroscopic anatomy can be approached in different ways. Regional anatomy, as the name implies, deals with all the structures, such as nerves, bones, muscles, blood vessels, etc., in a defined region such as the head or hip. Systemic anatomy entails the study of a given organ system, such as the muscular or skeletal system. It also involves the study of organ systems that are groups of organs that work together for a specific function, such as the digestive or urinary system. Surface anatomy looks at the markings that are visible from the outside. These may include knowledge of the muscles, such as the sternocleidomastoid muscle, in order to be able to find another structure, such as the carotid artery.

Microscopic anatomy includes cytology and histology. Cytology is the study of the structure of individual cells that constitute the smallest units of life. Histology is the study of tissues. Tissues are a collection of specialized cells and their products that perform a specific function. Tissues combine to form organs such as heart, liver, brain, etc., and will be explained in greater detail in Chapter 4.

Developmental anatomy is the study of the changes in structure that occur throughout life. Embryology is a subdivision of developmental anatomy that traces the developmental changes prior to birth. Many systems of the body are not completely developed at birth, hence the need to continue to follow their development after parturition.

Physiology is the study of the function of living systems. While various systems will be presented separately throughout this book, it must be recognized that all systems work together to maintain the normal functioning of an animal. Therefore, the cardiovascular system does not work in isolation from the respiratory or nervous system; instead, systems work in unison to coordinate the distribution of oxygen and removal of carbon dioxide throughout the body. Like anatomy, there are levels of complexity.

Cellular physiology is the study of how cells work. This includes the study of events at the chemical, molecular, and genetic level. Organ physiology includes the study of specific organs, i.e., cardiac or ovarian. Systems physiology includes the study of the function of specific systems, such as the cardiovascular, respiratory, or reproductive systems.

As one studies anatomy and physiology, it will become apparent that structure and function have evolved to complement each other. The complementarity of structure and function is an essential concept to grasp in order to understand how an animal works, and its limitations. The relationship between form and function is evident beginning at the cellular level. For example, the epithelial lining of the small intestine has tight junctions in order to restrict the movement of materials into the body from the gastrointestinal tract, whereas the epithelial lining of capillaries lacks such junctions. The lining of capillaries must be more porous so as to allow solutes to move readily in either direction across the capillary wall in order to nourish the tissue and remove waste products.

As another example, there are structural differences between birds and mammals that allow flight. Birds contain pneumatic bones, i.e., bones that are hollow, which are connected to the respiratory system. These bones include the skull, humerus, clavicle, keel, sacrum, and lumbar vertebrae. In addition, the lumbar and sacral vertebrae are fused as an adaptation for flight.

Levels of organization

The animal body has a complex organization extending from the most microscopic up to the macroscopic (Fig. 1.1). Beginning with the smallest microscopic units of stability, the levels of organization are as follows:

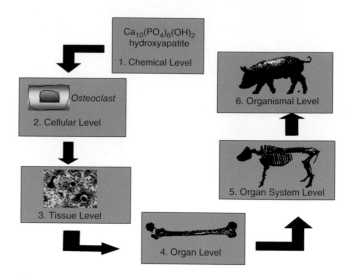

Fig. 1.1.   Levels of organization. 1) Atoms interact to form molecules, which combine to form complex chemicals. 2) Chemicals combine to form cells that can display specific functions depending on the proteins expressed. 3) Cells having a common function combine to form tissue. 4) Tissues combine to perform a common function. 5) Organs can work together for a common function. 6) All the organ systems combine to produce a living animal.

- Chemical level. Atoms are the smallest units of matter that have properties of an element. They combine with covalent bonds to form molecules such as molecular oxygen (O_2), glucose ($C_6H_{12}O_6$), or methane (CH_4). The properties of various chemicals have a major influence on physiology. For example, at a low pH, a chemical may not be ionized and can thus cross a cellular membrane, whereas above a certain pH, the same molecule may be ionized and thus unable to cross a lipid bilayer.
- Cellular level. As the smallest unit of life, cells have various sizes, shapes and properties that allow them to carry out specialized functions. Some cells have cilia that allow them to move materials across their surfaces (i.e., the epithelial lining of the bronchioles), whereas other cells are adapted to store lipid, produce collagen, or contract when stimulated.
- Tissue level. A tissue is a group of cells having a common structure and function. The four types of tissue include muscle, epithelia, nervous, and connective.
- Organ level. Two or more tissues working for a given function form an organ. All four tissue types combine to form skin, the largest organ of the body, or the cochlea in the ear, the smallest organ of the body.

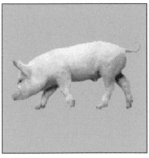

a. IntegumentarySystem: Forms the external covering of the body providing protection, preventing desiccation, supplying sensory information about the environment, synthesizing vitamin D.

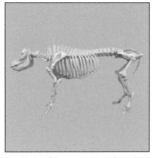

b. Skeletal System: Functions in support, protection, and movement. Also important in blood cell formation and mineral storage.

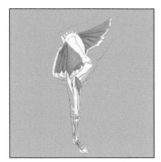

c. Muscular System: Functions in movement, maintains posture, and generates heat.

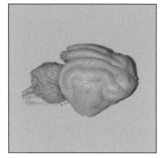

d. Nervous System: Through its functions of sensory input, integration, and motor output, it quickly helps the animal interact with the internal and external environment.

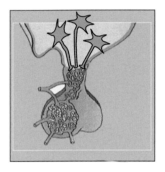

e. Endocrine System: Collectively, all the endocrine-secreting cells; these produce hormones that help maintain the internal environment.

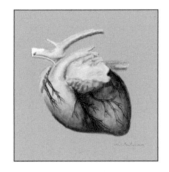

f. Cardiovascular System: Includes blood vessels and the heart, which function to carry nutrients and waste throughout the body

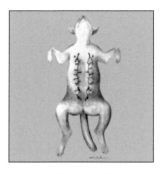

g. Lymphatic System: Returns excess interstitial fluid to the blood and contains phagocytic cells involved in immunity.

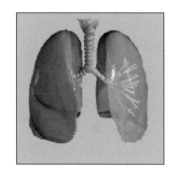

h. Respiratory System: Provides oxygen and eliminates CO_2.

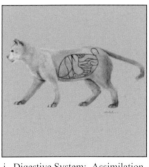

i. Digestive System: Assimilation, breakdown, and absorption of nutrients. Provides important immunological barrier against external environment.

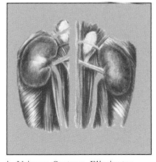

j. Urinary System: Eliminates nitrogenous wastes, maintains fluid and electrolyte balance, and has an endocrine function.

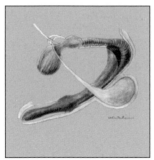

k. Reproductive System: Functions to produce offspring.

Fig. 1.2. Organ systems. The body consists of eleven major organ systems, shown above with examples of their components.

- Organ system level. Organs can work together for a common function. For example, the alimentary canal works with the liver, gall bladder, and pancreas to form part of the digestive system. The pancreas also functions as part of the endocrine system. The organ systems include the integumentary, skeletal, muscular, nervous, endocrine, cardiovascular, lymphatic, respiratory, digestive, urinary, and reproductive systems (Fig. 1.2).
- Organismal level. The organismal level, or the whole animal, includes all of the organ systems that work together to maintain homeostasis.

Homeostasis

The 19th century French physiologist Claude Bernard (1965) coined the term *milieu interieur,* which referred to the relatively constant internal environment, i.e., extracellular fluid, in which cells live. Walter Cannon (1932), a 20th century American physiologist later coined the word *homeostasis,* meaning "unchanging internal environment." While the concept of homeostasis is fundamental to understanding physiology, the term is better understood as a relatively steady state that is maintained within an animal despite a wide range of environmental conditions. In this way, various internal conditions, such as plasma glucose or electrolyte concentrations, or body temperature are maintained within narrow limits through homeostatic mechanisms.

Homeostasis is maintained at all levels of life. Individual cells, for example, control their internal environment via selectively permeable membranes. These membranes will allow the selective movement across the membrane based on such factors as pH, size, or whether there is a specific transport system for that compound. Whole animals maintain their internal environment by a host of behavioral and physiological mechanisms. A behavioral method of regulation may include moving from a sunny area to a shady area in order to decrease body temperature, whereas a physiological method may involve an increase in sweating or panting to accomplish the same goal.

Homeostatic regulatory mechanisms

Elaborate regulatory mechanisms exist to maintain homeostasis. Homeostasis is maintained by the actions of the nervous and endocrine systems that communicate changes in the internal and external environment. The two systems work in conjunction to make relatively rapid or slow changes, respectively. The nervous system responds to immediate, short-term needs such as seen in a reflex arc in which an animal withdraws its foot after stepping on a sharp object. In contrast, the endocrine system generally elicits responses that last hours or days, such as the release of insulin in response to a rise in blood glucose levels.

When regulation occurs at either the cellular, tissue, organ, or organ system level, it is termed autoregulation. For example, the presence of tryptophan in the small intestine will cause the local release of cholecystokinin (CCK), which will cause the pancreas to secrete enzymes. Extrinsic regulation, on the other hand, involves the coordinated action of both the nervous and endocrine systems. Such regulation occurs, for example, during prolonged stress where there is

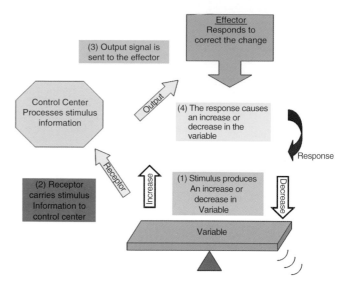

Fig. 1.3. Feedback systems. 1) A stimulus causes a change in a variable (i.e., plasma glucose, blood pressure, heart rate, etc). 2) A receptor senses the change in the variable and sends that information to the control center. 3) The control center compares the level of the variable to a set point, and then initiates appropriate responses to change the variable. 4) The actions of the effectors bring about a change in the variable.

release of norepinephrine, epinephrine, and corticosteroids from the adrenal glands. This results in an increase in blood pressure and a change in blood flow such that there is an increase to skeletal muscle and a decrease to the digestive tract.

The factor being regulated is the variable. The regulatory mechanisms involve a receptor, a control center, and an effector. The receptor is a neuron that senses a change in the environment, called a stimulus. In response to the stimulus, the receptor carries an afferent signal to the control center. The control center has a set point around which the variable is maintained. When the input signal is outside of the range of the set point, an appropriate response is elicited to correct the variable. An efferent signal is then sent to the effector. The effector induces a change in the controlled variable to bring it back to the set point (Fig. 1.3).

Feedback systems

Homeostatic regulatory mechanisms consist of either negative or positive feedback systems. Negative feedback systems are far more common than positive feedback systems.

Negative feedback system

In negative feedback systems, the control system initiates changes that counteract the stimulus (Fig. 1.4). This either reduces or eliminates the stimulus thereby

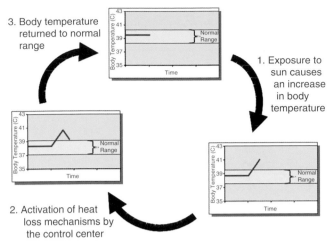

Fig. 1.4. Negative feedback systems. 1) A stimulus causes a change in a variable, in this example an increase in body temperature. 2) Information regarding the increase in body temperature is carried to the control center, which activates appropriate heat loss mechanisms to decrease body temperature toward the set point. 3) As a result of the heat loss mechanisms, body temperature is returned to the set-point value, and homeostasis is maintained.

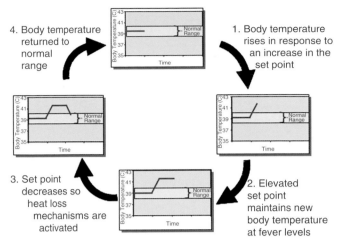

Fig. 1.5. Alterations in the homeostatic set points. The set point for a variable can change. For example, the development of a fever involves a change in the body temperature set point. 1) The control center responds to an increase in the set point for body temperature caused by a pyrogen (i.e., something that causes a fever) and activates heat production pathways. 2) After being raised to the elevated set point, body temperature is maintained at this new level. 3) The set point decreases either because the animal fights off the cause of the fever or has been given an antipyretic, so the set point decreases to the original value. The control center now detects that body temperature is elevated, and it activates heat loss mechanisms. 4) Body temperature is returned to normal.

reestablishing the variable near its set point and maintaining homeostasis. Using body temperature regulation as an example, every animal has a set point for body temperature, with the control center residing in the hypothalamus, a region of the brain. When the body temperature of an animal rises, possibly due to exposure to the sun, the warm receptors located in the skin and hypothalamus sense a rise in temperature and send a signal to the hypothalamus. The hypothalamus compares these signals to the set point, and then activates heat loss mechanisms (effectors) such as sweating and vasodilation. Sweating results in evaporative cooling while vasodilation increases the blood flow to the skin where heat is lost to the environment through radiation, conduction, and convection. The effector response results in a decrease in temperature back toward the set point.

While the negative feedback system acts to correct changes from the set point, it is also common for the set point to change under various conditions periodically throughout the day. When an animal gets a fever, the set point for body temperature increases. This results in the activation of heat production pathways, including shivering and vasoconstriction (Fig. 1.5). When the set point returns to normal, the animal activates the heat loss mechanisms.

Positive feedback system

In response to a stimulus, the animal elicits regulatory mechanisms that augment or exaggerate the effect.

This creates a regulatory cycle in which the response causes an augmentation of the stimulus, which further increases the response. While positive feedback systems are rare, there are situations where they prove beneficial. In the case of blood clotting, an injured blood vessel secretes factors that attract platelets to that site. These platelets secrete factors that attract more platelets, and thus a positive cascade begins to occur. While this is beneficial in preventing the loss of blood, if left unchecked, the clotting process would continue until all the blood in the body was clotted, resulting in death.

Childbirth is another classic example of a positive feedback system. Near the time of parturition, oxytocin is produced by the fetus, which, along with prostaglandins, initiates uterine contractions. The uterine contractions cause the hypothalamus of the mother to release more oxytocin causing greater uterine contractions. Thus a positive feedback loop is initiated.

Anatomical nomenclature

As with any field of science, anatomy has its own language. It is necessary to know this language in order to describe structures and events. When trying to describe the location of the femur, simply saying

Table 1.1. Directional and positional terms.

Term	Meaning	Example
Dorsal	Toward the back; also, below the proximal ends of the carpus and tarsus, dorsal means toward the head (i.e., *dorsal* replaces *cranial*)	The vertebral column is dorsal to the sternum.
Ventral	Toward the belly	The udder is ventral to the tail.
Cranial	Toward the head	The neck is cranial to the tail.
Caudal	Toward the tail	The tail is caudal to the head.
Rostral	Part of the head closer to the nose	The beak is rostral to the ear.
Proximal	Near the trunk or origin of the limb	The elbow is proximal to the ankle.
Distal	Farther from the trunk	The ankle is distal to the elbow.
Palmar	Below the proximal ends of the carpus, *palmar* replaces *caudal*	The dewclaws are on the palmar surface of the forelimb.
Plantar	Below the proximal ends of the tarsus, *plantar* replaces *caudal*	The dewclaws of the hindlimb are on the plantar surface of the foot.
Medial	Toward the longitudinal axis (midline)	The sternum is medial to the limbs.
Lateral	Away from the longitudinal axis	The scapula lies lateral to the spine.
Superficial	Nearer the body surface	The skin is superficial to the ribs.
Deep	Farther from the body surface	The heart is deep to the ribs.
Axial and abaxial	Restricted to the digits, these terms indicate position relative to the longitudinal axis of the limb; axial and abaxial are closer and further to the longitudinal axis, respectively	The lateral edge of the hoof is abaxial to the phalanges.

that it is "in the back leg and located before the tibia and fibula" will not suffice.

Directional and positional terms

Anatomical terms are used to describe an animal that is in the anatomical position. In the case of humans that are biped (i.e., walk on two legs), this means standing with the arms hanging by the side and the palms rotated forward. For animals that are quadruped (i.e., walk on four legs), anatomical position entails standing on all four limbs.

Directional and positional terms are presented in Table 1.1. The use of such terms allows for more precision while using fewer words to describe body structures. For example, one might say, "The knee is located on the front leg approximately halfway between the trunk and the hoof." With directional and positional terms, one can say "The knee is located distal to the femur and proximal to the tibia and fibula."

These terms can have different meanings when referring to humans as opposed to animals. While dorsal and posterior mean toward the back or spinal column in humans, dorsal means toward the spinal cord in a quadruped and posterior means toward the tail.

Body planes

When talking about anatomical locations, it is necessary to take into account the three-dimensional nature of an animal. The body can be sectioned, or cut, in all three planes. Knowing which plane one is observing when looking at a cross section gives knowledge of the location of various structures. Using the horse as an example, the terms are further depicted in Fig. 1.6.

A sagittal plane divides the body into right and left parts along the longitudinal axis (Table 1.2; Fig. 1.6). If the plane is exactly along the midline of the longitudinal axis, it is said to be a median, or midsagittal, plane. Any sagittal plane other than the midsagittal is said to be a parasagittal (*para* = near) plane.

A frontal (dorsal) plane runs longitudinally and passes through the body parallel to its dorsal surface and at a right angle to the median plane. In other words, it divides an animal into a dorsal and ventral portion and runs parallel to the ground. In humans, such a plane runs perpendicular to the ground.

A transverse plane runs perpendicular to the long axis of the structure. A transverse plane can divide an animal into a cranial and caudal half, or it can divide a limb into a proximal and distal section.

Table 1.2.   Body planes.

Orientation of Plane	Plane	Description
Perpendicular to long axis	Transverse	Divides the body into cranial and caudal parts; also crosses an organ or limb at a right angle to its long axis
Parallel to long axis	Median (midsagittal)	Divides body into equal right and left halves
	Sagittal	Divides body into unequal right and left halves
	Frontal (dorsal)	Longitudinal plane passing through the body parallel to dorsal surface and at right angles to the median plane

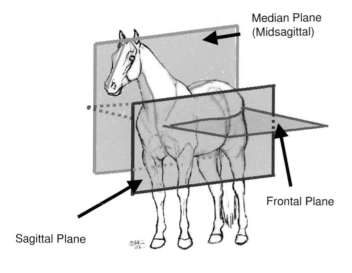

Median Plane (Midsagittal)

Frontal Plane

Sagittal Plane

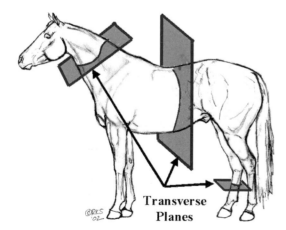

Transverse Planes

Fig. 1.6.   Planes of the body. The three major planes (frontal, transverse, and sagittal) are shown.

Body cavities and membranes

A median view of an animal will reveal two cavities, the dorsal and ventral. The dorsal cavity protects the brain and spinal cord and contains the cranial cavity within the skull and the vertebral, or spinal, cavity that is found within the vertebral column. The brain and the spinal cord are continuous; therefore, the cranial and vertebral cavities are also continuous.

When looking down the longitudinal axis, the trunk of the animal can be divided into three cavities. The thoracic cavity is surrounded by the ribs and muscles of the chest. It can be further subdivided into the pleural cavities, each of which houses a lung, and the mediastinum, which is located medially between the lungs and contains the pericardial cavity. The mediastinum also houses the esophagus and trachea.

The abdominopelvic cavity is separated from the thoracic cavity by the diaphragm. The abdominopelvic cavity has two components: the abdominal cavity that contains, among others, the stomach, intestines, spleen, and liver, as well as the more caudal pelvic cavity. The pelvic cavity is surrounded by the bones of the pelvis and contains the bladder, part of the reproductive organs, and rectum.

The walls of the ventral body cavities, as well as the surface of the visceral organs, are covered by a thin, double-layer membrane called the serosa, or serous membrane. The portion of the serosa lining the body cavity is called the parietal (*parie* = wall) serosa and the portion lining the organ is the visceral serosa.

The best way to visualize the relationship between the two layers of the serosa is to imagine pushing your fist into an inflated balloon. The layer of the balloon closest to your fist would be equivalent to the visceral serosa; that part of the balloon on the outside would represent the parietal serosa. The two serosal membranes each secrete serosal fluid into the space between the two layers. This fluid acts as a lubricant so as to reduce the friction between the parietal and visceral serosa as they slide across one another. This is important when one considers how often the heart beats or the lungs inflate, during which time the visceral and parietal serosa slide across one another.

The serosa membranes have specific names depending on their location. When found surrounding the heart, it is called the pericardium (*peri* = around + *kardia* = heart). Therefore, the parietal pericardium lines the pericardial cavity while the visceral pericardium adheres to the heart. The pleura adheres to the lungs and lines the thoracic cavity whereas the peritoneum lines the abdominopelvic cavity and adheres to the visceral organs.

References

Bernard, C. 1965. An Introduction to the Study of Experimental Medicine. Great Books Foundation, Inc., Chicago.

Cannon, W.B. 1932. The Wisdom of the Body. Norton, New York.

2 The cell: the common physiological denominator

Contents

All of the physiological systems, e.g., digestive, respiratory, or cardiovascular depend on the actions and activities of cells. Groups of cells and their products coalesce to create the four basic tissue types [epithelial, neural, muscular, or connective tissue]. Attributes of these tissues will be discussed in detail in Chapter 4. Combinations of these tissues produce organs. Functionally related organs are arranged into physiological systems. To illustrate, the digestive system includes the mouth and oral cavity, esophagus, stomach, small intestine, and large intestine. This tube-within-a-tube organization allows for acquisition of food, physical mastication, chemical digestion, and ultimately absorption of nutrients across the lining of the GI tract into the blood stream. The mature GI tract has elements of each of the four major tissue types.

The internal lining, the mucosa (an example of epithelial tissue), is composed of a layer of specialized epithelial cells called enterocytes. Enterocytes rest upon a thin layer of extracellular proteins, the basement membrane. The mucosal layer also includes other specialized connective tissue elements, including the structurally important proteins collagen, elastin, and protein-carbohydrate hybrid molecules, called proteoglycans. This tissue region also has a population of scattered smooth muscle cells, the muscularis mucosa, and a distinctive connective tissue called the lamina propria. The submucosa appears between the enterocytes and the next major tissue layer, the muscularis, and provides a passageway for capillaries and lymphatic vessels. Exocrine glands, which produce secretions destined for the lumen of the GI tract, also reside here. Closer to the outer circumference of the tract, there are two closely aligned, dense layers of smooth muscle cells called the muscularis externa. The innermost layers of smooth muscle cells are arranged around the circumference of the GI tract and the outer layers oriented along the longitudinal axis of the GI tract. The coordinated contraction and relaxation of these smooth muscle cell layers provide for mixing and movement of gut contents. A thin layer of epithelial cells called the serosa covers the outside of the GI tract. This layer is continuous with the mesentery, which provides a means for entrance of veins, arteries, and nerve fibers into the muscularis externa and submucosa and for general support via attachment to ligaments.

Despite the complexity of tissue and cell types in the GI tract, and requirement of multiple cell and tissue types for maximum efficiency, the essential feature of the GI tract depends on the actions of the lining cells of the mucosa, the enterocytes. Consequently, understanding physiological systems and principles ultimately should begin with an appreciation of cellular physiology and function. A common theme that we will emphasize repeatedly is that structure and function go together. This idea will become apparent at multiple levels of organization—molecular, cellular, organ, and system. Our story begins with a discussion of the cell.

Once past the primordial stem cell stage of the embryo, cells acquire varying degrees of differentiation. Differentiation produces structural and functional changes in the cells to better equip them for their particular function. For many years dogma was that once cells became differentiated it was impossible to reprogram them so that these cells or their daughters could be induced to follow a different path. Under usual circumstances this likely is true; however, it is also evident that advances in cell and molecular biology have called this dogma into question. Development of the cloned sheep Dolly in 1996 was achieved using cultured fibroblasts. Other examples of animals cloned from fully differentiated cells have been recently reported. These examples serve to emphasize an unexpected plasticity of cells. It may be possible in the future to bioengineer replacements for damaged or diseased organs or tissues as more is learned about the rules governing cell growth and differentiation.

Cellular organelles

Because mammals are composed largely of water (~70%), cellular biochemistry is governed by interactions of physiologically important molecules and water of the cell cytoplasm, the water surrounding the cells (interstitial fluid), or the aqueous environment of various cellular organelles. We all appreciate, at least in a general sense, that water is essential to our survival. But remembering some of the physical-chemical attributes of water will emphasize its physiological relevance. Water is an excellent solvent for many, but not all, physiologically important molecules. Blood

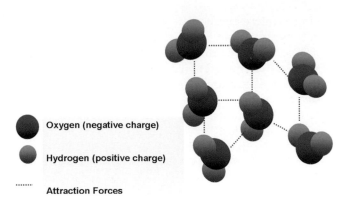

Oxygen (negative charge)

Hydrogen (positive charge)

······ Attraction Forces

Fig. 2.1. Hydrogen bonds and water. Because of its dipole moment there is a net negative charge associated with the oxygen atoms of the water molecule. This charge separation allows water molecules to organize to form attractant bonds with other water molecules. This property explains many of the attributes of water as the so-called universal solvent and the ability of other polar molecules to readily dissolve in water.

plasma (about 90% water) transports a myriad of dissolved nutrients (e.g., glucose, amino acids), minerals (e.g., Na, Cl, K) and gases (e.g., O_2, CO_2). Intra- and intercellular water is similarly filled with solutes. The urinary system maintains body water reserves to insure that blood pressure and volume are adequate as well as proper osmolarity. Water is touted as the biological universal solvent—but why? The answer is the abundance and structure of the water molecule. The chemical formula for water (H_2O) is well known, but Figure 2.1 illustrates that water has a distinct dipole moment. This means that there is unequal sharing of electrons between the oxygen and hydrogen atoms of the molecule so that the molecule is polarized. The oxygen atom, because of its greater capacity to attract electrons, has a slight negative charge. The hydrogen atoms therefore have a slight positive charge. This polarity causes the water molecules to arrange themselves so that they form hydrogen bonds (opposite charges attract). Hydrogen bonds, while weak compared with covalent chemical bonds, are very important physiologically because of their abundance. They also are important in attractions between many macromolecules. For example, the two strands of intact DNA are held together by hydrogen bonds between base pairs.

This feature explains the common sense example of oils not dissolving in water. Most common oils or lipids are composed of hydrocarbon chains that exhibit equal sharing of electrons between atoms and therefore there is no polarity. Nonpolar molecules cannot associate with water and are described as hydrophobic (water-fearing). Polar molecules associate with water and are described as a hydrophilic (water-loving). Interestingly, many macromolecules have both hydrophobic and hydrophilic regions. For example, the three-dimensional shape of a protein in the cell is determined by physical-chemical forces that act to shelter groupings of hydrophobic amino acids away from water while at the same time allowing hydrophilic amino acids hydrogen-bonding interactions with water. This fundamental property of water means that it can form highly oriented layers or shells around charged areas of large macromolecules, e.g., nucleic acids, proteins, or proteoglycans, and thereby impact structure and organization. Biochemists can take advantage of these properties to isolate macromolecules from homogenates of tissues or cells. For example, if the shielding of protein or nucleic acid charges by water is reduced by adding a watermiscible solvent that reduces hydrogen bonding, protein-protein or nucleic acid interactions are enhanced and precipitation of the macromolecules occurs. This is often achieved by the addition of ethanol or acetone.

Other physiologically important properties of water include specific heat, thermal conductance, and surface properties. Briefly, water can absorb substantial amounts of heat energy without a drastic change in temperature. Alternatively, a significant amount of heat energy can be lost without a dramatic effect on temperature. This buffering capacity is important since many biochemical processes are temperature sensitive. Evolutionarily, the greater success of warm-blooded mammals compared with cold-blooded animals reflects the appearance of physiological mechanisms to maintain body temperature, and therefore water temperature. Since the water content of animal tissues is so high, the total capacity to store heat energy is correspondingly high. Energy needed to vaporize water is also relatively high. Think of how quickly you feel the cool effect of an alcohol swab on your skin compared with a simple water-moistened swab. This property can be viewed as both an advantage and a disadvantage, depending on the physiological circumstances. In hot environments or with excessive work, thermoregulation depends on sweating or panting in many animals to reduce the thermal load. Too much loss and there is dehydration. New visitors to hot, dry desert environments must be admonished to drink often to make up for unrecognized insensible water losses. Many animals have adapted specialized physiological mechanisms and behaviors to minimize insensible water loss and to maximize efficient use of water. As another example, seal pups reared in polar seas (in many respects a "desert" environment with regard to water availability), depend on water derived from the metabolism of high-fat milk to supply much of their water requirement. Consider the impact of water in accumulation of milk in the mammary gland, blood in the cardiovascular system, or perhaps urine production. There are numerous moist surfaces on many organs. The surface properties of water affect fluid movement and the capacity of tissue surfaces to interact. This phenomenon is evident in the meniscus characteristic of a test tube filled with water. Another common sense example is the appearance of beads of rainwater on the surface of a waxed car; the wax is very hydrophobic so the molecules of water in the droplet are much more attracted to one another. The spherical shape is a reflection of the physics of attractions between the molecules and the fact that the sphere is the optimal shape to minimize forces. Surface tension describes these forces and is expressed in force per length or Newtons (N) per meter. Pure water has a surface tension of 7 N/m, but dilute detergent reduces this to about 4 N/m. Surface properties of water play a critical role in many physiological processes. Surface acting amphiathic molecules reduce surface tension. These molecules have distinct polar and nonpolar domains. When placed onto a moist surface environment, the molecules disrupt association between water molecules, and at liquid-vapor interfaces limit water-to-water connections and thus the strength of the surface tension. For example, the capacity of the lung alveoli to expand in the newborn requires that the surfaces of the epithelial cells lining the internal surface of the alveolar air sacs be coated with a surfactant. This minimizes the attraction of the surfaces and therefore allows expansion. In fact, the surface tension of lung extracts can be as low as 0.5 N/m. Specialized alveolar cells (Type II cells) scattered among the normal epithelial cells secrete surfactant. Production is stimulated by the secretion of glucocorticoids (steroid hormones produced in the adrenal gland), near the time of parturition. Animals that are born prematurely often have respiratory problems because of failed surfactant production.

Membrane structure and organization

Structures found inside cells are called organelles. Examples include the nucleus, mitochondria, and ribosomes. Most organelles are membrane covered. Other organelles, secretory vesicles, and lysosomes, for example, are unique because of their membrane-bound contents. Thus, understanding membranes is important to understand physiology. We begin with lipids and especially phospholipids. Lipids are very heterogeneous but common attributes include: 1) being practically nonsoluble in water but 2) soluble in nonpolar organic solvents such as ether, ethanol, or chloroform. Lipids include fats, oils, waxes, and related

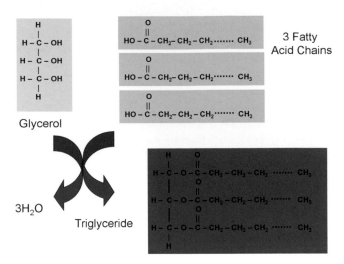

Fig. 2.2.   Triglyceride synthesis and structure.

Table 2.1.   Common saturated fatty acids.

Fatty Acid	Formula	Attributes
Acetic	CH_3COOH	Major end product of rumen fermentation, energy source for ATP production
Propionic	C_2H_5COOH	End product of rumen fermentation, major precursor for gluconeogenesis
Butyric	C_3H_7COOH	Major end product of rumen fermentation
Caproic	$C_5H_{11}COOH$	Minor end product of rumen fermentation
Caprylic	$C_7H_{15}COOH$	Small amounts in many fats
Palmitic	$C_{15}H_{31}COOH$	Common in all animal and plant fats
Stearic	$C_{17}H_{35}COOH$	Common in all animal and plant fats

compounds. Figure 2.2 shows the general structure of molecules necessary to produce common fats called triacylglycerols or triglycerides.

Neutral fats are esters composed of two building blocks, glycerol and fatty acids. Glycerol is a 3-carbon alcohol that is most often derived from the catabolism of the common hexose sugar glucose. Fatty acid molecules are linear hydrocarbon chains with a carboxylic acid moiety at one end. This residue is the most reactive or functional group of the molecule. Fatty acids vary in length, but the glycerol backbone of the triglyceride is constant. Fatty acids also vary with respect to the number of double bonds between carbon atoms. Those with no double bonds are called saturated fatty acids, those with a single double bond are monosaturated, and those with more than one are polysaturated fatty acids. The degree of saturation and length of the fatty acids affect their properties. For example, the shorter chain members <6 carbons are water soluble and volatile, but longer fatty acids are neither soluble nor volatile. Table 2.1 gives a listing of some of the common saturated fatty acids, structural formulae, and common features. Common names of many of the fatty acids are widely used, but systemic names make deduction of structure easier. To illustrate, palmitic acid is the common name for the 16-carbon fatty acid hexadecanoic acid. This indicates the carboxylic acid of hexadecane (*hexa* meaning 6 and *dec* meaning 10 and *ane* indicating an alkane). This fatty acid is also written as $C_{16:0}$, which means there are 16 carbons and 0 double bonds. Formally, triglycerides are called triacyl esters and are created from the alcohol glycerol and any of a number of particular fatty acids. The reaction involves a dehydration synthesis reaction (water is liberated, e.g., remember the earlier comment about seal pups getting water from milk fat catabo-

lism) between a carbon of the glycerol and the carboxylic acid residue of each of the fatty acid chains to create the ester linkage illustrated by this equation:

$$R-\overset{\overset{\text{O}}{\|}}{C}-OH + HO-R \longrightarrow R-\overset{\overset{\text{O}}{\|}}{C}-O-R$$

Carboxylic Acid   Alcohol   Ester

Fluid mosaic model

Glycerol linked with three fatty acids creates a triglyceride, two fatty acids create a diglyceride, and a single fatty acid creates a monoglyceride. Only a few naturally occurring triglycerides have the same fatty acid in all three ester positions. Most are mixed acylglycerols. Phospholipids demonstrated by the general formula shown in Figure 2.3, also contain a phosphoric acid residue. The alcohol moiety in many of the phospholipids is also glycerol, but for others, e.g., the sphingophospholipids, the alcohol is sphingosine. Phospholipids are often drawn in the form of a ball to represent the polar head of the molecule and two trailing tails to represent the nonpolar hydrocarbon chains of the fatty acids. Along with associated proteins and some other lipids, the capacity of the phospholipids to spontaneously form bilayers is essential to understanding the formation of all of the cellular membranes. The now-classic organization of the plasma membrane is described as a fluid mosaic model. This consists of a mosaic of globular proteins suspended in a sea of phospholipids. Membranes are organized with the polar heads of two layers of phospholipids oriented either toward the aqueous environment of teins associated with the membranes are oriented within either the outer or inner membrane leaflets. Other proteins completely span the membrane. Whatever their specific arrangement these proteins are called integral membrane proteins. Those that span the membrane are positioned so that fewer polar amino acids occur within the central hydrocarbon tails of the fatty acid chains, with polar amino acids located with the polar heads or aqueous surfaces of the membrane. Examples of complex plasma membrane proteins include receptors for hormones or growth factors and those required for transport of metabolites and nutrients.

Cellular membranes are fluid, dynamic, and active structures. Membrane components are also interchangeable between many cellular components. For example, in the mammary gland of a lactating mammal, milk components are packaged into secretory vesicles within the Golgi apparatus. These product-containing vesicles progressively make their way to the apical surface of the cell where their contents are released into the storage spaces of the mammary gland by the process of exocytosis. The membrane surrounding the vesicles becomes part of the plasma membrane. Furthermore, lipid droplets synthesized in the cells progressively enlarge and also migrate to the apical surface of the cells for secretion. However, in this case the droplets literally begin to protrude from the cells and become surrounded by the plasma membrane. This continues until droplets pinch off with the former plasma membrane now encapsulating the droplet. The membrane is now referred to as a milk fat globule membrane but its origin was the plasma membrane of the cell. Figure 2.4 illustrates the organelles and secretion activity of such a mammary epithelial cell. Similar events would be occurring in many other secretory cells, e.g., pancreas, liver, salivary gland, pituitary gland.

Microscopy techniques

Beginning with invention of the light microscope in the 1600s and progressive improvements in cell preservation, techniques to embed tissue in materials for sectioning, and staining to identify specific cellular components, much has been learned about cell structure and function. However, even simple smears of dislodged isolated cells can be very useful in physiological or clinical situations. The Pap smear is routinely used in women's health to monitor the cells of the cervix. The morphology of the cells is classified to determine whether any of the cells appear to have precancerous attributes, e.g., altered nuclear morphology or staining characteristics. Another example is the blood smear, i.e., a small sample of blood is spread and dried on a microscope slide and then stained.

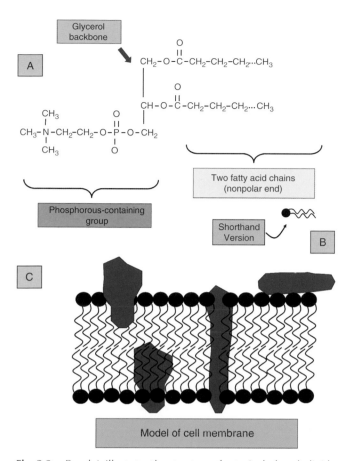

Fig. 2.3. Panel A illustrates the structure of a typical phospholipid. Similarity to triglyceride structure is apparent. Panel B gives a common shorthand version of the phospholipid structure that is often used to demonstrate the arrangement of phospholipids to create the bilayer organization of cellular membranes. Panel C shows the organization of both phospholipids and proteins within a typical membrane. The polar phospholipid heads are oriented toward aqueous environments either outside the cell or toward the cytoplasm of the cell. In contrast, the hydrophobic, hydrocarbon tails of the phospholipids interact with each other in the center of the bilayer. Various membrane-associated proteins (indicated by the dark blue structures) orient either with the hydrophobic center of the bilayer or with the more hydrophilic outer region of the membrane, depending on the nature of the protein.

the interstitial fluid or toward the aqueous environment of the cytoplasm. The hydrophilic hydrocarbon chains of the fatty acids interact so that the membrane has a trilaminar appearance, phospholipid heads on either side with fatty acid tails in the center. This organization is apparent in well-preserved tissues, embedded in plastic resins thinly sectioned (~900 nm) and prepared for examination in an electron microscope. This is sometimes likened to a peanut butter sandwich with the peanut butter as the tails and the two slices of bread the phospholipid heads. This fundamental structure is true for all cellular membranes, but there are differences in the specific composition, e.g., the Golgi membranes versus the plasma membrane. Pro-

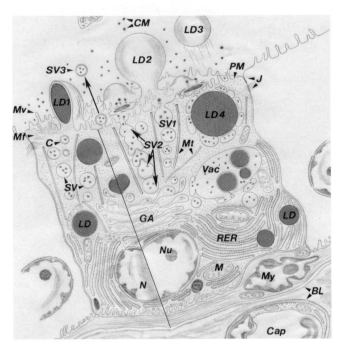

Fig. 2.4. Diagram to illustrate major pathways for cellular synthesis and secretion. Milk precursors in capillaries (Cap) are transported across the endothelial cells and basal lamina (BL) to the interalveolar connective tissue. Nutrients pass across the alveolar BL and/or myoepithelium (My), across the basal plasma membrane (PM), and into the cytoplasm. Milk proteins are synthesized in the rough endoplasmic reticulum (RER), enter the RER lumena, and are transported to the Golgi (GA) for processing and packaging. In typical exocytosis the secretory vesicles (SV) with casein micelles (CM) and lactose leave the Golgi, translocate to the apical PM, and release contents of the vesicle (SV1). Alternatively, vesicles can fuse to form chains for secretion (SV2) or fuse with release of double membrane bound micelles (SV3). Milk lipid is synthesized in the region of the RER and as droplets grow they also translocate to the apical PM. These droplets are enveloped by PM and protrude from the cell (LD1), and are pinched off from the cell into the lumen (LD2) and into the lumen (LD3). It is also possible that SV can fuse around lipid droplets, with other droplets, and with the apical PM in groups (LD4). Lipid droplets might also be released via coalesced secretion vacuoles (Vac). Other features include mitochondria (M), nucleus (N), nucleolus (Nu), microtubules (Mt), microfilaments (Mf), coated vesicles (C), and tight junctions (J). Diagram modified from Nickerson and Akers, 1984.

Such smears are cover-slipped and a differential count performed. In this procedure, the slide is scanned in a set pattern and the first 100 white blood cells encountered identified (lymphocyte, neutrophils, etc.) and tabulated. This information is used to produce a distribution profile of the types of leucocytes in the sample. For example, the horse averages about 55% neutrophils, 35% lymphocytes, 5% monocytes, 3% eosinophils, and 1% or fewer basophils. Changes in these proportions can reflect various diseases. What would be your prediction about a classmate with mononucleosis or a cat with leukemia?

Table 2.2. Relationship between MSCC, DHI cell counts score, and milk production in dairy cows.

MSCC	DHI Score	Milk Yield Daily (kg)	Milk Yield 305 d (kg)
12,500	0	29.2	8906
25,000	1	28.6	8723
50,000	2	28.0	8540
100,000	3	27.4	8357
200,000	4	26.9	8205
400,000	5	26.2	7991
800,000	6	25.4	7747
1,600,000	7	24.6	7503
3,200,000	8	23.6	7198
6,400,000	9	22.5	6863

Adapted from Jones et al., 1884.

In dairy animals, mastitis status (mastitis is inflammation of the mammary gland) is evaluated by the presence and number of leukocytes in the milk. The technology used is based on a well-characterized relationship between cell number and the amount of a specific dye that binds to DNA. As the cell number increases in the milk sample, the amount of dye binding increases proportionally. Although these assays are now automated, the milk smear is used to calibrate these machines. Table 2.2 illustrates the relationship between milk somatic cell count and milk production.

In some experimental situations, it is useful to know the stage of the estrus cycle. For many laboratory animals it is problematic to collect a sufficient number of repetitive blood samples to measure reproductive hormones (estrogen, progesterone, follicle-stimulating hormone, luteinizing hormone) for this purpose. However, daily vaginal smears can be used to evaluate the stage of the estrus cycle. The number of cornified epithelial cells and leukocytes varies according to the stage of the estrus cycle, so changes in these cellular profiles can be used to determine the stage of estrus cycle.

Although information obtained from smears of various cells is useful, the technique is limited because most cells are part of tissues. More importantly, the organization and differentiation of the various cell types and their products is fundamental to understanding the physiology of a tissue or organ. For this evaluation it is necessary to infiltrate the tissue and cells with a medium that is sufficiently solid to allow sections thin enough for light to penetrate to be prepared. The most common embedding medium is paraffin wax. Since tissues and cells are largely water based, fresh tissues are first preserved or fixed in an aqueous solution containing chemicals that cross-link major cell structures and macromolecules. These include formalin, formaldehyde, glutaraldehyde, and others. After a period of fixation, the tissues are dehydrated by transferring the tissue through a series of increasing concentrations of ethanol, and then into xylene—a mixture of xylene and paraffin—and finally into pure paraffin. This gradual process allows the water to first be replaced by ethanol, and then the ethanol by xylene, and finally the xylene by paraffin. The tissue blocks are submerged in additional paraffin in a mold and allowed to harden. This can be imagined by thinking of the wick in the center of a candle as being the processed tissue. If the candle is carefully sliced in cross section a piece of the wick would be in the center of each slice, representing the fixed embedded tissue. The slicing of the tissue blocks needs to be relatively precise and uniform. Embedded blocks of tissue are sliced in a machine called a microtome. The machine uses a thin steel blade, much like a razor blade, and the sections, which are cut one at a time, usually come off in a ribbon. The sections are floated on a water bath and then transferred to a microscope slide. Once the sections are dried, the slides are generally dipped in xylene and processed back to an aqueous environment to allow the sections to be stained. The staining allows structures to be seen in a standard bright field microscope. H&E or hematoxylin and eosin are very common stains. This technique makes the cell nuclei dark blue, the cytoplasm various shades of blue to pink, and extracellular components pink to red. Most histological slides used in physiological classes are H&E stained. Many other stains have been developed for specific uses and examples are given in various sections of the text. One especially exciting recent innovation in tissue staining is the use of specific antibodies to localize proteins within particular cells or even within particular cellular organelles. Figure 2.5 shows tissue blocks, molds, and processed sections for tissue embedded in paraffin.

Despite the widespread use of paraffin-embedded tissue sections and the rich experimental and pathological history with this technique, there are serious limitations. One of these is that tissue sections thinner than about 5 microns cannot be easily prepared. A reasonable approximation of an epithelial cell is about $10 \times 10 \times 10$ microns. This means that for the study of intracellular organelles the sections are too thick and it becomes difficult to distinguish these structures. These limitations allowed for the development of plastic resins that could be used for embedding cells and tissues. With subsequent development of specialized microtones designed to use pieces of fractured glass or even diamond knives, it became possible to section fixed tissues embedded in plastic very thin indeed. In fact, for light microscopic study, sections of 0.5 to 1 micron in thickness can be easily prepared. To distinguish these sections from the paraffin blocks these are often called semithin sections.

Perhaps more importantly these breakthroughs allowed even thinner sections to be examined using the electron microscope. While a detailed consideration of the electron microscope is beyond the scope of our text, some analogy with the readily understood light microscope is useful. The standard compound microscope is essentially a two-part magnifying system in which the specimen is first magnified by the lens in the objective barrel and second by the lens of the eyepiece or ocular. The total magnification is the product of the magnification of the objective lens used and that of the eyepiece. For example, using a 20× objective lens with a typical 10× eyepiece produces an image that is 200-fold greater than the original. The specimen is placed on a stage below the objective lens. Light is then directed from a light source, through an aperture, and then a substage condenser and through the specimen. Light rays from the specimen pass through the objective lens and are focused for view through the eyepieces. This is accomplished mechanically by raising or lowering the position of the objective lens relative to the specimen. Resolution is the degree of separation that can be seen between adjacent points in a specimen—in other words, the degree of detail. The smaller the distance that can be distinguished between two points, the greater the detail in the image. With the unaided eye, points appear as independent structures only if a distance of 0.2 mm or 200 µm separates them, but with a good microscope points as close as 0.25 µm can be distinguished. Ultimately resolution of the brightfield microscope is limited by the wavelength of light and sample preparation. The maximum useful magnification of the light microscope is about 1400-fold. Images can be reproduced to larger sizes in the printing process, but this does not increase true resolution.

In the electron microscope, a beam of electrons replaces the beam of light. The sample (now only about 900 nanometers in thickness) is positioned on a copper grid and the grid is inserted into a sealed chamber and placed under vacuum. A beam of electrons passes through the sample. To increase the electron density of the sample, the tissue is treated with heavy metals (usually lead citrate or uranyl acetate), which bind with macromolecules in the sample and improves sample resolution. The electron beam penetrates the tissue located in the open spaces of the grid, and the image produced is brought into focus by altering the voltage applied to a series of electromagnets located on either side of the column that houses the electron beam. The image is viewed first on a phosphorescent screen and the image is saved by positioning and exposing film. The film is developed and images of the specimen are prepared by making

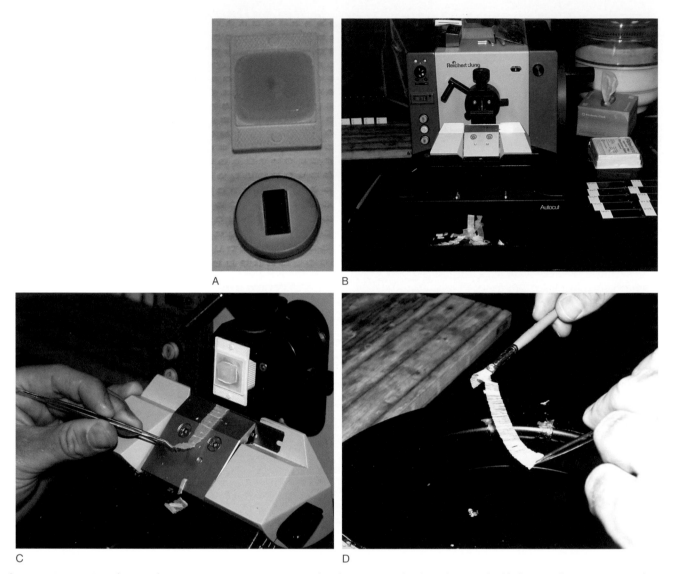

Fig. 2.5. Preparation of tissues for microscopic examination. Panel A shows tissues that have been embedded in paraffin (upper) or in plastic (lower) for preparation of sections for light microscopy. The tissue in the paraffin block is visible as a faint yellow mass in the center. The width of the block is about the size of a U.S. quarter. The tissue in the lower plastic block is not visible but occupies a position near the center of the block. Panel B shows a view of a typical microtome for preparation of paraffin-embedded tissues. Panel C shows a paraffin-embedded tissue block mounted in the microtome. With each up-and-down motion of the microtome, the block of tissue moves past a stationary knife so that a ribbon of serial sections (typically, 5 μm thick) is cut. The ribbon of sections is transferred to a water bath (Panel D) and ultimately floated onto a microscope slide. The sections are allowed to dry, and then the paraffin is removed, and the sections are hydrated, stained, and subsequently cover-slipped for examination. Processing of tissue embedded in plastic resins follows a similar procedure but thinner sections (~0.5 μm) can be prepared for light microscopy, and with the proper microtome, sections thin enough for electron microscopy can be prepared.

photographic prints from the film. The process as described is called transmission electron microscopy. A similar process called scanning electron microscopy relies on images produced by coating surfaces, often with a thin layer of gold. Detailed images of intracellular structure became possible only with electron microscopy; several examples are included along with descriptions of cell organelles. Figure 2.6 shows a block of tissue prepared for study in an electron microscopy; one of the small copper grids; and an example of an exposed, developed photographic plate.

Organelles of the cytoplasm

While many complete texts are devoted to aspects of cell and molecular biology, a basic appreciation of cell structures is important in understanding cellular physiology and ultimately tissue, organ, and systems level physiology. It is imperative to appreciate that essentially all organelles are found in all cells. However, the total number and arrangement of these organelles vary markedly from cell type to cell type. Numbers can also change dramatically within a given cell type

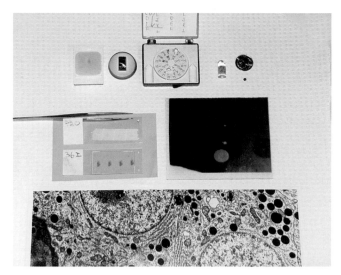

Fig. 2.6. Comparisons between tissue preparation for light microscopy and transmission electron microscopy. The upper row shows samples prepared for paraffin, plastic, and electron microscopy. The holder in the center of the upper row is designed to hold a series of small copper grids (just below the coin to the right) that have very small ribbons of plastic-embedded tissue. The tissue fragment is first embedded in a bullet-shaped mold that is filled with plastic resin. Once the plastic is polymerized, the mold is removed and the hardened plastic with the tissue, now located at the end of the bullet (upper) is sectioned. The ribbon of sections is then floated onto the copper grid. As can be appreciated from the scale offered by the coin, these ribbons must be maneuvered via a dissecting microscope attached to the microtome. The middle row shows a slide with a ribbon of unstained tissue compared with deparaffinized, stained tissue. The plate to the right of the middle row is an exposed, developed film plate (negative) from the electron microscope. The lower portion of the figure shows a part of a glossy print made from this negative (the tissue is from the pituitary gland).

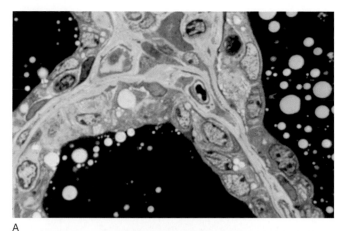

A

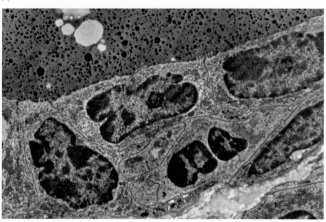

B

Fig. 2.7. Cellular differentiation examples. Shown are companion light (A) and transmission electron microscopic (B) images of bovine mammary tissue of a nonlactating cow in late gestation. Note the relatively large proportion of cell area occupied by the nuclei of the cells, relative lack of cellular organelles, absence of cellular polarity, and minimal evidence of secretion. These cells are minimally active, so there is a correspondingly minimal complement of cellular organelles.

depending on the activity of the cell. This is often described as the "degree of differentiation of the cell." For example, mammary secretory cells taken from a nonlactating pregnant animal have a very different complement of cellular organelles than cells collected during lactation. This is a reflection of differences in activity between these stages of development.

Certainly, biochemical differentiation of the secretory cells is required for onset of milk secretion. However, the cells must also acquire the structural machinery needed to synthesize, package, and secrete milk constituents. When alveolar cells first appear during midgestation, they exhibit few of the organelles needed for copious milk biosynthesis or secretion. The cells are characterized by a sparse cytoplasm with few polyribosomes, some clusters of free ribosomes, limited rough endoplasmic reticulum, rudimentary Golgi usually in close apposition to the nucleus, some isolated mitochondria, and widely dispersed vesicles. Individual cells often contain large lipid droplets (especially during later stages of gesta-

tion) that, along with irregularly shaped nuclei, account for much of the cellular area. Electron microscopy studies solidified the dramatic structural changes in the alveolar secretory cells at the onset of lactation. These differences are illustrated in Figures 2.7 and 2.8. Also it is important to appreciate that similar changes in cell differentiation occur in many epithelial cells, i.e., various glands, intestine, pancreas, etc.; the mammary gland makes a convenient example.

Mitochondria

Called the powerhouses of the cell, mitochondria provide most of the ATP necessary for energy requiring reactions. Two membranes enclose the generally elongated thin hot dog–shaped mitochondria. The outer membrane smoothly encapsulates the organelle, but the inner membrane is thrown into multiple folds

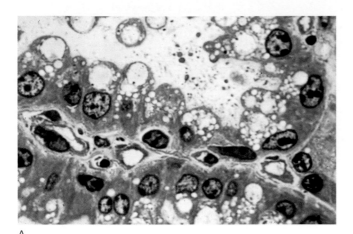

A

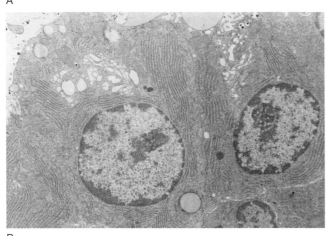

B

Fig. 2.8. Examples of light and transmission electron microscopic images of lactating bovine mammary tissue. The cells typically have rounded basally displaced nuclei, scattered fat droplets, and evidence of secretions (A). Note the lacy appearance of the apical ends of these well-differentiated, polarized cells. Confirmation that the lacy appearance indicates the presence of abundant secretory vesicles is evident in the EM view of portions of two secretory cells in Panel B. Image A is unpublished and image B is adapted from Nickerson and Akers, 1984.

that form partitions called cristae. Surfaces of the cristae are studded with embedded enzymes that interact with the internal gellike matrix of the mitochondria. Although details are discussed in subsequent chapters, as energy-yielding nutrients are metabolized, intermediate products from the digestive process, e.g., glucose, amino acids, fatty acids are converted into compounds that enter the mitochondria. These compounds are catabolized to carbon dioxide and water by the action of the mitochondrial enzymes, and a portion of the bond energy is captured and used to attach phosphate groups to ADP to generate ATP. This is called aerobic respiration because it requires oxygen. Essentially the need for oxygen is explained by the fact that it is required for production of adequate amounts of ATP.

Mitochondria are very complex organelles. They have their own DNA (derived incidentally from the mother) and RNA. As energy demand increases, mitochondria increase the density of cristae or undergo fission to create new mitochondria. Active cells like those in muscle, pancreas, or the lactating mammary gland may have hundreds of mitochondria, but inactive cells (nonlactating mammary gland) or quiescent lymphocytes, for example, have only a few. In living cells the mitochondria can also change shape. Regardless of its particular morphology, the emergence of mitochondria was a major evolutionary event. Figure 2.9 illustrates typical mitochondria. It is widely believed that mitochondria arose from bacteria that invaded the ancestors of plant and animal cells.

Ribosomes

These small dark-staining organelles are composed of proteins and a class of RNA called ribosomal RNA. Each of the ribosomes has two subunits identified based on size as 18 and 28s RNA. Ribosomes can appear singly as free structures in the cytoplasm or sometimes arranged along coiled loops of mRNA called polyribosomes. Alternatively, especially in cells that are synthesizing abundant amounts of protein for secretion, ribosomes are often attached to membranes to create rough endoplasmic reticulum (RER) (Fig. 2.10). As subsequently discussed, the ribosomes are the sites of protein synthesis. Fig. 2.10 illustrates relationship between endoplasmic reticulum and the Golgi apparatus. Ribosomes of the RER allow for newly manufactured proteins to be packaged in secretory vesicles for secretion from the cell. Free ribosomes in the cytoplasm function to synthesize proteins destined to act within the cell.

Endoplasmic reticulum and golgi apparatus

The endoplasmic reticulum (ER) is an interconnected network within the cytoplasm of the cell. It is a system of interconnecting membrane tubes or sheets that enclose fluid filled spaces that appear in two variations, smooth or rough ER. It is also continuous with the nuclear membrane. Protein synthesis depends on three forms of RNA. These are 1) transfer RNA (tRNA), 2) ribosomal RNA (rRNA), and 3) messenger RNA (mRNA). When the mature mRNA reaches the cytoplasm, it binds to a small ribosomal subunit by base pairing to rRNA. The tRNA transfers amino acids to the ribosome. There are approximately 20 different types of tRNA, each capable of binding a specific amino acid. The linkage process is controlled by a synthetase enzyme whose action depends on the cleavage of ATP to form the peptide bonds between amino acids of the growing peptide chain. Once its

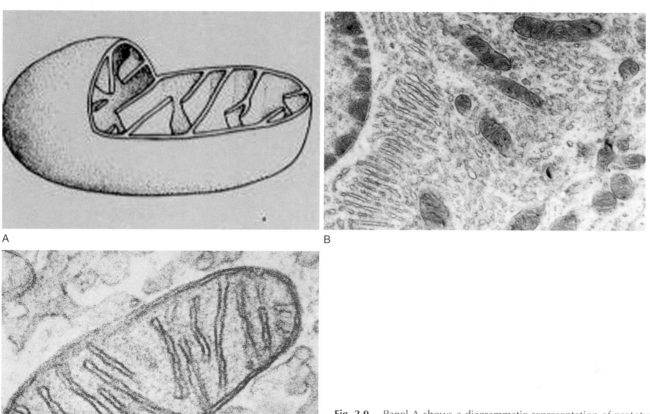

Fig. 2.9. Panel A shows a diagrammatic representation of prototypical mitochondria. The structure is clearly bounded by a double membrane with the inner membrane thrown into distinct folds, or cristae. Panel B shows a group of mitochondria in the basal region of a bovine kidney cell, and Panel C illustrates a high-resolution image of mitochondria from the bovine ovary.

amino acid is loaded, the tRNA migrates to the ribosome, where it moves the amino acid into position, based on the codons of the mRNA strand. The amino acid is bound to one end of the tRNA (the tail) but the other end of the molecule (the head) has a three-nucleotide base sequence (anticodon), which is complementary to the codon of the mRNA. For a given strand of mRNA, multiple ribosomes can become attached and as the ribosomes move along the molecule, many chains of new protein can be made simultaneously. In fact, it is not uncommon to find polyribosomes in the cytoplasm. These are represented in transmission electron microscopic views of active cells by chains or coils of ribosomes seemingly organized in the cytoplasm.

However, proteins destined for secretion from the cell are synthesized by ribosomes attached to the endoplasmic reticulum. The mRNA for these proteins codes an initial short peptide sequence (signal peptide), which directs the growing peptide chains into the cisternal space of the endoplasmic reticulum. Because this space is continuous with the Golgi apparatus, proteins destined for secretion are vectored into Golgi for packaging into secretory vesicles and secretion from the cell by exocytosis. After synthesis in the RER, modifications to secretory proteins may also occur in the Golgi apparatus. These posttranslational modifications can markedly affect the structure of the protein. Common modifications include the addition of sugar or phosphate groups. Other components can also be added to developing secretory vesicles in the Golgi. For example, in the mammary gland the milk sugar lactose is synthesized within the Golgi apparatus by the action of galactosyltransferase and α-lactalbumin.

Lysosomes and peroxisomes

Peroxisomes are intracellular vesicles containing a mixture of enzymes, namely oxidases and catalases. Oxidases depend on the presence of oxygen to detoxify various noxious substances, e.g., alcohols and aldehydes. They also convert toxic free radicals into hydrogen peroxide for neutralization by catalase. Free radicals are very reactive substances known to alter the structure and function of a variety of regulatory molecules. Thus the peroxisomes are essential to limit

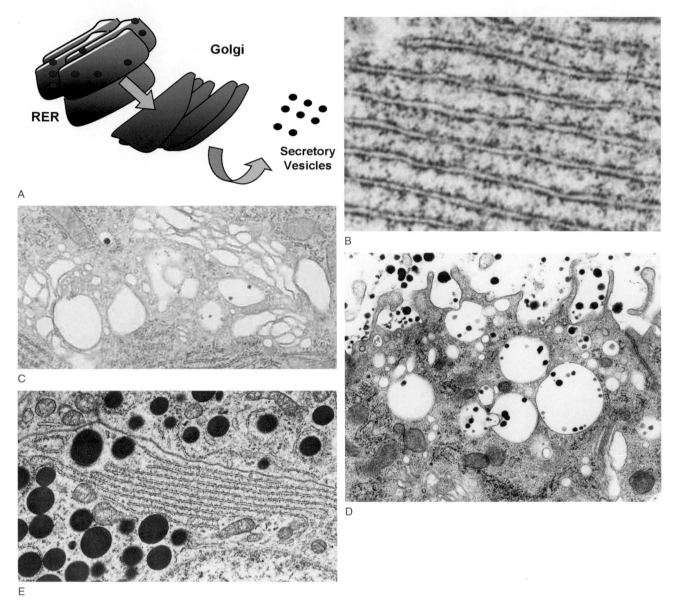

Fig. 2.10. Relationships between RER, Golgi, and secretory vesicles. Panel A shows the arrangement between ribosomes (red dots) on RER and movement of newly manufactured proteins into the cisternal space of the RER and then to the Golgi for packaging and appearance of secretory vesicles. Panel B shows a transmission electron microscopic view of RER, and Panel C shows an array of Golgi membranes. Panel D shows secretory vesicles from epithelial cells in a mammary gland of a lactating animal. The dark black granules are the casein micelles. Since lactose is also produced in the Golgi and packaged for secretion along with specific milk proteins, the vesicles appear swollen. This is because lactose cannot pass across the vesicle membrane, and so water is drawn osmotically into the vesicle. For other protein synthesizing and secreting cells, the secretory vesicles more often appear densely compacted with the vesicle membrane directly adjacent to the product. Panel E shows secretory vesicles and Golgi area from bovine anterior pituitary cells. Notice the close apposition of the membrane surrounding the secretory granules.

the free radical accumulation. Peroxisomes are abundant in liver and kidney cells, two organs recognized for their capacity to detoxify harmful substances.

Lysosomes also contain hydrolytic enzymes that are capable of digesting many cellular proteins. Known as suicide bags or sacs, inappropriate release of the contents of these organelles could destroy the cell. In fact, rupture of activated lysosomes is believed to be involved in some aspects of programmed cell death or apoptosis. Lysosomes are present in all cell types, but they are especially plentiful in neutrophils, macrophages, and other leucocytes. The acid hydrolases within the lysosomes function best in an acidic environment. Consequently the lysosomal membrane contains hydrogen transport proteins that sequester hydrogen ions from the cytoplasm to maintain a low pH. Many cells are capable of capturing materials from near the cell surface by endocytosis. Vesicles produced in this manner can then fuse with lysosomes. Captured molecules can be digested by the acid hydrolyses and released into the cytoplasm for use by the cell or for excretion. This digestion process is especially important in macrophages and neutrophils since these cells actively engulf potentially harmful bacterial and other toxins. Destruction of these agents by the lysosomes is protective and in the case of processed foreign proteins, fragments of the digested proteins are presented to other cells of the immune system to allow development of specific immunity. Lysosomes are also critical in the recycling of worn-out or nonfunctional organelles as well as a variety of metabolic actions—for example, release of thyroid hormones from storage.

Microfilaments, microtubules, and intermediate filaments

It was originally assumed that the cytoplasm of the cell was essentially a water-filled space with multiple dissolved substances. However, appropriate fixation and embedment techniques for electron microscope led to the realization that the cytoplasm contains an elaborate array of structures that make up the cytoskeleton of the cell. This does not mean that cells are rigid, but microtubules, microfilaments, and intermediate filaments of the cytoskeleton provide an unexpected structure and organization to the cell cytoplasm. Some of these organelles are for communication between the cell surface and interior, for transport of vesicles to be secreted, for cell division, or for cell adhesion.

Microtubules are the largest of these organelles and as the name suggests are hollow tubes composed of α and β subunits of the globular protein tubulin. They are slender with an outside diameter of 25 nm. When cut in cross section they appear as small circles with 13 subunits of tubulin around the circumference. Its cylindrical structure develops as heterodimers of tubulin pack around a central core, which appears as a space in electron micrographs. At 37°C, purified tubulin polymerizes into microtubules in vitro in the presence of Mg and GTP. Several antimitotic cancer drugs (colchicine and its relatives) act by interfering with tubulin polymerization. Another antimitotic drug, taxol, stabilizes microtubules and arrests cells in mitosis. These effects demonstrate the critical role of microtubules in cell division. Polymerization of tubulin to form microtubules occurs initially in a region near the nucleus called the centrosome. This has been demonstrated most clearly in cultured cells first treated with colchicine to disrupt the microtubules. After various periods of time groups of cells were fixed and the microtubules stained by using fluorescent-tagged antibodies against tubulin. When the

Table 2.3. Microtubules in mammary cells.

	Nonlactating	Lactating
Location		
Apical	4.6 ± 0.9	17.4 ± 2.1
Basal	0.9 ± 0.2	3.7 ± 0.8
Orientation		
Apical-Basal	4.2 ± 0.8 (50.3%)	18.9 ± 2.1 (65.6%)
Lateral-Lateral	4.1 ± 0.6 (49.7%)	9.9 ± 1.5 (34.4%)

Average number of microtubules in the apical or basal cytoplasm observed in an apical-to-basal or lateral-to-lateral orientation with respect to the plasma membrane in mammary epithelial cells of nonlactating and lactating cows. Adapted from Nickerson, Akers, and Weinland, 1982.

drug is removed new microtubules can be seen growing out from the centrosome to create a starlike structure called an aster. The microtubules then elongate toward the outer regions of the cell to reestablish the microtubule network.

It is also known that disruption of microtubules dramatically impairs cellular secretion. For example, intramammary infusion of colchicine into the lactating mammary gland virtually stops milk secretion, but once the treatment is ended milk secretion rapidly returns to normal. This demonstrates the requirement for microtubules for trafficking and exocytosis of secretory vesicles. An increase in the relative abundance of microtubules in mammary epithelial cells corresponds with increased milk secretion following parturition or increased secretory activity in other epithelial cells. Two families of microtubule-dependent motor proteins, kinesins and dyneins, are involved in organelle transport in the cytoplasm, in mitosis, and in movement of vesicles of the neurotransmitter from sites of synthesis in the cell body to sites of release at the ends of axon terminals. Table 2.3 provides an example of changes in microtubule number and orientation related to cell function and Figure 2.11 shows the appearance of microtubules in the mammary cells of a lactating cow.

Microfilaments are the smaller, thin components of the cytoskeleton composed of the protein actin. In many cells actin accounts for 5% or more of the total protein in the cell. Actin can exist as a monomer or, similar to the tubulin of microtubules, can polymerize to form thin threadlike structures (~7 nm in thickness) called filamentous actin. In most cells about half the actin is in the monomeric conformation because of its binding to the regulatory protein thymosin. Rapid changes in rates of polymerization-depolymerization produce changes in the cell surface that produce lamellipodia (essentially cell projections) and ultimately cell movement and migration. Specific arrangements of microfilaments within the cytoplasm can be induced

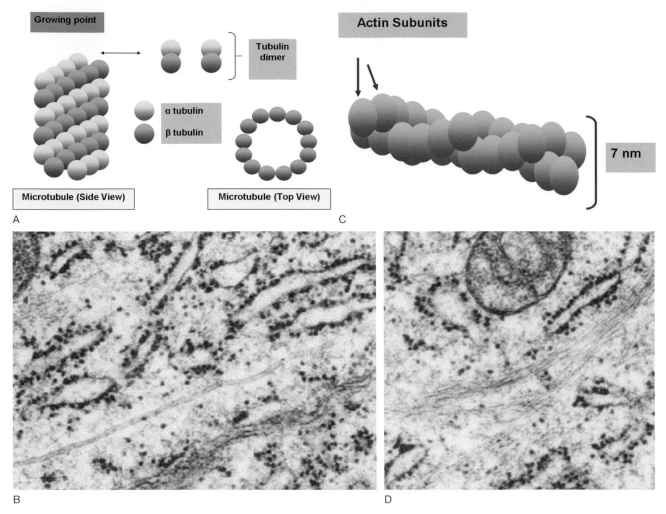

Fig. 2.11. Microtubules and microfilaments. Panel A illustrates the organization of a microtubule, and its development from dimers of α and β-tubulin. Panel B shows a transmission electron microscopic view of the apical region of an epithelial cell from the mammary gland of a lactating cow. Microtubules that have been cut longitudinally appear underneath the RER of the upper cell. Panel C shows the helical organization of monomers of actin arranged to create microfilaments. Panel D shows bundles of microfilaments in secretory epithelial cells.

by the activation of cell surface receptors. This is important for the action of highly mobile phagocytic cells of the immune system. Bundles of microfilaments are also found near cell surfaces and are highly ordered within the microvilli of absorptive epithelial cell layers. In this way bundles of actin filaments provide structural integrity for the microvilli. This is functionally significant because the adaptation of having the microvilli on the surface of an intestinal epithelial cell, for example, markedly increases the surface area available for absorption. A single intestinal enterocyte has several thousand microvilli. Actin filaments do not act independently; rather a variety of actin binding proteins control rates of filament formation and creation of the specific types of filament groupings. For example, cross-linked microfilaments can form loose gels or rigid bundles to anchor plasma membranes.

Intermediate filaments are less labile than microfilaments or microtubules and are more elemental members of the cytoskeleton. The protein structure of these filaments can vary between cell types, but the proteins are bound together something like a braided, woven rope. These filaments are called neurofilaments in nerve cells and keratin filaments in many epithelial cells. Regardless, they provide additional support for the cell. They are especially important in the creation of desmosomes. Desmosomes are a type of anchoring junction that serves to hold adjacent epithelial cells together. In these regions the plasma membranes of the neighboring cells do not touch, but linker proteins (cadherins) extend outward from the desmosomal plaque of each cell. On the cytoplasmic side of the plaque in each cell, intermediate fibers extend into the cytoplasm of the cell to provide interactions with other cytoskeletal elements and additional support.

Types of cell junctions will be considered in other chapters.

Centrioles

These structures are composed of a short cylindrical arrangement of microtubules. They occur as a pair near the center of the centrosome. The centrosome acts as an organizing center for building microtubules and serves as the spindle pole during mitosis. The pair of centrioles is oriented in an L-shaped pattern with the two centrioles at right angles to each other. The centrosome duplicates and divides into two equal parts during the interphase period of cell division so that each half contains a duplicated centriole pair. The daughter centrosomes migrate to either side of the nucleus at the start of mitosis to form the two poles of the mitotic spindle. The granular appearance of the cytoplasm in the region surrounding the centrioles is believed to be from a complex of proteins and fibers involved in the movement and duplication of the centrioles. Each centriole resembles a pinwheel made of each of nine triplets of microtubules arranged to form a hollow tube. They also form the basal structures of cilia and flagella and are usually called basal bodies based on the original interpretation that they were different from centrioles. It is now known that the structures are related. However, whereas the centriole has the pattern of nine microtubule triplets, the basal bodies have an arrangement of nine pairs of microtubules oriented around a single pair of microtubules in the center. Although each of the central microtubules is complete the outer doublets are fused so that the pair shares a common layer. This 9 + 2 organization is characteristic of most if not all types of cilia and flagella. The bending of the central core of the structure, which is called the axoneme, produces the movement of the cilia or flagella.

Figure 2.12 illustrates a cross section through the tail of a bovine sperm cell. The arrangement of doublets of microtubules around a central pair of microtubules is apparent. The diagram shows that the microtubules are linked with molecules of the protein nexin to form the circular array. The doublets are decorated with inner and outer arms composed of the protein dynein and anchorage proteins that position the outer doublets around the central core. In sperm cells, the asymmetric arrangement of filaments around the outside of the axoneme, allows the movement of the tail to follow a figure-eight pattern of motion characteristic of bovine sperm cell motility.

Nuclear structure

With the exception of mitochondrial DNA, the majority of the DNA in eucaryotic cells is confined to the

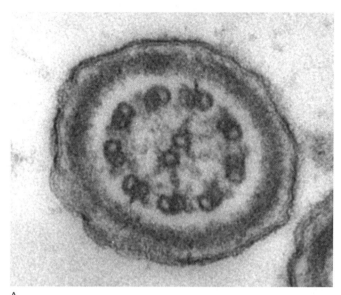

A

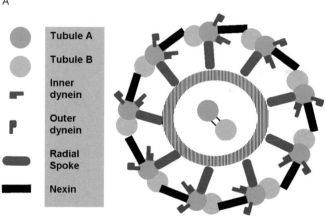

B

Fig. 2.12. Centrioles and cellular movement. Panel A shows a cross section through the tail of a bovine sperm cell. Panel B gives a diagrammatic representation of the molecular and associated proteins.

nucleus. Comparable to the double membrane of the mitochondria, the nucleus is delimited by a double membrane called the nuclear envelope. Unlike mitochondria, these membranes are interspersed with nuclear pores. A complex of proteins populates these areas and acts to control passage of molecules into the nucleus. This is important since the DNA or genes must be transcribed to generate molecules of messenger RNA. Newly synthesized mRNA molecules are processed and transferred to the cytoplasm for translation by the ribosomes to create the myriad of proteins needed by the cell. The presence of the nucleus in eucaryotic cells allows processing related to DNA synthesis and gene activation to be localized away from other activities in the cytoplasm. This likely serves to minimize possible disruption of these critical gene-related activities. In short, the eucaryotic cells have evolved with the creation of numerous membrane-bound organelles that allow for segregation of many specific, divergent, biochemical reactions. This is believed to increase metabolic and biochemical efficiency of eucaryotic compared with prokaryotic cells.

The nucleus houses all the chromosomes and therefore the genes. Fortunately for most cells, only a fraction of the total DNA is being actively utilized at any given moment. For example, although all cells would contain the gene copies for making the milk proteins or for synthesizing lactose, these genes would only be activated in the epithelial cells of the lactating mammary gland. Many other genes are activated only at a particular developmental period or in response to very specific stimuli. Consequently, much of the DNA is tightly compacted in the nucleus.

Most cells have a single nucleus but there are exceptions. Skeletal muscle cells, bone osteoclasts, cardiac cells, and some liver cells are multinucleated. This is usually associated with cells that have a larger-than-normal cytoplasmic volume. With the exception of mature red blood cells of mammals, all cells are nucleated, and even these cells have the nucleus until late in their developmental sequence. Of course without the nucleus and the genes necessary for protein synthesis, these cells cannot replace proteins that are progressively degraded by normal functioning. Although it is expected that the appearance of the nucleus would change dramatically during cell division, even in non-dividing cells (so-called "interphase" or "G_0 phase" of the cell cycle) there are distinct differences between cell types. These differences can be useful to identify some cell types. For example, plasma cells have a distinct pattern of condensed chromatin around the periphery of the nucleus resembling a clock face. Neutrophils have elongated, lobed nuclei that make the appearance of these cells unique.

Figure 2.13 shows an electron microscopy section through the nucleus of an epithelial cell. During most of the life of the cells the DNA is in a complex with strongly basic proteins called histones, some non-histone proteins, and a small amount of RNA. This combination of proteins and DNA is called chromatin. While the double helix structure of DNA is widely familiar, the degree of order or compaction of the DNA within the chromatin matrix varies. Compaction is extreme in cells that are preparing for the final stages of mitosis as the chromatin appears as distinct pairs of chromosomes. However, even in cells in G_0 degrees of chromatic condensation can be seen. Dark-staining areas indicate regions containing condensed, presumably inactive, chromatin. Lighter areas contain more active, extended chromatin. Clumps of condensed chromatin often appear around the periphery of the nucleus (peripheral chromatin) along with scattered

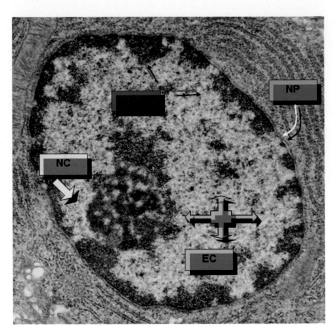

Fig. 2.13. The nucleus of an epithelial cell is shown. Regions of condensed (CC) and extended chromatin (EC) are indicated along with nuclear pores (NP) and the nucleolus (NC).

islands of condensed chromatin throughout the nuclear space. The interphase nucleus also has a protein network called the nuclear matrix. Much of this material appears as a thin, interwoven layer (the nuclear lamina) that adheres to the internal surface of the nuclear envelope. This provides support and anchorage for the nuclear pores. An extension of the nuclear lamina radiates into the interior of the nucleus. This layer also interacts with a similar lamina that surrounds the nucleolus. Together they regulate nuclear shape, reinforce the inner membrane of the nuclear envelope, secure the location of nuclear pores, and anchor condensed chromatin to the nuclear envelope. This organization is maintained except during mitosis. It is accepted that maintenance of the nuclear matrix is essential for routine gene transcription.

Nucleoli

The nucleoli (little nucleus) are dark-staining, generally oval bodies located within the nucleus (see Fig. 2.13). They are not membrane-bound and are sites for ribosome synthesis and assembly. The size and number of nucleoli vary between cells. Cells that are very actively synthesizing and secreting large amounts of protein are more likely to have a large nucleus and/or multiple structures. The nucleoli are closely linked to segments of chromatin (nucleolar organizer regions) that contain the genes that code for synthesis of ribosomal RNA (rRNA). As the rRNA is synthesized, proteins previously made in the cytoplasm are combined in the nucleus to create one of the two subunits of the ribosomes. These subunits are transported out of the nucleus into the cytoplasm where they are combined to make mature ribosomes. The primary rRNA transcript has a sedimentation coefficient of 45 S (Svedberg units) that corresponds to 13,000 nucleic acid base pairs. From this precursor molecule, a 28 S (5,000 base pair) rRNA molecule is created and combined into the larger (60 S) ribosomal subunit. A smaller 18 S (2,000 base pair) rRNA moiety is also generated. It is incorporated into the smaller (40 S) ribosomal subunit. Two additional smaller rRNA molecules are also synthesized and incorporated in the larger ribosomal subunit in its final mature state. The four primary rRNA molecules needed to manufacture the complete ribosome are all formed from the same primary transcript. This ensures that all of the pieces necessary for ribosome synthesis will be available when the process is initiated.

Chromatin structure

DNA and its associated proteins, the chromatin, are organized into a complex structure with varying degrees of condensation. In its most available open state the DNA strands are unwound as transcription occurs. At other times the fundamental basic structural units of chromatin are the nucleosomes. These highly repetitive units are made of clusters or cores of eight histone proteins oriented in repeating fashion along the DNA strand. If the DNA strand is envisioned as a ribbon, the histone clusters can be imagined as large Velcro-covered beads attached to the ribbon. Now imagine the ribbon with attached beads being wound into a repeating coil. This highly ordered structure allows a physical mechanism for the very long linear arrays of DNA to be compacted inside the nucleus but at the same time maintain critical orderliness. In addition to the physical aspects, the histones are also important regulators of gene expression. For example, changes in the methylation or phosphorylation of the histones bound to the DNA modify their capacity to sequester or bind the DNA. If the histones in a particular nucleosome become dissociated with the DNA this would increase the opportunity for the DNA in that region to be available for transcription. Responses of some target cells to hormone stimulation are known to cause the synthesis of new proteins. Corresponding with this, many of these hormones are known to alter rates of methylation of nuclear proteins. This suggests that gene activation must ultimately depend on regulatory molecules that can modify interactions between the histones and other nuclear proteins that function to control chromatin structure. The organization is illustrated in Figure 2.14.

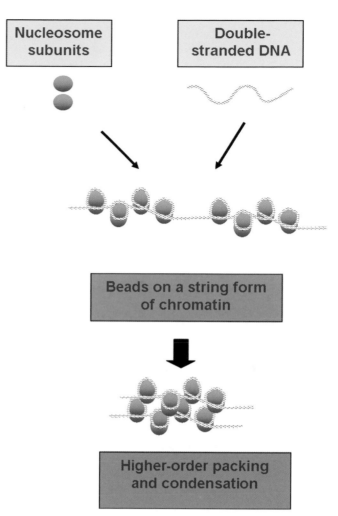

Fig. 2.14. DNA and histone relationships. DNA binding proteins as well as the histones and non-histones form complexes (nucleosome subunits) that allow the coiling of DNA into compact particles that make up chromatin. This can be envisioned first by the formation of subunits to create the core particle followed by the coiling of DNA around the structure. This produces a structure described as beads on a string. Further packing and condensation leads to a higher order of structure and the remarkable organized packaging of DNA.

Cell growth and differentiation

While a definition of growth might seem to have a common sense answer, characterizing growth is not simple. The question is what do we mean when we say growth? The simple answer might be—it got bigger. However, it is important to understand that changes in mass can occur for a variety of reasons. For example, under some circumstances it is possible to accumulate fluids in the interstitial spaces between cells so that edema occurs. This can occur in female humans as the stages of the menstrual cycle wax and wane. Another example is the mammary edema that frequently occurs as cows or goats approach parturition or the facial edema that can occur as a side effect of steroid treatments. But these increases in size would not be considered growth. In most instances, growth depends on an increase in cell number. This is called hyperplasia. It is also possible for cells to increase in size this is called hypertrophy. Both of these processes are involved in growth. It is also possible to increase the noncellular constituents between cells (extracellular proteins and complex carbohydrates) and affect an increase in tissue mass. This can be considered growth as well. This suggests that really understanding growth requires an understanding of the specific types of cells that might be dividing to affect an increase in tissue or organ mass as well as products that these various cells might be synthesizing.

In many cases it is possible to obtain a more detailed view of growth by measuring specific tissue components. For example, at any given moment only a small fraction of the total cells in a tissue or organ are actively synthesizing DNA in preparation for cell division. For a brief period just before the cell divides it will have duplicated its chromosomes so that it will have twice (2n) the normal complement of DNA. However, since this typically is occurring in only a small fraction of cells, measuring the total tissue content of DNA is an effective, quantitative way to determine changes in growth. After all, an increase in the DNA content of a tissue or organ can usually be explained only by an increase in cell number. Realization in the early 1960s that the DNA content of cells is essentially constant (with the exception of the generally small proportion of cells that are undergoing DNA synthesis in preparation for cell division at a given moment) ushered in a host of studies to estimate numbers based on total DNA content. Techniques to accurately and easily measure DNA have evolved so that assay of DNA is now a primary means used to determine whether growth is due to an increase in hyperplasia. Data in Table 2.4 illustrate the dramatic changes in mammary growth from birth to lactation in Holstein heifers and crossbred ewes. Measured as trimmed udder weight or parenchymal DNA, mammary growth is greatest

during gestation. However, relative lack of change in DNA from late gestation into lactation compared with trimmed udder weight suggests that DNA is a better measure of cell growth, since increased weight may be accumulated secretions. This method is especially valuable when combined with careful dissection of the mammary gland to distinguish the parenchymal portion (regarded as the function tissue of an organ) from the stromal tissue of the mammary gland. Even with careful dissection of the mammary gland to remove apparent connective tissue, there are clearly nonglandular cellular elements, i.e., blood vessels, lymphatic vessels, nerves, fibroblasts, adipocytes, and white blood cells, which contribute to the DNA content of the parenchymal tissue compartment. This illustrates the difficulty of accurately and precisely estimating growth at the tissue level. Regardless, classic studies in a variety of lactating species give direct evidence that the number of mammary epithelial cells is proportional to milk production. Indeed, the correlation between total parenchymal DNA and milk production averages about 0.85.

A more acute, dynamic means to evaluate cell proliferation utilizes either radioactively tagged thymidine (a nucleotide base that is unique to DNA) or the analogue bromodeoxyuridine (BrdU), which also incorporates into growing DNA strands like thymidine). In these cases, animals to be tested are injected with the test substances or in vitro experiments with cells or tissue incubated in culture are exposed to radiolabeled thymidine or the BrdU. After an appropriate period of time tissues are removed and the quantity of incorporation measured. The greater the rate of incorporation the greater the growth rate since only cells in the S phase (period of DNA synthesis prior to cell division) of the cell cycle accumulate these compounds. Figure 2.15 provides an example of changes in mammary tissue cell growth induced by the treatment of heifers with bovine growth hormone (bST) and shows that the effect is primarily in the epithelial cells of the mammary gland. However, other components may well be excellent measures of growth.

Table 2.4. Mammary parenchymal growth in heifers and ewes.

Measure	Stage of Development				
	Prepuberty	Postpuberty	Mid Gest	Late Gest	Lactation
Heifers					
DNA (g)	1.1	2.6	16.3	39.3	38.8
Wt. (g)	495.0	957.0	5,110.0	8,560.0	16,350.0
Ewes					
DNA (g)	0.02	0.09	1.3	2.3	2.6
Wt. (g)	15.00	78.00	557.0	1,057.0	1,340.0

Data adapted from Smith et al., 1989; Keys et al., 1989; McFadden et al., 1990; and Sejrsen et al., 1982, 1986.

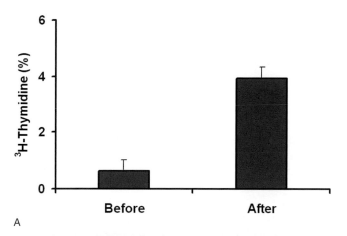

A

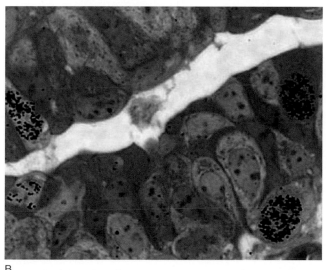

B

Fig. 2.15. Proliferation and cell growth. Panel A shows proliferation of bovine mammary epithelial cells indicated by the percent of epithelial cell nuclei incorporating tritiated thymidine in prepubertal heifers before or after a 1-week treatment with bovine growth hormone. Panel B shows a histological section of mammary tissue from a heifer that was injected with BrdU 2 hours prior to tissue collection. Cells that have incorporated BrdU (indicating these cells were in the S phase of the cell cycle) have been detected by immunocytochemistry using a specific antibody. Several cells that were synthesizing DNA are indicated by the presence of dark granules over the cell nucleus.

For example, an increase in muscle tissue would be an evident desirable attribute for a lamb producer. Quantification of such an effect might be better confirmed by measuring total muscle protein rather than DNA.

Clearly, the question of growth is complex, but understanding and regulating rates and types of tissue growth are key elements of many aspects of animal agriculture. For example, lamb or beef producers are concerned with getting their animals to market weight at an appropriate body composition as rapidly and cheaply as possible. However, at a whole-body level, the integration of multiple organ systems ultimately explains the rate of growth and tissue composition of individual animals. It is also apparent that growth of all but the simplest life forms is irregular. All tissues do not grow at the same rate or at the same times for that matter. Commonly observed changes in stature, degrees of fatness, or morphology (secondary sex characteristics, for example) are familiar when we consider aging. The evident differences in rates and patterns of growth among different tissues or organs are the essence of development.

For many tissues not only must new cells be created but these cells must acquire the capacity to carry out specific functions. The changing growth and development of the mammary gland or uterus during the reproductive cycle provide excellent examples of cellular differentiation. Analysis of mammary tissue at the light microscopy level, especially if the tissue is embedded in a plastic resin (compared with more traditional paraffin), allows an estimation of the proportion of alveolar epithelial cells, which fall into various classes of structural differentiation. Table 2.5 gives data to illustrate how evaluation of cell differentiation can be physiologically relevant. In this experiment the effect of arresting cell growth and cell differentiation was studied. Two diagonal mammary glands of each of two pregnant Holstein heifers were infused with colchicine every second day from 1 week prior to parturition until calving. Twice-daily milking began at calving and the drug treatment was discontinued.

Table 2.5. Effect of colchicine on structural differentiation of mammary alveolar epithelial cell.

	Milk Yield[a]	Light Microscopy[b]			Electron Microscopy[c]	
		% Undiff	% Inter	% Full	% RER	% Golgi
Control	60	7	12	81	18	25
Treated	17	49	46	6	7	9

[a] Milk yield is given as kg produced per udder half during week 3 postpartum.
[b] Light microscopy data is the percentage of epithelial cells classified as undifferentiated, intermediately differentiated, or fully differentiated.
[c] Electron microscopy data is the percent of cellular area occupied by rough endoplasmic reticulum or Golgi membranes and vacuoles.
Data adapted from Nickerson and Akers, 1983, and Akers and Nickerson, 1983.

Data for mammary biopsies obtained on day 21 of lactation is given. Clearly, measures of mammary epithelial cell structural differentiation correlate well with function. In this experiment, treatment with colchicine during the period just before calving prevented the normal structural differentiation of the epithelial cells. This in turn markedly impaired the functioning of the mammary gland, despite the fact that drug treatment was discontinued immediately after calving. The point of this is to illustrate how changes in cell differentiation are closely related to cell function.

Stages of the cell cycle

The cell cycle is a description of the events the cell undergoes from the time of its initial creation until it divides. However, there is a great deal of variation between cell types as to how quickly they progress through the cell cycle. Some cells divide very rapidly indeed. For example, once stem cells of the immune system are activated, clones of lymphocyte cells can be generated in a matter of days. Other cells—for example, neurons—are believed to almost never divide. Although early cytologists thought that cells that were not in the mitotic phase of development were inactive because of the absence of marked visual changes, this is not true. Cells without apparent mitotic figures or morphological changes were said to be in a resting or interphase period. It is now appreciated that these interphase cells carry out the normal functioning of tissues, e.g., secretion of pancreatic enzymes or excretion activity of the kidney. The only "rest" at this time is from activities directly leading to cell division. As a general rule, once cells acquire their terminal functional activity—as for example, many glandular epithelial cells—they effectively cease dividing and are referred to as G_0 cells. These cells are progressively degraded and lost but are replaced by the daughters of undifferentiated cells within the tissue. Dogma suggests that G_0 represents a terminal state, so these cells cannot be induced to return to a path leading to cell division; however, control of cell growth is an active area of research.

For cells that are not terminally differentiated, the interphase period encompasses three subperiods. After the initial division to create the cell, it enters G_1. During this time, the cells are metabolically active, rapidly synthesizing proteins and creating new cellular organelles. However, the time that the cell spends in G_1 can vary from a few hours in rapidly growing tissues to periods of weeks or even years. Once signals are produced to continue toward cell division, the cell enters the S or DNA synthesis phase. As G_1 ends, the centrioles begin to replicate. During the S phase the cell DNA is replicated and the cell produces new his-

tones and chromatin so that the cell has two complete copies of each of chromosomes. As indicated in our discussion of growth, incubating cells with radioactivity tagged thymidine and measuring the rate or degree of incorporation provides a valuable tool to study cell growth. This is because appreciable amounts of thymidine are incorporated only into cells that have entered the S phase of the cell cycle. Once duplication is completed the cell enters G_2. This is generally the shortest of the interphase periods, lasting only a matter of minutes. During this time the cells complete synthesis of enzymes and other proteins required for chromosomal migration, and the active process of mitosis is the last stage of the cell cycle. Figure 2.16 illustrates the sequence of stages in the cell cycle as well as changes in cellular DNA content during the cell cycle.

Stages of mitosis

The pattern of cell division is virtually identical among all cell types. The process begins at the end of G_2 as chromosome condensation becomes apparent and ends with cytokinesis, the physical separation of daughter cells into two independent cells. Simply stated, mitosis is a coordinated series of events that allows the duplicated DNA produced during the S phase of the cell cycle to be divided between two identical daughter cells. Once begun mitosis typically lasts less than 1 hour. For this reason in histological sections of most tissues it is relatively rare to observe mitotic figures. Exceptions are in samples of very rapidly growing tissues, e.g., tumors or perhaps the crypts of the small intestine. On the other hand, if rapidly growing tissues are treated with colchicine or some other microtubule-disrupting agent, the number of dividing cells will become more apparent since the cells become arrested in various stages of the mitosis. This has been especially useful for the study of cells grown in culture.

It is reasonable to ask how cells in different phases of the cell cycle can be identified and whether the duration of phases are different for different cell types. Because cells require a period of time for growth, even the cells in rapidly developing tissues require several hours to complete the cell cycle. For many mature tissues a cycle time of 16 to 24 hours is typical. An extreme example of short duration occurs in early embryonic cell growth. Because the cells spend little time in G_1 or G_2 cell hypertrophy does not occur and the time spent in a combination of S and then M phase may be only a matter of 60 minutes or less. The rate of proliferation in these cells can approach rates usually only observed for bacterial cells. This process serves to essentially subdivide the fertilized oocyte into many smaller cells. As for tracking cells in phases dense into recognizable chromosomes. In the prior S phase the chromosomes were duplicated. In this new configuration, each chromosome is made up of two identical arms or threads called chromatids. Each chromatid pair is held together by a small dense structure called a centromere. Newly duplicated centrioles separate in the cell to become polarized at opposite ends of the cell to create the spindle poles. This occurs as the nucleus disappears and the nuclear matrix and envelope dissembles. As the chromosomes condense and become visually apparent, each of the polarized centrioles become a focal point for the creation of a new assembly of microtubules. This growth of microtubules mimics a starburst pattern and is aptly called aster formation. These events occur during early prophase. Late in prophase elongating microtubules attach to protein-DNA complexes (kinetochores) in the region of the centromere of each chromatid pair. The kinetochore microtubules are critical for the role they play in subsequent separation and migration of chromosome pairs. Other microtubules create the mitotic spindle to maintain the polar orientation of the centrioles. Metaphase is the next well-defined event in mitosis. It is characterized by the appearance of the chromosomes aligned along the center or equator of the spindle. The organization of chromosomes in a plane between the poles is called the metaphase plate creation and is one of the more distinct, readily recognizable phases of mitosis.

Sudden separation of the sister kinetochores demarks anaphase. Within minutes, each of one chromatid pair (now called a chromosome) is pulled to one of the spindle poles. The arrival of all of the daughter chromosomes at each pole and dissolution of the kinetochore microtubules marks the beginning of telophase. Remaining polar microtubules elongate; a new nuclear envelope coalesces around each polarized cluster of chromosomes; and the compacted, dense chromatin expands and nucleoli reappear. The final stage of mitosis cytokinesis is characterized by appearance of a cleavage furrow between the cells. This narrows and, finally, the remaining elements of the mitotic spindle are broken and two independent cells are created.

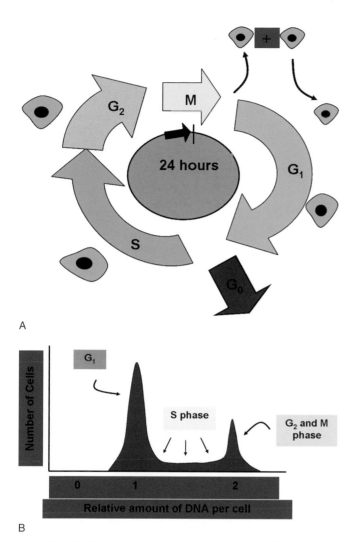

A

B

Fig. 2.16.   Cell cycle analysis. A typical cell cycle is divided into 4 phases (A). Following division the cell enters a phase called G_1 (G = gap). In most cases the cell undergoes hyperplasia at this time, and when appropriately signaled it passes into the S phase for replication of the DNA. Notice that the cell illustrated increases in size as it progresses through the cell cycle. Once synthesis is completed the cell enters G_2, which allows for completion of the final steps before the cell begins mitosis (M) and the creation of two daughter cells. Many cells can also enter a somewhat quiescent phase (G_0) during which time the cell carries out its usual functions but remains in a nondividing state.

Regulators of cell division

It is difficult to study the details of cell division and especially regulation in intact tissues or whole animals. Thus much of the detailed understanding has come from cell culture experiments. When normal mammalian cells are maintained in culture they usually can be propagated only for about 50 cell divisions. After this, the cells enter a senescence period and eventually die. Despite the obvious limitations, study of culture cells has been scientifically invaluable.

of the cycle, those in S phase can be identified by supplying them with labeled molecules of thymidine (some DNA repair occurs even in nondividing cells). The label is often radioactive, in the form of ^{3}H thymidine, or chemical in the form of bromodeoxyuridine (BrdU), a synthetic analog of thymidine (see Fig. 2.15). Figure 2.17 outlines the events and stages associated with mitosis.

From microscopic study, the passage from the last period of interphase (G_2) into prophase is gradual. Chromatin, which is relatively diffuse, begins to con-

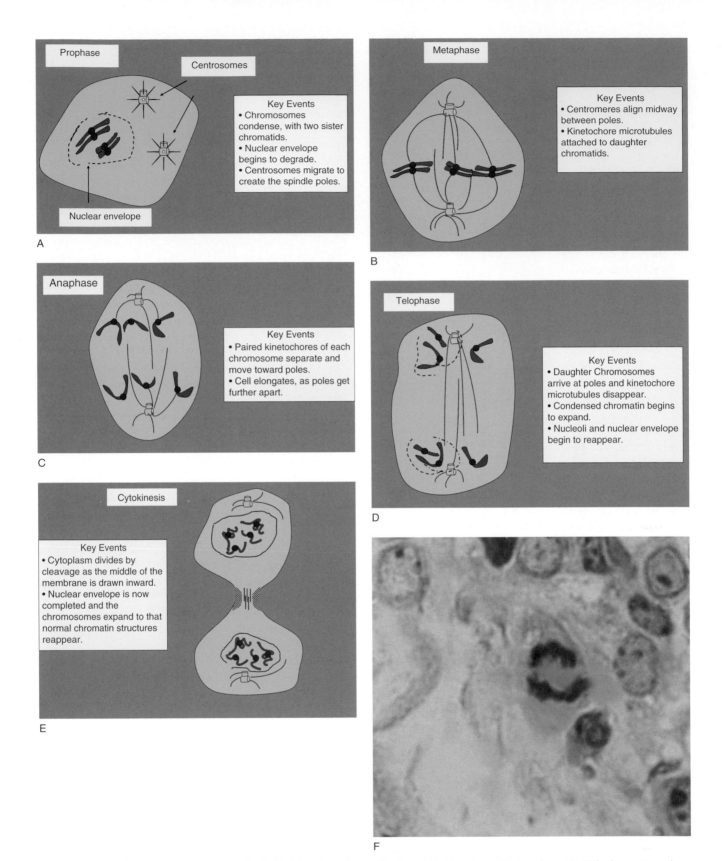

Fig. 2.17. Stages of mitosis. Mitosis is typically divided into four phases: Prophase (A), Metaphase (B), Anaphase (C), Telophase (D), and Cytokinesis (E). These involve first the condensation of chromatin into chromosomes, and then formation of spindle pole, division and migration of daughter chromatids, and finally cleavage to create daughter cells. The final panel (F) in this figure shows a dividing mammary cell caught in anaphase.

Mammalian cells were first cultured in clotted blood and for many years, efforts to routinely grow cells in culture failed, despite efforts to supply well-recognized nutrients. Cells could be maintained only if serum was included with the nutrients. In the absence of serum, cells would typically stop growing and become arrested in G_0. It is now known that serum supplies critical growth factors (GF), and even now for routine growth of cells, fetal bovine serum is often added to cell cultures. Platelet-derived growth factor (PDGF) was one of the first GF discovered. Like many GF, its existence was hypothesized from effects observed with cells in culture. Specifically, it was found that fibroblasts would proliferate in culture if serum were added but not with addition of plasma. Since serum is the liquid that remains after the blood clots, this suggested that the clotting process liberated a soluble agent from the blood cells or platelets that are contained within the clot. Subsequent experiments showed that extracts prepared from isolated platelets were also able to stimulate growth of fibroblasts. These observations eventually led to the isolation, purification, and identification of PDGF. In a physiological sense it is easy to visualize a role for PDGF in wound healing. With clot formation following an injury, liberation of PDGF at the site acts to stimulate the proliferation of fibroblasts in and around vessel walls. Since fibroblasts synthesize and secrete collagens, their role in healing and scar tissue formation is obvious. More than 50 proteins are now known to function as growth factors. However, it is important to appreciate that not all cells respond to this entire myriad of possible stimulators. Only those cells that express receptor proteins for a given GF are capable of responding. However, it is also possible to crudely divide GF into those that affect a broad spectrum of cells—for example, insulinlike growth factor one (IGF-I)—from those that impact only a specific population of cells—for example, erythropoietin, which stimulates proliferation of cells that are the precursors for red blood cells. We will discuss some of these specific GF in subsequent chapters.

Regardless of external agents that act to initiate cell division, this must involve the activation of specific genes that control DNA synthesis. Cell-cycle control relies on two classes of proteins. The first, cyclin-dependent protein kinases (Cdk) cause phosphorylation of selected enzymes. As we will see in our study of cell metabolism, a general feature of many regulatory proteins is that either adding or deleting phosphate groups dramatically alters function. The second class of proteins, the cyclins, bind to the Cdk proteins and thereby regulate their enzymatic activity. Cyclins get their name from the fact that they undergo a cycle of synthesis and degradation with each cell division. This means that the periodic assembly, acti-

vation, and disassembly of cyclin-Cdk complexes are critical elements in cell proliferation. Like most cellular activities, understanding the details of gene expression is central to understanding cellular function; for cyclins it is easy to visualize the significance of synthesizing these proteins at just the ideal moment during the cell cycle. Conversely, inappropriate synthesis or failure of disassembly, is likely important when cell growth becomes uncontrolled, i.e., tumor formation.

Macromolecules and cellular physiology

Although we have considered some aspects of lipid structure, especially related to membrane structure, it is apparent that normal cellular function depends on a myriad of biochemical reactions and macromolecules. First, the number of biologically relevant molecules in cells seems overwhelming. However, some relatively simple combinations of atoms—methyl ($-CH_3$), hydroxyl ($-OH$), carboxyl ($-COOH$), and amino ($-NH_3$) groups—appear repeatedly in biologically important molecules. Second, repeating combinations of relatively simple compounds creates most of the large complex macromolecules. Most of the organic molecules in cells are derived from four major groupings of molecules. These are simple sugars or carbohydrates, amino acids, fatty acids, and nucleotides.

Major phases of metabolism can be subdivided in a variety of ways, but a simplistic view would consider activities that build new cellular components (anabolism) compared with those that break down various cellular elements (catabolism). Interestingly, both processes are occurring simultaneously. For example, catabolism of various nutrient compounds by digestive tract tissues provides the structural building blocks for other tissues to grow or synthesize and secrete products (anabolism). Other nutrients are catabolized to provide elements needed for energy production (usually ATP). We begin our study of cellular physiology by first considering major classes of macromolecules. However, our discussion is no substitute for related classes in chemistry and biochemistry. Our goal is to provide enough of an overview and reminder to aid your understanding of physiological processes.

Proteins

In the absence of disease or trauma, most cellular proteins are synthesized from free amino acids or peptides absorbed from the blood stream. The cell membrane (and associated carrier proteins) regulates the uptake of these molecules from the interstitial fluids. Understanding of amino acid transporters is an area of active research but many features are common between tissues. Some of these transporters show an ion dependence (e.g., Na^+, Cl^-, and K^+) or use an H^+-gradient to drive transport. The Na^+-dependent system A transporters for neutral amino acids are believed to regulate the accumulation of neutral amino acids within the cells when compared with plasma concentrations. There is much interest in regulation of amino acid uptake to better understand factors limiting milk and meat protein synthesis. From an animal production viewpoint much of the value of animal products resides in the protein content, e.g., meat, milk, and eggs.

While the significance of proteins as important building blocks in anabolism is easily appreciated, the enzymes that are vital for cell function are also proteins. Like most biologically critical macromolecules, linking together subunit monomers—the amino acids—in this case, allows a large variety of proteins to be generated. Individual amino acids share the common structure illustrated in Figure 2.18. The R (or residual group) is attached to the α carbon and is unique for each amino acid. For the simplest, the amino acid glycine, the R is a hydrogen atom. Individual amino acids are bound together by a dehydration synthesis reaction (named because water is liberated in the process). Newly created covalent bonds between amino acids are called peptide bonds.

There are 20 common amino acids. Some are considered essential amino acids because they must be supplied in the diet. Others can be created by intermediary metabolism. However, specific amino acids considered essential vary between species, especially in ruminants compared with nonruminant species. This is because the bacteria and protozoa of the ruminant can generate amino acids not initially available in the diet fed to the animals. As illustrated in Figure 2.18, all amino acids have two functional (or reactive groups), an amine (—NH_2) and a carboxylic acid residue (—COOH). Differences in the number and arrangement of atoms in the R group give each of the amino acids its unique chemical attributes. For example, if the side group is a simple string of hydrocarbons (leucine, for example), this region of the amino acid will be very hydrophobic, much like fatty acids tails of a phospholipid. Other side groups, for example the inclusion of an additional amine group (lysine, for example), would make the amino acid very hydrophilic and more basic. The various amino acids can be categorized based on the properties that the R groups give to the molecule. These categories are acidic, basic, uncharged polar, or nonpolar attributes. In addition to the common names, the amino acids are also denoted

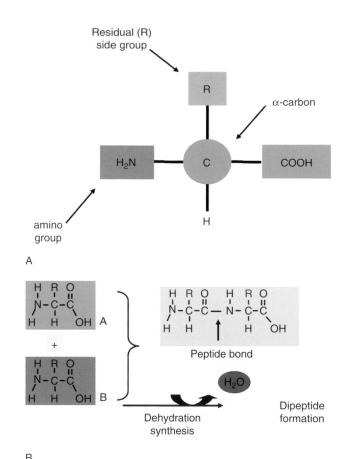

Fig. 2.18. Structure of amino acids. The upper panel shows the general structure of an amino acid. Formation of a dipeptide is illustrated in the lower panel. Two amino acids (A and B) are linked by the formation of a peptide bond between the carboxylic acid moiety of one amino acid and the amine group of the other amino acid. In this process a molecule of water is produced. The reverse reaction, hydrolysis, requires the addition of water to cleave the peptide bond.

by simple abbreviations or a single letter code. Other important amino acids or their derivatives, e.g., ornithine, 5-hydroxytrytophan, L-dopa, and thyroxine are found in the body but these molecules do not typically occur in proteins. Interconversions between some of the amino acids, as well as between amino acids and intermediates of carbohydrate metabolism associated with Krebs cycle reactions also occur, as part of normal cellular activity. Transamination reactions allow the conversion of selected amino acids into their corresponding keto acid and the simultaneous conversion of another keto acid into an amino acid. Oxidative deamination of amino acids occurs primarily in the liver. This initially leads to the generation of ammonia, which is highly toxic to cells. Fortunately, most ammonia is rapidly converted into urea, which can then be excreted. Some of the properties of the amino

Table 2.6. Characteristics of common amino acids.

Name	Abbreviation	Single Letter	R Group Class
Alanine	Ala	A	Nonpolar side chains
Arginine	Arg	R	Basic side chains
Asparagine	Asn	N	Uncharged polar side chains
Asparatic	Asp	D	Acidic side chains
Cysteine	Cys	C	Nonpolar side chains
Glycine	Gly	G	Nonpolar side chains
Glutamic acid	Glu	E	Acidic side chains
Glutamine	Gln	Q	Uncharged polar side chains
Histidine	His	H	Basic side chains
Isoleucine	Ileu	I	Nonpolar side chains
Leucine	Leu	L	Nonpolar side chains
Lysine	Lys	K	Basic side chains
Methionine	Met	M	Nonpolar side chains
Phenylalanine	Phe	F	Nonpolar side chains
Proline	Pro	P	Nonpolar side chains
Serine	Ser	S	Uncharged polar side chains
Theronine	Thr	T	Uncharged polar side chains
Tryptophan	Trp	W	Nonpolar side chains
Tyrosine	Tyr	Y	Uncharged polar side chains
Valine	Val	V	Nonpolar side chains

acids are given in Table 2.6. These properties explain much of the physical-chemical properties of proteins.

Proteins are long chains of amino acids linked by peptide bonds. Two amino acids create a dipeptide, three a tripeptide, and so forth. By definition, 10 or more linked amino acids are called polypeptides, and those with greater than about 50 amino acids are simply called proteins. Since each of the amino acids have unique properties because of variation in the R groups, the sequence of amino acids produces polypeptide and protein chains with correspondingly varied and complex properties. With the availability of 20 different amino acids, the variation of possible structures and therefore functional properties is very large. This is analogous to the huge number of words that can be created with the 26 letters of the alphabet.

Structurally, proteins are described at four levels of organization. The linear sequence of amino acids in a protein is called the primary structure of the protein. This can be thought of like beads on a string. However, proteins in solution do not simply exist as a long strand. Instead, variations in the properties of the R groups allow interactions between the protein and other molecules in the local environment as well as interactions between other amino acids of the same protein chain. This twisting and bending produces a more complex secondary structure. One of the more common results is the formation of coils that can be imagined like a coiled telephone cord. Portions of a protein organized in this way are called α helix segments or regions. The α helix configuration is stabilized by hydrogen bonds that occur between NH and CO groups of amino acids of the primary chain that are spaced about 4 amino acids apart along the series. To reinforce the significance of the primary sequence, this interaction can only occur if the particular side groups of the amino acids allow hydrogen bonds to form. The α helix formation only occurs within a single protein chain. In contrast, the formation of the β-pleated secondary structure can occur via interactions with amino acids within the same protein or by interactions between independent proteins. In this secondary structure arrangement, the amino acids are oriented side by side to produce a layer somewhat like a pleated ribbon. A given protein can exhibit both α helix and β-pleated sheet structure in different regions of the protein. A further or tertiary structure occurs when α-helical or β-pleated regions of a protein twist or fold upon one another to create a globularlike structure. To maintain this complex array, both hydrogen bonds and covalent bonds are required. When two or more independent protein chains interact to produce larger aggregates, the protein(s) is said to have quaternary structure. Examples include the 4 chains that create functional hemoglobin or the 12 proteins that create the enzyme fatty acid synthetase.

As the discussion suggests, the three-dimensional structure of a protein is critically important in allowing the protein to carry out its function. Since much of the secondary, tertiary, or quaternary structure depends on interactions between amino acids and creation of hydrogen and or ionic bonds, it is easy to see that changes in the local environment of the protein can markedly impact function. For example, changes in pH or aqueous conditions can markedly alter interactions that depend on ionic or hydrogen bonds. These changes in protein structure are called denaturation. Depending on the degree of insult and the particular protein involved, when conditions return to normal the protein can return to its appropriate, functional state. As an example of irreversible denaturation, consider what happens to the jellylike albumin of the egg when it is heated or is mixed with a bit of vinegar to make a sauce.

Proteins can also be divided into fibrous or globular classifications. Fibrous proteins are usually elongated and relatively insoluble. Examples include structural proteins found in the connective tissues of blood vessels, subcutaneous regions, surrounding muscles, or other glandular structures, and in tendons and ligaments. The most abundant of these is collagen, which is made by fibroblasts located throughout the body. Collagen begins with the synthesis of a monomeric form, helical tropocollagen. These precursor molecules are modified and packaged side by side to yield strong ropelike structures. Other types of collagen occur in the basement membrane just underneath epithelial cells. In fact, collagens are the most abundant proteins in the body. Other examples of fibrous proteins include other connective tissue proteins, elastic, keratin, and the contractile proteins of muscle cells, actin and myosin.

Globular proteins, by contrast, are generally very soluble, compact, and spherical. These proteins are reactive and therefore more fragile than the fibrous proteins. Since their functionality depends on their three-dimensional shapes and high degree of structural organization, disruption or denaturation effectively destroys function. Enzymes, antibodies, and protein hormones are examples of globular proteins. Adequate functioning of globular proteins depends on the maintenance of active site(s) of the protein. The consequence of denaturation of such a globular protein is illustrated in Figure 2.19.

Classic autoradiographic studies, which traced the movement of radiolabeled amino acids through the secretory cells, established that the site of protein synthesis was the RER. For example, after rats were injected with [³H]-leucine or tissue explants were incubated with a bolus of radiolabeled leucine, the percentage of label in the RER subsequently fell with a following peak in labeling of the Golgi region of the secretory cells. Within 30 min of exposure, label began to decrease in the Golgi but increase in the alveolar lumen. These simple but convincing studies demonstrated that after synthesis in the RER, proteins are rapidly transported to the Golgi for packaging into secretory vesicles and subsequent exocytosis.

Steps for protein synthesis are essentially the same for all cells, although final packaging and fate of new synthesized proteins varies between cells and tissue

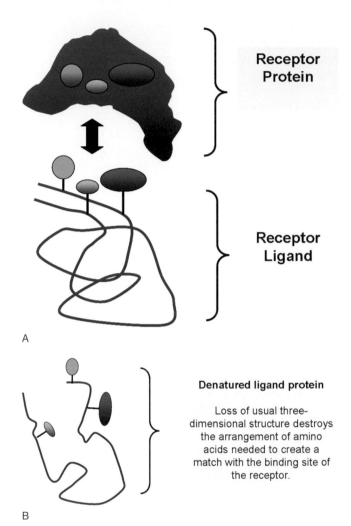

Fig. 2.19. Protein structure and function. Protein interactions and significance of secondary and tertiary structure is illustrated. Functional binding between a hormone receptor and the binding hormone or ligand requires that the ligand achieve the correct shape and orientation so that the amino acids that make the binding site match the active site of the receptor. This is illustrated by the correspondence between the two proteins (Panel A). When the ligand protein becomes denatured these critical amino acids lose their alignment so that the hormone can no longer bind to the receptor and function is lost (Panel B). Similar protein interactions are required in biochemical reactions, e.g., substrates binding to active sites of enzymes, neurotransmitters binding to their receptor, antibodies binding to antigens, or molecules binding to protein transporters in the cell membrane.

types. Aside from directing its own replication, DNA also directs protein synthesis by its capacity to generate mRNA. Each gene is composed of a segment of DNA, which carries the chemical instructions for synthesis of one polypeptide chain in its arrangement of nucleotide bases (adenine, thymine, cytosine, and guanine). Each sequence of three bases—the triplet code—directs the joining of a specific amino acid in the mature mRNA molecule. Although one half of the double-stranded DNA serves as a template for synthesis of the mRNA (transcription), not all of the nucleotides in the gene appear in the final mRNA blueprint. The genes of higher organisms contain exons, the amino-acid specifying sequences, separated by introns. These noncoding introns range from 60 to 100,000 nucleotides in length. Transcription of a particular gene depends on the binding of a transcription factor to a site on the DNA adjacent to the start sequence for the gene. This region is the promoter. The transcription factor mediates the binding of the enzyme RNA polymerase. This enzyme acts to open the DNA helix, and the DNA segment coding for the protein is uncoiled. Only one strand of the DNA, the sense strand, serves as the template for creation of a complementary mRNA. However, before the mRNA can direct protein synthesis, the noncoding introns are enzymatically removed before the newly made mRNA exits the nucleus for translation. Single-stranded RNA also differs from double-stranded DNA in having the sugar ribose instead of deoxyribose and the base uracil instead of thymine. This feature provides a ready means to access the ability of cells for proliferation or synthesizing of proteins by measuring the incorporation of radiolabeled thymidine or uracil.

While it is beyond the scope of this book, elegant molecular studies have confirmed that the specific proteins for secretion are synthesized by membrane-associated ribosomes and that the newly made proteins have short sequences of amino acids, which serve as signals to allow binding and vectoring of the nascent protein into the cisternal spaces of the RER. The signal peptide is ultimately cleaved as the protein progresses to the Golgi apparatus for possible posttranslational modification, i.e., enzymatic addition of sugar residues or phosphate groups. The proteins are ultimately released from the Golgi as secretory vesicles. From here they migrate to the apical membrane of the cell where they are released by exocytosis (see Fig. 2.4). Thus mechanisms of protein synthesis are essentially the same in all cell types. However, total protein synthesis and the degree to which proteins are manufactured for secretion varies markedly from cell type to cell type.

Carbohydrates

As with proteins, carbohydrates are utilized as both structural components in cells and as precursor molecules for energy production. The primary dietary carbohydrates are polysaccharides, disaccharides, and monosaccharides. Carbohydrates are classified according to size and relative solubility. For example, monosaccharides are more soluble than the larger polysaccharides. In both plants and animals, polymeric forms of carbohydrates are stored as relatively insoluble granules, i.e., starch in plants and glycogen in animals cells. Common monosaccharides include those with 3, 4, 5, 6, or 7 carbons; these are trioses, tetroses, pentoses, hexoses, and heptoses, respectively. Derivatives of trioses are generated when the enzymes of the glycolysis biochemical pathway break down the common hexose sugar glucose. These molecules are used by the cells for various catabolic and anabolic activities. For example, trioses are used to produce glycerol needed to create the backbone for the attachment of fatty acids in triglycerides (see Fig. 2.2). Understanding this biochemical pathway is critical to gain an appreciation of cellular energy production. Pentose sugars (ribose and deoxyribose) are key components of nucleotides, nucleic acids, and several coenzymes. The hexose monosaccharide, glucose, plays an especially critical role in intermediary metabolism particularly as an energy source. For the hexose sugars, glucose, galactose, and fructose, are especially important. These monosaccharides serve as the monomers of building blocks for generation of more complex carbohydrates needed by the cells. Many glycoproteins (proteins with attached sugar residues) appear on cell surfaces. Other complex polysaccharides are secreted into the connective tissues, e.g., the glycosaminoglycans where they serve important roles in maintenance of tissue structure and hydration.

Carbohydrates contain carbon, hydrogen, and oxygen, with the hydrogen and oxygen occurring in a $2:1$ ratio as in water. This explains the word *carbohydrate*, i.e., hydrated carbon. Structurally these simple sugars can be represented as chains, but more often a cyclic ring structure is preferred. Figure 2.20 illustrates the formulae and structures of some of these common simple sugars. Compounds that have the same structural formulae but have different spatial arrangement of their atoms are called stereoisomers. The presence of carbon atoms attached to four different atoms or groups, known as an asymmetric carbon, allows for the formation of isomers. The number of possibilities depends on the total number of asymmetric carbons in the molecule (n) and is determined by the following expression: 2^n. Glucose with its 4 asymmetric carbons has 16 possible spatial isomers. Furthermore, the orientation of the H and OH groups around the carbon adjacent to the terminal primary alcohol residue (OH group) determines whether the sugar is a D or L isomer. Nearly all monosaccharides in mammals are D isomers.

Whether they are created via dehydration synthesis or as a consequence of digestion from larger polysaccharides, disaccharides are physiologically important. One of the most common is lactose or milk sugar. It is produced by linking glucose and galactose. For most mammals lactose supplies much of the energy needed

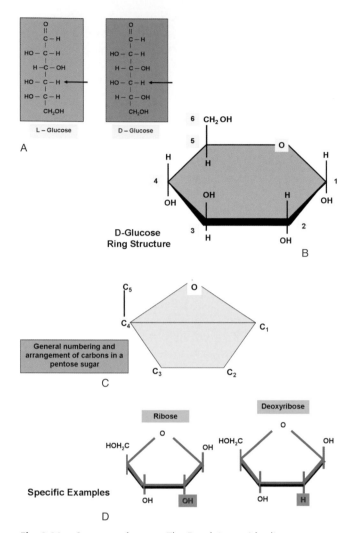

Fig. 2.20. Structure of sugars. The Panel A provides line structures for two structural isomers of the common hexose monosaccharide, glucose (arrows). Panel B gives the cyclic structure for α-D glucose. The arrangement and numbering of carbons in a pentose sugar appears in Panel C. Panel D shows the difference between ribose and deoxyribose, the sugar residues present in RNA and DNA, respectively.

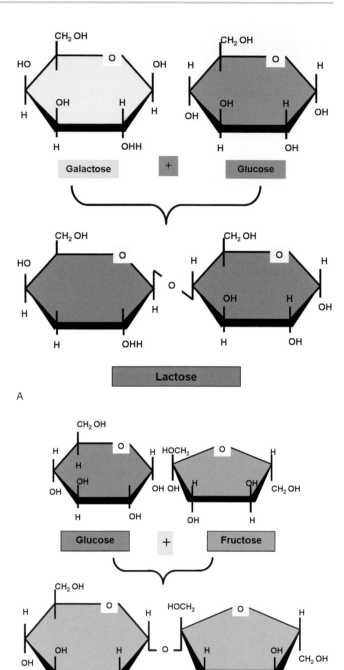

Fig. 2.21. Structure of disaccharides. Panel A shows the combining of galactose and glucose to produce the disaccharide lactose or milk sugar. Panel B depicts the creation of the disaccharide sucrose from the combination of glucose and fructose. Maltose, a disaccharide composed of two molecules of glucose, follows a similar pattern.

by the suckling neonate as well as the monomeric building blocks needed for rapid tissue development. Maltose, which derives from two glucose molecules, is a common cleavage product generated by the hydrolysis of starch. Table sugar, sucrose, is a combination of glucose and fructose. As the name suggests, 6-carbon fructose is a common fruit sugar. It also is a component in reproductive tract secretions. Figure 2.21 illustrates the structures of some of these common disaccharides.

Whether a plant starch or glycogen, both are polymers of glucose and are the essential sources of the glucose that is used throughout the body in monogastric species. Although glucose is also essential for ruminants, fed starches are fermented by rumen microorganisms so that little if any glucose is available

for absorption across the small intestine. For these animals, the primary fermentation products—acetate, butyrate, and propionate—supply the precursors for fatty acid synthesis and energy production. In

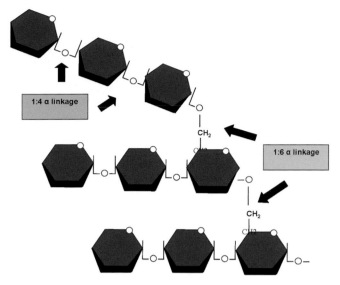

Fig. 2.22. Structure of glycogen. A simple example of the structure of a portion of glycogen is illustrated. Repeating glucose monomers are linked together to form large branched chain polymers. These relatively insoluble molecules serve as ideal storage products and appear in liver and muscle cells as dense granules. Cleavage of the 1 : 4α linkages that produce the linear chains and the 1 : 6α linkages that make branches depend on two different enzymes when glycogen is hydrolyzed for use by the cell.

particular, portal blood supplied to the liver from the small intestine allows for the conversion of most of the absorbed propionate to glucose for use by the cells. This is called gluconeogenesis. It is important in all animals at times, but it is especially critical in ruminants since glucose from the diet is essentially nonexistent.

Dietary starches are first attacked for hydrolysis by α-amylase in the saliva. This initial breakdown is suppressed by the reduced pH of the stomach, i.e., α-amylase pH optima is near neutrality. However, hydrolysis of starches increases again as starch reaches the small intestine and additional amylases from the pancreas and small intestine appear. Glucose is stored primarily in liver and muscle cells in the form of glycogen. This reserve of glycogen can then be mobilized to supply glucose when needed. When ATP is plentiful and stocks of glycogen are sufficient, additional energy reserves produced by the conversion of glucose to acetate and ultimately fatty acids are stored as triglycerides in adipocytes. Figure 2.22 illustrates the structure of glycogen. Subsequent chapters describe the biochemical reactions and pathways involved in catabolism of glycogen and other carbohydrates to supply the energy needs and building blocks for synthesis of important macromolecules.

Lipids

Although we have discussed triglycerides and phospholipids related to membrane formation, other lipids are also important. Some are messenger molecules. Details of endocrine and other aspects of cell signaling will be considered in subsequent chapters, but some appreciation of these special lipids is warranted. Steroids are structurally very different from triglycerides. They are derived from the parent molecule cholesterol. Despite its "bad press," cholesterol is nonetheless essential. In addition to serving as the parent molecule for steroid hormone production it is also a vital element in membranes, where it acts to increase membrane fluidity. It is also essential for the production of vitamin D and production of bile salts.

Unlike the hydrocarbon chain of the fatty acids, cholesterol is composed of a series of interlocking rings with a side chain. Specifically, the four interlocking A, B, C, and D rings of the cholesterol core contain the cyclopentanohydrophenanthrene nucleus that occurs repeatedly in all of the steroid hormones. For example, two structural types of steroid hormones are made in the cortex of the adrenal gland: those that have a 2-carbon side chain attached at position 17 of the D ring for a total of 21 carbons, the C_{21} steroids, and those that have a keto or hydroxyl group at position 17 for a total of 19 carbons, the C_{19} steroids. Most C_{19} steroids have a keto group at position 17 and are often simply called 17-ketosteroids. The C_{19} steroid hormones have androgenic or testosterone-like effects or actions. The C_{21} steroids of the adrenal gland are either mineralocorticoids or glucocorticoids. The mineralocorticoids have primary effects on sodium and potassium excretion. The major hormone in this class is aldosterone. The glucocorticoids, as you might guess from the name, have predominate effects related to glucose and carbohydrate metabolism. Examples of specific steroids in this class are cortisol and corticosterone. Other sex steroids, for example, estrogen and progesterone will be discussed in subsequent chapters. A major point of our discussion at this point is to appreciate the fact that despite the seemingly small differences in structure between, for example, estrogen and testosterone, these two steroid hormones have markedly different effects. This is directly related to the specificity of hormone receptors that are expressed in various target cells. That is, estrogen molecules bind very poorly to androgen receptors, and conversely testosterone binds very poorly to the estrogen receptor.

The eicosanoids are a diverse family of lipids generated from a 20-carbon fatty acid called arachidonic acid. Arachidonic acid is plentiful in the plasma membrane of the cell. The four major groups of eicosanoids include prostaglandins, prostacyclins, thromboxanes, and leukotrienes. A commercial preparation of prostaglandin F$_2\alpha$, luteolyse, is familiar to many dairy and beef producers because it is used in a management scheme to synchronize estrus in cattle. The product acts to cause early dissolution of the corpus luteum on the ovary. Various eicosanoids are important in the control of blood pressure, gastrointestinal tract motility, vasoconstriction, and blood flow.

Since the major lipids in plasma do not circulate freely in the aqueous environment of the blood, fatty acids and other important lipids are transported bound to carrier molecules. Free fatty acids are bound to albumin (a major protein produced by the liver). Most of the cholesterol, triglycerides, and phospholipids are in a complex with lipoproteins for transport. There are five families of lipoproteins that vary with respect to the ratio of protein to lipid in the complex. They can be distinguished based on the position they migrate to following high-speed centrifugation. Those with greater lipid contents (less density) orient closer to the top of the centrifuge tube and those with less lipid further toward the bottom of the tube. This is somewhat like the cream rising to the top of a container of nonhomogenized milk. This explains the description of the lipoproteins as very low- (VLDL), intermediate- (IDL), low- (LDL) or high-density (HDL) lipoproteins. The other class includes the chylomicra that are produced in the intestinal villi and are critical in initial packaging and transport of digested triglycerides. Lipoproteins are topics in the popular press because of their involvement with lipid and cholesterol transport in the blood and relationship with health. For this purpose, usually only the major classes, HDLs and LDLs, are distinguished. The amounts and ratios of these in the blood are important diagnostic tools related to cardiovascular health in humans and animals. Cells can take up cholesterol and other lipids from the blood. Most of the cholesterol is associated with LDLs. When cells need cholesterol to make new membranes or for other purposes, they synthesize transmembrane receptors for the LDL proteins. These receptor proteins migrate within the membrane until they become localized in clathrin-coated pits. These are areas of the cell membrane that are destined for endocytosis. LDLs that bind to the receptors are subsequently taken into the cells as part of an internalized vesicle. These coated vesicles are processed by interactions with lysosomes to release the cholesterol for use by the cell. Interestingly, more than 25 different receptors are processed via this clathrin-coated pit pathway. In the case of cholesterol, if the LDL receptor-mediated uptake of cholesterol is blocked, this leads to excess accumulation of cholesterol-laden LDL in the blood, and this excess cholesterol is believed to contribute to production of atherosclerotic plaques and consequently cardiovascular disease. The study of families with strong genetic links to cardiovascular disease initially led to discovery of this relationship. That is one mechanism responsible for some metabolic diseases, specifically a mutation that prevented normal expression of the LDL receptor. Structures of some selected lipids are illustrated in Figure 2.23.

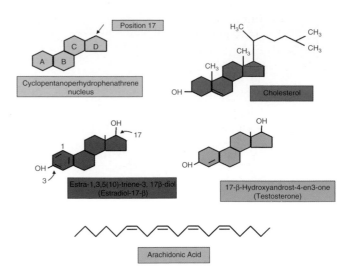

Fig. 2.23. Structure of specialized lipids. Structures of some of the specialized lipid molecules are illustrated. Cholesterol and the steroid hormones and their relatives have the cyclopentanohydrophenanthrene nucleus with four hydrocarbon rings in common (upper panel). Additions of side chains to the 17-carbon, methyl or hydroxyl groups, or addition of double bonds in the A ring lead to production of cholesterol, estradiol, testosterone, and other steroids. The relatively linear hydrocarbon chain of the 20-carbon arachidonic acid becomes folded and modified to yield various prostaglandins, thromboxanes, or leukotrienes.

Nucleic acids

Understanding DNA or RNA requires an appreciation of the molecules that compose these macromolecules. These nucleic acids are produced from combinations of nucleotides but nucleotides are in turn a combination of three elements: 1) a phosphate group, 2) a pentose sugar (either ribose or deoxyribose), and 3) a nitrogen-containing base (either a purine or a pyrimidine). There are three types of pyrimidines: cytosine (C), thymine (T), and uracil (U). The two types of pyrimidines are adenine (A) and guanine (G). Thymine is unique to DNA and uracil is unique to RNA.

Variation between DNA strands, or in other words between different genes, depends on the particular sequence of nitrogenous bases that occur. A combination of either deoxyribose or ribose and one of the bases is called a nucleoside. Include the phosphate group (sugar + base + phosphate) and you have a nucleotide. The phosphate groups are joined to the hydroxyl group on the C$_5$ carbon of the sugar residue. Moreover, as you will see related to ATP production it is not uncommon to find mono-, di- or triphosphates attached to many nucleotides. To illustrate, a combination of the purine adenine + deoxyribose + one phosphate makes adenosine monophosphate or AMP. The same base and sugar with two phosphates makes ADP, or adenosine diphosphate. If a third phosphate is added adenosine triphosphate, ATP, is generated.

Single strands of DNA or strands of RNA are produced when a phosphate group from one nucleotide (attached to the C_5 carbon of the pentose sugar) links with the hydroxyl group located on the C_3 carbon of the pentose sugar of another nucleotide. Thus the nucleic acid chain grows in a 3′ to 5′ direction. This means that along the course of a growing nucleotide chain, the nitrogenous bases are not directly linked with other bases in the same chain. For DNA this arrangement allows for complementary base pairing occurring between adjacent chains. This is the essence of creation of double-stranded DNA. The DNA molecule is most easily imagined like a ladder. The outside supports of the ladder are represented by the covalently linked, pentose sugars and phosphate groups of the nucleotides. Complementary bonding between bases creates the rungs of the ladder. Now if the ladder is imagined as being twisted like a spiral staircase, this gives a reasonable approximation of the DNA.

However, it is important to remember that while linkages between sugars within a chain are maintained by strong covalent bonds, the interactions between nitrogenous bases between two DNA chains depends on simple hydrogen bonding, similar to the interactions between adjacent water molecules (see Fig. 2.1). These hydrogen bonds, while not strong individually, are critical because of their abundance, this also allows the double-stranded DNA to readily unzip as required for gene transcription. Once this is accomplished, the strands can then readily rejoin. Interactions between bases allows for bonding between adenine and thymine, cytosine and guanine. These linkages, A + T and C + G, are called complementary bonds or complementary bases. However, the strands are oriented so that one is oriented in a 5′ to 3′ direction and the other 3′ to 5′ (the numbering is based on the orientation of phosphate groups linking the 3 or 5 carbons of the pentose sugar). In single-stranded RNA molecules, the bases are A, G, C, and U (which replaces the T found in DNA). The pentose sugar is ribose instead of deoxyribose. Examples of nucleic acid structures and components are illustrated in Figures 2.24 and 2.25.

Cellular biochemistry

The cell theory, the idea that cells arise only from other cells, was first proposed in the late 1800s. This now

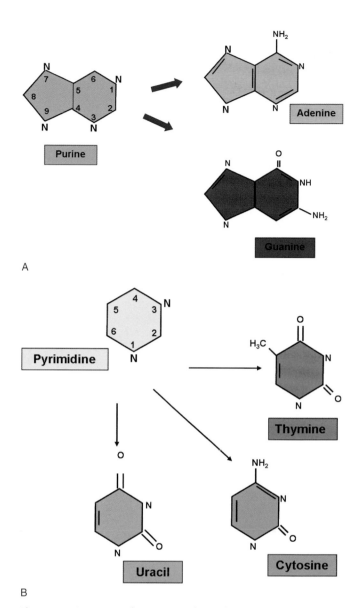

Fig. 2.24. Structures of nitrogenous bases found in DNA and RNA. Structures of the parent nitrogenous bases, purine (A) and pyrimidine (B), and specific bases occurring in DNA and RNA are illustrated.

seems elementary, but in the 1600s Robert Hooke based it on initial observations of plant samples, which showed that tissues were composed of cells. This was followed by studies by the German scientists Schleiden and Schwann who insisted that all living things were composed of cells. This idea flew in the face of the notion of spontaneous generation, which suggested that organisms arose from debris or other inert nonliving materials. The following are four ideas inherent in the cell theory:

1. The cell is the fundamental structural and functional unit of living organisms.
2. The function of organisms depends on activities of cells both individually and collectively.

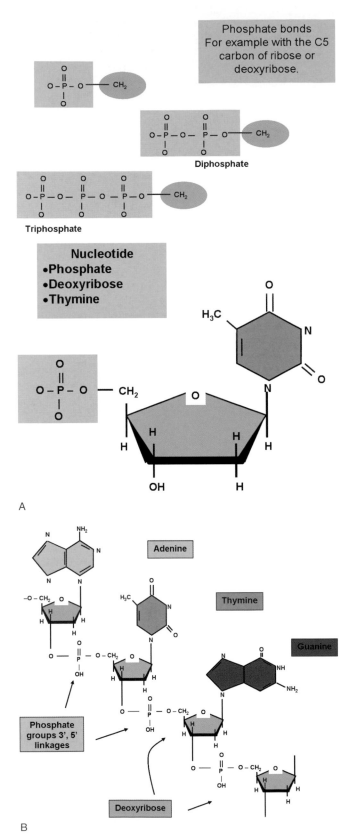

A

B

Fig. 2.25. Structure of a single strand of DNA. Bases shown are adenine, thymine, and guanine (A). The repeating pattern with the backbone of deoxyribose and phosphate groups is apparent with a variable sequence of nitrogenous bases (B).

3. The biochemistry of cells is dictated by the subcellular organelles present in the cell.
4. Propagation of life is based on cellular activity.

Despite the relevance of the cell in physiology, chemistry, physics, and biochemistry are at the center of all catabolism and anabolism. In other words, it is reasonable to think of the cell as the core-organizing element that allows for control and coordination of the myriad of chemical and physical reactions that constitute life and living. Understanding physiology requires an appreciation of these other scientific disciplines. Be advised that our discussions of specific chemical reactions, biochemical events, or physical properties are no substitute for specific classes in physics, chemistry, or biochemistry. However, we believe that a sincere, thoughtful study of physiology provides an opportunity to integrate the fundamentals gained from study of these disciplines. What could be more interesting than learning how our bodies and those of our animals function?

Chemical bonds

Cellular activity is tied to both the creation of complex macromolecules, which requires combining other simpler molecules and creation of new bonds or catabolic activity to break the bonds in nutrient molecules to supply the building blocks for these new creations. Some of the energy derived from breaking chemical bonds is also captured for future use by the cells. Enzymes catalyze nearly all cellular chemistry. As you learned in general chemistry, attractive forces maintain orientations between atoms in molecules to produce chemical bonds. Three major types of bonds are hydrogen bonds, ionic bonds, and covalent bonds. In addition, Van der Waals forces, similar to hydrogen bonds, are important in maintenance of the structure of complex biological molecules where charge differentials aid maintenance of structural relationships. We have already discussed hydrogen bonds in our description of how water behaves (see Fig. 2.1). Hydrogen bonds are produced when a hydrogen atom is covalently bound to an electronegative atom. The most common examples are oxygen and nitrogen. When these groups are positioned close to other strongly electronegative atoms, this produces a kind of tug of war as the two electronegative atoms "fight" for dominion of the hydrogen atom. These reactions create attraction forces that link or bridge the molecules. Hydrogen bonds are particularly important as intramolecular forces that act to mold the three-dimensional shape of many macromolecules. Much of the folding of proteins that defines their tertiary structure depends on hydrogen bonds. Another example is the interaction between complementary strands of the DNA molecule. Despite the relative weakness of individual hydrogen bonds, they are collectively critical for normal cellular functioning.

Ionic bonds are produced when the transfer of electrons from one atom to another generates attractive forces between atoms. This happens because the usual balance between + and − charges is lost and ions are formed. The atom that accepts electrons acquires a net negative charge and is called an anion. The electron donor, now called a cation, has a net positive charge. Atoms with opposite charges attract. This is the basis of the ionic bond. A commonly used example of ionic bonds is table salt or sodium chloride. As you may recall from general chemistry, sodium has an atomic number of 11 and therefore has only one electron in its third or outer shell. To achieve stability the atom would have to acquire an additional seven electrons (the third orbit around the nucleus can accept eight electrons). Stabilizing this outer orbit is more likely to happen by shedding the single electron so that the second orbit (filled) becomes the valance shell around the nucleus of the atom. Chlorine has an atomic number of 17. The outer valance shell needs only one electron to fill its valance orbit. When it accepts an electron, stability is increased, but the atom acquires a net negative charge and becomes an anion. As you would suspect, ionic bonds are common between atoms with one or two valance electrons (metallic elements, sodium, calcium, and potassium, for example) and elements with seven valance electrons (chlorine, fluorine, and iodine). The majority of ionic compounds exist as salts. When dry they form highly organized crystals as a consequence of their ionic bonds. In aqueous environments, salts dissociate to produce ions. Many more common ions (Ca^{+2}, Na^+, K^+, Cl^-) are critical to normal cellular physiology because of their roles in regulation of activity of many enzymes (Ca^{+2}) and significance in maintenance of polarity across cell membranes. Calcium, which is the most abundant essential mineral in the body, is especially important. It not only is critical for the activation of various cytoplasmic kinases, it is essential for muscle function, and in a more stable form—hydroxyappatite, $Ca_{10}(PO_4)_6(OH_2)$—it is a fundamental part of the inorganic, extracellular structure of bone. This likely explains the reason for lack of finding shed antlers or skeletal remains of animals in rural areas. Other animals, especially rodents, use these materials to supply their mineral needs.

About one-third of basal energy (ATP hydrolysis) is used to maintain an ionic gradient across the plasma membranes through the activity of Na-K ATPase protein transporters in the plasma membrane. Specifically, these proteins move Na^+ and K^+ against their concentration gradients (energy requiring) so

that concentrations of intracellular Na are about tenfold lower inside than outside the cell (~15 versus 150 mEq/l) with the opposite for K^+ ions (~14 versus 140 mEq/l). Since these ions passively move down their concentration gradients, the ATPase pumps must be constantly active. Somewhat like the bilge pumps of a boat that act to constantly remove water that leaks or splashes into the boat. The transporter couples sodium and potassium transport so that each action of the protein ejects $3Na^+$ out of the cell and carries $2K^+$ ions into the cell. Coupled with the fact that the membrane is slightly more permeable to K^+ than Na^+ under basal conditions, the action of the ATPase protein maintains the ionic and electrical gradient across the cell membrane. These actions combined with the accumulation of cellular proteins causes the production of an electrical gradient across most cells of about −40 mV (inside relative to outside). Many cells, especially nerve cells take advantage of changes in ion concentrations or polarity for cell signaling. The activity of chemical- and voltage-regulated gates for sodium and potassium (transporter proteins) are altered to explain the abrupt changes in membrane potential that occurs during nerve transmissions.

Aside from transferring electrons, atoms can also be stabilized by the sharing of electrons between nuclei. In these cases the valence orbits of the sharing atoms are also shared so that stability of both atoms is achieved. This is the essence of covalent bonds. If a single pair of electrons are shared this creates a single covalent bond. For illustrative purposes this is usually shown as a single line connecting two atoms. In other cases, atoms can share two or three electron pairs; this produces double or triple covalent bonds that are illustrated by double or triple lines between atoms ($O{=}O$), as in O_2 gas or ($N{\equiv}N$) in N_2 gas (see Fig. 2.18). Some atoms are considered relatively reactive and others relatively inert. As Figure 2.26 shows, a look at the atomic structure of some example atoms explains the reason for these differences.

Carbon is an especially abundant cellular atom. It has four electrons in its outer or valence orbit, but stability is achieved when the orbit is filled to capacity (eight electrons). This means that there are numerous possibilities of sharing electrons to achieve stability. One possibility is to create sharing of four electrons from four distinct neighbors. This would be the case in the creation of methane gas (CH_4). Since hydrogen needs either to lose an electron or gain another to complete its outer valence orbit, sharing between the single carbon atom and four hydrogen atoms satisfies both atoms. Numerous examples of covalent bonds involving carbon atoms are shown in the structures of neutral lipids (essentially hydrocarbon chains), carbohydrates, and proteins (see Figs. 2.2, 2.18, and 2.20). By convention, in drawings carbon atoms are not

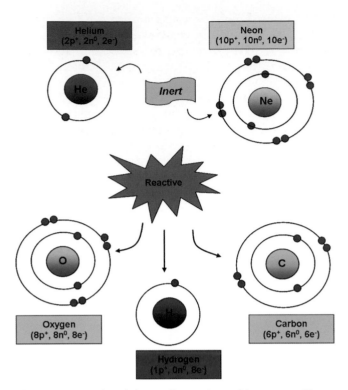

Fig. 2.26. Examples of chemically reactive and inert atoms. The red balls depict electrons in orbit around the nucleus of each atom. Helium and neon with completely filled valence orbits have little incentive to interact with neighboring molecules. In contrast, oxygen, carbon, and hydrogen need a change in the number of valence electrons to complete their outer shell of electrons and maximize stability.

explicitly shown but are understood to be positioned at line intersections. A simple example of double bonds is sharing of electrons between a carbon atom and two oxygen atoms. In carbon dioxide (CO_2 or $O{=}C{=}O$) sharing of electrons is equal between the atoms. Because of this there is no separation of charge so this covalent bond is also called a nonpolar covalent bond. Nonpolar covalent bonds are common. For example, consider the fatty acid tails of the phospholipids in cellular membranes (see Fig. 2.3). Our prior discussion of water (see Fig. 2.1), illustrates an example of a polar covalent bond. In these instances, like spoiled children, one or more atoms of the bond unit has a greater capacity to attract the shared electrons. Since the electrons spend more of their time in orbit near the stronger partner, these covalent bonds produce a separation of charge. In other words on average there is a separation of charge, one area of the new molecule has a net negative charge (shared electron[s] more often in this region) and a net positive charge (shared electrons more often playing next door). As a general rule small atoms with six or seven valence electrons (oxygen, nitrogen, chlorine) are better able to attract electrons, so they are described as being strongly electronega-

tive. These atoms favor "hogging" shared electrons to complete their valence orbital shells. Atoms with only one or two valence electrons are more likely to relinquish control of shared electrons and are called electropositive atoms. Examples of these include: hydrogen, potassium, and sodium. If you ponder the difference between polar and nonpolar covalent bonds, it should be easy to imagine why molecules with an abundance of polar covalent bonds easily dissolve (associate) with water. Conversely, molecules with few or any polar covalent bonds—lipids, for example—have little capacity to interact with the abundant polar water molecules in our cells and bodies.

Chemical reactions

It is apparent that living processes depend on an almost bewildering array of chemical reactions. Molecules in our food or in the rations of our animals are destroyed (chemical bonds broken) to supply intermediate molecules for building blocks, e.g., consider hydrolysis of plant starches to supply glucose for production of glycogen in liver cells. Some of the glucose is oxidized to produce ATP needed to supply cellular energy. DNA and RNA is synthesized as our cells flourish and grow. How do we organize and make sense of all of these reactions? Fortunately, despite the number of individual molecules involved, patterns begin to evolve. For example, the breaking down of bonds between the glucose and fructose in the disaccharide sucrose or of the peptide bonds between alanine and lysine in a protein molecule are both hydrolysis reactions. Chemical reactions occur when chemical bonds are created between atoms, chemical bonds between atoms are broken, or chemical bonds are rearranged. A common illustration is to denote the reactions in simple symbolic expressions as chemical equations. For example, the combination of carbon and oxygen to create carbon dioxide could be written in the following manner:

$$2O + C \longrightarrow CO_2$$
$$\text{(reactants)} \qquad \text{(product)}$$

This is an example of a synthesis reaction that requires the formation of new chemical bonds. This could be generally indicated by the following expression: $A + B \rightarrow AB$. Simplistically, such reactions explain the anabolic side of metabolism. Figure 2.18 shows an example of a synthesis reaction between two amino acids to create a dipeptide. The opposite of this is a decomposition reaction. These are often hydrolysis reactions because of the addition of water to complete the reaction. The expression $AB \rightarrow A + B$ gives a generic example of such a reaction. Specific examples would include the cleavage of glucose monomers from glycogen, the cleavage of peptides from a dietary protein by enzymes in the intestinal lumen, or the initial reactions of beta-oxidation—the process that acts to catabolize 2 carbons at a time from fatty acids chains. These are all examples of catabolic reactions.

Another type of reaction is the exchange reaction. As the name suggests, in this situation a functional group is moved from a donating molecule to a receiving molecule. This is indicated by these expressions: $AB + C \rightarrow AC + B$ or $AB + CD \rightarrow AD + CB$. Such reactions are common. For example, the nucleotides ATP or GTP are frequent donors of a phosphate group to another molecule. Kinases, a very large family of enzymes, catalyze these phosphorylation reactions. As we will see in our discussion of cell signaling, many important regulatory enzymes are themselves controlled by their phosphorylation state. Some of these proteins are activated when a phosphate group is added and others are inhibited. Other examples also abound. For example, the first step in the catabolism of glucose in the biochemical pathway, glycolysis, involves the introduction of phosphate to produce glucose-6-phosphate catalyzed by the enzyme hexose kinase. Other exchange reactions transfer amino groups to allow generation of nonessential amino acids. For example, the enzyme, alanine-pyruvate transaminase, functions to promote the transfer of amino groups from most amino acids to generate alanine by adding the amino group to pyruvate.

A final class of reactions to consider is the oxidation-reduction reactions. These reactions are central to catabolism of nutrients to manufacture ATP. Failure of these reactions, as occurs in the absence of oxygen, results in death. The essence of the reactions is the exchange of electrons between reactants. The molecule or atom that loses the electron (electron donor) is characterized as having become oxidized. The reactant that accepts the electron is said to become reduced. Many of these reactions involve the transfer of hydrogen (which, of course, includes the electron). These reactions will be considered in greater detail in our discussion of aerobic respiration.

Significance of enzymes

It is difficult to overstate the importance of enzymes in cellular metabolism. Without the presence of enzymes to catalyze the myriad of biochemical reactions required for anabolic and catabolic activities, life would cease. All enzymes are globular proteins that act as promoters of various but specific chemical reactions. Reactants must be present in the cell but rates of reaction for virtually all biologically relevant processes are nonexistent if the required enzymes are absent or defective. As catalysts, enzymes accelerate reaction rates but do not become altered in the process. The enzyme can be thought of as a kind of biochemical matchmaker. Binding sites for substrates allow for close association of the substrates, a lowering of activation energy, and an enhanced opportunity that the reaction will take place. Because of the critical nature of the substrate binding sites on the enzyme, even small changes in conditions can perturb the arrangement of amino acids around the binding site, rendering the enzyme ineffective (see Fig. 2.19). Because of the unique nature of the binding site, enzymes are highly specific. For example, the enzyme hexose kinase, which adds a phosphate group to glucose, has no capacity to add a phosphate group to fructose, despite the fact that both molecules are similar hexose sugars.

Some enzymes are functional just as they are synthesized, that is, the protein alone. Other enzymes require the presence of a particular ion (often a trace mineral, e.g., Mg, Co, Cu, Mn) in their environment. These ions are thought to maintain the active binding site of the enzyme in the appropriate conformation for reactants to be able to bind. These aids to enzyme function are called cofactors. Still other enzymes operate in combination with organic molecules called coenzymes that are essential for the enzyme to carry out its function. Coenzymes assist some groups of enzymes by acting as carriers of various specific functional groups or of electrons (hydrogen atoms). Many coenzymes are derived from vitamins, which explain the need for these substances to be present in the diet. For example, the B vitamins riboflavin (B_2) and niacin give rise to flavin adenine dinucleotide (FAD) and nicotinamide adenine dinucleotide (NAD), respectively. These cofactors become reduced as a consequence of carbohydrate catabolism. When membrane bond enzymes in the mitochondria subsequently oxidize them, a portion of the energy associated with these electron transfers is utilized to drive the synthesis of ATP. Finally, some enzymes are composed of more than one protein. Some enzymes are first synthesized as pro- or precursor enzymes that become active only when they reach the area where they are to be used. For example, digestive enzymes synthesized by pancreatic cells are secreted into ducts where the enzymes are mixed with alkaline secretions and dumped into the lumen of the small intestine. The enzymes become functional only when they enter the lumen of the intestine. This is an important safety mechanism. Since these enzymes are capable of hydrolyzing a wide array of cellular proteins, inappropriate activation of the enzymes at the time of synthesis and secretion could virtually cause degradation of your own pancreatic tissue. This is clearly undesirable.

Most enzymes are named based on the reactions they catalyze or the substrates upon which they act.

Table 2.7.   Enzyme classifications.

Enzyme Class	Action	Example
Oxidoreductases	Oxidation–Reduction reactions (electron–hydrogen transfer)	Lactate dehydrogenase
Transferases	Transfer of groups (other than hydrogen between substrates)	Hexose–6–phosphotransferase (Hexose kinase)
Hydrolyases	Cleaves ester, peptide, and other types of bonds	Amylase
Lyases	Removes groups leaving behind double bonds	Aldolase
Isomerases	Interconversions of optical or geometric isomers	Phosphohexose isomerase
Ligases	New bonds to link together two substrates	Glutamine synthase

For example, enzymes that cleave starch molecules are called amylases, those that cleave proteins are called proteases, lipases break down lipids and so forth. Others are designated as dehydrogenases because they act to remove hydrogen atoms or decarboxylases for removal of carboxyl groups. Unfortunately, there are often multiple names applied to the same enzymes and traditional names remain in usage. For example, the small intestine enzyme chymotrypsin is described as a hydrolyase, but more specifically as a proteinase, and further as a serine proteinase because this defines the catalytic mechanism by which the enzyme cleaves proteins. The International Union of Biochemistry promotes a very systematic nomenclature for the naming of enzymes. However, in much of the physiological literature common and general names for enzymes abound. Table 2.7 provides a six-level classification of enzymes along with examples.

Three steps occur in enzyme action. Step one is binding of substrates to the active site of the enzyme (formation of the enzyme substrate complex). This binding induces a conformation change in the protein that allows rearrangement of the substrates and formation of the product (step two). The third step is release of the products from the enzyme. This happens because the newly created product no longer has a shape that is compatible with the active site of the enzyme. Enzymes function by reducing activation energy. Some chemical reactions can be promoted in

the test tube by heating the reactants. This increases kinetic and thermal energy and makes collisions between substrates more frequent, thereby reducing the required activation energy. Lower activation energy in this manner in cells is not feasible. For example, one of the consequences of a high fever is the degradation of some proteins. By specific mechanisms that are poorly understood, binding of a substrate(s) to its specific enzyme lowers activation energy. The significance is profound. Compared with noncatalyzed conditions, rates of reaction are increased a millionfold or more. Just as remarkable, once the product is released, the enzyme is free to repeat the process thousands of times. Indeed some cellular enzymes remain in the cell for extended periods before they must be replaced. Figure 2.27 illustrates the idea of lowered activation energy and mechanisms of enzyme action.

Extracellular environment and cell function

As mentioned earlier, animal cells are continually bathed in the extracellular liquid interstitial fluid, which is mostly derived from blood. In many ways it is similar to blood plasma but contains few, if any, blood cells (some wandering leucocytes are sometimes present), and blood clotting factors are absent. Other electrolytes, nutrients, and water are abundant. The movement of these compounds into and out of cells is controlled by both passive and active mechanisms. Health of the cells depends on the fact that the plasma membrane is semipermeable and selective. This means that some substances are allowed to pass across the membrane, but others are not. As you might guess, nutrients are readily captured, waste products are secreted, and many potentially harmful substances are excluded. The purpose of this section is to characterize some fundamental properties related to cellular transport and maintenance of the cellular environment within appropriated boundaries. As noted previously, maintenance of normal concentrations of nutrients and ions in body fluids is an important part of homeostasis.

Osmosis

The diffusion of solvent—water, for example—through a selective or semipermeable membrane is called osmosis. Water transport occurs when there is a difference in the relative concentration of water molecules across the membrane. If both sides of a water permeable membrane are exposed to distilled water, there is no net move of water molecules, just as many

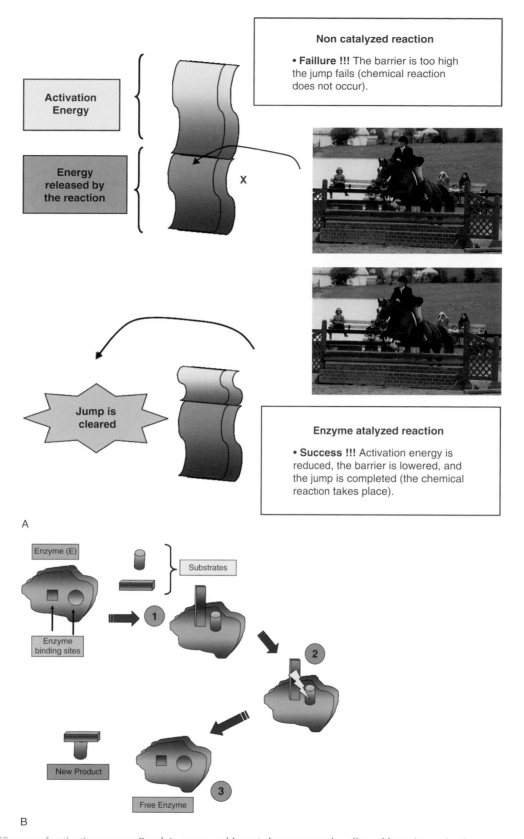

Fig. 2.27. Significance of activation energy. Panel A, upper and lower) demonstrates the effect of lowering activation energy on the chemical reactions. Enzyme catalyzed reactions are markedly enhanced. In Panel B the mechanism of enzyme action is depicted. Each enzyme is highly specific; only substrates capable of binding to the active sites will be affected. In step 1, the enzyme-substrate complex is formed. In step 2, internal rearrangements occur and substrates are covalently linked. In step 3, the new product is released and the enzyme is free for another round of activity.

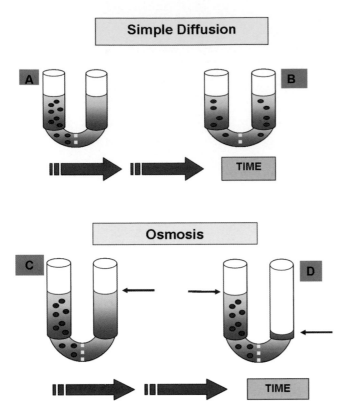

Fig. 2.28. Diffusion and osmosis. The Panels A and B illustrate the process of simple diffusion. At the beginning (A) two sides of a u-tube are separated by a membrane that is permeable to the solute (red particles) in the left arm of the tube. Over time (B) the solute molecules diffuse down their concentration gradient to areas of lower concentration. With sufficient time the solute molecules become equally dispersed throughout the entire solution. Panels C and D demonstrate osmosis. Two sides of the u-tube are separated by a semipermeable membrane that is permeable to the solvent (indicated by the green coloring) but not the solute (red) molecules (C). Since the right side of the tube has a greater concentration of solvent molecules, they move from the right side through the membrane. Migration continues until the hydrostatic pressure equals the osmotic pressure (D). Note the difference in the levels of liquid (arrows) after the experiment has continued for a period of time.

molecules would randomly move in either direction across the barrier. If on the other hand, a substance were dissolved in the water on one side of the membrane but not the other, the relative number of water molecules per unit volume would be decreased on the side of the membrane with the solute. If the membrane were impermeable to the dissolved substance (solute), but permeable to the water, then water molecules would begin to leave the area with the higher concentration of water molecules and pass across to the opposite side. Osmosis is the movement of solvent in this manner. Figure 2.28 illustrates the effects of membrane permeability on diffusion and osmosis. In the open system illustrated in the figure, differences in

osmolarity drive the movement of water molecules until hydrostatic pressure becomes sufficiently high to resist the further movement. Movement of water molecules to a region of greater solute concentration can be prevented by applying pressure. The pressure required to prevent migration of solvent molecules is the effective osmotic pressure of the solution.

If we consider the cytoplasm of the cell (or the aqueous environments of many cellular organelles), there are multiple opportunities for varying concentrations of solutes and corresponding differences in osmolarity across these membranes as well as between the cytoplasm and the outside interstitial fluid. Since these membrane-bound compartments are permeable to water, osmosis has dramatic effects. For these reasons it is important that the osmolarity of interstitial fluids and consequently blood be maintained within relatively narrow boundaries. Changes in the osmolarity of the solutions bathing cells can cause cells to either shrink or swell. The capacity of a solution to affect the tone or shape of cells by modifying the internal water volume of the cell is called tonicity. A typical value for blood plasma or interstitial fluid is about 300 mosm l/liter. Cells exposed to solutions with the same osmolarity or tonicity as blood plasma will retain their normal shape. Such solutions are described as isotonic. Examples include 0.9% saline (NaCl) or a 5% glucose solution. These solutions are routinely used for preparation of intravenous treatments because the solutions have no impact on normal cell volume. Solutions with a greater effective osmotic pressure than blood are hypertonic and those with lesser effective osmotic pressures are hypotonic. Cells that are placed in a hypertonic solution lose water and shrink or crenate. Cells that are placed in dilute (hypotonic) solutions swell. As an extreme example, if cells are placed in distilled water, there are no dissolved substances, so water molecules enter the cells until the cells rupture. Figure 2.29 illustrates the responses of red blood cells incubated in isotonic, hypotonic, or hypertonic solutions.

Osmotic pressure (P) is related to temperature and volume, similar to the pressure of a gas as described in the following equation:

$$P = \frac{nRT}{V}$$

In this expression n is the number of particles, R is the gas constant, T is the absolute temperature and V is the volume. In usual physiological circumstances, R, T, and V are essentially constants. This means that the primary factor affecting osmotic pressure is the number of particles or solute molecules per unit of solvent. With ideal solutions, the osmotic pressure can be easily predicted. For example, if the solute under

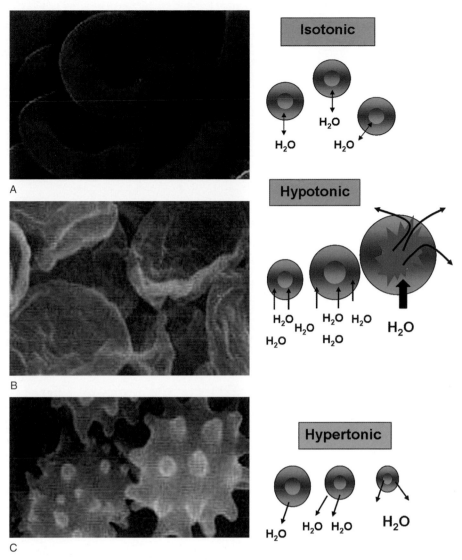

Fig. 2.29. Significance of tonicity. The consequence of placing red blood cells in solutions with differing tonicity values is illustrated. In the upper panel, cells are in an isotonic solution. Since the relative number of water molecules is the same inside and outside the cell, there is no net movement of water molecules and no change in cell volume. In the middle panel, cells are placed in a hypotonic solution. Here, the number of water molecules outside is much greater than on the inside, so water enters and rapidly swells the cells. In fact, if the solution is sufficiently hypotonic the cells will rupture. This is shown on the left. These are remnants of red blood cell membranes. The lower panel shows the effect of suspending cells in a hypertonic solution. Since the relative numbers of water molecules are greater inside, the cells lose water and they shrink. This is called crenation and is characterized by the spikes of cell membrane shown on the left.

consideration ionizes completely, each molecule or particle is osmotically active. For example 1 mole of NaCl per liter of water (58 g) would yield a 2 osm or 2,000 mosm solution. This is because NaCl dissociates completely so that each Na and Cl ion exerts an osmotic effect. By contrast 1 mole of glucose (180 g) per liter would produce a solution with an osmotic pressure of only 1 osm or 1,000 mosm. For solutes that do not ionize, the molarity and osmolarity of the solution are the same. However, it is important to consider whether the solute under consideration is penetrating or nonpenetrating relative to the cell membrane. If cells are exposed to a 300 mosm solution of a penetrat-

ing solute, the solute will enter the cells, the relative water concentration outside the cell increases proportionally, and water then enters the cells. The solution effectively becomes more hypotonic over time. In addition biological fluids are not ideal solutions. Interactions between molecules or partial dissolution of ionizing substances means that simply knowing the concentrations of various substances in blood, lymph, or urine, for example, cannot be used to accurately calculate osmolarity. Fortunately, it is possible to measure osmolarity by indirect means. The temperature at which a fluid freezes is directly related to the osmolarity of the solution. Thus the effective osmotic

Table 2.8.   Summary of transport processes used by cells.

Transport Type	Energy Source	Description	Example
Passive			
Simple diffusion	Kinetic energy	Movement of molecules down a concentration gradient (higher to lower)	Transfer of oxygen, lipids, and some ions
Facilitated diffusion	Kinetic energy	Like simple but substance is bound to a carrier protein	Transfer of glucose into cells
Osmosis	Kinetic energy	Basically simple diffusion of water through a semipermeable membrane	Water transport
Filtration	Hydrostatic pressure	Movement of water and solutes through a semipermeable membrane by a pressure gradient	Transfer of water and solutes from capillaries or renal filtration
Active			
Active Transport	ATP	Move of a solute against a concentration gradient	Recovery of glucose from kidney filtrate or uptake of amino acids
Exocytosis	ATP	Secretion of cellular products via fusion of membrane-bound secretory vesicles	Secretion of milk proteins and lactose
Phagocytosis	ATP	So-called cell-eating amoeboidlike engulfing of extracellular materials by pseudopodia	Removal of foreign debris or dead cell fragments by macrophages
Bulk-phase endocytosis	ATP	So-called cell-drinking, involves appearance of depression of the plasma membrane and progressive incorporation of fluid-filled vesicles	Occurs essentially in all cells
Receptor-mediated endocytosis	ATP	Ligand binding to surface receptors causes clustering of bound receptors in clathrin-coated pits, which are then taken into the cells for processing by lysosomes	Uptake of cholesterol and iron; down-regulation receptors

pressure of even complex solutions can be determined by measuring freezing point depression.

Transport mechanisms

Passage of molecules into and out of cells and across organelle membranes occurs by either active or passive transport. For passive mechanisms, there is no direct energy expenditure by the cell. Active mechanisms, in contrast, require metabolic energy. Table 2.8 provides a listing of the membrane transport processes.

As illustrated in Figure 2.30, simple diffusion is the tendency for molecules to disperse evenly throughout a solution. Substances that are small, nonpolar, and lipid-soluble readily pass across cell membranes. Examples are oxygen and carbon dioxide. Since oxygen concentrations are virtually always higher in the blood and interstitial fluid than in the cytoplasm, oxygen continually diffuses into cells. Similarly, carbon dioxide is nearly always higher inside the cells, as a consequence of metabolic activity, so carbon dioxide is continually diffusing out of the cells. Most water-soluble molecules cannot simply diffuse through the cell membrane. This is because these polar molecules cannot "dissolve" in the fatty acid tails of the phospholipids of the lipid bilayer. However if the substance is small enough, it can pass through the plasma membrane by passing through water-filled pores. Integral membrane proteins that span the entire width of the cell membrane create these pores. This means that substances sufficiently small and polar can essentially diffuse across the membrane by interacting with the water associated with these membrane-spanning proteins. Some of the pores are always available, but others can be regulated. For example, in the cells of the kidney tubules, specifically the collecting ducts, permeability of the cells to water uptake by osmosis is variable. This reflects changes in the conformation of these pore-forming proteins. When antidiuretic hormone (ADH) concentrations are elevated, the pores are widely available so that much of the water in the kidney filtrate is recovered. When secretion of ADH is inhibited, more of the pore-forming proteins acquire a conformation that impairs water movement, so urine production increases and the urine that is produced is more dilute.

Many important nutrient molecules, glucose and certain amino acids, are too polar to dissolve in the lipid bilayer for diffusion and too large to pass into the cells by passage through the plasma membrane pores or channels. These substances nonetheless pass into the cell by diffusion because they can interact with carrier proteins located in the plasma membrane. Precise mechanisms for this transport process are not well understood. But it is generally believed that binding of the substance to be transported causes a conformational change in the protein carrier that acts 1) to shield the molecule from interactions with the lipid bilayer and 2) to simultaneously move the molecule across the membrane. With the change in conformation the carrier protein no longer can bind the molecule, so it is released to the inside of the cell. This type of transport is called facilitated diffusion because substances transported still must pass down their concentration gradients but presence of the carrier proteins are required to mediate the transport. Unlike with simple diffusion, there are limitations. First, the carrier proteins themselves are typically highly specific. For example, carrier proteins that facilitate the diffusion of glucose would not be expected to also transport ribose. Second, the process can be saturated. This is essentially the reason why diabetic animals have glucose in their urine. Under normal conditions, a combination of facilitated diffusion and active transport are capable of removing and recovering all of the glucose molecules that appear in the kidney filtrate. However, concentrations of glucose in the blood and consequently the urinary filtrate of an animal with diabetes can be many times higher than normal. Since the number of transport proteins in the membrane of the kidney tubule cells is limited and the rate of transport finite, not all of the glucose can be removed before the fluid passes out of the nephron and into the renal pelvis. This is an example of saturation. Simply stated, when all of the binding sites are occupied, the rate of transport is maximized. This rate of transfer, called the V_{max}, is unique for each class or type of carrier protein. The capacity of the carrier to function is also affected by the relative ability of the binding site on the carrier protein to attract and hold the molecule for transport. This attraction is described as affinity. Carrier proteins with high affinity for their transport partner are able to sequester, bind, and transport their partner molecules even when concentrations are very low. Estimating the K_M or binding constant for this interaction provides a quantitative measure of affinity. The K_M is the molar concentration at which half of the carrier proteins are occupied. The lower this value, the greater the affinity.

Carrier proteins may also be affected somewhat like enzymes. Competitive inhibitors are able to block binding of the ligand (molecule to be transported).

These inhibitor molecules essentially compete for the same binding site. In some cases the competing molecule is transported, but in other cases it is not. Some inhibitors can bind to regions other than the ligand-binding site of the carrier protein and induce a change in conformation that then makes the usual binding site incapable of interacting with the transport molecule. These effects are similar to the actions that serve to modulate enzyme activity. Carrier proteins that facilitate the transport of a single molecule or class (single binding reaction) across the membrane are called uniporters or uniport transporter proteins. Their V_{max} and K_M values determine the rate of reaction for these carriers. Other transporters are more complicated because the transfer of one solute depends on the simultaneous binding and transport of another molecule. If the molecules to be transported both move in the same direction, the carrier is called a symport (something like a symbiotic relationship) but if the molecules move in opposite directions, the carrier is called an antiport. Clearly, the kinetics that affect the actions of symport and antiport carriers is more complex than for simple uniport carriers. As an example, consider the uptake of glucose. Most animal cells have uniport carriers that take up glucose from the extracellular fluids where its concentrations are usually higher than in the cytoplasm. This is passive transfer that depends on facilitated diffusion. However, intestinal and kidney cells continue to take up glucose even when concentrations are low. These cells actively sequester glucose across their membranes via a symport carrier linked with the diffusion of Na into the cell. In other words, the movement of Na down its concentration gradient allows for the coupled transport of glucose into the cell. While cellular energy is not directly needed, maintenance of an affective concentration gradient for Na does require energy. Figure 2.30 illustrates differences between simple diffusion and carrier-mediated diffusion as well as theoretical models of three types of carrier proteins.

Filtration is the physical process whereby water and solutes are forced through a membrane or a capillary wall by simple hydrostatic pressure. Despite the non-selective nature of this type of transport, it is critical for many physiological functions. Creation of urinary filtrate or movement of fluids across capillary beds throughout the body demonstrates physiological filtration. Filtration is considered a passive process, but it is obvious that pressure in the cardiovascular system depends on continued cardiac activity and muscle tone of arteries.

Hydrolysis of ATP and release of chemical bond energy that fuels transport of substances across membranes is active transport. Mechanisms are variable but fall into two broad groups. The first, like facilitated diffusion, depends on specific membrane carrier pro-

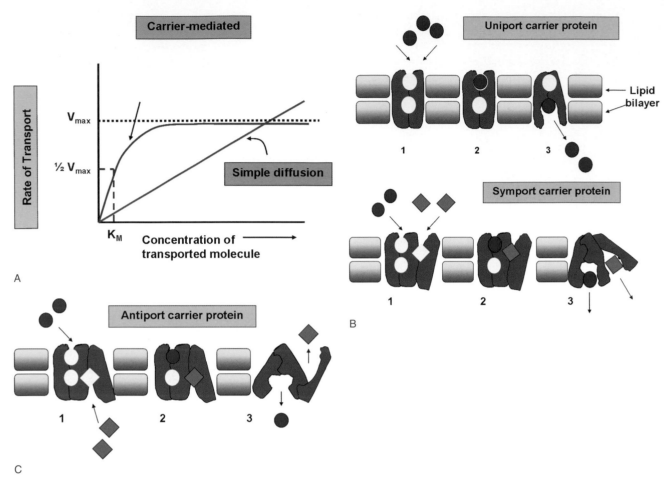

Fig. 2.30. Carrier protein–mediated transport properties. In Panel A the kinetics of simple diffusion compared with carrier-mediated transport are shown. For simple diffusion, the rate is directly proportional to the concentration of the transported molecule. Carrier-mediated transport shows a maximal rate (V_{max}) regardless of further increase in concentration. The concentration at $1/2\ V_{max}$ is an estimate of the binding affinity (K_M). Panel B illustrates the action of a uniport carrier protein. Step 1 shows binding of the transport molecule to the protein, followed by a change in carrier conformation (2), and then release (3) of the molecule to the inside of the cell. Symport carriers (Panel B) follow a similar pattern except that solute molecules (red and green symbols) bind and are transferred simultaneously in the same direction. In antiport carriers (Panel C) transport of one molecule depends on the simultaneously binding and transfer of another molecule in the opposite direction.

teins. The second is the formation and uptake of vesicles. Carrier-mediated transport is specific but unlike diffusion processes, moves molecules against their concentration gradients. In primary active transport, ATP is used to phosphorylate the carrier protein. Binding of the phosphate group to the protein alters its conformation. This causes the transport molecule to be shuttled across the cell membrane and released. One of the best studied of these carriers is the sodium-potassium ATPase pump. The carrier in this instance is a membrane-bound enzyme that cleaves ATP and functions to maintain steep gradients for Na (~tenfold higher outside) and K (~tenfold higher inside) relative to the plasma membrane. These ion gradients are essential for normal signaling in nerve cells and initiation of muscle contractions. Another example of active transport is closely linked with muscle activity. When muscle contraction occurs, the cytoplasm of the

cell is flooded with calcium. To regulate contraction events, calcium ions are pumped uphill back into storage inside the sarcoplasmic reticulum or back out of the cell in some situations. The working of the sodium-potassium ATPase pump is illustrated in Figures 2.31 and 2.32.

In addition to its relevance maintaining Na and K gradients and osmotic balance, the sodium-potassium ATPase pump is also responsible for transport of a number of important molecules. This is called secondary active transport. With greater concentrations outside the cell and the fact that the inside of the cell has a net negative charge, there is a continuous electrochemical gradient that promotes the diffusion of Na ions back into the cell. This is a bit like filling a pond behind a dam. Open a sluice and water pours out. The energy of the water flow can be used to spin a turbine to produce electricity or, as in the 1800s, to

---

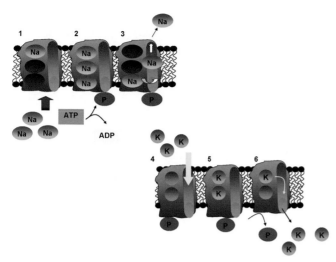

Fig. 2.31.   Action of ATPase pumps. At step 1, Na ions from the cytoplasm bind to three sites on the protein. In step 2 complete loading stimulates the hydrolysis of ATP and phosphorylation of the protein. Phosphorylation causes a conformation shift and unloading of Na ions to the outside of the cell (step 3). Unloading of Na exposes two K binding sites available to K ions from the extracellular space (step 4). Complete loading of K ions (step 5) triggers release of the phosphate group and release of K ions to the inside of the cell (step 6). Once K ions are released, the protein returns to the conformation as in step 1 and is ready for loading of Na ions once again.

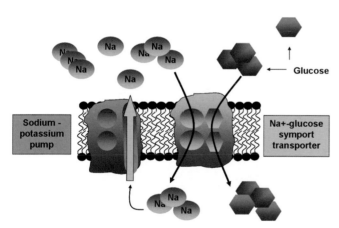

Fig. 2.32.   The sodium-potassium ATPase pump and sodium-glucose symport. As detailed in Figure 2.31, the Na-K pump maintains a gradient so that concentrations of Na are higher outside the cell. Na ions enter the cell because of an electrochemical gradient. The inside of the cell has a net negative charge and the concentration of Na ions is also lower. Moreover, transport of Na is directly linked with the simultaneous transfer of glucose into the cell (transporter on the right). With respect to glucose uptake, this is sometimes called secondary active transport, since ATP is not directly required for action of the glucose-Na^+, symport but it is needed to create and maintain the Na^+ gradient across the cell membrane.

turn grinding wheels to produce corn meal or flour. The cell can take advantage of energy from this downhill diffusion of Na by linking it with the uptake of other important molecules. For example, recovery of glucose and some amino acids, against their concen-

tration gradients, can be achieved in this manner. This is illustrated in Figure 2.32. Ion gradients are critical for the actions of many different membrane transport systems. Some of these are similar to the symport for glucose. For example, other specific symport carriers also linked with the electrochemical gradient for Na^+ cotransport uptake of some amino acids and other sugars. Ion gradients are also important in the operation of the antiport carrier that operates in the membrane of cells in the gastric pits in the stomach to regulate the pH of gastric juices by secretion of HCl.

In addition to the transport involving specific membrane carrier proteins, substantial numbers of molecules associated with the cell surface or molecules simply positioned near the surface can be moved into the cells by either pinocytosis (engulfment of fluids) or endocytosis (engulfment of particles). Both of these processes require energy. Control of endocytosis is complex and poorly understood. In some cases the process is receptor-mediated. That is, the binding of a specific ligand to proteins on the cell surface initiates a cascade that leads to endocytosis of the receptor and associated ligand. This process often begins in areas of the membrane containing clathrin-coated pits. These endocytosed receptor proteins can be processed in at least three different ways, depending on the particular receptor-ligand combination and cellular conditions. Multiple vesicles are believed to fuse to create a larger membrane structure called an endosome, from which smaller vesicles bleb or bud. A common fate is for receptors to be either recycled to the same region of membrane (recycling), to another area of membrane (transcytosis), or to be shuttled to lysosomes for destruction. As for pinocytosis, it is generally believed that essentially all cells continually ingest bits of their plasma membrane along with fluids via the continuous generation of these very small vesicles. Specialized blood-related cells; especially neutrophils and macrophages actively undergo phagocytosis. This process is familiar from our images of amoeba surrounding food particles. In similar fashion, these leucocytic cells send pseudopods around cell debris or bacterial cells and engulf the material. The ingested material is captured in a membrane-bound body called a phagosome. Most often this is followed by fusion with lysosomes to degrade the material. Interestingly, in some cases, protein fragments from the degraded material, especially in the case of foreign substances, are returned to the cell surface so that other leucocytes can detect them. Macrophages that carry out this activity are called antigen-presenting cells. This process allows other immune cells to generate memory cells and initiate the production of antibodies against the foreign invader. Figure 2.33 illustrates types of endocytosis and the trafficking associated with endocytosis.

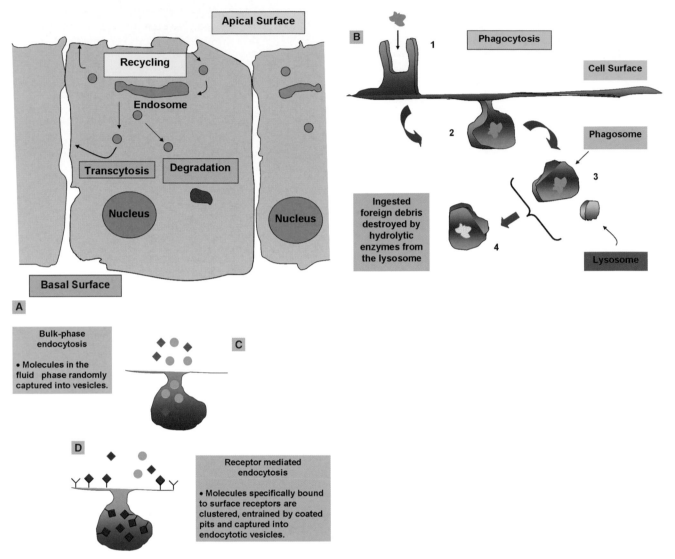

Fig. 2.33. Processing of vesicles derived from receptor-mediated endocytosis. Processing of vesicles derived from receptor-mediated endocytosis is illustrated in Panel A. Once vesicles enter the cell, they fuse to produce the endosome. Vesicles that bleb from the endosome are subjected to one of three fates. Many of the receptor proteins are returned to the plasma membrane to be reused at the original site (recycling) or in a different location of the plasma membrane (transcytosis). Other vesicles along with their proteins (receptors and/or ligands) are degraded by lysosomal enzymes following fusion. Panel B illustrates a specialized type of endocytosis (phagocytosis) that is employed by certain white blood cells. Macrophages, for example, identify cellular debris or perhaps bacterial cells for engulfment. Cytoplasmic extensions called pseudopods extend and surround the targeted particle (1). The material is engulfed and captured in a vesicle called a phagosome (2). Fusion between the phagosome and lysosomes (3) lead to destruction of the captured material (4). The next two panels (C and D) illustrate differences between pinocytosis and receptor-mediated endocytosis. Pinocytosis is more random since the cell has no control over specific molecules that can be secured.

References

Akers, R.M. and S.C. Nickerson. 1983. Effect of prepartum blockade of microtubule formation on milk production and biochemical differentiation of the mammary epithelium in Holstein heifers. Int. J. Biochem. 15: 771–775.

Jones, G.M., R.E. Pearson, G.A. Clabaugh, and C.W. Heald. 1884. Relationships between somatic cell counts and milk production. J. Dairy Sci. 67: 1823–1831.

Keys, J.E., A.V. Capuco, R.M. Akers, and J. Djiane. 1989. Comparative study of mammary gland development and differentiation between beef and dairy heifers. Domestic Anim. Endocrinol. 6: 311–319.

McFadden, T.B., R.M. Akers, and A.V. Capuco. 1988. Relationships of milk proteins in blood with somatic cell counts in milk of dairy cows. J. Dairy Sci. 71: 826–834.

McFadden, T.B., T.E. Daniel, and R.M. Akers. 1990. Effects of plane of nutrition, growth hormone, and unsaturated fat on mammary growth in prepubertal lambs. J. Anim. Sci. 68: 3171–3179.

Nickerson, S.C. and R.M. Akers. 1983. Effect of prepartum blockade of microtubule formation on ultrastructural differentiation of the mammary epithelium in Holstein heifers. Int. J. Biochem. 15: 777–788.

Nickerson, S.C. and R.M. Akers. 1984. Biochemical and ultrastructural aspects of milk synthesis and secretion. Int. J. Biochem. 16: 855–865.

Nickerson, S.C., R.M. Akers, and B.T. Weinland. 1982. Cytoplasmic organization and quantitation of microtubules in bovine mammary epithelial cells during lactation and involution. Cell and Tissue Res. 223: 421–430.

Nickerson, S.C. and J.W. Pankey. 1983. Cytological observations of the bovine teat end. Amer. J. Vet. Res. 44: 1433–1441.

Sejrsen, K., J. Foldager, M.T. Sorensen, R.M. Akers, and D.E. Bauman. 1986. Effect of exogenous bovine somatotropin on pubertal mammary development in heifers. J. Dairy Sci. 69: 1528–1535.

Sejrsen, K., J.T. Huber, H.A. Tucker, and R.M. Akers. 1982. Influence of plane of nutrition on mammary development in pre-and post-pubertal heifers. J. Dairy Sci. 65: 793–800.

Smith, J.J., A.V. Capuco, W.E. Beal, and R.M. Akers. 1989. Association of prolactin and insulin receptors with mammogenesis and lobulo-alveolar formation in pregnant ewes. Int. J. Biochem. 21: 73–81.

3 Fundamental biochemical pathways and processes in cellular physiology

Contents

Although our focus is physiology, as we have already seen, understanding physiological function requires an appreciation of various aspects of chemistry, bio chemistry, physics, and other disciplines. The purpose of this chapter is to introduce you to some of the basics of how cells carry out essential steps to obtain the energy needed for various activities and to generate the building blocks required for growth and development. Please appreciate that in many respects our discussions are rudimentary. However, this foundation will give you the tools and concepts to understand the roles and actions of each physiological system, and to excel in advanced courses in nutrition, reproduction, lactation, or other biological and animal-oriented courses.

Metabolism and energetic definitions

We have all heard the expressions, "there are no free rides" or "no free lunches." This is certainly true when it comes to living our lives but also a physiological truth. For example, acquiring the energy to maintain the ionic gradients we discussed in Chapter 2 depends on the hydrolysis of one of the phosphate bonds of ATP. The question becomes: Where did the energy needed to produce the ATP in the first place come from? This is the crux of the problem; some molecules are catabolized so that others can be created. Simply put, living systems are in a constant thermodynamic battle. As the second law of thermodynamics suggests, the natural tendency is production of equilibrium with dispersion of energy and increasing disorder, or in thermodynamic terms, increased entropy. Living systems, cells, tissues, organs, systems, and organisms are characterized by just the opposite. The degree of complexity and organization in living systems is antithetical to this law. Unlike most of the nonliving universe, open biological systems are able to exchange matter and energy with their surroundings. This allows living systems, while they are alive, to move away from the dispersion and energy equilibrium that the second law of thermodynamics dictates. The first law of thermodynamics is familiar as the maxim that energy can neither be created nor destroyed. More formally, it is expressed in this way: The total energy of a system plus its surroundings remains constant. Thus, the exquisite organization and complexity that characterizes living systems is at the expense of free energy from the environment. That is, energy that can be harnessed to do work. Thus, living systems are analogous to an oasis in the desert. The oasis, often short-lived in a geological sense, provides a place of relief for the weary traveler. Living systems represent transient conditions during which time nonequilibrium conditions related to energy-matter circumstances exist.

A fundamental postulate of theoretical biology is that life processes can be explained in terms of chemistry and physics—in other words, in terms of matter and energy. Following this idea, it can be reasoned that life processes are represented by the myriad of chemical (enzymatic and nonenzymatic) and physical reactions that occur within cells and tissues—in other words, metabolism. The yin and yang of metabolism are anabolism and catabolism. Our discussion begins with catabolism.

The phrase *intermediary metabolism* is often used in nutrition and biochemistry texts. This refers to the many steps of reaction between the initiation of a biochemical process and its completion. For example, the complete oxidation of the critical nutrient glucose begins with uptake of the glucose into the cell and entry of the molecule into a sequence of reactions called glycolysis. This is an example of a biochemical pathway. The steps in the pathway detail the reactions that are required to convert this 6-carbon hexose sugar into two 3-carbon molecules of pyruvate. This process is also called anaerobic respiration. The various molecules that are temporarily produced in the 10 steps of glycolysis are called intermediates. Other biochemical pathways would generate their own specific family of intermediate molecules. Consequently, intermediary metabolism refers to the creation and existence of the hundreds of molecules that are fabricated as various molecules progress toward their final biochemical destination. Finally, although we typically describe important biochemical pathways singly, it needs to be emphasized that a host of biochemical reactions or pathways are occurring simultaneously. Intermediates from one pathway often also supply materials that can be used in other pathways. For example, one of the intermediate steps in glycolysis produces triose phosphate. This molecule can continue to supply the carbon atoms to make pyruvate or alternatively be shuttled out of the glycolysis pathway to produce glycerol, which is needed in the anabolic pathway to make triglycerides. A key idea is that regulation and control of the rates of activity of these various, often competing biochemical pathways is critical. Resources must be used effectively and efficiently.

Given the importance of energy to fuel the biochemical reactions in cells, it is fitting that we consider some definitions. What do we mean by energy? Are all forms of energy equally valuable from a physiological viewpoint? We often say that the diets we supply to our animals give them the energy they need for productive functions—for example, to allow draft horses to pull wagons, thoroughbreds to race, or cows to produce milk. Our animals do not consume energy directly but rather it is the digestion of foodstuffs that liberate the nutrient molecules that can then be oxidized in a controlled, deliberate fashion to provide the energy needs. In physics, energy is described as the capacity to do work. In biological systems, energy is sometimes expressed as heat units or calories. A calorie (cal) is the amount of energy needed to increase the temperature of 1 gram of water 1 degree at a pressure of one atmosphere. Other related terms are the kilocalorie (1,000 calories) or the megacalorie (Mcal = 1,000,000 calories) often used in descriptions of the energy content of animals feeds. Other measures of energy are also frequently used. For example, 1 joule (J) is the work done by a force of 1 Newton working over a distance of 1 meter ($m^2 \times kg \times sec^{-2}$). Other measures of energy can be derived as well (1 cal = 4.187 J or 0.004 British Thermal Units (BTU)).

It is also clear that not all of the bond or chemical energy that is available in food molecules can be captured for use by tissues or cells. If a known quantity of a food material or nutrient is completely combusted or oxidized in an oxygen atmosphere and the heat generated measured, this provides an estimate of the gross or potential energy of the substance. This process is called calorimetry. This technique is valuable because it provides a measure of the potential energy available in a particular nutrient or other substance. However, as another old expression says, "it takes money to make money"; there are costs involved in acquiring the energy that is potentially available in various nutrients. Just as there are overhead costs in running a business or a university, there are physiological costs that must be paid to capture the energy available in nutrients. For example, consider feeding your horse a carrot and the steps needed to capture the energy in the starch. For processing there is mastication and swallowing, transport to the small intestine, secretion of gastric and intestinal enzymes, and transport of digested glucose molecules across the epithelial cells. All of these events can be thought of as overhead or maintenance costs associated with the physiological processing of the carrot.

Thus the amount of energy present in the diet does not equal energy that is ultimately available to the animal. Animal science nutritionists often conduct feeding trials to evaluate the practical value of different feedstuffs. These feedstuffs are often complex mixtures. Consider total mixed rations that are often fed to dairy cows with various combinations of forages and concentrates. In such studies, great care must be

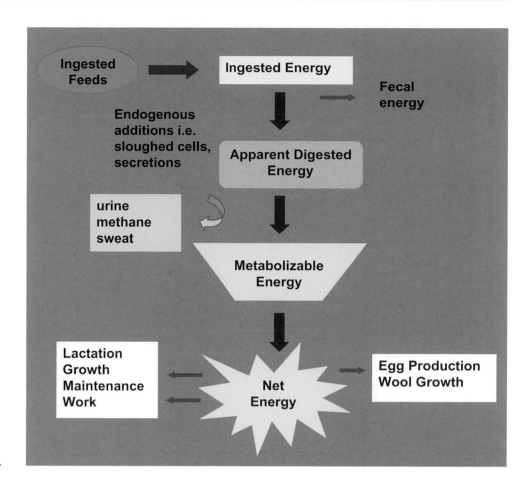

Fig. 3.1. Processing of feedstuff energy. Compared with the total estimate of gross energy in consumed feeds, the amount of energy ultimately available to cells and tissues is substantially reduced.

taken to account for measurement errors, e.g., spilled feed, variation in the efficiency of digestion and ingestion. Particularly for complex rations, the gross energy content of the diet, gives only a broad indication of how valuable the diet is to the animal. What happens if one of the components in the diet cannot be digested? What if there are interactions so that the breakdown of one dietary component affects the microorganism population of the GI tract so that normally effective nutrients are lost. Even under the best conditions, especially for animals fed fibrous feeds, a part of the feed is not digested and contributes to the energy content of the feces. The difference between the gross energy content of the diet and the portion of the energy that is available to the animal is called digestible energy. Various rations can then be compared based on their digestibility energy, often expressed as a fraction or percentage of the gross energy. From measurements made over the course of several days and sometimes weeks, average daily energy consumption minus the energy content of the feces and urine is called the apparent digestible energy. It is called apparent because some, generally small portion of fecal energy comes from sloughed intestinal epithelial cells, bacteria cells, and substances that have been excreted by way of the feces.

For nutrients that are ultimately absorbed, the energy content still does not match energy that ultimately becomes available to the animal. However, the fraction that is represented by digested and absorbed nutrients is called the metabolizable energy. This is the fraction of total or gross energy fed that is directly available to the tissues and cells to be processed. This energy can be used for maintenance, heat generation (sometimes considered a waste product), or for more recognizable practical productive functions, i.e., muscle growth, egg production, or milk production. Metabolizable energy is less than digestible energy, typically about 80%, because of other losses in addition to the fecal losses. This fraction would be lower still if the heat that is generated is considered a waste product. The additional losses include materials that are lost in urine in all species as well as gaseous products from gut fermentation that are expelled. These products are especially plentiful in herbivores and particularly ruminants. The fraction of energy that is ultimately used for physiological activities is called net energy. Figure 3.1 illustrates the processing of dietary energy.

It is common to characterize energy that is needed for basal or resting life activities in animals as the energy of maintenance. These energy costs do not reflect energy that is needed for productive work in a production agriculture sense—for example, work done by a draft horse or racehorse or energy recovered from such products as meat, milk, or eggs. These are critical physiological functions, action of the Na-K ATPase pump, cardiac function, and so forth. As Figure 3.1 illustrates there are additional energy costs associated with acquiring feed and assimilating nutrients themselves. Ideally, maintenance activities are stated as the energy costs of preserving an adult animal under resting or sedentary circumstances, in the absence of weight gain or loss, in thermoneutral conditions. In practical terms, this ideal status is rarely obtained, but it does give a framework to understand the meaning of maintenance energy costs. In humans the term *basal metabolic rate* may be more familiar and is determined for subjects in a quiet, thermoneutral environment, about 12 hours after a meal.

Basal energy needs are determined indirectly by measuring oxygen consumption under these conditions. This is effective because the amounts of oxygen needed to completely oxidize fats, proteins, or carbohydrates are known. If CO_2 production is simultaneously measured, the respiratory quotient can be calculated (moles of CO_2 exhaled divided by the moles of O_2 consumed). These data can then be used to estimate the nature of the nutrients (protein, carbohydrate, or fat) being oxidized for energy production. The alternative to indirect calorimetry is to measure heat production along with complete collection of gases and other wastes. This is clearly a difficult and expensive undertaking with large domestic animals. However, Table 3.1 shows an example of calorimetry data from a study by Tyrrell et al., (1988) designed to determine in part, if the metabolic rate of dairy cows treated with bovine somatotropin (bST) was increased compared with controls. Briefly, nine cows received bST (51.5 IU/d) or a daily control injection in a single reversal design, which utilized 14-d treatment periods. With increased milk production after bST (22% increase), cows already in a negative tissue nitrogen balance (–21 g/d) tended to become more negative during the bST treatment period (–34 g/d). Energy and nitrogen balances were measured in open-circuit respiration chambers. As predicted from increased milk production, there was corresponding greater heat energy losses and increased milk energy secretion after bST treatment. Tissue energy balance was – 1.1 Mcal/d during the control treatment period. Increased use of energy reserves with bST treatment decreased tissue energy balance to –9.8 Mcal/d. These researchers concluded that much of the effect of bST to increase milk production in dairy cows is related to increased use of tissue reserves and altered partitioning of nutrients rather than dramatic effects on digestibility of nutrients or apparent changes in maintenance

Table 3.1. Effect of bovine somatotropin (bST) in lactating dairy cows on milk production and energy metabolism parameters.

	Treatment	
	Control	bST
Variable		
Milk yield (kg/d)	26.0 ± 0.5	31.8 ± 0.5*
O_2 consumption (L/d)	5345 ± 58	5562 ± 58*
CO_2 production (L/d)	5391 ± 82	5454 ± 82
	—— % intake ——	
Fecal energy	33.9 ± 0.5	35.2 ± 0.5
Digestible energy	66.04 ± 0.5	64.81 ± 0.5
Gaseous energy	5.29 ± 0.1	5.78 ± 0.1*
Urinary energy	3.22 ± 0.05	3.33 ± 0.05
Heat energy	34.65 ± 0.66	37.62 ± 0.66*
Retained energy	22.88 ± 0.92	18.08 ± 0.92*
Milk energy	24.24 ± 0.95	31.66 ± 0.95*
Tissue energy	–1.55 ± 1.58	–13.71 ± 1.58*

* Indicates a statistically significant difference between treatments P ≤ 0.05.
Data adapted from Tyrrell et al., 1988.

requirements of the animals. Simply, the increases observed would have been expected with the degree of increased milk production, regardless of the specific reason for increased production.

Production of ATP

For essentially all physiological activities, the most useful and available form of energy comes from ATP or adenosine triphosphate. When the terminal phosphate group is cleaved to produce ADP (adenosine diphosphate), each mole of ATP yields 7,400 calories. There are other similar high-energy–yielding molecules, but most are similar to ATP—for example, GTP or creatine phosphate. Indeed the creation of creatine phosphate (which acts as a storage form of energy in muscle cells because of its capacity to regenerate ATP from ADP) gains this capacity only when ATP is produced in excess of immediate demand as in the following reaction:

ATP + Creatine ↔ ADP + Creatine phosphate 3.1

This means that production of ATP is vital. The structure of ATP is shown in Figure 3.2. Mitochondria are critical because the final stages of oxidation of several coenzymes occur within these organelles. When the reduced coenzymes are oxidized, a portion of the energy produced is utilized to drive the synthesis of ATP from ADP, as shown in the following equation:

ADP + Phosphate + Energy → ATP 3.2

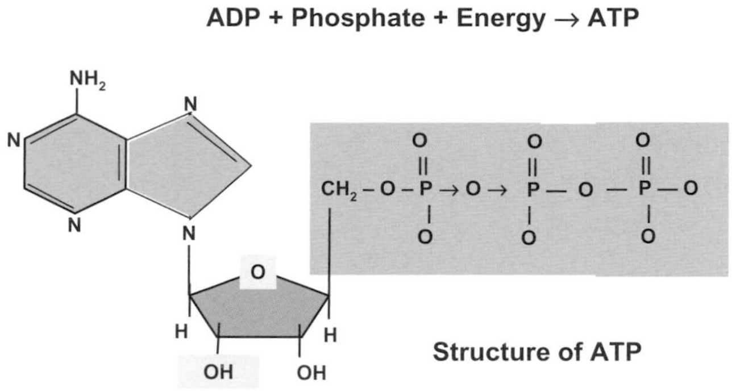

ADP + Phosphate + Energy → ATP

Structure of ATP

Fig. 3.2. Structure of adenosine triphosphate (ATP). It is the most important labile energy carrier in the body. Hydrolysis of the terminal phosphate bond yields an exceptionally high level of free or (available) energy. The nitrogenous group should be familiar as adenine, linkage with the ribose produces adenosine, addition of a single phosphate moiety gives adenosine monophosphate or AMP and two adenosine diphosphate or ADP.

Table 3.2. Common terms associated with the metabolism of carbohydrates.

Term	Definition
Glycolysis	Anaerobic oxidation of a molecule of glucose via 10 enzymatic reactions to produce 2 molecules of pyruvate. The reactions occur in the cytoplasm.
Glycogenolysis	The breakdown of the glycogen to produce glucose for utilization in the glycolysis catabolic pathway.
Glycogenesis	Synthesis of glycogen from glucose. Occurs in times of energy abundance.
Gluconeogenesis	The formation of glucose from noncarbohydrate substrates. Important in times of stress, makes glucose available from nonessential amino acids. Critical in ruminants due to fermentation of dietary carbohydrates.

As you might guess, since many different feedstuffs can be used to produce energy, a host of nutrient molecules under the appropriate circumstances can be modified to enter the biochemical pathway for ATP production. Although some ATP can be generated in the absence of oxygen through substrate level phosphorylation (essentially the regeneration of ATP from ADP, as with creatine phosphate), production rates are minor compared with oxidative phosphorylation. In a nutshell this explains the critical need for oxygen. Within the mitochondria, where reduced coenzymes are oxidized, oxygen serves as the final acceptor of electrons in this cascade of reactions. Without oxygen available, the electron transport chain fails, and the energy normally available to drive phosphorylation of ADP to regeneration of ATP also fails. Needs for continuous supplies of ATP are so acute that unless oxygen is quickly returned, death occurs in a matter of minutes. To understand the pathways for ATP generation we will focus first on the catabolism of carbohydrates and specifically with the catabolism of glucose. Once we have this core of information we will then discuss how other nutrients can be diverted for use as fuels to drive ATP generation.

Glycolysis

We begin our quest to understand energy production with glucose because it is typically the most common nutrient used for acute energy production. The initial processing of glucose molecules begins in the cytoplasm of the cell. Once inside the cell, 6-carbon glucose is converted in a series of reactions into two 3-carbon molecules of pyruvate. As mentioned before, the 10 linked reactions responsible for this conversion are collectively called glycolysis or anaerobic respiration. This process is also called the Embden-Meyerhof pathway. It is typical to describe carbohydrate catabolism beginning with glucose, but you should remember that polymers of glucose (glycogen in animal cells) can be cleaved to provide the glucose monomers to enter the glycolysis pathway. Thus the cell may well contain stores of glycogen that can be cleaved to supply glucose aside from the uptake of glucose across the plasma membrane. Table 3.2 provides a listing of some often confusing, similar sounding terms that have to do with carbohydrate metabolism. It may be useful for you to periodically refer to this table as you study this important topic. Figure 3.3 provides an outline of each of the steps in glycolysis. We have purposefully not given all of the chemical structural detail showing changes in carbons and functional groups as glucose is modified through glycolysis. If this is needed, it is available in any introductory biochemistry book. Our goal is for you to appreciate the highlights, the overall chemical events, and most importantly the physiological relevance. Although each of the reactions of glycolysis is enzyme-mediated we have focused on two glycolysis reactions and their associated enzymes along with one other reaction that is not strictly part of glycolysis. These are 1) the conversion of glucose to glucose-6-phosphate (step one of glycolysis, catalyzed by hexokinase), 2) step three, the conversion of fructose-6-phosphate into fructose 1,6-diphosphate, catalyzed by phosphofructokinase and 3) the conversion of pyruvate into lactate, catalyzed by lactate dehydrogenase. Some specific reactions and molecules associated with glycolysis are provided in Figure 3.4. At this point it is worth remembering the significance of the glycolysis. This pathway allows the

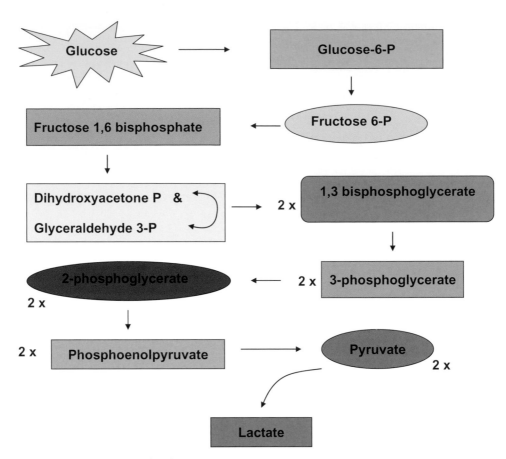

Fig. 3.3. Chemical steps and intermediates in glycolysis.

conversion of the nutrient glucose into molecules that can then be shuttled into the mitochondria for use in the process of oxidative phosphorylation. However, as we indicated above, oxidative phosphorylation (simply the production of ATP linked to a series of oxidation-reduction reactions) requires oxygen. In addition to preparing molecules for entrance into the mitochondria, a small amount of ATP is produced during the glycolysis reactions. In contrast with mitochondrial activity, this occurs via substrate level phosphorylation. As you will see, the amount of ATP made in this manner is very small compared with that which occurs with the complete catabolism of the glucose (glycolysis reactions + mitochondrial activity), but it is nonetheless essential. This is because production of ATP via glycolysis alone can occur in the absence of oxygen. For this reason it is called anaerobic respiration.

Let's outline the steps of glycolysis. Typically, glucose is captured by the action of membrane transporters and passed into the cytoplasm. At this juncture, a phosphate group is added to the 6th carbon of the glucose. This then produces glucose-6-phosphate. Somewhat ironically, even though the glycolysis ultimately leads to energy production, in the first step of

glycolysis ATP is actually used. This is because the phosphate group added to the glucose is donated from ATP, as illustrated in Figure 3.4. In the next step glucose-6-hosphate is converted into another hexose sugar by the action of the enzyme phosphohexose isomerase, namely fructose-6-phosphate. Step 3 again utilizes another molecule of ATP as the enzyme phosphofructokinase (PFK) catalyzes the addition of another phosphate group to produce fructose 1,6-diphosphate. Step 4 is a cleavage reaction catalyzed by the enzyme aldolase, which produces two 3-carbon molecules: dihydroxyacetone phosphate and glyceraldehyde 3-phosphate. In step 5 the enzyme phosphotriose isomerase converts dihydroxyacetone into a second molecule of glyceraldehyde 3-phospate. There are now two identical molecules to continue through glycolysis so that products made from this point are doubled. Step 6 depends on the enzyme glyceraldehyde 3-phosphate dehydrogenase. As we will discuss in more detail relative to mitochondrial activity, this enzyme depends on the oxidized form of the coenzyme nicotinamide adenine dinucleotide or NAD^+. During this reaction the NAD^+ becomes reduced (NADH) and inorganic phosphate is added to the substrate to produce 1, 3-bisphosphate glycerate. The first

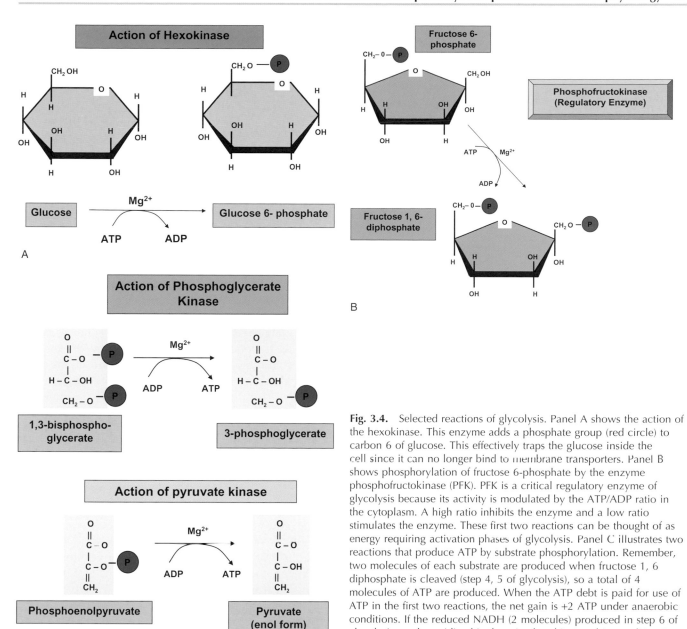

Fig. 3.4. Selected reactions of glycolysis. Panel A shows the action of the hexokinase. This enzyme adds a phosphate group (red circle) to carbon 6 of glucose. This effectively traps the glucose inside the cell since it can no longer bind to membrane transporters. Panel B shows phosphorylation of fructose 6-phosphate by the enzyme phosphofructokinase (PFK). PFK is a critical regulatory enzyme of glycolysis because its activity is modulated by the ATP/ADP ratio in the cytoplasm. A high ratio inhibits the enzyme and a low ratio stimulates the enzyme. These first two reactions can be thought of as energy requiring activation phases of glycolysis. Panel C illustrates two reactions that produce ATP by substrate phosphorylation. Remember, two molecules of each substrate are produced when fructose 1, 6 diphosphate is cleaved (step 4, 5 of glycolysis), so a total of 4 molecules of ATP are produced. When the ATP debt is paid for use of ATP in the first two reactions, the net gain is +2 ATP under anaerobic conditions. If the reduced NADH (2 molecules) produced in step 6 of glycolysis can be oxidized in the mitochondria (aerobic conditions), an additional 6 ATP are generated as a consequence of glycolysis.

direct production of ATP occurs in step 7 as a phosphate group is cleaved and the energy is utilized to simultaneously add a phosphate group to ADP. This is an example of substrate phosphorylation to produce a molecule of ATP, and the reaction is catalyzed by phosphoglycerate kinase. Step 8 depends on phosphoglycerate mutase to induce a rearrangement of the 3-phosphoglycerate made previously to yield 2-phosphoglycerate. Step 9 is the conversion of the 2-phosphoglycerate into phosphoenolpyruvate catalyzed by enolase. Step 10 is another ATP-making event as the enzyme pyruvate kinase acts to transfer a phosphate from phosphoenolpyruvate to ADP as pyruvate is also created. At this point the pyruvate is at a cross-

roads. The redox state of the tissue determines which of two alternative paths will be followed. If oxygen is available the pyruvate is shuttled into the mitochondria as subsequently described. If, however, oxygen is limited, i.e., there are anaerobic conditions, pyruvate is reduced by the action of lactate dehydrogenase and the coenzyme NADH becomes oxidized again. This is a critical process under these conditions. You may recall that step 6 of glycolysis requires the oxidized form of this coenzyme (NAD^+). Although only a small amount of ATP is derived directly from glycolysis, even this would be lost were it not from the action of lactate dehydrogenase. As an aside, there are also several isozymes of lactate dehydrogenase that are important clinically. For example, the unique structure of the LDH isozymes from heart muscle can be detected in blood serum in animals that have suffered cardiac injury (Fig. 3.5). Table 3.3 summarizes ATP production that is associated with glycolysis.

The Cori cycle

Most carbohydrates in the diet can be readily converted into glucose, galactose, or fructose when digested. These molecules are absorbed into the portal vein that drains the intestinal tract for use by the liver and other tissues. There are various other compounds that are considered glucogenic. These are molecules that can readily be converted into glucose to be processed via glycolysis for subsequent ATP production or for use in other biochemical pathways. For example, propionate, which is derived from fermentation of dietary carbohydrates in ruminant animals, is an essential substrate to allow ruminants to synthesize

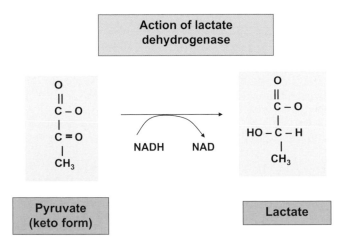

Pyruvate (keto form) → **Lactate**

Fig. 3.5. The action of lactate dehydrogenase (LDH). After an initial spontaneous rearrangement of pyruvate from the enol form to the keto isomer, LDH catalyzes the conversion of pyruvate to lactate. Most important in anaerobic conditions, this is linked with the simultaneous oxidation of reduced NADH. This newly produced NAD is essentially for glycolysis to continue under these conditions. This is because NAD^+ is required for step 6 of glycolysis.

the glucose they need. These glucogenic compounds can be divided into two groups: 1) those that are essentially direct conversions into glucose without a significant amount of recycling, propionate and certain amino acids, for example, and 2) products of partial metabolism of glucose, in particular molecules that are then transported to the liver or kidney for generation of glucose, lactate for example. In all animals there are times when oxygen is locally limited so that anaerobic respiration is favored and lactic acid accumulates. For example, the accumulation of lactic acid occurs in active muscle tissue and produces the sensation of muscle fatigue. In addition, since erythrocytes lack mitochondria, they rely on glycolysis for all of their ATP needs and consequently continually produce lactic acid regardless of oxygen availability. Most of the lactic acid from muscle or erythrocytes diffuses into the bloodstream. Fortunately it is transported to the liver and, to a lesser extent, the kidney where it can be converted into glucose. At this point it can be stored as hepatic or renal cell glycogen or released back into the bloodstream for use by muscle or other tissues (see Fig. 3.10, later in this chapter). Cycling of lactic acid from muscle (or other tissues) to liver and the return of glucose is called the Cori cycle and is outlined in Figure 3.6.

Krebs cycle

Let's now trace the fate of pyruvate that is produced at the end of glycolysis under aerobic conditions. Remember our goal here is to understand how the catabolism of glucose and other carbohydrates is used to generate the ATP that is essential to cells and tissues. Once this foundation is established we will then be able to understand how other nutrients can also be used for energy production. The next major biochemical pathway for this processing is called the citric acid or Krebs cycle. These reactions occur inside the mitochondria, so before pyruvate can be modified it has to pass across the mitochondrial membrane.

This occurs via the action of a specific membrane transporter. The pyruvate is then quickly oxidatively

Table 3.3.   Summary of ATP production in glycolysis.

Reaction	ATP Production Type	Number Formed per Mole of Glucose
Glyceraldehyde-3-P dehydrogenase	Creation of reduced NADH (2)	6
Phosphoglycerate kinase	Substrate level phosphorylation	2
Pyruvate kinase	Substrate level phosphorylation	2
Subtract ATP used by hexokinase and phosphofructokinase		−2
		Net gain 8 (aerobic)
		Net gain 2 (anaerobic)

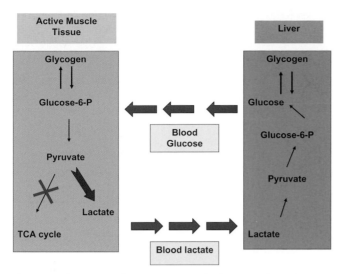

Fig. 3.6. The Cori cycle. In active muscle (for example, with anaerobic conditions) the conversion of pyruvate into acetyl CoA and processing via the TCA cycle is blocked (red X). This leads to lactate or lactic acid production. The lactate diffuses out of the muscle tissue into blood where the liver and kidney can convert lactate into glucose-6-phosphate for storage as glycogen or conversion to glucose-1-phosphate and then glucose. Muscle or other tissues in the body can then use this regenerated glucose.

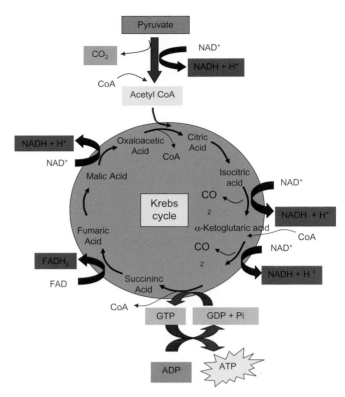

Fig. 3.7. Outline of the Krebs cycle reactions. Since each glucose molecule yields 2 pyruvate molecules (in the presence of oxygen), this allows two turns of the cycle. With each turn, 2 carbons are removed from the citric acid (6 carbons) by decarboxylation reactions; this leads to the production of the 4 carbon intermediate oxaloacetic acid. Oxaloacetic acid initiates the cycle as it condenses with acetyl CoA (2 carbons) to produce citric acid. Although the pyruvate that entered the mitochondria had 3 carbons, remember that 2 carbons were lost as CO_2 to generate acetyl CoA. Although not "officially" part of Krebs cycle, at the time of decarboxylation of the pyruvate, NAD^+ is simultaneously reduced. Four additional oxidations by the removal of hydrogen atoms occur during the cycle. This yields four molecules of reduced coenzymes (3 NADH + H^+) and 1 $FADH_2$). One ATP molecule is made with each turn of the cycle due to the initial creation of GTP, which then provides the phosphate group to make ATP from ADP. As in glycolysis this is another example of substrate level phosphorylation.

decarboxylated (removal of CO_2) to produce acetyl CoA. This reaction is catalyzed by the action of the multienzyme complex pyruvate dehydrogenase. The product, acetyl coenzyme A (acetyl CoA) plays an especially central role in energy metabolism. This overall reaction involves two coenzymes:

$$\text{Pyruvate} + NAD^+ + CoA \rightarrow \text{Acetyl-CoA} + NADH + CO_2 \qquad 3.3$$

The oxidized-reduced NAD^+ and NADH are familiar from the action of glyceraldehyde 3-phosphate dehydrogenase or lactate dehydrogenase and reactions of glycolysis. Now a description of coenzyme A is in order. Coenzyme A (CoA) is a complex molecule derived from pantothenic acid (common in meats and grains), thioethanolamine, and ATP. The essential feature is that CoA acts as a carrier of acyl groups. Specifically the thiol group of the thioethanolamine residue of the molecule functions in this manner in a variety of reactions involved in fatty acid oxidation and fatty acid synthesis and acetylation reactions. The molecule is also important in oxidative decarboxylation reactions, as with pyruvate. A common convention is to abbreviate the structure of the reduced form of the molecule as CoA·SH, which designates the reactive SH group of the molecule. So the acetyl group is now part of acetyl CoA is derived from the catabolism of pyruvate (2 carbons remaining after decarboxylation of pyruvate). As we will see, acetyl CoA is at the confluence of a variety of major metabolic pathways.

Almost all of the many specific carbohydrates and fats that are catabolized for energy production form acetyl CoA. In addition a number of the nonessential amino acids from degraded proteins also are cannibalized to generate acetyl CoA. As a special case in ruminants, one of the major products from fermentation of dietary carbohydrates is acetate, which is readily converted to acetyl CoA for subsequent processing through the mitochondria.

Back to our story, at this point the 2 carbons of the acetyl group of acetyl CoA and the 4-carbon molecule oxaloacetate condense to create the 6-carbon compound citrate. This is the first step of the Krebs cycle, as outlined in Figure 3.7. There are two critical physiological points to the Krebs cycle reactions. The first is that some ATP is produced directly via substrate level phosphorylation of ADP similar to that which occurs in glycolysis. The second and most important is that with each turn of the cycle, reduced forms of the coenzymes NAD and flavin adenine dinucleotide (FAD) are produced. When enzymes of the electron transport chain, also located in the mitochondria, subsequently oxidize these molecules, this yields the energy for synthesis of the vast majority of ATP that can be created from overall catabolism of glucose. We have provided only a skeleton outline showing the names of the intermediates of the Krebs cycle reactions and locations of specific events. Remember that each molecule of glucose generates two molecules of pyruvate so there are two turns of the cycle for each glucose molecule. As was the case with glycolysis, the coupled oxidation-reduction reactions are a critical part of the processing. The combination NAD+ and NADH appears again along with FAD and FADH. The enzymes that catalyze these oxidation reactions by removal of hydrogen atoms are dehydrogenases, for example, lactate dehydrogenase whose action is illustrated in Figure 3.9. For these reactions to take place the enzymes require the assistance of coenzymes that act to hold or carry these hydrogen atoms. It can be a source of confusion, but transfer of the hydrogen atom, with its lack of a neutron but paired electron and proton is effectively viewed as an electron transfer. Thus oxidation-reduction reactions defined by either electron acceptance or electron donation are often linked with movement of the hydrogen atom. This explains the abbreviations related to FAD versus $FADH_2$ or NAD^+ versus $NADH + H^+$ in the Krebs cycle reactions outlined in Figure 3.7. Figure 3.8 gives an example of this type of reaction.

At this point you might be wondering just how much ATP gets generated from glucose catabolism and when this actually occurs. As we have seen, each turn of the Krebs cycle generates only two molecules of ATP via substrate level phosphorylation. The key depends on a cluster of interrelated membrane bound enzymes that make up the electron transport chain. The activity of these enzymes also account for essentially all of our need for oxygen. As the electron chain enzymes function, the hydrogen atoms (electrons) that are removed as various intermediates of glycolysis and the Krebs cycle are oxidized and are progressively passed along until they are combined with oxygen. Oxygen is the final electron acceptor in the chain so that water is formed. The reduced forms of both NADH and $FADH_2$ that were generated in the Krebs cycle become oxidized again as their hydrogen is donated to the electron chain enzymes. Energy that is produced as electrons passes ultimately to oxygen is indirectly used to power the attachment of inorganic phosphate groups to ADP to create ATP. The enzyme responsible for this final step is ATP synthase, whose activity is linked to the movement of hydrogen atoms down a concentration gradient across the membrane of the mitochondria. Some of the energy from the action of the electron transport chain acts to transport hydrogen ions out of the mitochondrial matrix space. The resulting electrochemical gradient drives hydrogen ions back across the membrane in conjunction with ATP synthase leading to ATP generation. Because of the need for oxygen as the final electron acceptor in the electron transport chain, making of ATP in this manner is called oxidative phosphorylation.

Interestingly, the position along the electron transport chain at which $FADH_2$ or $NADH + H^+$ donate their electrons differs. Because of this, the amount of energy that is produced is greater for NADH compared with $FADH_2$. Specifically, each pair of hydrogen atoms from $NADH + H^+$ supplies energy for creation of three ATP, but the two hydrogen atoms from $FADH_2$ yield only two ATP. Most of the proteins of the electron transport chain are closely linked clusters within the inner mitochondrial membrane along with more mobile proteins (coenzyme Q and cytochrome C) that act as carriers between complexes. Figure 3.9 illustrates the release of energy associated with oxidation of NADH or $FADH_2$ in the electron transport chain, and Table 3.4 summarizes ATP production from completed catabolism of glucose.

Under ideal conditions, the complete oxidation of one glucose molecule to CO_2 and water yields 36 to 38 ATP. Alternative figures come from uncertainty about the energy yield of reduced NAD^+ that are produced from glycolysis. For these molecules to be utilized they must be passed across the mitochondrial membrane by active transport. An estimate of this "expense" is that the net ATP gain from reduced NAD^+ derived from the cytoplasm is only 2 ATP per molecule instead of the usual 3 ATP for those created inside the organelle. Since two of these molecules are produced in the cytoplasm during glycolysis the total yield is reduced to 36 ATP per molecule of glucose. Regardless, when

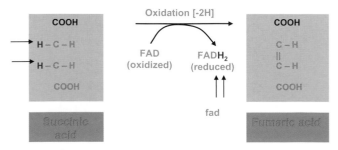

Fig. 3.8. Reduction of FAD. Coupled reduction of FAD in conjunction with the conversion of succinic acid to fumaric acid as occurs in the Krebs cycle is shown. Arrows indicate the fate of hydrogen atoms (electrons).

oxygen is available, energy capture from the biological oxidation of glucose is highly efficient. If a mole of glucose is completely combusted, as in a calorimeter, it yields 686 kcal. Energy obtained in the creation of high-energy ATP bonds equals 262 kcal for an efficiency of 38% [262/686 × 100]. This is markedly more efficient than most machines. Energy not captured in the formation of ATP is liberated as heat.

Intermediary metabolism—processing and pathways

Now that we have an appreciation for the processing of glucose to make ATP, we will explore some of the alternatives for storing glucose for situations when it is not immediately required for ATP generation, as well as pathways involved in mobilizing carbohydrate reserves. Similarly, we will also consider pathways that allow other important nutrients, i.e., proteins and lipids to be processed for ATP production. As we shall see, the glycolysis, Krebs cycle, and electron transport chain are central to the capacity to catabolize many different nutrients.

Glycogenesis, gluconeogenesis, and glycolysis

Although much of the available glucose is used to produce ATP, when energy demands are reduced, ATP production also declines. Cells have little capacity to "store" ATP; in fact as ATP concentrations in cytoplasmic rise, this produces allosteric inhibition of the regulatory enzyme PFK. So what happens to excess glucose? Fortunately this rise in ATP stimulates reaction pathways that act to convert excess glucose molecules into glycogen and into fat. Our animals have much more capacity to store fat than to store glycogen, but glycogen stores are nonetheless critical, especially for acute energy demands. We will consider fatty acid synthesis (lipogenesis) and catabolism (lipolysis) in a subsequent section.

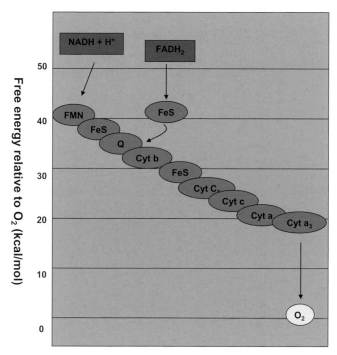

Fig. 3.9. Electron transport chain and reduced coenzymes. Each linked protein oscillates between reduced and oxidized states. As an upper protein is reduced, its capacity to hold the electron is lowered and the next protein in the cascade captures the electron. This continues until the oxygen atom at the end of the cascade captures the electron. The overall reduction in energy for electrons passed from NADH to oxygen is 53 kcal/mol, but the energy is captured stepwise. Since electrons from FADH$_2$ enter the chain further down, less energy is available so fewer ATP molecules are created.

Table 3.4. Summary of ATP production from Krebs cycle and electron transport chain reactions.

Reaction	ATP Production Type	Number Formed per Mole of Glucose
Pyruvate to acetyl CoA	Creation of reduced NADH (2)	6
Isocitrate to α-ketoglutaric acid	Creation of reduced NADH (2)	6
α-ketoglutaric acid to succinyl-CoA	Creation of reduced NADH (2)	6
Succinic acid to fumaric acid	Creation of reduced FADH$_2$ (2)	4
Malic acid to oxaloacetic acid	Creation of reduced NADH (2)	6
Succinyl-CoA to succinic acid	Substrate phosphorylation GTP and then ADP to ATP	2
Total from Krebs and electron transport chain		30
		8
Grand Total		38

When glycolysis is inhibited but glucose is available, this initiates glycogenesis (*glyco* = sugar + *genesis* = origin). Like the case with glycolysis, the first step depends on the uptake of glucose and conversion to glucose-6-phosphate by the ubiquitous enzyme hexokinase. However, instead of progressing through the glycolysis pathway, the glucose-6-phosphate is converted to its isomer glucose-1-phosphate by the action of glucose-6-phosphomutase. Interestingly, the ability of this enzyme to bind glucose to its active site is substantially less than for hexokinase. In other words its binding site has much less affinity for glucose. This means that when concentrations of glucose are low (likely also associated with a need for energy), the hexokinase reaction pathway is favored because of the higher affinity binding site. Of course high concentrations of ATP also allosterically inhibit PFK. As glucose concentration increases the law of mass action promotes the activity of the mutase enzyme, thus favoring the path toward glycogen synthesis. The enzyme glycogen synthase catalyzes the attachment of glucose-1-phosphate molecules to growing glycogen chains (see Fig. 2.22).

As energy demands increase, stored glycogen molecules can then be hydrolyzed to cleave glucose molecules for use by the cells. This process is called glycogenolysis and is catalyzed by the enzyme glycogen phosphorylase. This regenerates glucose-1-phosphate, which can then be converted to glucose-6-phosphate and processed for glycolysis. In most tissues (muscle cells, for example), the glucose-6-phosphate is effectively trapped in the cells since it cannot interact with membrane carrier proteins. This means that for most cells, glycogenolysis can supply energy for specific cells with stored glycogen only. However, liver cells along with some intestinal and kidney cells express the enzyme glucose-6-phosphatase, which catalyzes the removal of the phosphate group. In these cells when intracellular concentrations of glucose are increased some of the glucose can pass back out of cells and into the bloodstream. The capacity of the liver to utilize some of its glycogen stores to replenish blood glucose is critical for homeostasis. Pathways associated with glycogenesis and glycogenolysis are illustrated in Figure 3.10.

Describing gluconeogenesis completes our discussion of glucose metabolism. As we have seen, glucose and its intermediates from glycolysis and the Krebs cycle are essential. As indicated above, maintenance of blood glucose concentrations within relatively narrow boundaries is vital to the homeostasis and health of our livestock and pets. However, in some situations (especially acute for ruminants) rations either do not supply sufficient carbohydrate or situations of high demand or depleted glucose reserves occur. Fortunately, there is a kind of metabolic backup

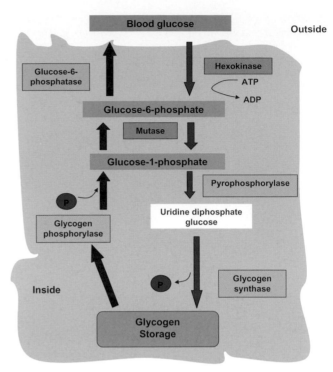

Fig. 3.10. Glycogenolysis and glycogenesis. Biochemical pathways for glycogenesis (red arrows) and glycogenolysis (black arrows) are illustrated. When glucose is abundant, some of the excess is converted into glycogen. When demand for ATP subsequently increases, glycogen is cleaved to provide glucose-6-phosphate for ATP generation. The conversion of glucose-6-phosphate to glucose that can then leave the cell occurs only in some cell types but is especially important in liver cells. Because of the mass of the liver and capacity to store glycogen, hepatocytes can be called upon to maintain blood glucose concentrations.

system. Gluconeogenesis effectively protects the body, and especially the nervous system, which has an absolute requirement for glucose, from hypoglycemia. Fortunately many nonessential amino acids and some other intermediates can be converted into glucose. This conversion is acutely driven by increases in stress-related hormones (epinephrine and glucocorticoids) and over longer periods by increased secretion of growth hormone and triiodothyronine. These topics will be covered in greater detail when we consider endocrinology.

Before we leave carbohydrate metabolism, it is worth considering one of the major pathways that is an offshoot of glycolysis. It's called the hexose monophosphate shunt or pentose phosphate pathway. Major functions are to provide NADPH (similar to NADH), which is needed for many reactions, particularly fatty acid synthesis, and to supply ribose that is essential for DNA and RNA synthesis. This sequence of reactions begins with glucose-6-phosphate, which is converted by the enzyme glucose-6-phosphate

Table 3.5. Activities of several enzymes involved in NADPH production and fatty acid synthesis in mammary tissue of cows 2 weeks before and 2 weeks after calving.

Enzyme	Prepartum	Postpartum
Glucose-6-phosphate dehydrogenase	7.8 ± 2.8	12.1 ± 3.1
6-phosphogluconate dehydrogenase	16.0 ± 5.3	39.5 ± 5.3
NADP-isocitrate dehydrogenase	98 ± 24	338 ± 100
Acetyl CoA carboxylase	0.1 ± .07	7.3 ± 0.9
Fatty acid synthase	0.7 ± 0.1	10.5 ± 1.8

The first two enzymes are part of the pentose phosphate shunt pathway and are involved in generation of NADPH that is required for fatty acid synthesis. Isocitrate dehydrogenase, one of the Krebs cycle enzymes, is also involved in NADPH production in ruminants. Acetyl CoA carboxylase catalyzes reactions between acetyl CoA and CO_2 to form malonyl CoA that is required for fatty acid synthesis. As the name suggests, fatty acid synthase is directly involved in condensation of malonyl CoA with acetyl CoA to add 2 carbons at a time to growing fatty acid chains. Data is adapted from Akers et al., 1981.

Table 3.6. Data for rates of acetate and glucose use for energy production (CO_2) and for fatty acid synthesis by bovine mammary tissue slices before and after calving.

Activity	Prepartum	Postpartum
Acetate incorporation into fatty acids	385 ± 137	2,428 ± 265
CO_2 production from acetate	168 ± 113	455 ± 127
CO_2 production from glucose	22 ± 14	92 ± 18

Rates of fatty acid synthesis or CO_2 production were calculated from rates of incorporated measured for radiolabeled [2-^{14}C]-acetate or radiolabeled [U-^{14}C]-glucose and are expressed as nmoles of substrate converted into product per hour per 100 mg of tissue. Data is adapted from Akers et al., 1981.

Lipogenesis and lipolysis

Although storage of glucose in the form of glycogen is critical, for longer-term energy needs, lipids sequestered in the adipocytes of adipose tissue supply the bulk of the fuel necessary for ATP synthesis. Depending on immediate needs, a variable amount of the carbohydrate of the diet is also converted into triglycerides before ultimately being catabolized. For many tissues, presentation of the fatty acids removed from storage provides the major carbon source for energy generation. As the principle form of energy storage in the body, triglycerides have distinct advantages over both proteins and carbohydrates. The first is that the caloric value ~38.9 kJ/g of a triglyceride is more than twice that of either glucose or protein. Second, storage in adipocytes is dense, compact, and occurs with much less water. Third, the catabolism of fatty acids provides metabolic water when oxidized, a distinct advantage to animals living in dry environments. The formation of triglycerides is called lipogenesis and the breakdown of triglycerides is called lipolysis. We will first consider how fatty acids are catabolized for energy production.

dehydrogenase into 6-phosphogluconate with the simultaneous conversion of $NADP^+$ (oxidized) into NADPH (reduced). The next step catalyzed by the enzyme 6-phosphogluconate dehydrogenase, produces another molecule of NADPH, frees CO_2, and yields a molecule of the pentose sugar ribulose 5-phosphate. This provides a direct precursor for ribose or deoxyribose synthesis. One way to appreciate the significance of these reactions is to consider how dramatically the activities of selected enzymes change with physiological conditions. For example, Table 3.5 shows the activity of several metabolically important enzymes in mammary tissue from cows just before and after parturition. Remember this is a time of dramatic changes in the synthetic activity of the mammary gland as lactation is initiated. The corresponding needs for energy and precursors for milk component biosynthesis are also elevated. Similarly, Table 3.6 shows metabolic flux data for bovine mammary tissue slices during the same period. Specifically, rates of oxidation of acetate and glucose, as well as use of these substrates for milk component biosynthesis, are shown. Do the changes in enzyme activities and metabolism reflect your reasoning of what the physiological status of the mammary tissue would be at these times? Remember this is just one selected example, during periods of rapid growth, work, etc. Many tissue would exhibit dramatic changes in tissue and cell activity. Our mammary gland example illustrates a major shift in organ function.

Whether they are derived from the diet or from storage, fatty acids are broken down into acetyl CoA, which as we saw with glucose oxidation, enters the Krebs cycle for subsequent processing. Fatty acid oxidation first requires activation of the fatty acid. This reaction occurs both inside the mitochondria and in the cytoplasm. If it occurs in the cytoplasm, activated fatty acids cross the membrane in a process that requires carnitine. Carnitine is a lysine derivative that markedly stimulates the oxidation of fats. The subsequent cleavage of the fatty acids takes place inside the mitochondria as 2-carbon units (essentially acetic acid or acetate molecules) are produced and fused with coenzyme A to produce acetyl CoA molecules. These acetyl CoA molecules transit the Krebs cycle to produce a small amount of ATP by substrate level oxidation but more importantly reduced coenzymes (NADH + H and FADH$_2$) as illustrated in Figure 3.7. This process is called beta-oxidation because the carbon atom in the third or beta position of the fatty acid chain is oxidized with each cleavage step. This reaction sequence is illustrated in Figure 3.11. Table 3.7 summarizes the total ATP produced from the oxidation of a common fatty acid, 16-carbon oleic acid. Although the most common fatty acids from stored triglycerides are typically longer than 6 carbons, even the oxidation of the 6-carbon fatty acid caproic acid is more efficient (44

versus 38 ATP) than the oxidation of glucose (also 6 carbons). Fatty acids are activated via hydrolysis of ATP coupled with coenzyme A. If first activated in the cytoplasm, the fatty acid is passed into the mitochondria by carnitine for further processing. With each cleavage cycle this generates one molecule of reduced NAD, one of reduced FAD and finally cleavage of the 2-carbon end group to produce acetyl CoA. This process repeats until the final 4 carbons of the fatty acid chain are cleaved to make two additional molecules of acetyl CoA. In this manner, long-chain fatty acids are degraded completely into these 2-carbon acetyl CoA units. The β-oxidation pathway oxidizes fatty acids with an odd number of carbon atoms until 3-carbon (propionyl CoA) residue remains. This compound is converted into succinyl-CoA, a constituent of the Krebs cycle. Of course the capacity for storing fat as an energy substrate is very large given the capacity of animals to deplete and replenish adipocytes.

As a dramatic example of utilization of body fat reserves, consider the capacity of high-producing dairy cows to mobilize fatty acids to supply the energy needed for milk production. Paradoxically, just at the time when the cow needs the most nutrients, there is routinely a decline in voluntary dry matter intake (VDMI) in the periparturient period. This decline begins in late lactation and continues into early lactation. For modern dairy operations, management of these transition cows is critically important. Most of the health problems, both of a metabolic or infectious nature, occur in early lactation. The typical decline in VDMI coincides with marked changes in reproductive status, body fat status, and the dramatic metabolic adjustments necessary to support energy, protein, and mineral demands of milk secretion. Just on the basis of energy needs the changes are staggering. For example, it is estimated that fetal development demands on day 250 of gestation (~3 weeks before calving) average 2.3 Mcal/d. The requirement for the lactating cow producing 30 kg of milk per day is estimated at 26 Mcal/d. Eating behavior and intake result from multiple interactions between neural inputs associated with the feed, feed presentation,

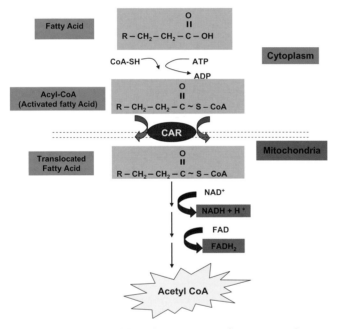

Fig. 3.11. Overview of β-oxidation. Fatty acids are activated via hydrolysis of ATP coupled with coenzyme A. If first activated in the cytoplasm, the fatty acid is passed into the mitochondria by carnitine (CAR) for further processing. With each cleavage cycle, this generates one molecule of reduced NAD, one of reduced FAD, and finally cleavage of the 2-carbon end group to produced acetyl CoA. This process repeats until the final 2 carbons of the fatty acid chain are cleaved to make two additional molecules of acetyl CoA.

Table 3.7. Summary of ATP production from β-oxidation of the 16-carbon oleic acid.

Reaction	ATP Production Type	Number ATP Formed
One cleavage cycle to produce acetyl CoA	Creation of reduced NADH (1) and reduced FADH$_2$ (1)	5
Each acetyl CoA through Krebs cycle	Creation of reduced NADH (3), reduced FADH$_2$ (1) and ATP	12
Total from cleavage reactions (8)		40
Total from processing acetyl CoA (8)		96
Minus ATP for activation		−1
Grand Total		135

management, metabolic conditions, and endocrine signals that are poorly understood but especially so in ruminants. Dramatic changes in VDMI occur both within and between lactations in dairy cows. Pregnant dairy heifers, for example, begin to progressively reduce their VDMI, beginning several weeks before calving, approximately 0.17 kg per week until 3 weeks before calving. For primiparous and multiparous cows given diets of constant composition, milk yield typically peaks at about 6 weeks postpartum but maximum intake is not achieved until 8 to 22 weeks postpartum. Indeed, the demands of lactation require that the high-producing cow mobilize body tissues through much of the first one-third to one-half of lactation so that the animals are in a prolonged period of negative energy balance. Difference in the rate of intake recovery postpartum depends on the diet fed in early lactation as well as the degree of fatness or body condition score (BCS) at the time of calving. The normal feeding behavior is also markedly impacted by both clinical and subclinical infections so that appetite and performance is reduced in sick animals.

As championed in a review by Bauman and Currie (1980) and emphasized recently by Ingvartsen and Andersen (2000), onset of lactation in high-producing dairy cows requires a coordinated physiologically mediated reallocation of biochemical resources—homeorrhesis—to allow high milk production while maintaining homeostasis. Because of the premium placed on glucose to supply precursors for lactose synthesis and the general energy requirements of the udder, changes in circulating nonesterified fatty acids (NEFA) and glucose are especially dramatic at calving. Concentrations of NEFA immediately postpartum are dramatically increased while glucose in the blood is reduced (Fig. 3.12). This reflects the mammary demand for glucose and the corresponding stimulation of lipolysis and use of lipids as an energy source.

Table 3.8 provides a partial listing of metabolic adjustments that accompany the onset of lactation. It

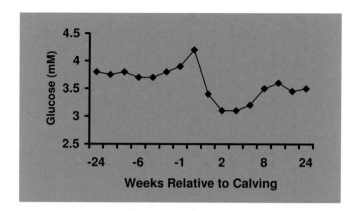

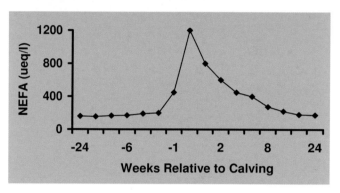

Fig. 3.12. Plasma glucose and nonesterified fatty acids. Changes in plasma glucose and nonesterified fatty acids (NEFA) in heifers in the period before and after calving are shown. Data is adapted from Ingvartsen and Andersen, 2000.

Table 3.8. Summary of major metabolic adjustments associated with the onset of lactation in high-producing dairy cow.

Physiological Process	Biochemical Adjustment	Tissue Affected
Milk synthesis	↑ Synthesis ↑ Blood flow ↑ Nutrient uptake	Mammary gland
Lipid metabolism	↑ Lipolysis ↓ Lipogenesis	Adipose tissue
Glucose metabolism	↑ Gluconeogenesis ↓ Glucose utilization	Other body tissues
Protein metabolism	↑ Proteolysis	Muscle and other tissues
Mineral metabolism	↑ Absorption ↑ Mobilization	GI tract bone
Intake	↑ Food consumption	Nervous system
Digestion	↑ GI tract hypertrophy ↑ Capacity of absorption	GI tract and liver

Data adapted from Bauman and Currie, 1980, and Ingvartsen and Andersen, 2000.

is important to appreciate that similar changes occur in all lactating mammals. We have used the dairy cow as an example because effects are especially dramatic because of selection for increased milk production. The increase in milk yield during early lactation precedes increases in appetite so that the animals are in negative energy balance, and thus there is dramatic lipid mobilization over the first 12 to 16 weeks of lactation. It is estimated that the body fat needed to meet demand is equivalent to more than 50% of the milk fat yield during this period. These animals typically mobilize 50 to 60 kg of fat, ~10% of body weight and likely 50% of body fat reserves. Figure 3.13 illustrates the mobilization of lipid to supply the demands of lactation in a high-yielding dairy cow. Similar responses occur in other lactating mammals. For example, Table 3.9 shows changes in mean adipocyte volume in sheep between late pregnancy and midlactation related to the number of suckling lambs. Clearly increased demand has a dramatic impact on adipose tissue metabolism.

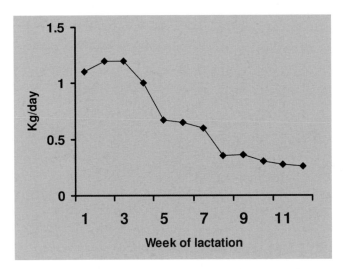

Fig. 3.13. Fat mobilization in lactating cows. The estimated amount of fat mobilized per day to meet the demands of lactation in a high-producing dairy cow is illustrated. The cows in this study averaged 9,534 kg of milk over a 305-day lactation. Adapted from Bauman and Currie, 1980.

Table 3.9. Changes in adipocyte volume of ewes between late pregnancy and mid lactation.

Sheep	Average Adipocyte Volume (pl)		
	Late Pregnancy	Peak	Mid
1 Lamb		423	476
2 Lambs	478 ± 31	293 ± 33	215 ± 28
3 Lambs		286 ± 63	199 ± 53

Data adapted from Vernon and Flint, 1984.

Let's now consider how fats are liberated from storage and the processing required for making the fatty acids from the triglycerides available. As you might guess, signals are required to stimulate the breakdown of triglycerides from storage in the adipocytes. Both the nervous and endocrine systems are involved. As a reminder, biologically important lipids fall into two broad classes: 1) structural lipids, e.g., phospholipids, and 2) neutral fat, e.g., triglycerides stored as an energy reserve. Blood plasma averages about 300 mg of lipid per 100 ml of blood. About 50% is typically phospholipid, 30% triglycerides, and 20% cholesterol and a variety of other lipids. Included in this fraction are the nonesterified or free fatty acids. These molecules have a rapid turnover and are the main form in which fatty acids are transferred from storage in adipocytes for oxidation in other cells. Interestingly, oxidation of fatty acids in the adipocytes of white adipose tissue is very limited. If you consider the structure of these cells, this is easy to explain. The cytoplasmic compartment of the cells is limited to a small crescent containing the nucleus, a bit of RER, and a few mitochondria. The bulk of the cell area is the stored lipid droplet. With a minimal number of mitochondria β-oxidation of fatty acids is limited. In contrast, a specialized type of adipose tissue, brown adipose tissue, has an abundant blood supply and numerous mitochondria. This type of adipose tissue contains adipocytes with many small lipid droplets. This tissue is vital for thermogenesis in many newborn animals as these cells oxidize large amounts of lipid and generate heat that is essential to the neonatal homeostasis. However, the white adipose tissue reserves are critical for maintenance of homeostasis or to meet energy demands—in particular, physiological circumstances. Figure 3.14 provides an overview of lipid synthesis and mobilization specifically oriented to ruminant adipose tissue and the significance of acetate availability. For monogastric species, little acetate appears in the blood, so glucose is the predominate substrate for lipid synthesis.

Given the need to carefully control release of fatty acids to supply critical energy needs, especially at times when the diet may be limited or demands are increased, it is not surprising that multiple regulators are involved. The neurotransmitter norepinephrine, locally released by nerves supplying adipose tissue, in conjunction with glucagon and epinephrine released into the circulation are major stimulators of lipolysis. As we will see in our discussion of the fight-or-flight reactions that occur with stimulation of the sympathetic division of the autonomic nervous system, making energy available in emergency or stress situations is critical. This means that the very rapid response that occurs with nervous system stimulation is reinforced by more prolonged secretion of the hormones

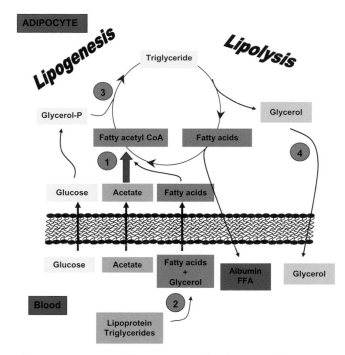

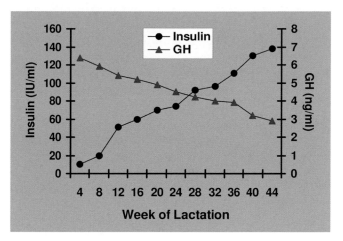

Fig. 3.15. GH and insulin in lactating cows. Data is adapted from Koprowski and Tucker, 1973.

Fig. 3.14. Overview of lipogenesis and lipolysis. Overall aspects of lipogenesis and lipolysis in a ruminant adipocyte. Included are de novo fatty acid synthesis (1), uptake of preformed fatty acids from blood (2), fatty acid esterification (3), and lipolysis (4). For nonruminants species uptake of acetate (red arrow) would be of minor importance. In these animals, glucose would act to supply the carbon skeleton for both glycerol and growing fatty acid chains. Adapted from Bauman and Davis, 1974.

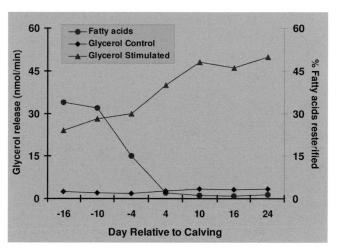

Fig. 3.16. Adipose tissue metabolism. Rate of glycerol release from adipose tissue explants incubated with or without norepinephrine and the proportion of fatty acids re-esterified (a measure of synthesis) in the absence of norepinephrine is illustrated. Notice that there is an increasing rate of stimulated lipolysis that begins before the actual onset of milking. Data is adapted from Metz and Van Den Burgh, 1977.

epinephrine and glucagon. An excellent example of an even more prolonged adjustment to promote lipid mobilization occurs at the onset of lactation in many mammals (see Fig. 3.13). It is now known that genetically superior dairy cows, for example, have an enhanced capacity to respond to the energy demands of lactation with a greater-than-average capacity to mobilize nutrients from body stores. It is hypothesized that this is in part due to enhanced secretion of growth hormone (GH) in these animals. Logically, changes in average circulating concentrations of GH and insulin (which promotes lipogenesis) are reversed during the course of lactation in dairy cows. During early lactation when the animals are in a net negative energy balance, concentrations of insulin are suppressed and those of GH enhanced. As the animals begin to consume more feed and milk production declines, after the peak of lactation, the situation is reversed. GH concentrations decline (less need for nutrient mobilization from storage) but insulin concentrations increase (to store excess nutrients). This is illustrated in Figure 3.15.

Not only are there adjustments in the secretion of hormones that affect lipid tissue metabolism, there are also modifications in the activity of the tissue itself.

For example, sensitivity of the tissue to the effects of epinephrine or norepinephrine also changes as cows enter lactation. Specifically, adipose tissue becomes more sensitive to these catecholamines and rates of fatty acid re-esterification (related to storage) drop precipitously. These responses are produced by changes in the number of hormone receptors expressed by the target adipocytes as well as alterations in the signaling pathways within the cells. As we will see in our discussion of endocrine system physiology, there are very complex, yet elegant interactions between the nervous system, endocrine system and cellular biochemistry to maintain homeostasis and to prepare for specific physiological events. The data illustrated in Figure 3.16 shows very clearly some of the adjustments in adipose tissue physiology that enable pregnant animals to prepare for the metabolic demands of lactation. In this experiment adipose tissue was collected by biopsy at varying times before and after calving. The tissues were minced and incubated in the absence (control) or the presence of norepinephrine. The rate of release of glycerol (a measure of the rate of lipolysis) was determined. Addition of norepinephrine markedly stimulated lipolysis, but tissue collected immediately after calving were more responsive. Furthermore, the rate of fatty acids synthesis (re-esterification) began to decrease before calving and was markedly inhibited after the onset of milk secretion. These metabolic adjustments in adipose tissue begin to occur before the actual onset of milk secretion after calving and the first milking. This suggests that changes in neural and endocrine signaling pathways act to anticipate subsequent needs. As an example, the supply of fatty acids to various tissues is regulated by two lipases: 1) the lipoprotein lipase that resides on the surface of the endothelial cells to cleave triglycerides from circulating chylomicra, and 2) hormone-sensitive lipase that exists inside the adipocytes. Hormones that increase intracellular concentrations of the cyclic AMP (cAMP), a second messenger molecule, in adipocytes increase lipolysis. This is because high concentrations of cAMP activate an intracellular kinase that converts the hormone-sensitive lipase from an inactive to an active conformation. Since this reaction is initiated by the binding of norepinephrine or epinephrine to β_1-adrenergic receptors on the surface of adipocytes, changes in receptor number or the concentration of their ligands in the fluid surrounding the cells impacts the rate of lipolysis. The relationship between receptor binding and lipolysis is illustrated in Figure 3.17.

Before we leave the topic of lipolysis, we should mention one of the more common disorders related to lipid metabolism—ketosis. For example, it is likely the most common metabolic disorder of lactating cows but can be a problem in many animals. Ketosis can be simply defined as the accumulation of excess concentrations of acetoacetic acid (AAA), β-hydroxybutyric acid (BHBA), and decarboxylation products acetone and isopropanol in various body fluids. In many tissues, acetyl CoA molecules can condense to form acetoacetyl CoA. The liver (unlike most tissues) expresses a deacylase enzyme that cleaves this to form acetoacetic acid. This material is converted to BHBA and acetone that then diffuses into the bloodstream. These compounds are called ketone bodies. Since these compounds are catabolized slowly, continuing production can eventually lead to metabolic acidosis, a condition that can be severe and even fatal. The fundamental problem is an impairment of the entrance of acetyl CoA into the citric acid cycle because of the

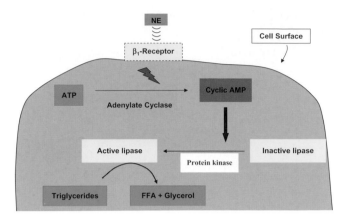

Fig. 3.17. Adipose tissue signaling. The association between binding of norepinephrine to the β_1-adrenergic receptor on the surface of an adipocyte and activation of an intracellular lipase is illustrated. The binding reaction promotes the activation of the enzyme adenylate cyclase, which converts ATP to cyclic AMP (cAMP). Increased concentrations of cAMP activates a protein kinase by adding a phosphate group to the inactive lipase enzyme, changing its conformation and thereby allowing the lipase to actively catalyze the cleavage of triglycerides into free fatty acids (FFA) and glycerol. This internal lipase is called hormone sensitive because of the ability of catecholamines and other hormones to induce the appearance of intracellular cAMP and therefore increase the rate of lipolysis.

relative lack of oxaloacetic acid. This leads to increased concentrations of acetyl CoA and ketone formation or ketogenesis. Three conditions that lead to low intracellular glucose supplies include starvation, diabetes mellitus, and feeding of a high-fat, low-carbohydrate diet (in monogastric species). In the case of diabetes, uptake of glucose by the cells is impaired so that signals are generated to supply energy demands by oxidizing fatty acids. This only exacerbates the problem and leads to even more accumulation of ketone bodies. When most of the energy is supplied by fat, (high-fat, low-carbohydrate diet), there is a carbohydrate deficiency because there is no major route for converting fats to carbohydrates. Liver cells are also likely to become engorged with fat (fatty liver syndrome), which impairs cellular functioning.

So what are some of the conditions that promote this chain of events? It is most likely to occur in dairy cows in early lactation (between 2 and 6 weeks postpartum). Symptoms can include decreased appetite, lethargy, decreased milk production, reduced body weight, and an acetonelike odor of milk or exhaled air. However, the disorder can be either subclinical or clinical. With clinical ketosis, the need for treatment and losses in milk production become readily apparent, but subclinical ketosis is much more problematic. In the absence of overt testing, these cows are often described as "not doing as well as expected."

Kronfeld (1982) distinguishes four classifications of ketosis:

- Primary underfeeding ketosis. Essentially a result of poor management, i.e., failure to offer enough acceptable feed to the cow.
- Secondary underfeeding ketosis. The cow's VDMI is reduced by disease.
- Ketogenic ketosis. The cow is consuming a diet with elements that promote production of ketones.
- Spontaneous ketosis. The cow is consuming an adequately balanced diet but ketosis occurs nonetheless.

Whatever the cause, lactation ketosis is a worldwide problem and is seemingly most prominent in high-producing herds. However, incidence, especially of subclinical ketosis can vary substantially between herds irrespective of average milk production. This suggests that its etiology is complex. Some common features are that ketotic cows are usually in negative energy balance and that frequency of clinical ketosis is often greatest at about the time of peak milk production postpartum. Two reliable biochemical changes are a reduction in blood glucose and increased concentrations of ketones in blood, urine, and milk. This has led to renewed interest in development of reliable screening methods to detect subclinical ketosis via monitoring of ketones, especially in milk samples. Animals destined to develop ketosis seemingly fail to maintain blood glucose concentrations, so the energy demands begin to be met by inappropriate overmobilization of adipose stores. Increased catabolism of the fat leads to elevations in blood lipids and transport of fatty acids into the liver in greater quantities than the liver can metabolize. Acute treatments typically involve glucose infusions or injections to provide alternative energy substrates and/or treatment with glucocorticoids to stimulate the cow's own capacity for gluconeogenesis. Reasons why some animals seemingly readily adapt to make the metabolic adjustments required for onset of lactation and high milk production are unknown. It is interesting, however, that genetically superior animals (with respect to milk production) often secrete more GH and that one of the salient properties of GH is to promote mobilization of nutrients.

Paradoxically, excessively overfeeding cows during the dry period, which would logically allow the accumulation of adipose tissue stores for use in lactation, actually impairs the capacity of the cow to mobilize tissue nutrients in early lactation. Most nutritionists recommend that cows be moderately fed during late lactation and that concentrated feeding be increased only just before calving and then into early lactation. Prevention of ketosis is focused on management of feeding practices in the dry period and in early lacta-tion. Since overfeeding and excessive weight gain in the dry period adversely affect the capacity of the cow to mobilize nutrients, attention to dry cow management is essential. Because of the economic problems associated with ketosis and the subtle nature of subclinical cases there has been increased attention directed toward development of easy-to-use cow-side tests. Blood concentrations of BHBA greater than 1,200 µmol/liter can be used to classify normal from subclinically ketotic cows.

Let's now consider some of the events associated with conditions when energy supplies are plentiful and excess nutrient resources are being used to "restock" adipose tissue. The fatty acids in the triglycerides of the adipocytes can be derived by de novo synthesis (within in the tissue) or can be "deposited" following digestion and absorption of dietary lipids. For the preformed dietary fats, this requires first the action of lipases in the GI tract and absorption of liberated fatty acids into the intestinal cells. As these dietary fats are hydrolyzed and emulsified by the actions of bile salts and phospholipids, particles called micelles are formed. These aggregates have the polar portion of the bile salts to the outside and the nonpolar cholesterol-like portion interacting with the fatty acids, monoglycerides, and cholesterol oriented to the center of the sphere. The cells absorb the micelles and process their contents. Fatty acids of 12 carbons or less can pass into the bloodstream to be transported as free (nonesterified) fatty acids. The larger fatty acids are reesterified to triglycerides and along with cholesterol become coated with a layer of lipoprotein and phospholipids to generate chylomicra, which leave the intestinal cells and enter the lymphatic drainage. Once they appear in blood circulation the chylomicra can be utilized to supply the fatty acids for regenerating adipose tissue fat. In monogastric species after a fat-rich meal so many of these particles can appear in the blood that the plasma can have a milky appearance (lipemia). The chylomicra are removed by the action of the enzyme lipoprotein lipase, which is sequestered on the surface of the endothelial cells of capillaries. When activated, the enzyme catalyzes the hydrolysis of triglycerides, making fatty acids and glycerol available to the surrounding tissues. In the case of adipose tissue, the fatty acids and glycerol is absorbed by the cells and reesterified to form much of the neutral fat stored in the cells.

The direct synthesis of fatty acids is called de novo synthesis. Since nutrients other than fats can be consumed or fed in excess, there are alternative methods of fat synthesis, which allow storage of carbohydrates and proteins as energy sources in the form of neutral fat. One of the more common fatty acids is palmitate ($C_{16:0}$). The overall reaction to produce palmitate is illustrated in the following equation:

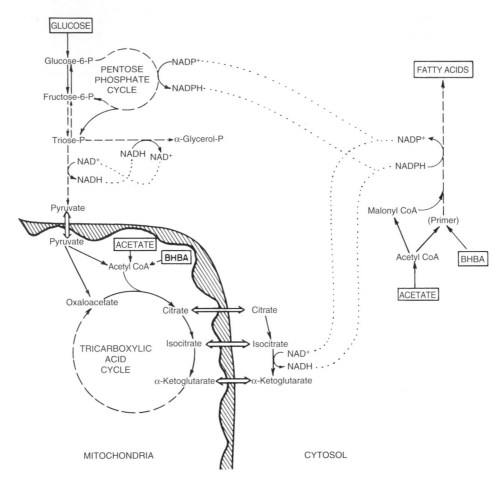

Fig. 3.18. Fatty acid synthesis in ruminant tissue. Biochemical pathways related to fatty acid synthesis in the ruminant mammary gland are depicted. Adapted from Bauman and Davis, 1974.

$$\text{Acetyl-CoA} + 7 \text{ malonyl-CoA} + 14 \text{ NADPH} + \text{H}^+) \rightarrow \text{Palmitate} + 7 \text{ CO}_2 + 14 \text{ NADHP+} + 8 \text{ CoA·SH} + 6 \text{ H}_2\text{O} \qquad 3.4$$

Let's consider the source for these ingredients. First, our discussion of carbohydrate metabolism provides a ready explanation for the source of the acetate to make acetyl CoA, i.e., the oxidation of glucose or other sugars. The malonyl Co-A can be produced from acetate or butyrate. The coenzyme NADPH is generated from the pentose phosphate shunt or in ruminants by isocitrate dehydrogenase in the cytoplasm. A number of amino acids can be catabolized to produce intermediates of glycolysis or the Krebs cycle that can be used to make acetate. Ruminants exhibit extensive fermentation of dietary carbohydrates and produce large amounts of the volatile fatty acids: β-hydroxybutyric acid (BHBA), acetate, and propionate. Some of this acetate is directly used for ATP production or shunted to fatty acid synthesis. Similarly, butyrate is readily used in fatty acid synthesis. Thus, availability of acetate is a key to fatty acid synthesis. Because rumi-

nants depend on gluconeogenesis to maintain blood glucose concentrations, they have evolved mechanisms to minimize the use of glucose for direct synthesis of fatty acids, a glucose sparing effect. In fact, in the case of lactating cows, the demand for glucose is even greater with the need for lactose synthesis by the mammary gland. Whereas in nonruminants glucose oxidation leading to pyruvate oxidation in the mitochondria produces citrate that can pass into the cytoplasm to be used to make acetyl CoA for fatty acids synthesis, this is minimal in ruminants. There are many details concerning fatty acid synthesis, i.e., control over the degree of desaturation and chain length that are beyond the scope of our text, but a rudimentary description of the process is in order. Figures 3.18 and 3.19 illustrate differences in fatty acids synthesis pathways in ruminants and nonruminants.

In cows and other ruminants, precursors for de novo fatty acids synthesis are acetate and BHBA. BHBA appears in the first 4 carbons of the majority of fatty acids made in the cells or the molecule is cleaved into 2-carbon units to be used as acetyl CoA. Acetate

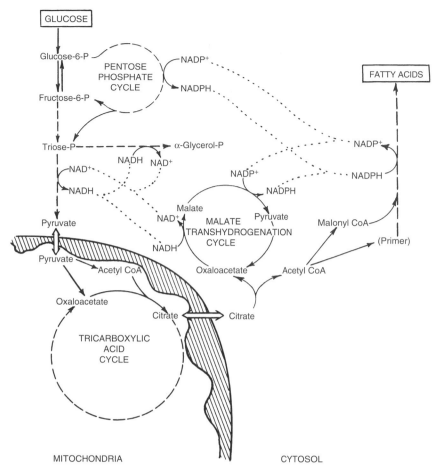

Fig. 3.19. Fatty acid synthesis in nonruminant tissue. Biochemical pathways for fatty acid synthesis in a nonruminant mammary gland are depicted. Adapted from Bauman and Davis, 1974.

yields the carbon for the shorter fatty acids (C4–C14) and some C16 fatty acids. The NADPH comes from the catabolism of glucose via the pentose phosphate shunt or the oxidation of isocitrate to α-ketoglutaric acid in the Krebs cycle. The malonyl CoA pathway, which sequentially adds 2 carbon units to the growing fatty acid chain, is the major synthesis pathway in the ruminant mammary gland and occurs in the cytoplasm. The first step depends on the regulatory enzyme acetyl CoA carboxylase and involves the addition of carbon from CO_2 to acetyl CoA and hydrolysis of ATP to form malonyl CoA. The second step is catalyzed by the enzyme fatty acid synthase. This complex enzyme controls growth of the growing fatty acid chain 2 carbons at a time. In most fat synthesizing tissues, fatty acid synthase produces mostly palmitic acid. However, the presence of the enzyme thioestearse II in mammary tissue induces the synthesis of more medium-chain fatty acids and fewer long-chain fatty acids. Thus, differences between fatty acid synthesis in ruminants and nonruminants primarily concern the sources of the acetyl CoA needed in the

initial step and generation of the necessary NADPH.

In nonruminants the acetyl CoA for fatty acid synthesis comes from the decarboxylation of pyruvate in the mitochondria but not directly. Since acetyl CoA does not easily pass across the mitochondrial membrane, citrate derived from the combination of acetyl CoA and oxaloacetate diffuses from the mitochondria and enters the cytoplasm. The citrate is broken down by ATP-citrate lyase to give acetyl CoA and oxaloacetate. The acetyl CoA provides the carbon skeleton for fatty acid synthesis, and the oxaloacetate enters the malate transhydrogenation cycle, which yields pyruvate and NADPH. The pyruvate subsequently enters the mitochondria.

In ruminants acetate and BHBA from the blood provide most of the carbon needed for fatty acids synthesis. In mammary cells, for example, glucose is largely spared from being used as a carbon source for fatty acid synthesis because of the near absence of the citrate lyase enzyme in the cytoplasm of the cell. The citrate that does leave the mitochondria is either converted to isocitrate and then α-ketoglutarate generat-

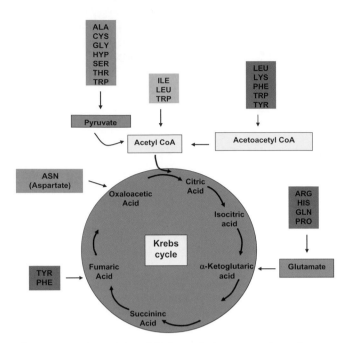

Fig. 3.20.   Amino acids and Krebs cycle. Interconversions of carbon skeletons of common amino acids to intermediates associated with Krebs cycle are illustrated.

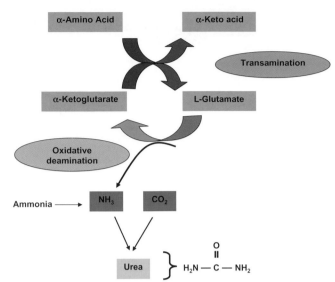

Fig. 3.21.   Amino acid nitrogen metabolism. A general overview of nitrogen flow in amino acid metabolism is shown. Transamination reactions provide a mechanism to catabolize a variety of amino acids by transfer of the amine group to pyruvate (alanine transaminase, i.e., alanine is produced from pyruvate in the transfer) or transfer of the amino acid amine group to α-ketoglutarate catalyzed by the enzyme glutamate transferase, i.e., glutamate is produced by the transfer. The ability to generate glutamate is especially important because it is the only amino acid in most mammals that readily undergoes oxidative deamination. This provides a mechanism to excrete the amine group in the form of ammonia, which is typically converted to the less toxic urea.

ing NADPH in the process, or it passes into the Golgi and is secreted into milk. Cow's milk is higher in citrate than nonruminants and concentrations of citrate increase with the final stages of lactogenesis. Indeed, this abrupt increase in citrate concentrations of mammary secretions can be used as a marker for lactogenesis and parturition.

Interconversions and catabolism of proteins

Just as there are multiple paths by which substrates can be supplied for fatty acid synthesis, there are also interconversions that are possible to allow nonessential amino acids to be used for ATP production. However, before amino acids can be used, they must be deaminated—that is, the NH$_2$ has to be removed. This remaining carbon skeleton can then be converted into pyruvate or one of the other intermediates of the Krebs cycle, as shown in Figure 3.20. A key to these reactions is glutamic acid, a common nonessential amino acid. Many amino acids are modified when their amine group is passed to α-ketoglutaric acid (one of the Krebs cycle intermediates). This produces glutamic acid from the former α-ketoglutaric acid, and the remaining carbon skeleton from the amino acid is converted into a keto acid (there is now an oxygen atom in place of the original amine group). This is a transamination reaction, literally the transfer of an amine group of an amino acid. The liver absorbs the glutamic acid and the amine group is removed as

ammonia (NH$_3$). This is called oxidative deamination. This reproduces the α-ketoglutaric acid, freeing it to be recycled in another round of transamination reactions. Because ammonia is toxic in mammals it is usually quickly carboxylated to produce urea and water. The urea diffuses into the bloodstream and after filtering in the kidney, large quantities of urea are excreted in urine. Thus the urea was derived from the catabolism of amino acids. The capacity of liver glutamic acid to shuttle amine groups from various amino acids for excretion as urea (urea cycle) is critical to animal well being. Some organisms (fish) actually excrete free ammonia. These species are called ammonotelic. Other animals (birds and amphibians) excrete uric acid and are referred to as uricotelic species; those that excrete urea are referred to as ureotelic species. Thus, ammonia is typically removed from the body after being converted into less toxic urea, often in the liver. Blood urea is cleared by urinary excretion. However, in ruminants substantial urea also is excreted into saliva. Once the urea reaches the rumen microorganisms it is hydrolyzed and the free NH$_3$ used by the microflora for protein synthesis. Much of this microbial protein passes to the small intestine where it is

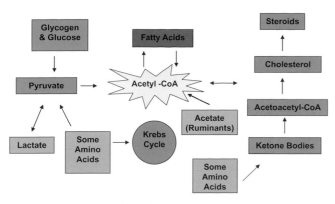

Fig. 3.22. Overview of acetyl CoA metabolism.

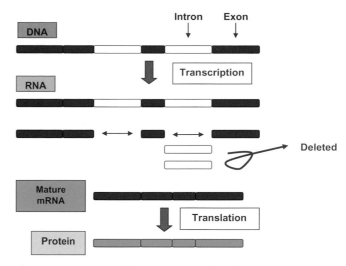

Fig. 3.23. Overview of transcription and translation and protein synthesis.

absorbed. Thus some of the absorbed proteins contain amine groups that were originally waste products. Figure 3.21 illustrates reactions associated with the catabolism of amine groups from amino acids.

As we have seen, glycolysis and the Krebs cycle reactions explain not only how glucose and other carbohydrates are oxidized to supply ATP, but also how both proteins and fats must be catabolized to enter this pathway for ATP production. Figure 3.22 provides an overview to emphasize the critical role that production of acetyl CoA has in schemes to produce the energy and provide building blocks that are needed to meet physiological demands.

Structure and function of DNA and RNA

As we have now learned essentially all of the biochemical reactions to produce energy or build cellular components depend on enzymes. Other proteins are critical components of various cellular organelles. This means it is nearly impossible to overestimate the importance of proteins. It follows then that the creation and activation of proteins must be carefully orchestrated so that the suitable enzymes are available when required and the proteins for organelle generation are present. In many respects cellular functioning follows the now popular business concept of on-time delivery. This ultimately goes back to regulation of gene expression and controls that affect transcription and translation (see the section "Proteins" in Chapter two). Although we have considered some of the basics of RNA and DNA structure, we will now review protein synthesis in a bit more detail. It is reasonable to think of cells as miniature protein factories and that the particular combination and number of proteins fashioned determine the functional attributes of the cell. For example, although all cells have common components it is logical to predict that the comple-

ment of proteins needed for adequate functioning of a fibroblast would be very different from the complement of proteins made by a secretory epithelial cell from the pancreas.

Protein synthesis

DNA not only provides the template to direct its own replication, it also provides the blueprint for the synthesis of proteins by its ability to direct the formation of mRNA. As you will recall, this process is called transcription. As a reminder, Figure 3.23 gives an overview of information transfer from DNA to RNA to proteins for a eucaryotic cell. An important aspect for eucaryotic cells compared with prokaryotic cells is the fact that the genes of higher organisms are interrupted by DNA sequences that do not code for the ultimate protein product. DNA sequences that do correspond with the protein are called exons and those that make the intervening sequences are called introns. A single gene may contain 50 or more introns. Moreover these introns contain from as few as 60 to more than 100,000 nucleotides. This means that the initial RNA strand must be processed to remove the introns before it can be used to accurately direct protein synthesis. One of the great puzzles of cell biology is the physiological significance of the introns. On the surface it seems wasteful for the cell to spend the biochemical resources to synthesize introns initially and then to re-create segments of the mRNA molecule that must be removed and discarded.

As you will recall, proteins are chains of amino acids. Genes can be viewed as the segment of DNA that provides the directions for construction. There are also a few genes that direct the creation of specialized variants of RNA, but certainly most genes direct protein synthesis. The nucleotide bases A, T, C, and G make up the foundation of the code for these assembly instructions. A sequence of three bases, or triplet, specifies a particular amino acid. For example, the sequence AAA indicates the amino acid lysine. This means that the sequence of triplets in the mature processed mRNA that leaves the nucleus (see Fig. 3.23), spells out the exact sequence of amino acids for a particular protein. These triplet sequences are the genetic code.

So what are the mechanics of protein synthesis? This requires the combined activities of three types of RNA molecules: 1) mRNA, rRNA (ribosomal), and tRNA (transfer RNA). The ribosomes are the cellular organelles that are the focus of actual protein synthesis. These organelles are composed of subunits derived from RNA and protein molecules and are fabricated by the nucleolus inside the nucleus of the cell. To use an automobile analogy, rRNA can be thought of as the factory that houses and organizes the needed components. Processed mRNA provides the blueprint for protein assembly. It could be thought of as the assembly line that is organized along the factory floor. The tRNA can be thought of as the forklifts and cranes that bring the components (in our case, amino acids) needed to make the car (protein, in our case). Of course with cars, the components are welded or bolted together by workers or workers driving machinery. In our analogy, as we have seen with other biochemical processes, the bolting or welding of the amino acids (peptide bond formation) requires energy supplied by ATP hydrolysis and is accomplished by enzyme activity. To summarize, polypeptide synthesis requires two fundamental steps: 1) transcription, during which time the DNA "information" is encoded into mRNA, and 2) translation, the process by which the "information" in mRNA is decoded and used to manufacture the proteins. This process is outlined in Figure 3.24.

Let's begin with detailing transcription. The first step involves the unwinding or unraveling of a segment of DNA that is destined for use. The cytoplasm contains specialized molecules (some of which are mediators of hormone action by the way) called transcription factors. These molecules have the capacity to bind to regions near the beginning or "start" sequence of a gene. This region, that is not part of the final mRNA product, is called the gene promoter. In simplistic terms, activation of this region sets in motion or promotes the subsequent transcription of a particular gene. As you may have guessed by now, a great deal of cellular activity is determined by the complex of particular transcription factors that are unleashed in a cell at a given moment and which promoter regions are available to be acted upon.

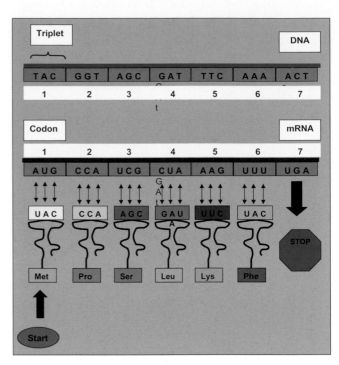

Fig. 3.24.   Information transfer from DNA to RNA. Processed mRNA is utilized to direct the fabrication of the growing protein chain via transfer RNA and their attached amino acids, which have complementary binding (anticodon) to the codons of the mRNA.

The transcription factor acts to mediate the binding and initiation of the enzyme RNA polymerase. RNA polymerase allows opening of the double-stranded DNA. One strand then serves as the template to produce the complementary mRNA molecule (sense strand). For example, if the triplet sequence were AGC, this corresponding mRNA would UCG. You might recall that RNA differs from DNA in that it is single-stranded, contains ribose instead of deoxyribose, and the base uracil (U) substitutes for thymine (T). This explains the U instead of T in the newly created RNA triplet. The strand of DNA that is not used as a template is called the antisense strand. Each triplet of the DNA corresponds with a three-base sequence of the mRNA called a codon. Since there are four different nucleotides in RNA or DNA, there are 4^3 or 64 possible codons. Three of these (UAA, UAG, and UGA) serve as stop signals and AUG, which codes for the amino acids methionine serves as a start signal. Since there are only 20 common amino acids, some amino acids are coded by more than one triplet sequence.

Once the mature or processed mRNA (introns removed) reaches the cytoplasm, it joins the smaller of the ribosomal subunits. At this point, the tRNA comes into action. Transfer RNA binds its amino acid and transports it to the ribosome. There are approximately

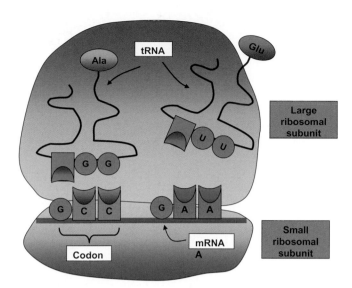

Fig. 3.25. Transfer RNA. Transfer RNA transports amino acids (alanine and glutamic acid), in this example, to the ribosome for interaction with the mRNA. The triplet codon of the mRNA strand corresponds with complementary binding of the anticodon of the tRNA. Following binding of adjacent amino acids, the enzyme aminoacyl-tRNA synthetase catalyzes the formation of peptide bonds. As the mRNA passes through the ribosome complex the protein chain continues to elongate until a stop codon is reached and the nascent protein chain is released.

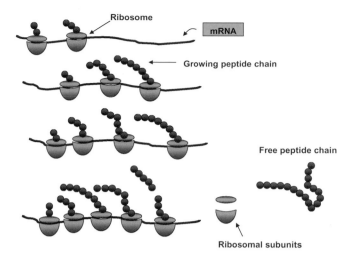

Fig. 3.26. Development of polyribosomes. Each polyribosome consists of a strand of mRNA that is being transcribed by multiple ribosomes. As the mRNA moves through the ribosome, each codon is sequentially read and peptide bonds formed between adjacent amino acids. Ribosomes that have been attached longer have the correspondingly longer peptide chains. This progression (left to right) continues until the stop codon is reached when the nascent peptide is released along with the ribosomal subunits.

20 different tRNA variants, which correspond with each of the different amino acids. Not only must the tRNA recognize its particular amino acid (by possessing a unique binding site), it must also recognize the triplet codon of the mRNA molecule. These tRNA molecules have a complex wire-hanger–like conformation that allows simultaneous recognition of the mRNA codon by complementary base pairing (anticodon) along with orientation of the attached amino acid into position to allow the enzyme aminoacyl-tRNA synthetase to catalyze formation of peptide bonds between adjacent amino acids attached to the mRNA (see Fig. 3.25). This is accomplished because of the elegant structure that is produced by the combination of the large and small ribosomal subunits attached to the mRNA molecule. There is a binding site for the mRNA and three sites for binding of the tRNA molecules. The charged tRNA (one that has its amino acid attached) binds to the A (attachment) site. As the peptide bonds are formed there is a shift to the P site, which holds the growing peptide chain. As newly charged tRNA molecules arrive at the ribosome, the old empty tRNA shifts to the E (exit) site and is released to capture another amino acid. As the mRNA codons are progressively read, the mRNA passes through the ribosome as the elongating amino acid chain appears. As the mRNA emerges, other ribosomes can attach and begin the process of translation. This means that

many protein molecules can be fabricated simultaneously. These complexes are called polyribosomes. This is illustrated in Figure 3.26. The mRNA strand continues to be read and the protein chain grows until its stop codon is reached. At this point the elongating protein chain along with the ribosomal subunits is freed from the ribosome.

References

Akers, R.M., D.E. Bauman, A.V. Capuco, G.T. Goodman, and H.A. Tucker. 1981. Prolactin regulation of milk secretion and biochemical differentiation of mammary epithelial cells in periparturient cows. Endocrinol. 109: 23–30.

Bauman, D.E. and W.B. Currie. 1980. Partitioning of nutrients during pregnancy and lactation: A review of mechanisms involving homeostasis and homeorrhesis. J. Dairy Sci. 63: 1514–1529.

Bauman, D.E. and C.L. Davis. 1974. Biosynthesis of milk fat. In *Lactation: A Comprehensive Treatise*, Vol. 2, edited by B.L. Larson and V.R. Smith. Academic Press, New York.

Ingvartsen, K.L. and J.B. Andersen. 2000. Integration of metabolism and intake regulation: a review focusing on periparturient animals. J. Dairy Sci. 83: 1573–1597.

Koprowski, J.A. and H.A. Tucker. 1973. Bovine serum growth hormone, corticoids and insulin during lactation. Endocrinol. 93: 645–651.

Kronfeld, D.S. 1982. Major metabolic determinants of milk volume, mammary efficiency, and spontaneous ketosis in dairy cows. J. Dairy Sci. 65: 2204–2212.

Metz, S.H. and S.G. Van Den Burgh. 1977. Regulation of fat mobilization in adipose tissue of dairy cows in the period around parturition. Neth. J. Agric. Sci. 25: 198–211.

Tyrrell, H.F., A.C. Brown, P.J. Reynolds, G.L. Haaland, D.E. Bauman, C.J. Peel, and W.D. Steinhour. 1988. Effect of bovine somatotropin on metabolism of lactating dairy cows: energy and nitrogen utilization as determined by respiration calorimetry. J. Nutrition 118: 1024–1030.

Vernon, R.G. and D.J. Flint. 1984. Adipose tissue: metabolic adaptation during lactation. Symposium Zoological Soc. Lond. 51: 119–145.

4 Tissue structure and organization

Contents

Introduction

Although the cell is considered a basic unit of life, complex functions in multicellular animals require interaction and cooperation between cells. With increased development, specialized functions appear in subpopulations of cells. Many of these activities are attributed to types of tissues. For example, nervous or neural tissue composed of neurons and supporting neurological cells allow generation, transmission, and interpretation of electrical signals. This is the hallmark of the nervous system. Another tissue type, epithelium, is widely dispersed in animals and generally is involved in covering surfaces, i.e., skin or peritoneum, in the development and function of various glands—mammary, pituitary, pancreas, and so forth. Muscle tissue is readily recognizable because of its capacity to generate motion and distinct appearance. It is worth remembering, however, that there are three classes of muscle tissue: skeletal or voluntary, cardiac, and smooth muscle. The final tissue type, connective tissue, is also very widely distributed and is usually found as a component of the other tissue types. This means that when you study preparations of various tissues, although there will be emphasis on particular cells (epithelial, muscle, or neural) various connective tissue elements are also present. Lastly, there are also subclasses of connective issues, i.e., bone, cartilage and blood. Our purpose in this chapter is to aid your activities in the laboratory, especially time spent looking at samples in the microscope, to reinforce your other reading and attendance of lectures, and to give you some rudimentary understanding of histology.

Microscope general points

Remember, your text cannot substitute for self-study. It will also become apparent that you simply cannot

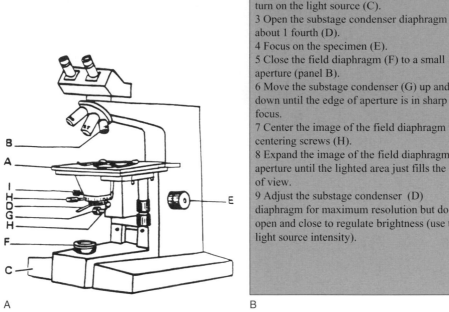

Alignment Steps
1 Carefully place a slide on the stage (A).
2 Swing the 10x objective (B) in to position and turn on the light source (C).
3 Open the substage condenser diaphragm about 1 fourth (D).
4 Focus on the specimen (E).
5 Close the field diaphragm (F) to a small aperture (panel B).
6 Move the substage condenser (G) up and down until the edge of aperture is in sharp focus.
7 Center the image of the field diaphragm with centering screws (H).
8 Expand the image of the field diaphragm aperture until the lighted area just fills the field of view.
9 Adjust the substage condenser (D) diaphragm for maximum resolution but do not open and close to regulate brightness (use the light source intensity).

A   B

Fig. 4.1. Microscope parts and use. The first step in getting the most out of your efforts is to make sure your microscope has the proper illumination: Place a prepared slide on the microscope stage (A) and carefully rotate the 10× objective lens (B) into position and then turn on the light source (C). You should then adjust the focus knob (E) to view the image. To get the best image, illumination should be centered on the specimen and the beam of light should completely fill the aperture of the objective lens. Examples of needed adjustment are detailed in Figure 4.2.

randomly view a microscope slide labeled, for example, "simple epithelium," and immediately see an image equivalent to what you would see as a text example. Samples are chosen because there is a predominate tissue or cell type, but this does not exclude others. Second, we have searched slides to find excellent examples of the features we want to illustrate. Some areas of even professionally prepared slides have artifacts, i.e., wrinkles, folds, areas of poor staining, and so forth. Consider yourself warned!

Although you will not likely spend lots of time at the microscope, the image you see is no better than your ability to handle the microscope and appropriately adjust the light source and various condensers and lens to get the best, brightest image with adequate resolution. Figure 4.1 (microscope parts and use) and Figure 4.2 (microscope alignment) describe some of the attributes of the typical brightfield microscope and how you can get the most out of the time you spend in laboratories at the microscope. The following are keys to good microscope use when examining prepared slides:

- Insure that the stage is lowered.
- Place a low-power objective (4 or 10×) in position for initial examination.

- Ensure that the slide is clean and the cover-slipped side is face up.
- Bring the specimen into proper focus and orient yourself to the entire sample.
- Close the field diaphragm to ensure proper alignment (see Fig. 4.2).
- Switch to the magnification of choice; if the objectives are parfocal on the revolving nosepiece, only small adjustments should be necessary when changed.
- Be careful not to smash the slide when focusing.
- Always lower the slide stage and place a low-power objective lens in position when you are finished.
- Turn off the power to the light source.
- Use only approved lens paper to clean any lenses.

Terminology and definitions

In any field of study there are terms and expressions that are common and allow easy communication. You have already been introduced to some basic physiology language in Chapter 1. As we begin to explore the

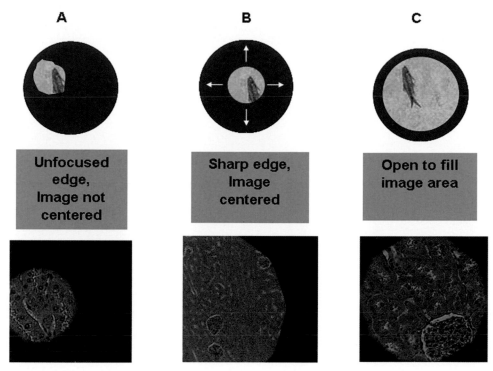

Fig. 4.2. Microscope alignment. In panel A the field diaphragm (F) has been closed to create a small aperture; however, the image is not centered in the field of view and the edge is not in focus. In panel B the edge was focused by carefully raising or lowering the substage condenser lens (G) until the image of the field of light is at its sharpest. The image has been centered by adjusting the two centering screws (H). In panel C, the field diaphragm has been opened further to expose more of the image. Lower panels (left to right) are images of a section of kidney tissue before centering, focusing the edge of the field diaphragm, and opening of the field diaphragm. Letters in parentheses refer to microscope parts in figure 4.1.

structure of tissues, it is important to appreciate some of the specific language and terms that apply. Here are some tissue-related definitions:

- Histology. Subspecialty of anatomy that deals with the microscopic structure of tissues.
- Tissue. A group of similar cells and intercellular materials specialized to carry out a specific activity. The four primary tissues are: epithelial, muscle, nervous, and connective.
- Organ. A discrete portion of the body composed of two or more tissue types dedicated to a particular function. For example, the heart is an organ of the circulatory system.
- Cytology. Subspecialty of anatomy that deals with the structure and functional differentiation of individual cells either as isolated cells or as part of a tissue.
- Pathology. Subspecialty of anatomy and physiology that deals with changes in gross anatomy, histology, or cytology associated with disease or injury.
- Necropsy. Refers to the gross and/or microscopic examination of organs, tissues, and cells after death. Most often associated with determinations of the cause of death.

- Parenchyma. Refers to the functional portion of a tissue or organ. For example, in the kidney the epithelial cells of the nephron are responsible for the formation of urine and recovery of important nutrients filtered into the lumen of the nephron. Thus these epithelial cells make up the critical functional structure of the kidney.
- Stroma. Refers to the support cells, e.g., connective tissue, blood vessels, nerves, etc., that are needed for the parenchymal tissue to carry out its functions.

Although the task of learning the rudimentary histology of various tissue and organs may seem daunting at first, the job becomes easier when the information is organized into more manageable blocks. For example, any cell or cellular product can be classified into one of four basic tissue types, listed here with their primary functions:

- Epithelium. Covering for protection, glandular activity
- Muscle. Movement, cardiovascular function, heat production
- Nervous. Signaling, control, integration of physiological systems
- Connective. Support, mineral storage, protection

We will cover the basics of each of these tissues in this chapter, but as we consider more of the physiology of various organ systems in subsequent chapters we will often return to discuss structural attributes of cells or tissues. This is because to a very large degree structure and function go hand in hand. In other words, the capacity of a tissue or organ to complete a specific function is directly dependent on the arrangement and organization of the cells within the tissue or organ.

Epithelial tissue

As illustrated in Figure 4.3, epithelial cells are classified based on the shape of the cells. In addition the number of epithelial cells in the layer adds an additional element of classification (Fig. 4.4). A single layer of squamous, cuboidal, or columnar cells is called simple epithelium. An alternative structure with several layers of cells is called stratified. These stylized images are oversimplified but you should get the idea of how these cells are classified. One of the tasks that

will take some practice is distinguishing epithelial cells from other cells present in tissues, i.e., connective tissue cells (fibroblasts, adipocytes), etc. One key is that the epithelial cells are often on a surface (even if the surface is internal, the lining of a duct for secretion onto the internal surfaces of body cavities). When the stratified type occurs, the shape classification is considered only for the single layer of cells on the outer surface. For example, in the stylized example given in Figure 4.4, the epithelium would be classified as stratified cuboidal epithelium.

Notice that the outer layers of epithelial cells in both examples in Figure 4.4 are classified as cuboidal. Second, the dark lines underneath the cells represent the basement membrane on which the epithelial cell layer rests. The is an unfortunate term, in that the basement membrane is not a true membrane in the usual sense, but is a complex of extracellular proteins (collagen, elastin, etc.), proteoglycans, and so forth that serve to support and anchor the epithelial layer. In some histological preparations these proteins may be apparent but not in others. This depends on the fixation process used to preserve the tissue and the particular staining process (see Fig. 2.5). Since most routine processing focuses on the cellular structure, do not be alarmed if the basement membrane is not also apparent.

Epithelial Classification

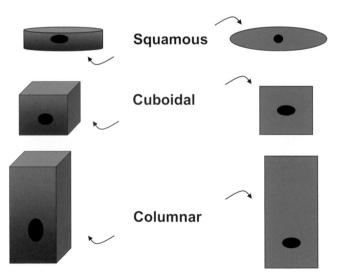

Fig. 4.3. Epithelial cell shape classifications. These stylized illustrations show three dimensional as well as surface views for three common shapes of epithelial cells. The cell nucleus is indicated by the black oval. Relatively flattened, thin cells are squamous. The one cell thick row of cells that line the internal surface of capillaries or the lung alveoli are examples of squamous cells. Cuboidal cells, as the name suggests, are similar to a child's set of ABC toy blocks. The cells approximate cubes. Such cells appear as part of the lining of many ducts in glandular tissues. Columnar cells, by contrast, are more elongated and can be likened to tiny skyscrapers. These cells appear on the surface of the lining of the intestinal tract, among other places.

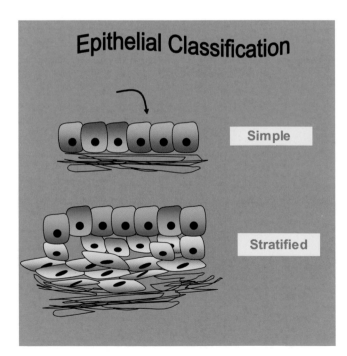

Fig. 4.4. Epithelial cells classified by number of strata. This classification is straightforward; a single layer of cells (arrow) constitutes a simple layer but when there are multiple layers of cells this is called a stratified epithelium. The black lines represent various extracellular matrix proteins that provide anchorage and support for the layer of epithelial cells.

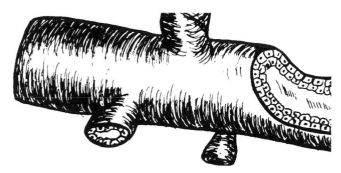

Fig. 4.5. Drawing of glandular duct. You can easily imagine that the structure illustrated in this drawing is essentially a large tube to transport secretions that empty from several other small tubes. As the cutaway area to the right suggests, the larger tube is lined by a double layer of cells, the small cross section of one of the smaller tubes (lower left) suggests it is lined by a simple layer of epithelial cells. How would the image of the larger structure appear if it were sectioned longitudinally? What if the structure was sectioned in a perfect cross section compared with an oblique angle? What would it look like? These are some of your concerns as you examine tissue sections. You need to strive to imagine the tissue in three dimensions.

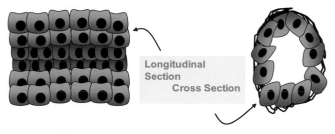

Fig. 4.6. Diagram of tubular structure. These simple drawings are an attempt to illustrate the appearance of an epithelial duct cut in either longitudinal or cross section. The cross-section profile is easier to imagine, but the longitudinal profile can easily seem like a simple mass of cells.

Tissue sections prepared for the light microscope are usually made from tissues that have been preserved in formalin, dehydrated in ethanol, and ultimately infiltrated with paraffin wax, as discussed briefly in Chapter 2. These tissue blocks are then placed in a machine called a microtome that is used to cut thin slices or sections that are then mounted on a microscope slide and stained. This is how the majority of tissues have been prepared since the late 1800s. Although this is a routine process, the sections prepared can be relatively thick, sometimes more than one cell in thickness, so that you are sometimes looking at parts of multiple cells. Just like problems with other artifacts, wrinkles, tears, and so forth, thickness has to be considered as you use the microscope or consider illustrations. A further problem concerns learning to recreate three dimensions from the flat images you will be studying. Take a moment to consider the examples of what the cutting angle does to the image you see in the microscope. Imagine a real organ with twisting and turning epithelial ducts or blood vessels and the possible variations. How would this equate to the two-dimensional image of tissue on the microscope slide? For many structures you need to consider whether the specimen has been cut longitudinally, in cross section, or perhaps at some odd tangent. All of these things impact the image that you see in the microscope. Consider the illustrations in Figures 4.5 and 4.6.

When you are interpreting what is seen in a single plane of section, it is important that you think about what might have been present either above or below a particular structure (Figs. 4.7, 4.8).

We will now consider the features of some of the more common epithelial types. Can you reexamine the tissue in Figure 4.7 and imagine the organization and three-dimensional structure of the tissue from the microscopic image?

Epithelial tissue characteristics

Epithelial tissue, or epithelium (the plural form is epithelia), occurs as a sheet of cells to cover an organ surface or line a body cavity. In other cases, epithelial tissue makes up the bulk of the cells in glandular tissues. The covering type of epithelium is abundant and widespread. These are the cells that make up the skin, the internal surfaces of the cardiovascular system, the digestive tract, the reproductive tract, and the respiratory tract. Epithelial tissue also covers internal body cavities. The functional cells of the accessory organs of the digestive system, i.e., liver, pancreas, and gall bladder, are mostly epithelial cells. Other glandular organs, i.e., pituitary, adrenal, thyroid, salivary, and so forth, are also composed of epithelial cells. Epithelial cells form boundaries between different regions of the body. For example, the epidermis of the skin creates a protective barrier between the inside and outside of the body. The same is true for the epithelial cells that line the internal surface of the respiratory or digestive tract. Other specialized epithelial cells include reproductive cells (ova and spermatozoa), rods and cones of the retina, and taste buds. This explains the myriad of functions attributed to epithelial tissues: 1) protection, 2) absorption, 3) secretion, 4) excretion, 5) filtration, and 6) sensory reception.

Distinctive features also contrast epithelial tissues from the other three tissue types. One of these is the degree of cellularity of the epithelial tissues compared with other tissues. Specifically, epithelial tissue is composed of cells that are very tightly packed together so that usually there is a minimal of space between the cells. In fact, for the epithelial cells to successfully

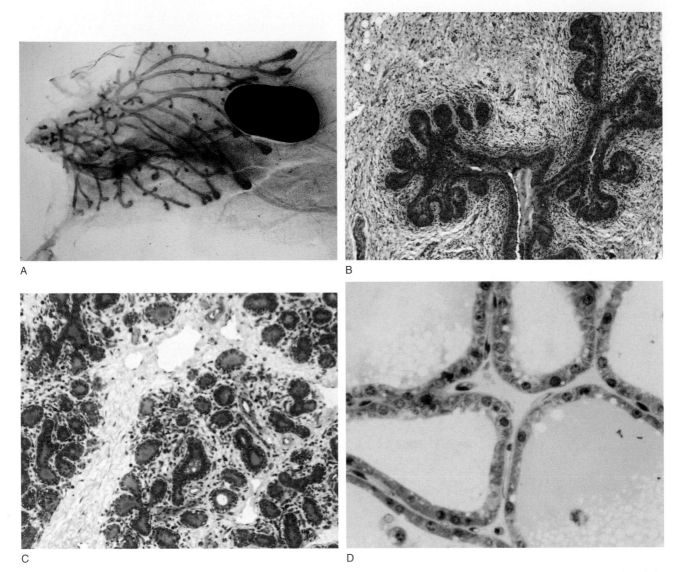

Fig. 4.7. Examples of epithelial structures. The four images shown in Figure 4.7 are actual mammary ducts. Panel A is a picture of a whole mammary gland taken from a prepubertal mouse after the gland was defatted and stained. The picture was taken with a dissecting microscope, so the ducts are intact and whole. Notice the elongated ducts with the bulbous endings (terminal end buds). Panel B is a section of mammary tissue from the mammary gland of a prepubertal Holstein heifer. Panel C is an image of mammary tissue from a pregnant heifer and Panel D is of mammary tissue taken from a lactating cow. Late in pregnancy the mammary ducts begin to develop alveoli. The alveoli are spherical, hollow structures lined by the epithelial cells that are responsible for the synthesis and secretion of milk (this is more evident from the drawing in Fig. 4.8). The epithelial cells that line the internal surface of the alveoli are simple cuboidal. Around the outside of the alveoli, specialized myoepithelial cells form a network around the circumference of the alveolus. These cells contract in response to oxytocin released from the posterior pituitary at the time of milking. This reduces the volume of the alveolus to force accumulated milk into larger ducts and then the nipple or teat. This is called milk ejection, or milk letdown. Somewhat similar structures are found in lungs, pancreas, and thyroid gland.

complete their roles as protective barriers, adjacent cells form specialized contacts. Epithelial cells acting to absorb or secrete products are described as being polar. This is most easily visualized for glandular secretory cells. The basal region of the cell (closest to the basement membrane and capillaries) can be thought of as the manufacturing site for the cell. Products to be secreted are packaged and processed in the Golgi for subsequent secretion from the cells in the apical region of the cell (Fig. 4.8). In other cases the apical end of the cell (near the free surface) is acting to absorb nutrients or move surface secretions. For example, the cells of the intestinal tract and kidney tubules have extensive microvilli. This markedly increases surface area to improve function. Other epithelial cells are even more specialized with cilia—for

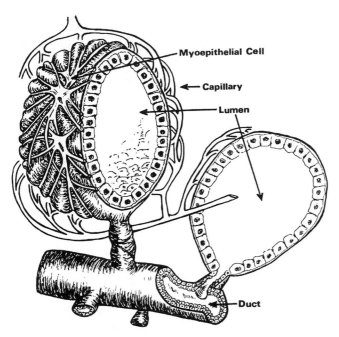

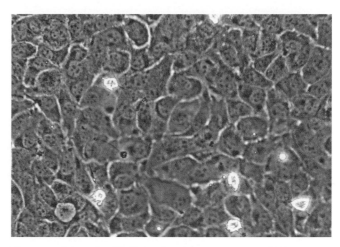

Fig. 4.9. Cultured epithelial cells. These mammary cells have formed a monolayer that is one cell thick. This is similar to the sheet of simple squamous epithelial cells that would line the surfaces of organs or surfaces of internal body cavities.

Fig. 4.8. Representation of the structure of mammary alveoli. As you can see, it takes experience and practice to discern the three-dimensional structure of tissues. One of the tissues for which this is very important is the kidney. Once you develop an appreciation of the structure of the kidney nephron it will be much easier for you to understand and appreciate the filtering, reabsorption, and excretion that occurs in the urinary system.

example, cells lining the ova duct or the respiratory tract that function to propel substances along their surfaces.

The epithelial cells, however, are not alone in carrying out their activities. The cells are attached to a thin supporting sheet or layer of nonliving material called the basal lamina. This layer is composed of proteins and glycoproteins that are produced by the epithelial cells. In some regions, e.g., Bowman's capsule of the kidney tubules, the basal lamina is particularly thick so that it acts as a filtration barrier to prevent the movement of plasma proteins into urinary filtrate. The reticular lamina appears beneath the basal lamina. This is an additional layer of more fibrous proteins, e.g., collagens and elastic that link the epithelial cells with the connective tissue underneath. These two layers or lamina (basal + reticular) are collectively called the basement membrane, as mentioned above. It defines the boundary between the epithelium and the connective tissue or stromal. Interestingly, although there are nerve fibers, i.e., sensory nerves that penetrate the epithelium of the skin or intestinal tract, the epithelium is avascular. That is, it does not contain blood vessels. These appear in the loose, more open spaces of the connective tissue. This means that both the nutrients that supply the epithelial cells and waste products depend on diffusion to pass between the tightly packed epithelial cells and the capillaries underneath. This likely explains why it is rare to find epithelial tissue that contains more than a few strata of living cells. A final property is the capacity of epithelial cells for rapid growth and regeneration. For example, notice how quickly skin abrasions heal. This may have a down side when you consider that most cancers are carcinomas, i.e., derived from epithelial cells.

Simple epithelium

As you will likely experience in a laboratory setting with a microscope and set of slides or in multimedia presentations, tissue samples contain multiple cell types and in the case of epithelial tissues often more than one type of epithelial cell. Thus, although the focus of a particular specimen may be on a specific cell or tissue, it does not mean this cell or tissue type is exclusive. Our first example (Fig. 4.9) shows epithelial cells growing on the surface of a cell culture dish. These cells have proliferated and arranged themselves into a pavement of cells one cell layer thick. If you imagined these cells growing on a flexible sheet that could be rolled into a tube, you would have a simple recreation of a capillary. Regardless, in this view you are looking directly down onto the surface of the cells. Each cell looks something like a fried egg, with the nucleus the yolk of the egg. The cells are flattened and closely packed together. They would be classified as simple squamous. As another way to visualize simple squamous cells, imagine the flattened floor tiles in a kitchen as single squamous epithelial cells all linked together to make the floor. The grout between the tiles would represent the membrane junction complexes that anchor epithelial cells together and create functional barriers between tissue compartments, i.e., the surface and the subflooring underneath. It is typical to find simple squamous epithelium in areas where absorption and filtration occur and a thin barrier is desirable, for example, capillaries or lining of alveoli of the lungs. Can you rationalize why simple squamous would be a poor choice for the surface of the body?

The image shown in Figure 4.10A is from the kidney and is mostly parenchymal tissue. It shows a series of cross-sectioned tubules from several nephrons. You should remember that epithelial cells are often found on free surfaces, even though some of the surfaces may be very minute internal surfaces, i.e., the inside of small vessels or tubules. Some of these tubules are lined by a single layer (simple) of squamous epithelial cells, but others are lined by a single layer of cuboidal epithelial cells. Can you find examples of each? Perhaps a hint is in order. For many of the squamous epithelial cells the cytoplasm is very thin, so the most prominent feature of the cells is the nucleus, which often seems to protrude in to the lumenal space of the tubule. Can you pick some of these out of the image?

In Figure 4.10B the arrows indicate several tubules lined by simple squamous epithelial cells. You should note that in many cases the nuclei of the cells seem to protrude into the lumen space of the tubule. Remember, the squamous cells are very thin with a relatively small amount of cytoplasm that often stains poorly. The oval indicates a collecting duct tubule lined by simple cuboidal cells.

Figure 4.11 shows a portion of this tissue taken at a higher magnification 1,000×. This is accomplished by use of the 100× objective lens of the microscope and the 10× eyepiece. This means that the magnification reaching your eye is a thousandfold. The camera used to take the photographs also utilizes a 10× lens mounted in position where the eyepieces would normally be located. There can also be additional magnification associated with printing or viewing, but this does not really increase true resolution. At this magnification, the difference in the cellular appearance of squamous and cuboidal epithelial cells should be apparent in the lower portion of the image. Many of the cuboidal cells have distinct pink staining around their borders, and the nucleus when present is generally oval-shaped and positioned in the center of the cells. Three of these cells are present near the center of the image. For the low squamous cells surrounding the lumen of a smaller duct (lower portion of the slide), the cells have only a thin rim of cytoplasm, but

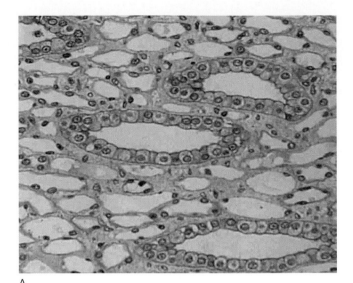

A

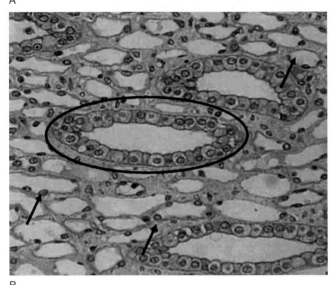

B

Fig. 4.10.   Kidney tissue. Multiple kidney tubules are cut in cross section. Some are thin-walled regions of the loop of Henle, lined by simple squamous epithelial cells; others are sections of capillaries, also lined by simple squamous epithelial cells (called endothelial cells). There are also a smaller number of cross sections through a portion of the nephron called the collecting duct. These are lined by simple cuboidal epithelial cells.

the nuclei are prominent and seem to protrude in to the lumen of the duct.

Figure 4.12 is taken with a 20× objective and is an image of a tangential section through a blood vessel, specifically a vein. You can see clusters of red blood cells in the lumenal space of the vessel and you can also distinguish a layer of simple squamous epithelial cells that line the internal surface of the vessel. The center of this section shows the lumen of a vein that has been cut at a tangent. Several red blood cells are clustered near the upper center of the vessel lumen.

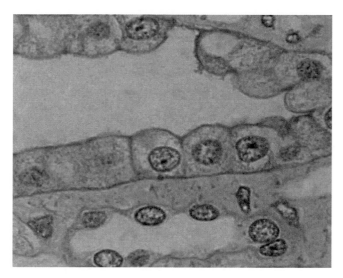

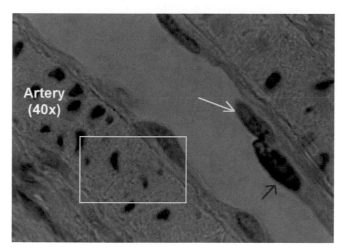

Fig. 4.13. Section of artery wall.

Fig. 4.11. High-power image of kidney tissue.

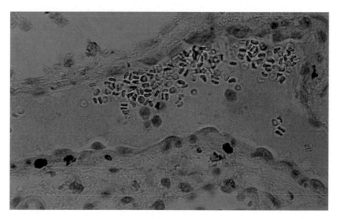

Fig. 4.12. Section through blood vessel.

The cells that line the side of the lumen are endothelial cells. Notice the difference in the staining compared with Figure 4.10. This means that you need to learn structures not based on color but on morphological characteristics.

Figure 4.13 shows a similar section through an artery at higher magnification. The box (yellow) in the figure indicates a portion of the tunica intima or interna, which is composed of simple squamous epithelial cells (also called endothelial cells) and the layer just under these cells, the tunica media, which has smooth muscle cells in arteries. The yellow arrow points to the nucleus of an endothelial cell. The adjacent structure is another endothelial cell's nucleus, which was synthesizing DNA at the time the sample was taken. The brown stain is due to the attachment of an antibody that is specific for presence of bromodeoxyuridine (BrdU), an analog of thymidine that is used to measure DNA synthesis. You should recall the

relevance of these analogs in the study of cell proliferation from your earlier reading.

Before we leave our discussion of simple epithelium, as you have likely gathered from the figure descriptions, some simple squamous epithelia have specialized names. The term *endothelium* (inner covering) is used to describe the lubricating cell covering for all vessels of the cardiovascular system, including the lymphatic vessels and the internal surfaces of the chambers of the heart. Capillaries specifically are made of endothelium. This structure promotes rapid easy movement of nutrients to the surrounding cells and the corresponding uptake of waste products. Similar simple squamous cells also make up the mesothelium (middle covering), the epithelium that makes the serous membranes of the body. These are the coverings of the internal organs and body cavities that are well lubricated to allow organs to slide past one another.

Figure 4.14 is an image from a tissue sample taken from a section of the small intestine. A portion of a villus is shown with a layer of simple columnar epithelial cells covering the outer portion. The nuclei appear mostly in a row in the lower third of the cell. Notice that the cells are tall and narrow (Fig. 4.15).

Although not apparent at lower magnification, the apical ends of the cells have many microvilli, which add capacity for absorption. This is also called the brush border. If you look closely, you should notice that the outer rim of the cells looks as if the cells have been slightly colored. This is because the microvilli clump slightly and trap proteins when the tissue is preserved. These associated proteins and carbohydrates are called the glycocalyx. The accumulated material and closely aligned microvilli allow staining and explains the darker rim.

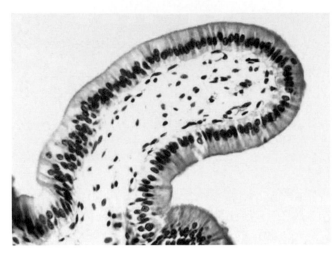

Fig. 4.14. Simple columnar epithelial cells from intestine. This tissue section is longitudinally cut through a villus in the intestine. The epithelial cells appear as a uniform row of cells that cover the surface. Notice the dark blue-purple nuclei, most of which appear lined up in the basal region of individual epithelial cells.

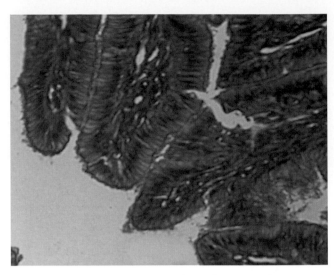

Fig. 4.16. Small intestine tissue artifacts. This image of a section of the intestine illustrates some of the problems that can be encountered in the study of typical histological sections.

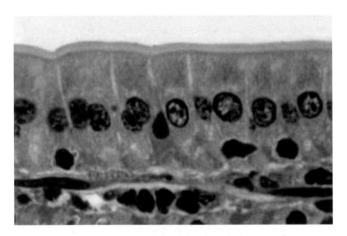

Fig. 4.15. High-power view of intestinal epithelium. In this image the outer layer of epithelial cells is clearly tall and slender with the round nuclei oriented toward the basal ends of the cells. There is a very evident brush border (outer thin layer of the cells) that results from staining of the abundant microvilli and associated proteins.

Can you distinguish individual epithelial cells? Columnar cells are usually associated with absorption and secretion and are found lining the intestinal tract from the stomach to the rectum. This epithelium has two modifications that greatly aid its functioning. The first is the presence of the microvilli that markedly increase absorptive surface, and the second is the presence of goblet cells. These unicellular glands produce mucus that is secreted on the epithelial surface. This increases lubrication and provides protection. These specialized secretory cells also appear in the respiratory and reproductive tracts. Although the images shown in Figures 4.14 and 4.15 are excellent, representative examples of the features of intestinal tract epi-

thelium, it is important to appreciate that not all histological sections are of such quality. Also as indicated previously, the plane of section can make it difficult to interpret a given tissue section.

The image in Figure 4.16 is also a section of the small intestine. It is still possible to distinguish the presence of villi and the appearance of the epithelium, but can you detect some of the problems? First, the image is a bit out of focus, and second, it is a bit too thick. This makes it difficult to distinguish individual cells. The villi have become pushed into one another during processing, so it takes some effort to distinguish individual structures. Finally, to the upper right and far right of the section there are some tears that have altered the orientation of the tissue.

Many other artifacts also can occur. The point is that section preparation is sometimes as much an art as a science, so patience is needed as you study even professionally prepared slides. Regardless, several villi have been sectioned roughly along their longitudinal axis. This simply illustrates what you can and will see when you examine actual slides. Since you know what you are looking for in columnar epithelial cells from Figures 4.14 and 4.15, you should still be able to distinguish several villi covered by a layer of columnar epithelial cells.

Figure 4.17 illustrates a similar section of the duodenum, but the sample is from a calf and the animal was injected with BrdU 2 hours before it was killed. Remember, this is the analog of DNA that gets incorporated into cells that are in the S-phase of the cell cycle. In this section many of the villi are cut at a tangent to the longitudinal axis, but you can see that there are many brown-stained nuclei (indicating that

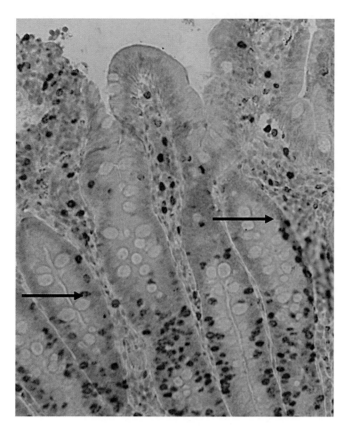

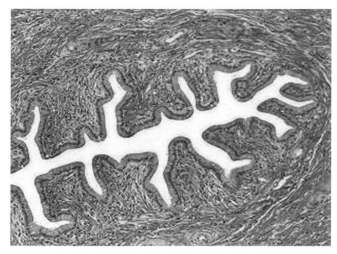

Fig. 4.18. Tissue from the anterior bovine vagina. This section illustrates the general structure of internal lining of a region of the bovine reproductive tract. The surface is thrown into folds and is covered by simple columnar epithelial cells. Notice the red-stained, dense connective tissue surrounding the epithelium.

Fig. 4.17. Section of duodenum from BrdU-injected calf. This section of intestinal tissue is processed to show the presence of BrdU-labeled cell nuclei. Several villi are closely aligned and some are cut at a tangent, but it is apparent that the number of BrdU-labeled cells (brown-stained nuclei and arrows) is markedly higher in the crypts of the villi. The pale globules indicate the presence of goblet cells. Image is courtesy of Dr. Anthony Capuco, USDA, Beltsville, MD.

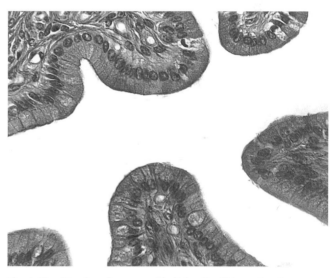

Fig. 4.19. Simple columnar epithelial cells. This section is a higher-power (40× objective) image of the epithelium shown in Figure 4.18. Note the layer of closely aligned epithelial cell nuclei and scattered goblet cells.

the cells were synthesizing DNA) in the lower regions of the villi. It is well known that the cells that populate the villus proliferate in lower crypts and are lost from the upper region of the villi as they age. To maximize the opportunity of detecting labeled cell nuclei but to also be able to distinguish basic tissue structure, the sample was only briefly counter-stained in hematotoxylin but without eosin. This gives the pale blue staining to the cells, but it is less distinct than in the H&E-stained sections of intestinal tissue (Figs. 4.14 and 4.15).

Subsequent Figures 4.18 and 4.19 give examples of simple columnar epithelial cells from the reproductive tract. The complex folding of the internal surface is evident (Fig. 4.18) and the regular arrangement of epithelial and goblet cells (Fig. 4.19).

Figure 4.18 shows a tissue section from the anterior (Fornix) vagina of a cow taken during the follicular phase of the estrus cycle. Notice the epithelium is on the internal surface, and as the higher magnification (40× objective) image (Fig. 4.19) shows the epithelium is also a simple columnar epithelium.

Stratified epithelium

To this point we have considered examples of simple epithelium with squamous, cuboidal, or columnar cells. Now let's consider stratified epithelium types. As you should surmise, the stratified types are better able to withstand physical trauma and wear and tear than simple epithelial but are much less efficient at absorption. This means these cells are also poorly adapted for secretion. When secretions are needed along a stratified epithelial surface, this is usually

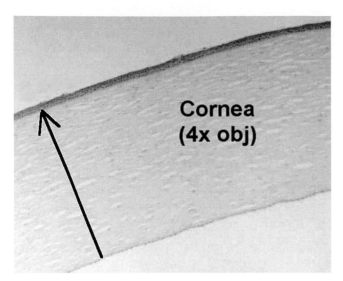

Fig. 4.20. Low-power image of sectioned cornea. At this magnification no cellular detail is visible, but it is apparent the outer cell layer is thicker than on the inside (stratified versus simple epithelial layers).

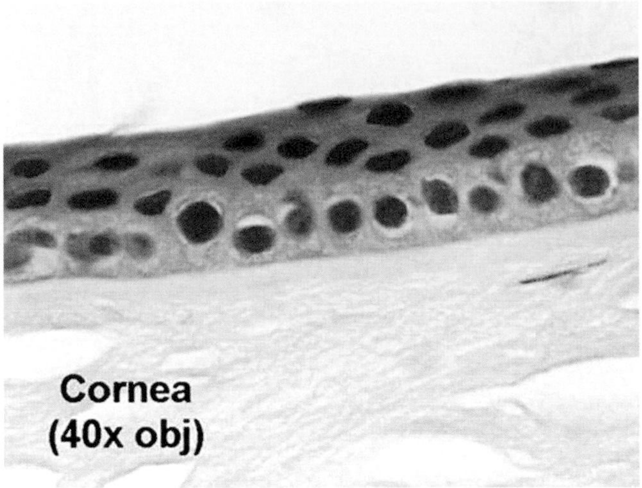

Fig. 4.21. Stratified squamous epithelium cornea. This higher-magnification view of the outside of the cornea shows several layers of epithelial cells. The outermost layers are highly flattened. Within the body of the cornea there is the faintly stained nucleus of a fibroblast (right).

accomplished by the presence of exocrine glands that are located inferior to the epithelial surface. Ducts that radiate from the glandular cells to the surfaces provide most needed secretions. However, most of the lubrication for these internal epithelial surfaces is provided by goblet cells. As mucus accumulates in the cells, they eventually rupture to release their contents.

Remember that with stratified epithelium, the classification depends on the shape of the epithelial cells on the outer surface, adjacent to the lumen or free surface. The first image in this series (Fig. 4.20) is a section through the cornea taken at very low magnification (4×) objective. The outside of the cornea is covered by a stratified squamous epithelium and the inside by a simple squamous epithelium. The bulk of the corneal structure (arrow) consists of collagen fibers arranged in lamella that are parallel to each other as well as scattered fibroblasts.

The outer stratified squamous epithelium of the cornea is about five cells thick (Fig. 4.21). The basal cells appear as cubes or polyhedrons, but the cells are progressively flattened as they migrate to the surface. Since the outermost cell layer is flattened, the classification is stratified squamous. Can you detect any of the fibroblast nuclei in the underlying bulk of the corneal tissue (substantia propria)? Figure 4.22 shows the epithelial layer on the inner surface, also at higher magnification. The cells are in a single layer and they are highly flattened, so it is an example of simple squamous epithelium. Other areas where this epithelial type would appear is on the internal surface of the lung alveoli. What better way to promote rapid diffu-

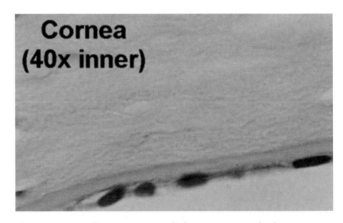

Fig. 4.22. Simple squamous epithelium cornea. At higher magnification only a single layer of highly flattened epithelial cells is apparent on the internal corneal surface. As above, there is also a faintly stained fibroblast nucleus within the lamellae of the cornea.

sion of gases than with a single layer of thin epithelial cells?

Figure 4.23 provides another very common example of stratified squamous epithelium. The section is from an internal body opening that is moist but requires protection. Examples for this type of epithelium would include the lip, mouth, posterior vagina, and anus. The bracketed area indicates the epithelial portion of the tissue; the lower portion of the slide is the connective tissue or stroma. Notice the multiple layers of cells but that the outermost layer of cells are flattened (arrows), thus, the stratified squamous classification. In contrast to areas that are moist, the skin also needs

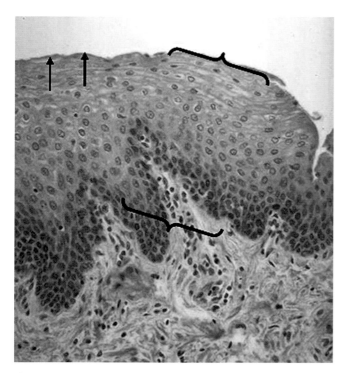

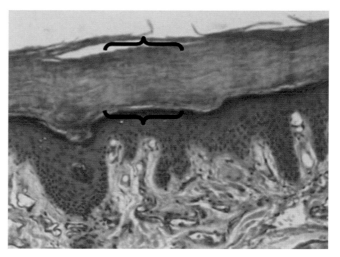

Fig. 4.25. Low-power section of skin. This low-power image shows a section of skin from a region with high friction and pressure. The outermost layer, called the stratum corneum (brackets), can account for 75% of the total epithelial thickness. It is composed of keratin and thickened plasma membranes from multiple layers of dead cells.

Fig. 4.23. Nonkeratinized stratified squamous epithelium. This tissue sample from just inside the bovine oral cavity shows the hallmarks of stratification, i.e., multiple layers of epithelial cells (bracket area). The outermost layers of visible cells are highly flattened (arrows), thus the squamous classification. The lower area of tissue is connective tissue.

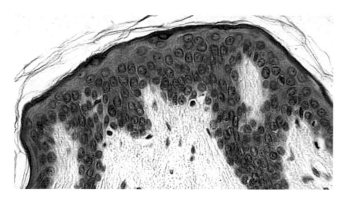

Fig. 4.24. Keratinized stratified squamous epithelium. This tissue sample from just inside the bovine reproductive tract shows the beginnings of keratinization. The outer visible layer of cells is highly flattened and more darkly stained. There are also strands of keratin fibers near the surface of the tissue.

the protection provided by multiple layers of cells, but excess loss of moisture can be a problem for many animals. Figure 4.24 shows the beginnings of the keratinization process. The number of cell layers and classification is similar except that there is now a layer of keratin (a cellular protein) and a layer of progressively dying cells. This keratin layer provides protection. As a specific example, the keratin that is produced in the

teat opening of lactating cows is a very important protection against mastitis. In experiments in which the keratin has been artificially removed, incidence of mastitis is markedly increased. Figure 4.25 shows a more extreme example of the protection that is provided by keratinization in the skin. Here, dead and dying cells form a very distinct outer layer that markedly increases protection against abrasion. The layer is especially increased in skin areas subjected to pressure. Figure 4.26 shows some of the cellular features of skin at higher magnification. Here, you can begin to see staining and morphological characteristics that allow the epithelial cells in varying strata within the epithelium to be distinguished. These will be described in more detail in our discussion of the integumentary system.

Other types of stratified epithelium occur on the internal surfaces of some of the larger tubular structures in the body, i.e., trachea, reproductive tract, and bladder. These will be considered in subsequent slides. Stratified cuboidal epithelium is usually associated with various exocrine glands in which secretions made by the secretory cells of the gland must be transported through ducts to be emptied. The cells, which compose the walls of the ducts, generally do not produce secretions themselves but provide a passageway for products to the site of secretion. Figure 4.27 illustrates a cross section through a duct leading from a sweat gland. Note the roughly double layer of epithelial cells. The tissue surrounding the duct is mostly collagen fibrils and other extracellular matrix materials, a few fibroblasts, and blood vessel cells.

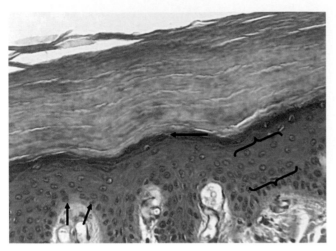

Fig. 4.26.   High-power section of skin. In this higher magnification you can see some of the morphological characteristics that distinguish other strata in the epithelium. For example, the dark-stained boundary (upper arrow) at the lower edge of the stratum corneum is called the stratum granulosum because of the presence of the keratohyaline granules. The bulk of the cells are in the stratum spinosum (brackets) and are bounded by the stratum basale (lower arrows), which appear as lighter, staining cells occurring just before the connective tissue in the dermis.

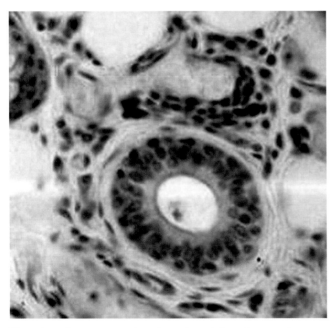

Fig. 4.27.   Duct cross section. A portion of tissue from a sebaceous gland. The cross-sectioned duct shows an example of stratified cuboidal epithelium. It is typical of the structure of various ducts of exocrine glands.

The cells in Figure 4.28 illustrate a type of epithelium found in the trachea and areas of the reproductive tract. These are pseudostratified because although the cells appear to be residing in multiple layers, in reality each of the epithelial cells is anchored to the

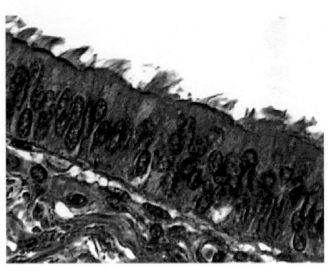

Fig. 4.28.   Pseudostratified columnar epithelium. This image is from a section of the oviduct of a cow. Only one side of the oviduct is shown, with the surface epithelial projecting into the lumen. The nuclei stained in dark blue-purple appear to be aligned in multiple layers. However, all of the individual cells are actually anchored in the region of the basement membrane. For this reason the cells are classified as pseudostratified (false stratification). The shape of the cells is columnar. In addition these cells exhibit a surface specialization, the presence of cilia. Here they were clumped into tufts when the tissue sample was processed.

Pseudostratified Epithelium

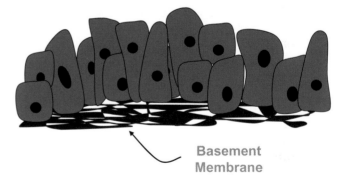

Fig. 4.29.   Drawing of pseudostratified epithelium.

basement membrane. This may be by only a thin projection of cytoplasm, but since all the cells are attached the layer only appears to be stratified. The sample is from the oviduct of a cow. Clusters of cilia are evident as tufts protruding from the apical ends of the cells.

The drawing provided in Figure 4.29 illustrates the arrangement of pseudostratified epithelial cells. Again, the nuclei appear at various layers, but all are attached to the basement membrane. It is also usual for this epithelial type to have goblet cells and cilia. Another

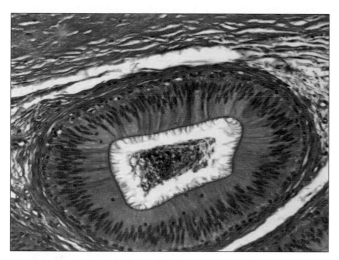

Fig. 4.30. Pseudostratified epithelium bovine epididymis. These epithelia have stereocilia that protrude from the apical cell surfaces into the lumenal space. The movement of these stereocilia maintains the flow of maturing sperm cells in the reproductive tract. Compacted sperm cells appear as the dark cluster in the center of the lumenal space.

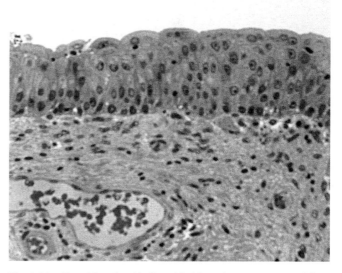

Fig. 4.31. Transitional epithelium bladder. The appearance of this epithelial layer changes related to the degree of stretch. As the bladder or other areas of the urinary tract expand, the apparent number of epithelial cell layers decreases until the pressure is relieved.

example of pseudostratified columnar epithelium is shown in Figure 4.30. This sample is a cross section through the epidymis of a bull. In this tissue, there is a more complex surface specialization, called stereocilia. These structures, similar but more elaborate than simple cilia, are evident as the elongated spikes that protrude into the lumenal space of the tubule. The center of the lumen is also filled with stored spermatozoa, a highly specialized epithelial cell.

A final epithelia type (Fig. 4.31) we will consider is transitional. This type appears in the lining of the bladder and is unique because its appearance changes as the bladder expands and contracts. When relatively empty the epithelium is similar in appearance to non-keratinized stratified squamous. As the bladder fills the expansion reduces the number of apparent cell layers. In the nondistended state the rounded surfaces of the epithelial cells seem to protrude into the lumenal space. Notice the cross section of the vein and artery just below the epithelium. The nuclei of the larger circumference of the vein (upper) also provide an excellent example of simple squamous epithelium.

Epithelial cell junctions

Along the adjoining borders of epithelial cells there are specialized cell junctions. These are regions or sites where some special contact between cells can be recognized. Three functional classes of junctional complexes include 1) occluding junctions, 2) anchoring junctions, and 3) communicating junctions. Some of

the communicating junctions, e.g., the gap junction, also appears in other cell types. However, because of the importance of epithelial tissue to create tissue compartments or barriers, it is important to understand the role of cell junctions in this process. To illustrate the idea of barriers consider the differences between milk and blood. It is clear that blood circulates throughout the mammary gland within the capillaries just underneath the secretory epithelial cells of the mammary alveolus (see Fig. 4.8). However the composition of blood or interstitial fluids and milk is very different. The same can be said for the environment of the gut lumen versus the interstitial fluid of the lacteals of the villi of the intestinal tract. How are these differences developed and maintained? This is where junctional complexes come into play.

In circumstances where it is necessary to maintain a seal between epithelial cells, the lateral margins of the cells become fused together along a system of membrane ridges between adjacent cells. These ridges extend completely around the perimeter of the cells to create a sort of belt located near the apical ends of the cells. These junctional complexes are called zona occludens (tight junctions) to indicate that they produce an effective barrier. For example, during the latter stages of mammary development in the pregnant heifer, the approach of parturition signals both the structural differentiation of the alveolar cells and maturation of tight junctions between the cells. Increases in circulating glucocorticoids along with declining progesterone seem to be especially important. Once this occurs, paracellular (transport of components between the cells) is dramatically reduced. This creates an effective blood-milk barrier so that transfer of serum components into milk or milk constituents into blood is minimized. This does not mean that transport cannot occur but that wholesale leakage is prevented. The effectiveness of this barrier function is readily apparent from study of secretions obtained from animals with acute mastitis or experimental treatments known to disrupt the tight junctions. One of the effects of this disruption is the appearance of serum proteins in milk, e.g., albumin. Conversely, these situations also allow abrupt increases in the appearance of lactose and α-lactalbumin (and likely other milk components) into serum.

Adhering junctions are a second class of membrane specializations that act to anchor epithelial cells together. These complexes also appear as bands or belts that circumnavigate the perimeter of the cells below the level of the tight junctions. In intestinal epithelial cells, for example, these complexes are called zona adherens. As you traverse along the lateral membrane toward the basal end of the cell, a second type of adhering junction, the desmosome or macula, adherens appears. Anchoring junctions are widely distributed and allow the epithelium to maintain structural integrity by linking cells together and by linking cells to the underlying extracellular matrix. These complexes are plentiful in tissues that are subjected to mechanical stress, e.g., skin. The adherens junctions are focal points where actin filaments attach to the junctional proteins. In general terms, there are two basic parts of these complexes. The intracellular attachment proteins create a plaque or thickening on the cytoplasmic side of the cell membrane and provide sites for attachment of cytoskeleton proteins and for transmembrane linker proteins. The transmembrane linker proteins have cytoplasmic tails that attach to the plaque structure, but the extracellular domains of the proteins interact with the extracellular domains of adjacent junction proteins or with other extracellular matrix proteins, i.e., hemidesmosomes. In the case of the adhesion belts in epithelial sheets, the complexes in companion cells are directly apposed. The transmembrane linker protein is a member of a family of Ca^{2+}-dependent proteins called cadherins. The plaque or adhesion belt through the actions of several linker proteins (catenin, vinculin, and others) binds bundles of actin fibers that radiate into the cytoplasm interacting with the cytoskeleton. It is thought that changes in the orientation and contraction of these bundles explain the folding of epithelial sheets to create tubular structures during tissue development.

Desmosomes, unlike the bands of the zona adherens, are limited to spots or patches of the membrane between adjacent cells. They could be envisioned as spot welds or small dollops of glue to help bind adjacent epithelial cells together. To carry this analogy a bit further, the zona adherens could be thought of as miniature packing straps that bind the epithelial cells. Both the zona adherens and desmosomes are closely associated with microfilaments within the cytoskeleton of two cells that are linked. A variant of the desmosome, the hemidesmosome, has the structure of only half a desmosome. This complex serves to anchor the epithelial cells to the underlying basement membrane. For desmosomes the transmembrane linker proteins also belong to the cadherins family of proteins, but the specific intracellular protein associated with the plaque varies. In most cells these are keratin filaments, but desmin filaments fulfill the same function in cardiac cells.

A final type of structure is the gap junction. In this instance proteins aligned in neighboring cells essentially create pores that pass from one cell to the other. This can be imagined as small pipes passing between two adjacent apartments. Gap junctions appear not just in epithelial tissue but are prominent in cardiac muscle, some types of smooth muscle cells, and between cells of the nervous system. Gap junctions allow for the direct passage of small molecules (typically less than 300 MW) between cells. This is important for cell-to-cell communication and rapid responses necessary for nerve function and muscle contraction. We will discuss the specific physiological events related to cell junctions in subsequent chapters. A stylized view of cellular junctions is provided in Figure 4.32. Figure 4.33 illustrates the structure of the gap junction.

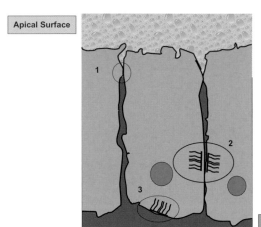

Fig. 4.32. Cellular junctions. Tight junctions (1) serve to effectively seal the apical from the basal surfaces of the epithelium. Notice that apical or basal molecules penetrate between the cells only to the region of the junction. Desmosomes (2) act to link cells together something like spot welds, while hemidesmosomes anchor the cells to extracellular matrix molecules. Adhesion belts are not illustrated but would typically occur in the region just below the tight junctions.

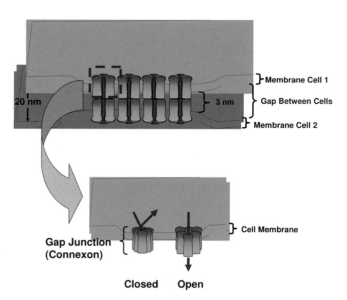

Fig. 4.33. Gap junction structure.

Gap junctions are composed of transmembrane proteins called connexins. When arranged to create a complex, six connexin proteins align to form a pore or channel called a connexon. As illustrated in the upper panel, when connexons of two adjacent cells become aligned they create an aqueous pore that connects the two cells. However, unlike tight junctions the outer leaflets of the adjacent cells are not fused. Gap junctions can also alternate between open and closed states. For example, a decrease in pH or increase in Ca^{2+} concentrations promotes closure. Thus, the function of gap junctions can be regulated.

Glandular epithelial types

Numerous glands serve multiple physiological functions. The simplest classification of glands is based on the number of cells. The single or unicellular gland represented by mucus-secreting goblet cells is the most rudimentary. Multicellular glands include two subtypes: 1) exocrine, and 2) endocrine glands. Exocrine glands are familiar examples, i.e., salivary or mammary glands, in which products or secretions made by the epithelial cells are transported via a duct to be emptied. Endocrine glands by contrast are ductless. Hormones produced from these secretory cells are captured by capillaries surrounding the tissue and transported to target tissues throughout the body. We will consider the structure and function of endocrine glands in subsequent chapters.

In addition to the structural organization of multicellular exocrine glands, there are also differences in how secretions are released from the cells. For example,

early anatomists tried to define the origin of the mammary gland by classifying the secretion mechanism for the secretory cells. To illustrate, sebaceous glands exhibit a holocrine mode of secretion in which cells are ruptured and sloughed to become a part of the secretion. Sweat glands follow an apocrine mode of secretion in which only portions of the cells are lost so that individual cells are capable of periodic secretion. Other glands follow a meocrine mode of secretion in which products are secreted but the secretory cells remain intact. Mammary cells follow both apocrine and meocrine modes of secretion. Specifically, as lipid droplets form in the cytoplasm of the cells these droplets progressively enlarge, migrate to the apical end of the cell, and protrude into the alveolar lumen until the membrane-bound droplets pinch off to become the butterfat of milk. Since the membrane surrounding the lipid droplet is derived from the plasma membrane of the cell, it is clear that a portion of the cell is lost to become a part of the cellular secretion. This is an example of an apocrine mode of secretion. For secretion of specific milk proteins and lactose, these products are packaged into secretory vesicles in the Golgi apparatus. These vesicles both singly or in chains fuse with the apical plasma membrane and release their contents via exocytosis. Since only the secretory vesicle contents are lost from the cell, this mode of secretion is meocrine. In reality, the details for secretion patterns of mammary cells were not settled until mammary tissue from lactating mammals was studied with transmission electron microscopy in the early 1960s. Thus, attempts to determine the phylogeny of the mammary glands based solely on the basis of the secretion pattern were futile. It seems likely that the primitive mammary gland arose from a hybrid combination of both types of glandular cells. Diagrams showing holocrine, meocrine, and apocrine modes of secretion are shown in Figure 4.34.

Epithelial glands follow several distinct patterns of development based on the arrangement of cells within the secreting unit of the gland. Simple glands have a duct that opens onto a surface. Usually cells that create the duct opening or neck are nonsecretory and serve as a passageway for products made deeper within the gland. The shape of the gland mimics the shape of tubes or rounded flasks called alveoli or acini. Presence of a single glandular unit denotes a simple gland. Depending on the shape of the secretory structure the gland is classified as simple tubular or simple alveolar. By contrast, compound glands are branched with multiple secretory units opening into a duct. Depending on the specifics of the secretory units, glands are classified as compound tubular, alveolar, or tubuloalveolar. Mammary glands for example are compound alveolar glands. Various arrangements of the cells within glands are illustrated in Figure 4.35.

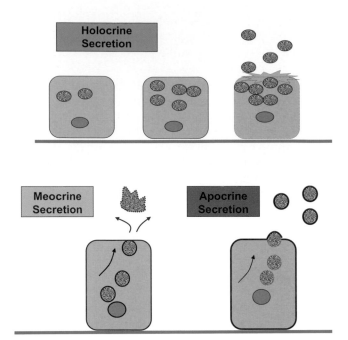

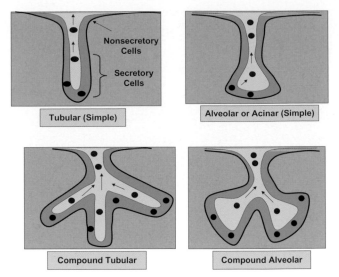

Fig. 4.34. Mechanisms of cellular secretion. In holocrine secretion, secretory products accumulate until the cell ruptures and secretions are released. In the meocrine mode, membrane-bound secretory vesicles move the cell margin, fuse with the plasma membrane, and release the contents by exocytosis so that only the contents of the vesicles are lost. In apocrine secretion, accumulating droplets of product protrude from the plasma membrane and are progressively lost as membrane-bound vesicles. Since the membrane is directly derived from the plasma membrane, a portion of the cell is lost in the secretion.

Fig. 4.35. Glandular structures. Simple tubular or simple alveolar glands (upper left and right) are essentially cellular pipes lined by epithelial cells (illustrated by the darker green). Cells near the opening that form the neck of the bottlelike structure are usually nonsecreting cells. They create the passageway for products to be secreted. Epithelial cells located deeper within the structure produce and secrete the glandular secretions (illustrated by the dark spots). Secretions are released in the lumen spaces of the glands (lighter green) to make their way out of the gland. Differences in the morphology of tubular versus alveolar glands indicate differences in the shape (tubelike versus flasklike) for the portion of the gland that contains secretory cells. Compound glands simply have multiple secreting units that empty into common ducts. Can you visualize the appearance of a compound tubuloalveolar gland?

The type of products they secrete also distinguish subclasses of exocrine glands. Mucus glands produce a viscous glycoprotein mixture called mucus. Serous glands produce a more watery or wheylike secretion that contains enzymes. The exocrine portion of the pancreas is an example. Some glands (the parotid salivary gland, for example) produce both types of secretions because they contain a mixture of mucus and serous cells. In typical H&E stained sections, mucous secretory units are very pale-staining compared with the serous secretory units. The serous cells usually have an intense basophilic staining of the basal areas of the cells. This is because of the abundant amounts of endoplasmic reticulum, as the cells are actively producing proteins for secretion. The pale-staining mucus-secreting cells typically have a flattened nucleus with most of the area of the cells packed with vacuoles containing mucus. Examples are illustrated in Figure 4.36.

Connective tissue

The term *connective tissue* is used in several contexts. First, it is a general name for a diverse collection of tissues with varying functions. This includes the connective tissues proper, outlined below, as well as several specialized tissues. Although connective tissue histology is extremely varied, there are nonetheless generalities that can be made to compare these tissues with others, for example, epithelial tissues. One of the most apparent is that the relative density of cells is much less than in epithelial tissue. As the name, implies connective tissues serve to support, unify, and "connect" other tissues to allow the creation of more complex tissues and organs. The "connecting" properties of connective tissues depend on products (largely proteins and complex carbohydrates) synthesized and secreted by connective tissue cells. Connective tissue cells (derived from the mesoderm germinal layer), become surrounded by their products so that they are "suspended" in a sea of their own making. In summary, connective tissue consists of cells and extracellular fibers (protein polymers) embedded in a matrix consisting of ground substance and fluid. These fibers are divided into one of three types: collagen, reticular, or elastic. If you imagine a gelatin dessert with bits of string, scattered hair, and perhaps some fine paper fibers you'll have a reasonable mental image of the

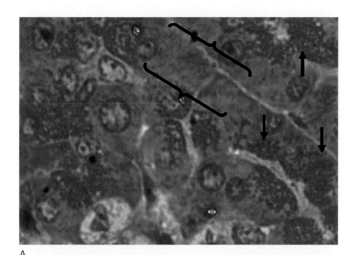

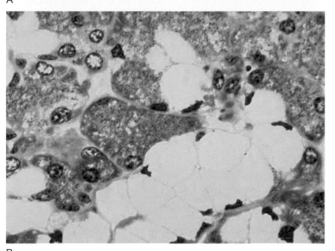

Fig. 4.36. Serous and mucus glands. A) An area of pancreatic tissue. These serous-type cells exhibit abundant red-staining secretory granules in the apical regions of the cells (arrows) as well as densely basal cytoplasm (brackets). B) A portion of salivary gland; the pale cells are mucus-secreting cells and the surrounding darker-stained cells are serous secretory units.

extracellular matrix of many connective tissues. Now in your imaginary connective tissue add a random suspension of small raisins to represent connective tissue cells (primarily fibroblasts) and you have an idea of the composition.

One final idea related to the cells that are present is that some are considered fixed, that is, they are always constituents of the connective tissue in question, i.e., fibroblasts or osteoblasts in bone, for example. Other cells called wandering cells, various blood derived cells, macrophages, neutrophils, plasma cells, and so forth may be present as well.

When tissues are fixed, embedded, and prepared for histological examination, the material between cells can sometimes appear as empty space, but this is far from the truth. When more specialized stains are used,

many of these specialized products can be readily visualized. Our purpose is to simply introduce you to the idea of connective tissues and to provide some examples of the many varieties of connective tissues.

Classification of connective tissue

It is not easy to formulate a classification of connective tissue that is completely adequate for all situations. However, some organization helps the learning process by producing at least a general frame of reference. General connective tissues, called proper connective tissues, are divided into loose, dense regular, and dense irregular types. The primary distinction here is with the arrangement and relative number of fibers between the connective tissue cells. The loose connective tissue contains aggregates of loosely arranged fibers and a relatively large number of cells. Loose connective tissues have many fibroblasts but many other cells as well. A major site of loose connective tissue is just below the various epithelial layers that cover internal and external body surfaces. These are sites where antigens and other foreign materials can be present; it should not be surprising that many of the other cell types in loose connective tissue are the "wandering" immune-related cells that migrate from local capillaries.

Dense connective tissue has more abundant, thicker fibers but not as many cells. The most abundant cell type is usually the fibroblast, the cell responsible for the synthesis and secretion of the proteins of the fibers. Dense irregular connective tissue is found in the protective capsules around organs and surrounding developing glands. Dense regular connective tissue is more specialized, in that the regular arrangement of fibers is important in providing strength as in tendons and ligaments. Other specialized connective tissues that will be briefly described and illustrated include cartilage, bone, adipose, and blood.

The first illustration in this section (Fig. 4.37) shows a simple mesenteric spread. This image of fixed stained tissue that anchors and protects the intestines demonstrates many of the general features of connective tissues, namely the presence of extracellular fibers, space between cells, and varying types of cells.

As might be expected there is some gray area in deciding the difference between loose and dense connective tissues. How compacted must the material be to be considered dense? The tissue just underneath many epithelial surfaces—for example, the skin or areas of the reproductive tract—is loose connective tissue, but there is certainly variation. The immature mammary gland provides good examples of this variation. The connective tissue immediately adjacent to the ducts (intralobular) is less dense than the

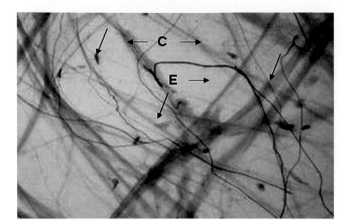

Fig. 4.37. Mesentery spread. The mesentery, which serves to anchor and support the loops of the digestive tract, is very thin. Many of the very thin fibers (E) are elastin fibers; the thicker pink fibers are collagen (C). Some of the dark specks are nuclei of fibroblasts (arrows).

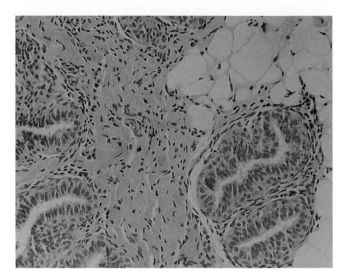

Fig. 4.39. Loose connective tissue bovine mammary. This image illustrates an area of loose connective tissue from the bovine mammary gland. Notice the similarity to the tissue from the pancreas. However, this section also shows an area with a cluster of adipocytes or adipose tissue, a specialized type of connective tissue, in addition to the band of pinkish connective tissue in the center of the image.

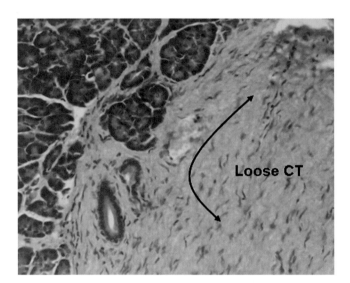

Fig. 4.38. Loose connective tissue. This image from the pancreas illustrates general features of the loose connective tissue present under the epithelial regions of many tissues. At the low magnification of this image of H&E stained tissue shows only the amorphous pink of faintly stained collagen fibrils and scattered fibroblast nuclei in the region adjacent to the glandular tissue.

connective tissue some distance away from the developing ducts (interlobular). Other organs also have abundant areas of connective tissue. Figure 4.38 shows a section from the pancreas. The epithelial tissue to the upper left is part of the exocrine glandular tissue of the organ. The pale pink tissue to the right is a region of loose connective tissue that supports and anchors the glandular structure. Notice that relatively little detail or apparent cells are evident in this region. Collagen fibrils and other extracellular matrix proteins and ground substance occupy most of the space. The

scattered fibroblasts and other cells only become apparent at higher magnification. Figure 4.39 illustrates an area of similar loose connective tissue from the bovine mammary gland.

At a higher magnification (Fig. 4.40) some of the fibroblast nuclei become apparent and the swirls of light pink-stained collagen fibrils and other more amorphous proteins can be seen. Many of the fibroblasts are so closely aligned with the collagen fibrils that it is difficult to distinguish between cell cytoplasm and the extracellular matrix. This is especially true for paraffin embedded tissues. However, the darkly stained nuclei of various cells stand out in the preparation. The next example (Fig. 4.41) shows a sample of dense and loose connective tissue in the same specimen. Another difference is the staining of the specimen. It has been stained with a dye called Sirus Red and counter-stained with another dye called Fast Green. In this preparation the collagen appears as bright red, wavy fibers and the epithelium is stained a faint bluish-green, but there is little detail for the epithelium.

The higher magnification image shown in Figure 4.42 also illustrates the difference between dense irregular and loose connective tissue. It is easy to see that it is largely a matter of degree. The red collagen fibers appear in both regions, but just underneath the epithelial surface of a large epithelial duct (to the upper left) the fibers are much more apparent. The very pale blue structures embedded in this dense collagen matrix are mostly the nuclei of fibroblasts.

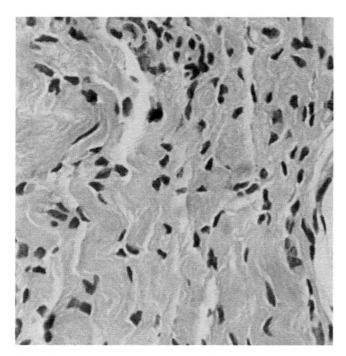

Fig. 4.40. Loose connective tissue detail. An example of loose connective tissue for the mammary gland of a cow is shown at higher magnification. Most of the darkly stained nuclei are from fibroblasts. The pink, somewhat wavy pattern is largely from collagen fibrils.

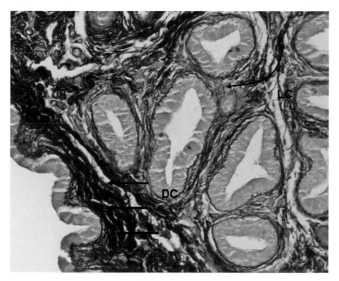

Fig. 4.41. Sirus Red–stained connective tissue. Examples of loose (LC), compared with dense (DC), irregular are indicated. Cross sections of epithelial ducts appear a faint pale bluish-green color.

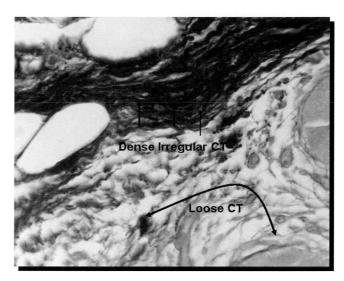

Fig. 4.42. Dense irregular connective tissue. Dense irregular tissue is contrasted with loose connective tissue in this image from the developing mammary gland of a heifer.

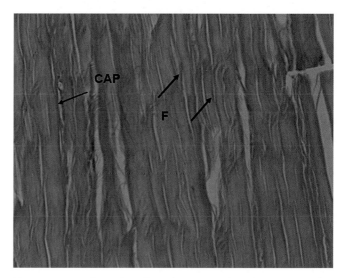

Fig. 4.43. Histology of tendon. This section through a portion of a tendon demonstrates the largely directional, parallel orientation of the fibers from top to bottom. This corresponds with the direction of greatest strength. Fibroblast nuclei (F) are very difficult to detect, and their pale blue–stained nuclei seem to blend with the general structure of the fibers. An approximate longitudinal cut through a capillary (CAP) is also indicated.

As you might suspect, dense connective tissue is especially strong because of the abundant fibers. A subclass of dense connective tissue, dense regular connective tissue, is found in tendons and ligaments. This tissue gets its name because of collagen and other fibers that are uniformly arranged. This is easy to imagine in a tendon or ligament where there is a need for great tensile strength, usually along a particular axis. In fact, injuries and tears to ligaments are especially common when forces are applied perpendicular to the direction in which the fibers are oriented. Figure 4.43 illustrates a histological section through a portion of a tendon. The staining is not specialized for detection of collagen or other fibers (H&E staining), so it is difficult to distinguish individual fibers or fibroblasts but the general regular

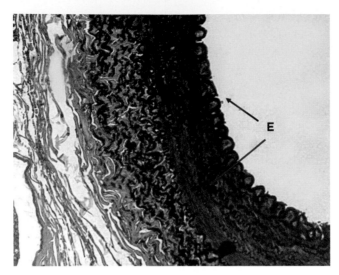

Fig. 4.44. Elastin fibers. This is a section through the wall of a large artery. In this specimen the sample has been stained with a special dye to emphasize elastic fibers. They appear as black wavy lines (E) oriented around the circumference of the artery. Given the need for many arteries to expand and recoil in response to changes in blood pressure, it is easy to rationalize the function of these fibers.

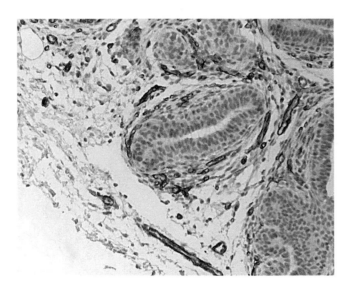

Fig. 4.45. Collagen immunocytochemistry. This specimen is an immunocytochemical preparation showing the expression of type IV collagen in the developing mammary gland. The brown staining (where antibodies against collagen type IV are located) indicates the location of this protein. Notice that it is almost exclusively located around blood vessel endothelial cells as part of the basal lamina of these vessels.

orientation of the fibers is evident from top to bottom in this image (Fig. 4.43) and the elastin of Figure 4.44.

The image in Figure 4.45 shows the result of immunostaining for the presence of one of the subclasses of collagen in the developing tissue. In this procedure an antibody specific for type IV collagen was incubated with the tissue section, and then the location of the

bound antibody detected by use of a secondary antibody linked with an enzyme. When the enzyme is activated in the presence of an appropriate substrate, a reaction product is deposited at the site(s) where the antibody is bound. In this specimen you can see that type IV collagen is almost exclusively located around the endothelial cells of blood vessels. Use of immunocytochemistry provides a powerful tool to study details of tissue development. If you compare the very evident red stain for "total" collagen fibers in Figure 4.41 and 4.42 with the restricted expression of collagen type IV in Figure 4.46, you can see that the distribution of type IV collagen is very concentrated or localized. In fact, type IV collagen is most often expressed in the basal lamina. This explains its abundance around the endothelial cells of the capillaries, but its apparent absence around the developing epithelial ducts in the tissue is surprising. It may be that basal lamina associated with epithelium does not fully develop until later. This is further suggested by the image shown in Figure 4.46, which shows staining for expression of type IV collagen in the mammary tissue of a lactating cow. In this case the expression occurs around the blood vessels as well as the secretory alveoli. This supports the idea that the basal lamina is not fully developed until major ducts and/or the alveoli are fully formed. Again the point here is showing how these histology techniques can provide information about tissue growth, development, and ultimately physiological function. Other collagens include types I, II, and III. Type I is associated with connective tissues of skin, bone, tendon, and ligaments. Type II is predominating in cartilage and type III in fetal tissues and connective tissue capsules around various organs.

Specialized connective tissues

Adipose tissue is a specialized connective tissue consisting of fat-storing cells called adipocytes. There are two types of adipose tissue, white (unilocular) and brown (multilocular). In well-nourished animals (or people) adipose tissue forms a nearly continuous layer within the connective tissue underneath the skin. It is called panniculus adiposus, and is part of the hypodermis. It is generally believed that adipocytes are derived from the mesenchymal cells of the mesoderm germinal layer. Unilocular adipocytes are often large cells 100 μm or more in diameter. The size is a reflection of the accumulation of a large lipid droplet that occupies most of the cell area. This causes the nucleus and most of the cytoplasm to be pushed to one side of the cell, so that the cells are often described as having a signet ring appearance when sectioned. In most histological preparations the lipid is lost because of the lipid solvents (ethanol and xylene) used to prepare

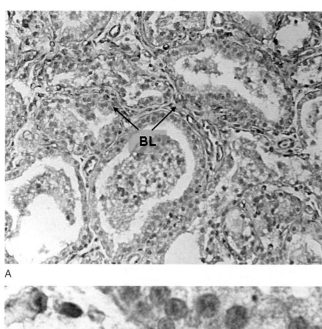

A

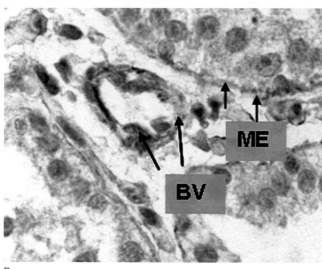

B

Fig. 4.46. Type IV collagen. Immunostaining for type IV collagen in mammary tissue from a lactating cow is shown. In this functionally and developmentally mature tissue, there is marked expression of type IV collagen in the area of the basal lamina (BL) immediately adjacent to the epithelial cells of the alveoli as well as blood vessels (A). The figure insert (B) at higher magnification (oil immersion) makes the expression around both regions evident. In the center of the figure there is a cross section through a capillary with each of three nuclei of endothelial cells evident (BV and arrows). Other arrows (ME and arrows) indicate staining associated with the basal lamina of the mammary epithelial cells.

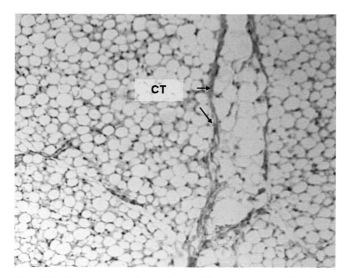

Fig. 4.47. Low-power adipose tissue. This is a low magnification view (10× objective with 10× eyepiece, i.e., hundredfold) view of white adipose tissue. The essential feature is the appearance of lots of seemingly closely packed, circular structures, which are the profiles of sectioned adipocytes. Remember, in the living tissue the spaces would have been occupied by lipid droplets. The other prominent features are several bands of connective tissue, which appear here as pink bands (CT). At higher magnification (Fig. 4.48) the cellular organization becomes more apparent.

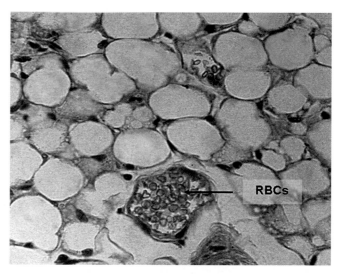

Fig. 4.48. Adipose tissue, paraffin, high magnification. Here, cellular organization becomes more apparent. There is only a small rim of cytoplasm and nuclei positioned at the periphery of the cells.

the tissue for embedding in paraffin or plastic. White adipose tissue is most abundant. Brown or multilocular adipose tissue is less common but is present in large amounts in hibernating animals. In other animals, it is relatively more common in newborn and young animals. Unlike much of the lipid that is mobilized by lipolysis to produce ATP from white adipose tissue, brown adipose tissue adipocytes have mitochondria that have evolved to use most of the mobilized lipid

to produce heat energy rather than ATP. This probably explains the importance of these specialized cells in hibernating animals and in newborns where maintenance of body heat is so critical.

The following series of slides show examples of white adipose tissue. Figures 4.47 and 4.48 illustrate the general structure of adipose tissue at a relatively low magnification. Both of these images are from

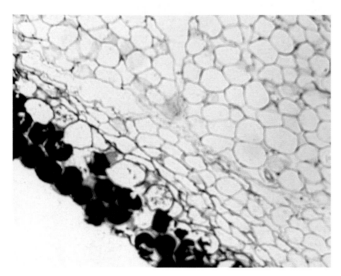

Fig. 4.49. Adipose tissue, low-power, osmium-stained. In this case, some of the lipid was retained in the cells during processing and the tissue was subsequently stained with osmium tetroxide. This chemical has a very high affinity for lipid and causes the appearance of a dense black product. Notice the darkly stained adipocytes in the lower left of this tissue section.

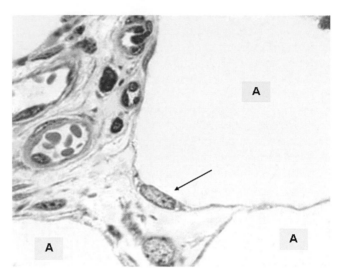

Fig. 4.51. Adipose tissue, high magnification. In this section, portions of four adipocytes (A) are visible. The large open spaces contained stored lipid. The nucleus of one adipocyte (arrow) appears at the rim of the cell. The upper left has cross-sectioned profiles of a small artery and companion venule. Red blood cells appear in the lumen of the artery.

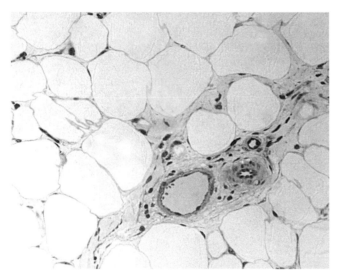

Fig. 4.50. Adipose tissue. Adipose tissue from a region of the mammary gland. The tissue was embedded in plastic, sectioned at about 2 μm in thickness, and stained with Azure II. Cell profiles are distinct but there is little cytoplasm.

samples embedded in paraffin. As indicated in an earlier section, samples prepared in this manner are usually relatively thick (4–7 μm), so some details of cellular structure are difficult to see. Figures 4.49 and 4.50 illustrate sections of white adipose from samples embedded in plastic. The stains used are different (H&E versus Azure II) but, more importantly, plastic embedded sections can routinely be cut at 1 μm or less. The difference in cellular detail between paraffin- and plastic-embedding is striking but especially so

with actively secreting epithelial cells, i.e., pancreas, liver, mammary gland, and so forth.

Figure 4.51 shows the structure of small parts of the four different adipocytes. This image also provides some perspective on the size of these cells. The connective tissue between the cells has cross sections of two vessels with several red blood cells. A reasonable estimate for an RBC is 7 μm across its widest dimension, so the adipocytes (A) in comparison are clearly many times larger. The nucleus of one of the adipocytes is also apparent compressed to one edge of the cell. Nuclei for the other adipocytes do not appear in this image.

Although the structure of other specialized connective tissues will be discussed as we consider specific systems, it is worth introducing bone and cartilage. In the case of the long bones of the limbs, e.g., tibia and humerus, they begin as cartilage models (essentially miniature versions) in the fetus. As the animal develops, the cartilage is progressively replaced by bone in a process called endochondral ossification. Three cartilage types can be distinguished. These are, in order of abundance, hyaline, fibrocartilage, and elastic cartilage. Hyaline cartilage is grossly characterized by the presence of a shiny, milk glass–like homogenous matrix. It should be familiar to you as the cartilage that appears at the end of a chicken leg or the gristle you sometimes bite into at the edge of a chicken breast. Cartilage very clearly illustrates the idea that connective tissues have relatively few cells but lots of extracellular matrix components. However, unlike many other connective tissues, which usually have a ground substance with an abundance of collagen fibrils, cartilage is also rich in three types of proteoglycans. These complex polymeric molecules are composed of a core protein with various attached glycosaminoglycan (GAG) chains. The three-dimensional shape of the molecule resembles a miniature bottlebrush, with the stem being the core protein and the bristles the GAG chains. The GAGS include hyaluronic acid, chondroitin sulfate, and keratin sulfate. These sugar chains are highly charged (polar) so that cartilage is very highly hydrated. This aids the cushioning associated with cartilage but the sparseness of cells in the mature tissue and relative lack of blood supply also explains the difficulty of repair to injured cartilage. Figure 4.52 is an example of hyaline cartilage from the trachea. In this instance these C-shaped rings of cartilage (with the opening of the C facing a dorsal direction) provide the rigid support to hold the entrance to the respiratory tract open. You may recognize the upper-right edge of the tissue as an epithelial layer. Although you could not identify its characteristics at this level of magnification, you might recall that pseudostratified columnar epithelial cells cover the respiratory tract above the level of the bronchioles. The cartilage appears as two "islands" within the connective tissue. As cartilage is created by chondroblasts, the cells progressively mature into chondrocytes as their own products trap the cells. These mature chondrocytes come to reside in spaces called lacunae.

The insert in Figure 4.52 shows a higher power image of hyaline cartilage, it appears as a largely avascular field of matrix with scattered chondrocytes. The chondrocytes produce this matrix so that in its fully mature state the cells are literally trapped. The spaces, lacunae, immediately surround the cells. This terminology also applies to bone but the cells within the spaces are called osteocytes. The outer covering of the cartilage is called the perichondrium and can be divided into an outer more protective, capsulelike protective layer and an inner region with more cells that are chondrogenic. That is, these cells can be induced to produce more active chondrocytes. Although the matrix surrounding the cells appears rather homogenous in typical H&E-stained sections, the matrix contains collagenous fibrils, which add strength. Often the chondrocytes appear very close together; these are called isogenous cell clusters because they arise from division from a single predecessor cell. Growth in this manner, with subsequent addition of more matrix material around the cells, allows for interstitial growth of the cartilage or growth within the substance of the cartilage. In contrast, development of additional cartilage in the outer perichondrium, leads to growth at the surface called appositional growth. This later style of development explains the continued lengthening of the long bones

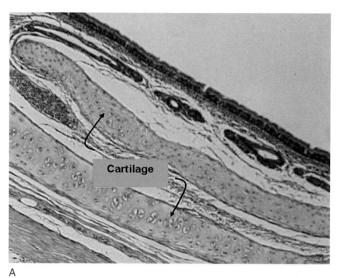

A

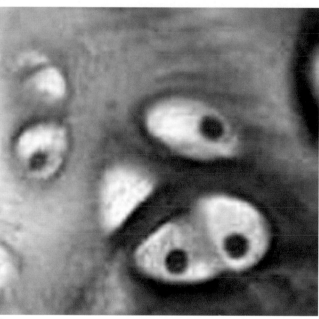

B

Fig. 4.52. Section of cartilage from trachea. This low-power image shows general features of the trachea. A) The internal surface of the trachea (upper right of the image) is covered by epithelial cells (pseudostratified columnar epithelial cells), and just underneath there are several mucus-producing glands. Further into the tissue, portions of sectioned hyaline cartilage appear (arrows). B) The inset shows a grouping of chondrocytes in greater detail. The cell structure is barely visible but the nuclei appear as distinct dots.

prior to the time of epiphyseal plate closure at puberty. At this time there is cessation of the generation of new cartilage needed for appositional growth and to provide the ground substance and matrix necessary for osteogenesis. Sections of the fetal mouse foot provide an excellent tissue sample to study the structure of cartilage and developing bone.

In mature bone, for example, the humerus, two types of osseous tissue can be distinguished. The outer

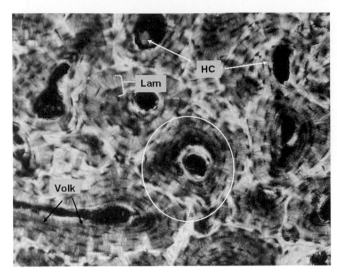

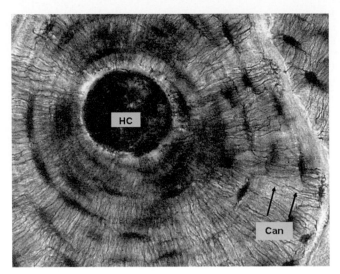

Fig. 4.53. Compact bone, low power. The structure of compact bone can be imagined as a series of miniature trees where in the center of the trunk is a canal called the Haversian canal (HC), and the rings or lamellae (Lam) represent the concentric growth rings. These Haversian systems, or osteons (circled area), generally align themselves along the longitudinal axis of the long bones. Other channels called Volkmann canals (Volk) pass perpendicular to intersect the central Haversian canal and link the central passageways to provide for entrance of blood vessels and nerves. In compact bone, the spaces between lamellae is occupied by the osteocytes, which come to be surrounded by the matrix they have produced and secreted, much like chrondrocytes in cartilage. Small fissures, called canaliculi (Can) also radiate out from the lacunar spaces that hold the mature osteocytes.

Fig. 4.54. Haversion canal. This high-power image of compact bone shows the ringlike lamellar structure surrounding the Haversian canal (HC). Each ring is a lamella. The dark areas are the lacunae. These spaces contain the osteocytes. Radiating away from the lacunae are small fissures called canaliculi (Can). These spaces allow for diffusion of nutrients and waste products.

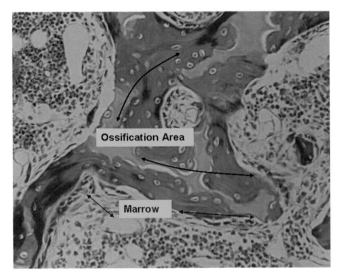

Fig. 4.55. Ossification. This image illustrates the process of ossification in a region of spongy bone. The center (blue-stained) area contains cartilage cells undergoing ossification to become osteocytes. The surrounding area will contain red bone marrow.

portion of the bone is called compact or dense bone and it has a very distinctive structure. At the microscopic level it is often viewed by preparing ground bone samples. Essentially preserved, fixed samples are cut into very thin wafers and mounted on slides. This allows an examination, primarily of the matrix structure. The center or medullary cavity, in addition to marrow components, is composed of an interlacing, spider-weblike component of bone called spongy or cancellous bone. Both types of bone have osteocytes and various other bone cells (osteoblasts, osteoclasts) but the organization of the matrix is much less regular. Figure 4.53 shows a relatively low-power image of a sample of ground bone to illustrate major features; Figure 4.54 gives a higher magnification to show some of the detail of osteocytes and lacunae.

At higher magnification (Fig. 4.54) structures of an individual Haversian system become apparent. The dark areas are the spaces that in living bone would contain the osteocytes. Other apparent structures are the canaliculi. Bone located between the circular osteons is called interstitial bone.

Figure 4.55 shows an area of ossification in a developing bone that is destined to be spongy bone. The irregular shape of the ossifying tissue and lack of orga-

nization with respect to lamella is evident. The area of ossification is stained pale blue, areas with lacunae containing trapped osteocytes are scattered in the matrix. Areas to the outside (stained red) are areas of bone marrow.

A final type of connective tissue to consider is blood. At first glance it seems odd to think of blood as connective tissue but once you consider that it consists of a matrix (plasma) with suspended cells, it matches our

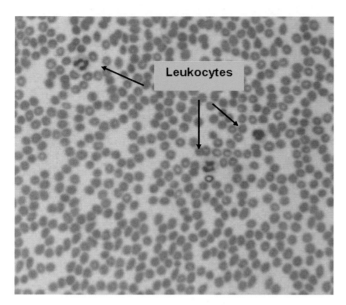

Fig. 4.56. Blood smear. This low-power image shows a field of pale-staining erythrocytes and several leukocytes (three neutrophils).

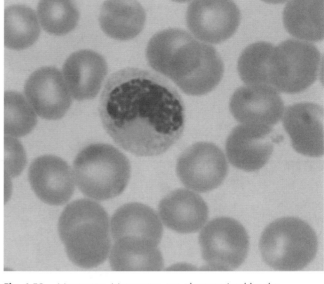

Fig. 4.58. Monocyte. Monocytes are characterized by the presence of a kidney bean–shaped nucleus and under normal conditions are relatively rare, ~2–8% of total.

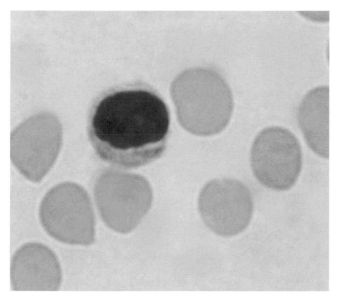

Fig. 4.57. Lymphocyte. Lymphocytes have a large nuclear to cytoplasmic ratio, i.e., typically only a thin rim of cytoplasm may be evident. The nucleus is uniformly stained roughly ovoid in shape, and cells are common in the circulation ~25% of the total.

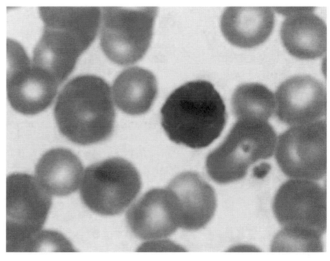

Fig. 4.59. Basophil. Basophils have abundant darkly stained blue or purple granules (with standard basic dyes), and the cells are smaller than neutrophils or eosinophils. The nucleus is typically lobed and numbers are usually very low ~1–2% of the total.

prior definition of connective tissue. Of course the majority of cells are erythrocytes or red blood cells, typically 4–5 million/mm^3. The white blood cells or leukocytes average 6,000 to 9,000/mm^3 and are divided into two subclasses based on the presence or absence of cellular granules, i.e., granulocytes versus agranulocytes. Agranulocytes include large and small lymphocytes (30–35% of the total white cells) and monocytes (3–7%). Granulocytes include neutrophils (55–60%), eosinophils (2–5%), and basophils (0–1%).

Platelets, also called thrombocytes, are small structures that average 200,000 to 400,000/mm^3). Figure 4.56 shows a relatively low-power image of a blood smear to provide some perspective. There are two neutrophils and one lymphocyte in the field. It is clear that RBCs greatly outnumber WBCs. Figures 4.57 through 4.60 show some of the features of various leukocytes. Specifically, Figure 4.57 shows a lymphocyte, Figure 4.58 a monocyte (these are the agranulocytes), Figure 4.59 shows a basophil and Figure 4.60

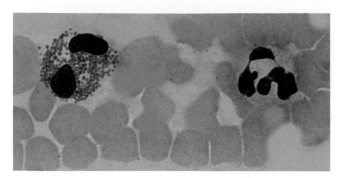

Fig. 4.60. Eosinophil and neutrophil. The eosinophil that appears to the left of the image, gets its name from the dark-staining of its granules with the red acidic dye eosin. The nucleus is lobed but relatively rare ~1–2% in the circulation. The neutrophil on the right is commonly ~50% of the total and, unlike other granulocytes, the granules stain poorly with either basic or acidic dyes, e.g., the neutral of the name. The nucleus has two to five lobes, a bit like beads on a string. Neutrophils are also called PMNs or polymorphonuclear leucocytes because of this characteristic.

Skeletal Muscle CT Layers

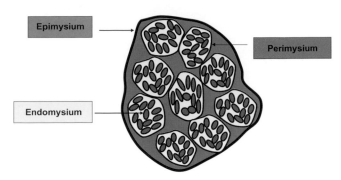

Fig. 4.61. Cross section, skeletal muscle. A thin layer of connective tissue, the endomysium, wraps each skeletal muscle fiber or cell. Bundles of muscle fibers called fascicles (outlined in yellow) are wrapped by the perimysium and the entire muscle by the epimysium that is continuous with the tendon that attaches skeletal muscles to bone.

has a neutrophil on the right and an eosinophil on the left.

Muscle tissue

Epithelial, muscle, and nervous tissues are sometimes called composite tissues. This simply means that although the tissue primarily is composed of the cells that give the tissue its name, there is also the incorporation of at least some connective tissue. For muscle tissue in particular, the connective tissue elements are essential for functioning of the tissue. First, because of the metabolic demands of the muscle tissue, availability of nutrients and capacity to get rid of wastes is critical. The connective tissue sheaths that surround skeletal muscles and the connective tissue layers that penetrate around even individual muscle cells (fibers) provide passageways for capillaries. Second, the various connective tissues sheaths from around the outside of a muscle to bundles of muscle fibers, to individual muscle fibers (epimysium, perimysium, and endomysium, respectively) means contractile elements are anchored together. This allows for unified, smooth functioning of the muscle.

There are three types of muscle cells. First, the familiar skeletal or voluntary muscle is named because its contraction is linked with movement of the skeletal system. A second, cardiac muscle, shares many features with skeletal muscle, including the presence of striations. The third type, smooth muscle, is very widely distributed and gets its name because it does not exhibit striations present in the other types. Like epithelial tissue, muscle tissues are highly cellular but

in contrast are also highly vascularized. Muscle cells have elegantly constructed myofilaments, primarily combinations of actin and myosin protein filaments, that allow for contract and tissue movement. Details of muscle cell structure and the sliding filament model for contraction will be described in a subsequent chapter. Our purpose in this section is to introduce the basics of muscle tissue histology.

Skeletal muscle

At a gross level each skeletal muscle is a distinct unit composed of several tissues. Of course the muscle cells or fibers predominate, but adequate functioning requires connective tissue sheaths, blood vessels, and nerve fibers. One of the most unusual features of skeletal muscle cells is that they are multinucleated, large elongated cells. Furthermore the internal volume of the cell is chiefly dedicated to the packaging of a complex array of myofibrils. These individual myofibrils are composed of overlapping thin filaments, primarily made of the protein actin, and the thick filaments made of the protein myosin. These myofibrils, like tightly packed wires in a telephone cable, are arranged along the longitudinal axis of the individual muscle cells. Let's consider organization of a common muscle (the bicep) cut in cross section across the belly or gaster of the muscle. Our examination would allow us to distinguish the three connective tissue sheaths as diagrammed in Figure 4.61. In this diagram the smallest circular units (dark pink) within the yellow background represent the individual muscle cells that have been cut in cross section. The

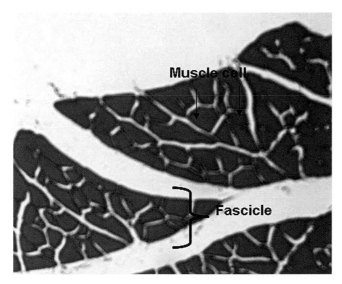

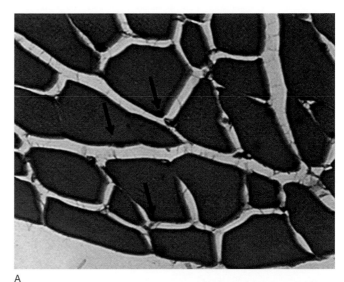

A

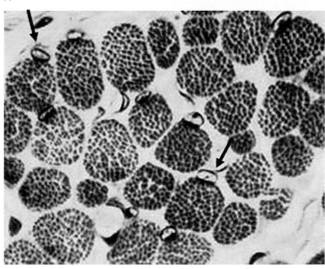

B

Fig. 4.62. Cross section, skeletal muscle. This image at very low magnification shows portions of several muscle bundles or fascicles; profiles of individual muscle cells or fibers appear as the irregular shapes within the muscle bundles.

Fig. 4.63. Skeletal muscle, cross section, high. At progressively higher magnification, it is possible to see profiles of individual muscle cells and the fact that many of the cells are multinucleated (arrows, A). Depending on the preparation, the myofibrils may also be discernable (B).

endomysium that surrounds individual cells is indicated by the black outline of each cell. The cells are grouped together in fascicles, outlined in yellow, and the perimysium that anchors these muscle bundles is distinguished by the black outline around each (Fig. 4.62). Groups of fascicles come together to create the muscle, which is surrounded by the epimysium. When skeletal muscle cells are sectioned along their longitudinal axis, the highly organized arrangement of the myofilaments is evident by distinct banding or striations. These alternating dark and lightly stained regions reflect areas in which only thin filaments, thick filaments, or both overlap. This explains why skeletal and cardiac muscle is also referred to as striated muscle. Some of the microscopic features of skeletal muscle are outlined in subsequent figures as well as the molecular organization of the contractile filaments.

At higher magnification with cells cut in cross section you can distinguish profiles of individual cells (Fig. 4.63) and in some preparations individual myofibrils within the cells. It also becomes apparent that there are multiple nuclei per cell and that they are located at the peripheral edges of the cell. It is only when cells are sectioned longitudinally that striations are seen (Fig. 4.64). However only at very high magnification is it possible to decipher the detail of the filaments responsible for the banding pattern of the muscle sarcomere (Fig. 4.65). A diagrammatic representation of the sarcomere is provided in Figure 4.66. Mechanics of muscle contraction will be discussed in a subsequent chapter.

At first glance the striations of the muscle cell fibrils seem to be repeating disks stacked along the length of the cell. However, when examined in the electron microscope (Fig. 4.65), the striations clearly appear only in the myofibrils but not within the cytoplasm of the cell. The alternating dark and light bands are due to the relative density in regions where there are only thin or thick filaments. Furthermore, the pattern is very highly ordered. This is because the fibers are linked together into a sarcomere, the organizing unit. The sarcomeres are linked together, something like train cars along the entire length of the myofilaments. The myofilaments are essentially repeating groups of linked sarcomeres. The contraction process is explained

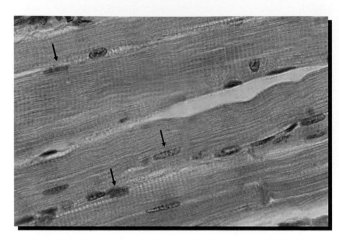

Fig. 4.64. Skeletal muscle, longitudinal. This section from the bovine tongue illustrates the peripheral location of nuclei (arrows) and the pattern of striations characteristic of skeletal muscle.

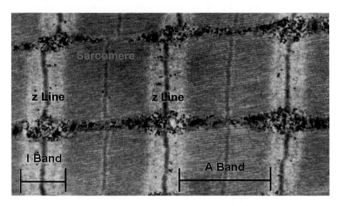

Fig. 4.65. Transmission EM image, skeletal muscle. This image shows portions of several sarcomeres. A single sarcomere is bounded on either side by the Z line, the site where the thin filaments are anchored. The region bounded by the pale band is the I band of the sarcomere. Notice that the I band at each end of the sarcomere also contains the I band for the adjacent sarcomere. The darker band is the A band. Depending on the degree of contraction, a lighter band (the H band) can be seen in the center of the A band. In this particular sample, because the muscle was contracted at the time it was prepared, the H band is barely visible as the thin pale stripe in the center of the A band. The darker stripe (M line) is the location where the thick myosin filaments are anchored.

Sarcomere Action

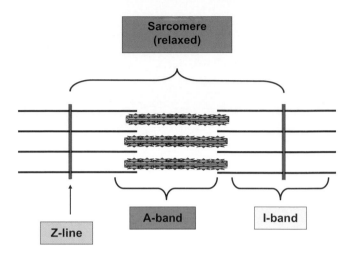

Sarcomere Action

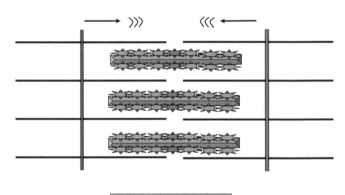

Fig. 4.66. Structure of sarcomere. A schematic view of sarcomere shortening is shown to illustrate changing relationships between I, A, and H bands as contraction occurs. The thick filaments are outlined as green bundles with protruding myosin heads, and the thin filaments as simple black lines. Note that the A band stays constant but that the H and I bands get smaller as the Z lines and ends of the thin filaments approach.

by the ability of the sarcomere to shorten and then relax. Regulatory details will be discussed in a subsequent chapter, but the fundamental process involved is the movement of the thinner actin filaments moving along the thicker myosin filaments. As indicated by the diagram in Figure 4.66, as pairs of thin filaments (attached at the Z line) on either end of the sarcomere move toward one another, the sarcomere shortens. Since the sarcomeres are linked and the myofibrils are anchored and cells are bound to other cells by the endomysium, this results in shortening of entire

bundles of muscle cells and, if stimulated sufficiently, the entire muscle.

Cardiac muscle

Skeletal muscle and cardiac muscle are very similar. Both have striations and essentially identical sarcomere structures. However, individual muscle cells (fibers) are typically shorter and contain fewer nuclei per cell, i.e., are often binucleated. There are also some

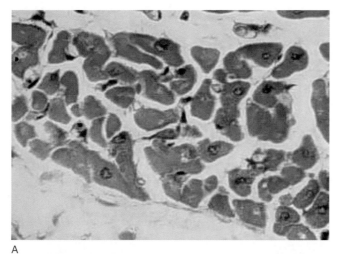

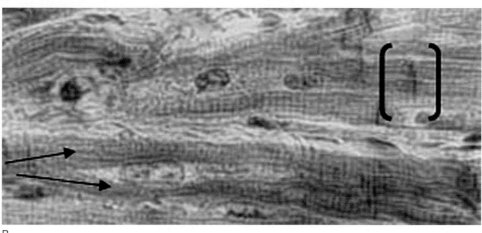

Fig. 4.67. Cardiac muscle. Panel A shows a group of cardiac muscle cells cut in cross section. In profiles where the nucleus is present, it is located toward the center of the cell, in contrast to skeletal muscle. Panel B shows a longitudinal section of cardiac muscle. Note the striations and, at the arrows, branching of a cell. The dark bars (brackets) are intercalated disks that join cells in series.

differences in the mechanics of contraction regulation. In skeletal muscle, the calcium needed for interaction between the actin and myosin, comes from storage within the muscle cells, the sarcoplasmic reticulum. For cardiac cells, extracellular calcium plays a more important role than in skeletal muscle. Also, although it is possible to learn to change heart rate under special circumstances, cardiac contraction is usually considered involuntary. Control of cardiac rate and force of contraction is clearly important to supply the oxygen and nutrients necessary for varying levels of activity. It should be no surprise that regulation involves close coordination between the nervous and endocrine systems, as discussed in our review of cardiovascular physiology.

At a histological level cardiac cells have striations but also frequently are branched, nuclei are located centrally within fibers, and groups of cells are linked longitudinally by complexes of gap junctions within regions called intercalated disks. These features allow skeletal muscle fibers to be distinguished from cardiac muscle fibers in histological sections, as illustrated in Figure 4.67.

Smooth muscle

Although it is common to describe all muscle cells as fibers, it is easier to think of the large multinucleated skeletal muscle cells or the cardiac cells linked by intercalated disks as fibers in a common sense view. Smooth muscle cells by comparison are small spindle-shaped cells that taper on either end. Like the cardiac cells, smooth muscle cells have a single centrally located nucleus. Despite their small size, groups of smooth muscle cells are physiologically vital. These cells are found in the walls of hollow viscera and in the walls of all but the smallest blood vessels. In the walls of many tubular visceral structures, the smooth muscle cells appear in two distinct layers. For example, in the muscularis externa of the GI tract there is an outer layer of longitudinally oriented cells and an inner layer that goes around the circumference of the tract. Smooth muscle cells that are arranged in these coordinating layers of cells are called single unit smooth muscle and are the most common type. In contrast, about 1% of smooth muscle cells act rather independently and are called multiunit cells. Both classes are involuntary. However, the single unit smooth muscle is more likely to be impacted by the secretion of various hormones than the multiunit cells that depend on neural input for contraction to occur.

For example, within the muscularis externa of the GI tract, groups of smooth muscle cells act as pacemaker cells for the tissue. When these cells spontaneously depolarize, this induces rhythmic contractions that pass through the tissue. The level of autonomic nervous system activity or secretion of some hormones (i.e., estrogen or progesterone influence on uterine smooth muscle) can also alter the normal pattern of spontaneous contractions that occur or the strength of contractions.

As the name suggests, there are no apparent striations in smooth muscle cells. There are however thin and thick myofilaments anchored to the cytoskeleton, that allow shortening of the cells. Since the cells are linked together (single unit cells) this allows the coordinated contraction of the tissue layer. Multiunit cells are typically anchored to extracellular proteins. Extra-

cellular calcium concentrations also have a greater impact on contraction of smooth muscle cells than skeletal muscle cells because of the lack of sarcoplasmic reticulum for intracellular storage of calcium. Differences in the appearance of cross-sectioned versus longitudinally sectioned smooth muscle cells are illustrated in the diagrams shown in Figure 4.68, and examples of smooth muscle tissue from the small intestine are shown in Figure 4.69.

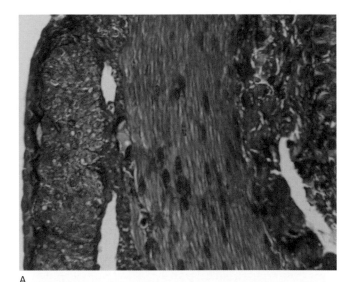

A

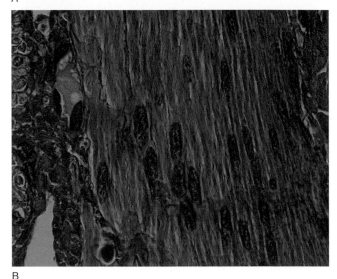

B

Fig. 4.69. Smooth muscle cells, small intestine. Panel A shows inner and outer layers of smooth muscle tissue in the muscularis externa of the intestine. The muscularis externa (to the left of the figure) has an inner circular smooth muscle layer that has been sectioned longitudinally and an outer layer of cells that are oriented lengthwise along the intestinal tract. This cell layer has been cut in cross section. Panel B illustrates some of the cellular detail. Notice how the cells cut longitudinally seem to "flow" together. It is difficult to distinguish individual cells.

Fig. 4.68. Diagram of smooth muscle. The upper panel illustrates the arrangement of smooth muscle cells in a longitudinal view. The spindle-shaped cells with a single central nucleus make a tightly compacted layer of closely adhering cells. The lower panel illustrates the appearance of cellular profiles cut in cross section (see dashed line). Since some of the cells would be cut near the center, these profiles would be relatively large ovals with the nucleus in the center. Other profiles would be smaller oval shapes because of sections through the more narrowed tapered ends of the cells.

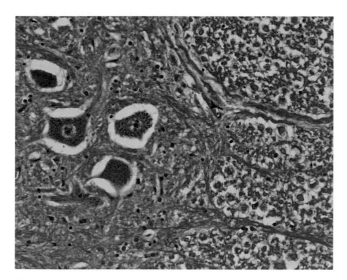

Fig. 4.70. Section of spinal core. A portion of the cell bodies of several motor neuron neurons appear to the left of the section. The dark spots are nuclei of smaller supporting cells.

Nervous tissue

Clearly the functional cell in the sense of impulse transmission is the neuron. Diagrammatic examples of various types of neurons are illustrated in Chapter 8. However, it is important to appreciate that neural tissue is more than simply collections of neurons. The health and functioning of neurons depends on many supportive cells called neuroglia or sometimes simply "glia." Four types of neuroglia appear in the central nervous system and two in the peripheral nervous system. Some of these cells produce growth factors and other agents that promote health and tissue development, and others are responsible for manufacturing the myelin sheath that acts to insulate many axons. The supporting cells of the CNS include astrocytes, microglia, ependymal cells, and oligodendrocytes.

Astrocytes are important in anchoring neurons and two of these cell types, Schwann cells in the peripheral nervous system and oligodendrocytes in the central nervous system, produce the myelin sheath that wraps many axons. Structure of neurons related to conduction of nerve impulses will be discussed in subsequent chapters. Figure 4.70 illustrates the appearance of neural tissue from the spinal cord. The most prominant feature is the profile of several neuron cell bodies in the left of the image.

It is important to realize that this brief chapter is meant simply to give you some of the basic histology for each of the fundamental tissue types. We focused a great deal of effort on epithelial tissue because epithelial cells (of one organ or another) are responsible for the synthesis and secretion of nutrients, signaling molecules, enzymes, etc.—in other words, the functional attributes of many vital organs. However, it should be clear at this point that each of the basic tissues must interact for physiological function and homeostasis to be maintained. You should appreciate that microscopic study of tissues and cells provides an important adjunct to a better understanding of physiology. In short, as we indicated at the beginning, structure and function are ultimately intertwined at multiple levels. As you learn the attributes of various organs and organ systems, consider the organization, development, and differentiation of the cells within the organ that make the physiology possible.

References

Ross, M.H. and W. Pawlina, 2005. Essential Histology, 5th Edition, Lippincott Williams & Wilkins, ISBN: 0781772214.

Junqueira, L.C. and J. Carneiro. 2005. Basic Histology—Text and Atlas, 11th Edition, McGraw-Hill Medical, ISBN: 007144091.

5 Integumentary system

Contents

Although we sometimes consider some of the agricultural products—e.g., leather or wool—derived from skin, we often fail to appreciate the physiological relevance of skin. The skin and its derivates (sweat and oil glands), hair (wool, fur), and nails (claws, hoofs) constitute a complex mix of tissues that together create the integumentary system. This system is critical to the health and well being of our animals and in many cases provides important economic assets. It is easy to appreciate that its primary function is protection. But it is more than a simple physical protective covering. Without skin our animals would quickly fall prey to environmental pathogens and rapidly die from dehydration and heat loss. Our major goal is to outline some of the physiological attributes of the integumentary system that are essentially for homeostasis. The following list illustrates critical functions of the integumentary system.

- Physical protection: barrier against the outside
- Prevention from dehydration
- Body temperature regulation
- Sensory information via cutaneous receptors
- Metabolic actions
- Excretion of wastes

The skin covers the entire exposed surface of the body and is continuous with the mucous membranes lining opening onto the body surface, for example, the digestive, respiratory, and urogenital systems. We'll begin by considering the structure of the skin.

Overview of skin structure

As you can appreciate, the thickness of the skin varies from region to region of the body. Consider our own bodies and the toughness of the skin on the plantar (sole) surface of our feet compared with the skin of our faces. Now imagine how tough the skin of a horse or cow must be to withstand the environmental and physical demands. This probably explains the durability of leather-covered furniture. However, no matter the location or thickness, skin is composed of two distinct tissue regions—epidermis and dermis. The epidermis is the outer layer and, as we'll see, it is composed of multiple layers of epithelial cells along with other specialized cells. The underlying dermis is largely composed of connective tissue and provides for the passage of blood vessels and nerves. The epidermis is also avascular. This means that nutrients must diffuse from capillaries located within the dermis. The tissue that lies just under the dermis is the hypodermis, often just called subcutaneous tissue. This subcutaneous tissue is not strictly part of the skin, but because the region primarily contains areolar connective tissue and adipose tissue, it serves to cushion and protect both the skin and underlying muscle and organs. A needle and syringe is often generically called a hypodermic syringe or "hypo." Penetrating the skin and releasing the material into the space just below the dermis constitutes a hypodermic injection, hence the name.

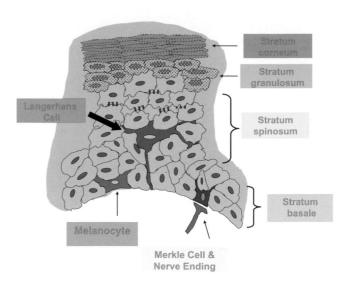

Fig. 5.1.   Diagram of skin cell types and layers.

Epidermis

The epithelium of the epidermis is a keratinized stratified squamous epithelium that consists of four cell types and four to five distinct layers (depending on location). The most common epidermal cell is the keratinocyte. As their name suggests, a major function of these cells is to produce keratin, a fibrous protective protein. Keratin acts to waterproof the skin and, along with secretions produced by accessory glands, protect the underlying tissues from heat, microbes, abrasion, and chemicals. Keratinocytes are closely connected by desmosomes, which serve to anchor the cells together to physically create a more protective barrier. The keratinocytes are first produced in the cell layer closest to the underlying dermis called the stratum basale. As the cells age, they are progressively pushed into layers closer to the surface of the body. By the time the cells reach the outermost layers they have accumulated large amounts of keratin. The turnover of epidermal cells is rapid. The entire epidermis can be replaced every 25 to 50 days. In areas subjected to abrasion, cell proliferation and replacement is even faster.

Essentially, new cells are formed in the stratum basale (or stratum germinativum). This is the deepest of the epidermal layers. It is composed of one row of cuboidal to columnar-shaped epithelial cells that divide rapidly to produce new keratinocytes that push up toward the surface and become part of the more superficial layers. In addition approximately 20% of the cells are melanocytes. As new cells push older cells outward these older cells become the stratum spinosum, which is typically 8 to 10 cells thick. These cells contain thick bundles of intermediate filaments (tonofilaments). In histological preparations, cells also often shrink. This causes the cells to have a prickly or spiked appearance. This explains the name of this layer, i.e.,

spinosum (little spine). Because the stratum germinativum and stratum spinosum are immediately adjacent to the dermis these are the only epidermal cells that receive adequate sustenance from diffusion of nutrients from the capillaries of the underlying dermis. With further degeneration and increased keratin accumulation the cells appear in the stratum granulosum. In this layer the keratinization process begins in earnest and the cells begin to die. This layer is called granulosum because the accumulation of keratin granules becomes more evident in dead cells. In areas of thick skin a layer called the stratum lucidum can be distinguished. Here a thin layer of cells (typically 2–3 cells in thickness) becomes translucent. With time the dead cells, accumulated keratin, and lipids combine to create the outermost layer of skin, the stratum corneum. The relative thickness of these layers varies considerably from region to region. Figure 5.1 provides a diagrammatic illustration of these tissue layers and Figures 5.2 and 5.3 provide histological examples.

There is much interest in the antimicrobial properties of molecules that accumulate in or are produced by the epidermis. For example, Schroder and Harder (1999) described an inducible, transcriptionally regulated antibiotic peptide produced by human skin. The peptide (named hBD-2: human beta defensin-2) was shown to be effective in killing Gram-negative bacteria. Such findings might well find application in the dairy industry. For example, the opening of the teat end of cows and other ruminants is lined by stratified squamous epithelium, which continues into the teat meatus as the streak canal. It is well known that the keratin and other molecules serve as a barricade to seal the streak canal of the teat and protect the mammary gland from mastitis. Much of the protection

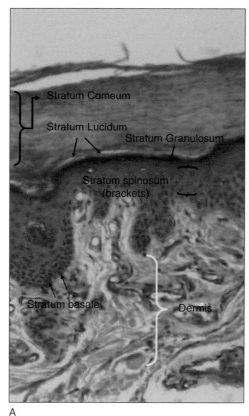

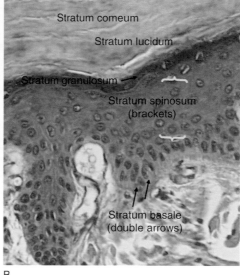

A   B

Fig. 5.2. Low-power view (A) of thick skin and cell detail (B).

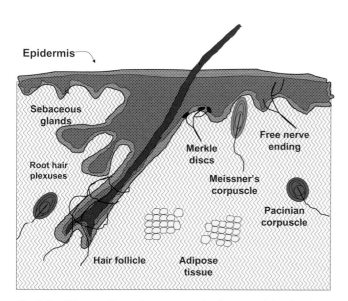

Fig. 5.3. Diagram illustrating some major features of the dermis.

involves the physical closure of the teat opening between milking episodes, but there is substantial evidence that specific components within the keratin layer can directly act as antimicrobial agents. Some of these substances are likely analogous to hBD-2, but others may be derived from mammary secretions that become trapped within the epithelium of the streak canal. Effects might involve the direct killing of microorganisms or perhaps the prevention of colony formation.

During machine milking, there are dramatic physical effects on the teat, the teat end, and the streak canal. Given that the rate of milk flow in cows is 7 to 8 m/s it is reasonable to expect that resulting shear forces might remove some of the protective keratin. It is also probable that some milk constituents are absorbed into the keratin during the time of milking or from milk droplets remaining after milking. If milking removes substantial amounts of the keratin and if renewal is delayed or changes in composition favor the formation of bacterial colonies or bacterial adherence, this could decrease the effectiveness of the streak canal as the primary defense against mastitis. In fact, experimental removal of streak canal keratin markedly increases the rate of intramammary infections. In Holsteins, keratin weight before milking was 1.6 times greater than after milking (3.1 versus 1.9 mg per teat). Jerseys by contrast showed little effect of milking (3.5 versus 3.1 mg per teat). There is a negative correlation between keratin loss at milking (r = 0.53, wet weight basis, or r = 0.65, dry weight basis) and milk production. Total lipid in the keratin is similar before and after milking. In addition, although the major aspects of the fatty acid profiles are also similar before and after milking, keratin after milking has more short-chain fatty acids. This is consistent with addition of milk-derived lipids to the keratin by contamination of milk droplets remaining in the streak canal. In the case of the Holsteins a greater proportion of the keratin is made up of these lipids after milking (Bitman et al., 1991). Although it was once thought that the keratin regenerated rather slowly, i.e., 2–4 weeks, detailed quantitative studies show that following an initial collection, the keratin regenerates at a rate of 1.5 mg (wet weight) or 0.6 mg (dry weight) per day per teat. This suggests complete restoration of the keratin occurs within 1 to 2.5 days (Capuco et al., 1990). Just as in human medicine there is considerable research interest in the identification of epidermal-keratin components that might act to protect the udder from infection. Clearly, techniques to enhance the protective function of the integumentary would find many animal agricultural applications.

While the keratinocytes are most plentiful, other cells also play important roles. For example, Merkel cells function as sensory receptors (touch). They orient with elements from the nervous system to create a disc-shaped sensory nerve ending called a Merkel disc. Other nerve endings and specialized receptor cells also occur in the skin, but these are located within the dermis.

A very specialized immune system cell type, Langerhan's cells, develops in the bone marrow but they migrate to the epidermis where they take up residence. They are also called epidermal dendritic cells and are essentially modified macrophages. Usually located within the stratum spinosum, they nestle between keratinocytes and send projections between the cells to create an extensive network. In this way the cells act as monitors to detect the presence of foreign debris, microorganisms, and other materials. When they are simulated they actively process these materials and function as antigen-presenting cells to induce activity of T- and B-lymphocytes. We have all experienced the results of immunological response in the skin after being exposed to irritants, the itch and rash. In fact, the skin is continually exposed to an incredible variety of antigenic stimuli. Consequently a wide array of immune responses occurs in part because of mediators secreted by keratinocytes, dendritic cells, and mast cells in the skin.

Melanocytes are the final cell type of the epidermis. They are located in the lowest layer, the stratum basale, where they function to produce the pigment melanin. As melanin is synthesized, it accumulates in secretory vesicles—melanosomes—that are sequestered in elongated processes that extend from the cells. The presence of these peripheral vesicles causes the cells to have a spiderlike appearance. Over time, melanin is released and taken up by surrounding keratinocytes. Once the concentration of melanin granules build up they become oriented on the surface of the cells that face the outside of the body. This pigment shields and protects the nucleus of the cell from ultraviolet radiation.

Dermis

The dermis, the second major subdivision of the skin, accounts for about 80% of the total mass. It is typical of many connective tissues. There are a variety of cell types present, but as you might expect fibroblasts are common along with their products, i.e., the collagen, elastin, and reticular fibers that provide essential strength and flexibility. Unlike most other connective tissues, there is also, seemingly, a dizzying array of specialized structures. Most of these are related to the sensory side of the nervous system. Since the integumentary is intimately associated with the external environment, various receptors provide the central nervous system information necessary to maintain homeostasis: external temperature, pressure and touch, and presence of noxious or damaging agents. There are also other specialized epithelial structures that assist maintenance of homeostasis: sweat and sebaceous glands and hair.

The dermis consists of two layers, the papillary layer and the reticular layer. The papillary layer is the outer region closest to the epidermis. In this area there are fingerlike projections called dermal papillae (these also give the layer its name) that indent into the epidermis. In some areas, for example, the palms of the hands or fingertips in humans and apes, or the pads of a cat's foot, the papillae are arranged on the top of larger structures called dermal ridges. This acts to increase friction and allow for an easier grip. The particular pattern of ridges is unique to each individual and is the basis for fingerprints in humans or other primates. These projections contain capillaries, and a variety of nerve endings and receptors. Three broad groupings of receptors include 1) exteroceptors, 2) interoceptors (sometimes called visceroceptors), and 3) proprioceptors. Exteroceptors are concerned with stimuli that arise from the outside. Most exteroceptors are located on or near the body surface. These are the focus of our study of the integumentary system. Interoceptors react to stimuli from within the body, for example, chemical signals, temperature, or gut motility. Proprioceptors also reflect internal responses but are specifically involved in relay of information concerned with muscle, tendon, or ligament movement or stretch. In other words they monitor the musculoskeletal organs. The latter two classes of receptors will be

Table 5.1.   Integumentary sensory receptors classified by structure and function.

Structural Class	Functional Activities	Location
Unencapsulated		
Free nerve endings	Pain (nociceptors); thermoreceptors; mechanoreceptors (pressure)	Most tissues
Modified nerve endings (Merkel discs)	Mechanoreceptors (light pressure)	Stratum basale
Root hair plexuses	Mechanoreceptors (hair movement)	In and around hair follicles
Encapsulated		
Meissner's corpuscles	Mechanoreceptors (light pressure, discriminative touch, vibration)	Dermal papillae, esp. face, fingertips
Krause's end bulbs	Mechanoreceptors (modified from Meissner's corpuscles)	Connective tissue of mucosae
Pacinian corpuscles	Mechanoreceptors (deep pressure, stretch) rapid adaptation	Widespread skin
Ruffini's corpuscles	Mechanoreceptors (deep pressure, stretch) slow adaptation	Deep dermis, joint capsules

discussed in subsequent sections. Our focus now is on exteroceptors of the skin. These receptors can also be classified based on their structural complexity. For example, free nerve endings are structurally very simple, especially when compared with receptors associated with the special senses (vision, hearing, olfaction, or taste). Even the relatively simple receptors of the integumentary can be divided into unencapsulated (free nerve endings, for example) and encapsulated groupings. Specialized Meissner's or Pacinian corpuscles are examples of encapsulated receptors. Pacinian corpuscles have a structure like the layers of an onion; pressure induces ion changes that are translated into graded potential in the associated nerve fibers (see Fig. 5.5). These impulses are interpreted as touch or pressure by neurons in the cerebral cortex. Table 5.1 summarizes the types and classes of sensory receptors within the skin.

The reticular layer is the thicker and deeper layer of the dermis. It is composed of dense irregular connective tissue and contains thick bundles of interlacing collagen fibers and some coarse elastic fibers. However, elastin fibers are typically only visible after special staining. These fibers run in several directions, which increases strength, but most are oriented parallel to the skin exterior. The fibers provide much of the strength and resistance to stretch in skin and the long-wearing attributes of leather. The reticular layer is also abundantly supplied with blood vessels and nerves. These elements of the dermis are illustrated in Figure 5.3. Figures 5.4 and 5.5 show histological examples of some of the other structures that occur within the dermis.

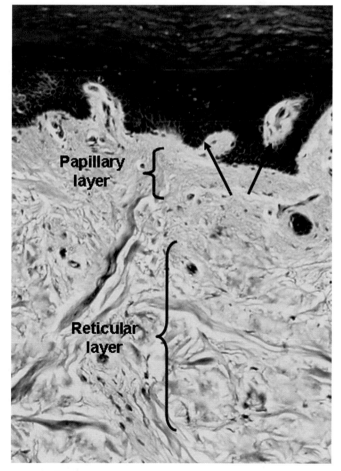

Fig. 5.4.   Example of thick skin. In this preparation the dermis is stained a pale turquoise and stands in sharp contrast to the epidermis. Arrows indicate dermal papillae.

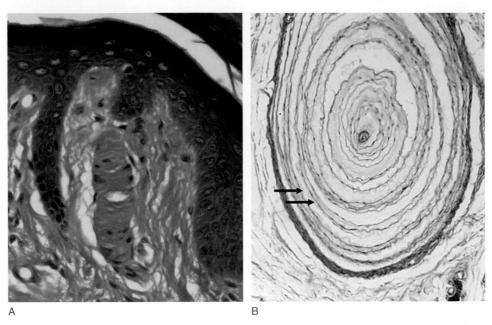

A   B

Fig. 5.5.   Structure of Meissner's corpuscle (A) and Pacinian corpuscle (B). Both of these sensory receptors are located in the dermis and are responsive to pressure and touch. Arrows indicate multiple layers of a Pacinian corpuscle.

Specialized structures

Sweat glands

The dermis contains a variety of glandular structures. Sweat glands in primates are plentiful and widely distributed. The most common type is the eccrine gland. These simple coiled glands open onto the surface in pores. They produce a hypotonic watery secretion that is derived from interstitial fluids. It is mostly water with some dissolved salts, lactic acid, and traces of other waste products. The rate of secretion is controlled by the activity of the sympathetic nervous system. In humans, a typical response occurs with overheating. Sweating induced in this way begins on the forehead and progresses downward. Emotionally induced sweating—fright, embarrassment, or nervousness—begins on the palms, soles, and armpits and spreads to other areas. Of course the primary function of sweat is to cool the body as a result of evaporation. A second type of sweat gland, apocrine glands, makes up a small proportion of the total. These glands are larger than eccrine glands and their ducts open onto hair follicles. They are primarily confined to the axillary and anogenital areas of the primate body. The secretions in addition to watery sweat also contain fatty acids and some proteins. The glands are affected by sex steroids, i.e., activity begins with the onset of puberty. For this reason apocrine glands are believed to be analogous to the scent glands of other animals. Eccrine sweat glands are sparse among domestic animals. For example, in dogs and cats they are located only on the footpad. This limited distribution means that these glands have virtually no effect on heat loss but they do act to moisten the surface and improve traction. We have all noticed the panting dog on a hot day or after exercise. Panting is an effective cooling mechanism because it moves greater amounts of air over moist surfaces. This extra water saturated air is exhaled and in the process body temperature decreases.

Although eccrine sweat glands are lacking, horses, cattle, sheep, swine, dogs, and cats have numerous apocrine glands. In the dog for example, the proteinaceous, whitish secretions from the apocrine glands mixes with the oily secretions of the sebaceous glands to form an emulsionlike coating on the skin. The characteristic dog, horse, or cow odor is primarily a result of bacterial action on these accumulated secretions. These secretions also impact heat loss, but this is likely most effective in horses, followed by cattle, sheep, dogs, cats, and swine. Regardless, of the evaporative effect of heat lost from sweat, the skin of these animals is nonetheless important in temperature regulation. This is because simply changing the rate of blood flow through capillaries in the skin alters the volume of warm blood near the surface of the body, thereby affecting thermoregulation.

Sebaceous glands

Sebaceous or oil glands also occur in mammals. These are simple branched areolar glands that release their products (holocrine mechanism) onto the hair follicles.

The secretion is called sebum, which is a mixture of cellular lipids and other cell components. Sebum is a natural skin cream and hair protector. It helps hair from becoming brittle, prevents excessive evaporation of water from the skin, keeps the skin soft, and contains a bactericidal agent that inhibits the growth of certain bacteria. This is closely related to lanolin that secrets onto wool fibers in sheep.

Other skin glands

Many animals have glands associated with the anal region. These glands are usually divided into three classes depending on specific location and orientation: 1) anal glands, 2) glands of the anal sac, and 3) perianal glands. Anal glands are found in dogs, cats, and pigs. They are modified tubuloalveolar sweat glands located in the submucosa of the anal canal and the opening of the anus. Carnivores secrete a lipidlike material, but pigs secrete a more mucuslike material from these glands. Clusters of lymphatic tissue, similar to the Peyer's patches in the intestine, often accompany the glands.

Anal sac glands sometimes called perianal sinuses occur in pairs and are essentially invaginations or diverticula of the anal surface. They are located between the outer and inner anal sphincters. Within each pocket or sac, glands embedded in the wall have openings that release the contents into the space of the sac. The anal sac is present in carnivores and rodents. In dogs the glands are arranged as compound tubular structures and exhibit an apocrine mode of secretion. In cats the glands are similar but apocrine and holocrine secretion occurs. Products from the glands open into secretory ducts in the neck of the anal sac. The excretory secretions of the anal sac glands, sloughed cells, and fecal material can block the openings of these anal sacs. When the sacs become blocked they may have to be manually expressed—not a pleasant experience.

Circumanal or perianal glands are anomalies, in the sense that they often appear as masses of epithelial cells within the submucosa that appear not to have functional ducts that lead to the surface. They are sometimes oriented adjacent to sebaceous glands, which suggests they may be related but this is far from certain. These nondescript masses of cells are frequently described as nonsecretory glands. Unfortunately, the solid masses of cells are believed to be especially prone to neoplasia.

The mammary glands are also skin glands but will be considered in greater detail in Chapter 12. Some other specialized glands include the infraorbital glands of sheep, the submental organ of the cat, and the scent or horn glands of goats. For example, the submental glands of the cat are located within the intermandibu-

lar space under the jaw. The "organ" is essentially a cluster of sebaceous glands. It is not uncommon to note domestic cats marking their territory by rubbing their chins. In goats this activity is a bit more apparent. The scent glands in the goat are located along the caudal to medial aspect of the base of the horns. Rubbing this area leaves sebaceous secretions that are apparent because they contain caproic acid. This is the short-chain volatile fatty acid that is responsible for the distinct odor of male goats. The uropygial gland of birds, also called the oil or preen gland, is the only skin gland that appears in birds. It is composed of a series of closely aligned sebaceous adenomeres (secretory units) that empty into a common space or sinus that ultimately empties onto a common papilla. The papilla has associated smooth muscle fibers that surround the duct opening. The opening is located above the last sacral vertebra.

Hair

Functions associated with hair include insulation, protection, and sensory reception. Hair or fiber production in domestic animals is directly related to the number and size of the follicles in the skin. As you might expect, various aspects of hair growth and development have been extensively studied in sheep and goats. Regardless of whether the animal in question is used for fiber production, unlike humans, the hair is especially important physiologically. We'll begin by first considering some of the basics of hair structure and properties. Hairs or pili are generated by hair follicles and are flexible strands that mostly consist of layers of dead keratinized cells. However, the keratin in hair is harder and more durable than the softer keratin of the epidermal cells. The parts are simple: 1) the shaft projects from the skin; 2) the root is embedded in the skin. In humans for example, if the cross section of the shaft is ribbonlike the hair is kinky. If the shaft in the cross section is oval, the hair is wavy. If the shaft is round, the hair is straight and relatively coarse. These basic relationships also apply to animal hair.

At a more detailed level, the hair shaft can be divided into three regions: 1) outer cuticle, 2) inner cortex, and 3) central medulla. The outer cuticle is a layer of cornified epithelial cell "husks" that closely interlink with the cuticle cells of the root of the hair. The cortex makes up the majority of the hair shaft and is composed of several layers of flattened cornified cells that have accumulated "hard" keratin. Pigments may also appear in these cells along with air spaces. The medulla contains cells that are more cuboidal. These layers are especially clear in cross-sectioned hair shafts. The hair terminates in the root or hair bulb. Essentially, the hair resides in an invagination of the surface of the epithe-

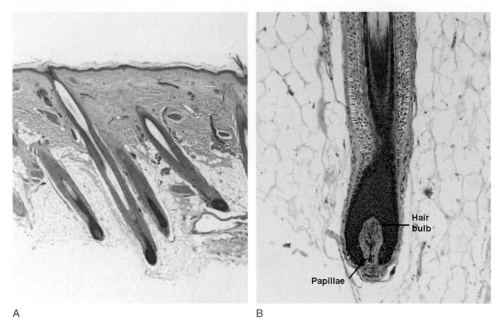

A   B

Fig. 5.6. Histology of hair follicles. Histological section of several hair follicles at low magnification (A) and of a single follicle at higher magnification (B) is shown. At lower power it is evident that the hair bulbs penetrate deep into the dermis and hypodermis.

lium that extends to the dermis. This is important because it allows ready transfer of nutrients and waste products from the hair bulb to the interstitial fluid of the dermis. Growth occurs when cells in the apex of the root bulb give rise to new medullary cells. Laterally positioned cells give rise to the cells of the inner cortex and outer cuticle, respectively. The growth of the hair then is analogous to the growth of the epidermis generally. Cells from lower depths progressively displace those above. See Figure 5.6 for examples of hair and hair follicle structure.

In many situations there is a sheath of smooth muscle, the arrector pili, that attaches to the connective tissue that surrounds the hair follicle and a portion of the hair shaft that is underneath the surface of the skin. The contraction of this smooth muscle causes the hair to stand on end and is likely associated with increased secretion of surrounding sebaceous glands. This is the basis of a hair-raising experience or the familiar Halloween cat with its arched back and raised hair.

In horses and cattle, the hairs are evenly distributed across the body, but in other species (dog, cat, and pig) the hairs are oriented into groups called hair beds. In the dog for example, each hair bed has a group of follicles that consist of one larger major hair (guard or principle hair) typically about 150 µm in diameter. A cluster of auxiliary hairs that are typically shorter and only about 75 µm in diameter surrounds the guard hairs. These hairs often exit the skin in the same opening as the guard hairs. In addition, the auxiliary hairs do not have a medulla. Clustering of hairs in

this manner can be extreme. For example the chinchilla, noted for its soft dense pelt, can have clusters that have 50 to 75 auxiliary hairs each. In this case the guard hair is also very fine and only slightly larger that the auxiliary hairs, i.e., 15 versus 11 µm in diameter.

Other specialized hairs include tactile or sinus hairs. These are familiar as cat's whiskers, for example. These hairs are usually longer and larger than normal but share similar structures to normal guard hairs. The roots of these hairs are highly innervated by free nerve endings and Merkel's discs.

The hair growth cycle is divided into three phases: 1) anagen, 2) catagen, and 3) telogen. Hairs are generated by the proliferation of cells within the hair bulb during anagen. The continuous addition of new cells to the shaft or the hair produces elongation. Termination of growth occurs when the mitotic activity of the basal cells decreases. Catagen is a transition phase. It is characterized by gradual transition of the bulb cells. The cells progressively convert into a solid, keratinized mass and the more distal region of the follicle thins. The bulb is forced toward the surface and the papilla is lost. In this condition the hair is referred to as a club hair. After a time a secondary germ structure develops deep under the club hair. The formation of the new germinal center marks the beginning of telogen, which can last for weeks or even months. During early anagen, the new hair bulb progressively elongates, and the shaft of the new hair displaces the older club hair. Figure 5.7 provides a diagrammatic illustration of the cycle of hair growth.

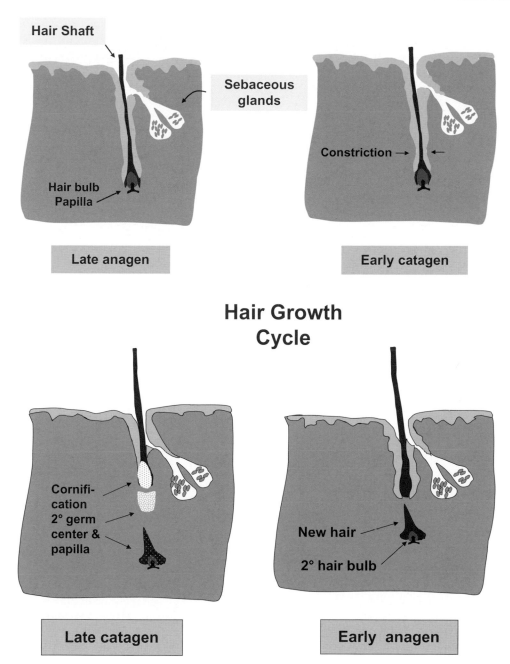

Fig. 5.7. Diagram of hair cycle events. Growth begins to slow in late anagen, followed by constriction of the follicle in early catagen. By late catagen, the hair is increasingly cornified producing a club hair that is progressively extruded. A 2° germ center and papilla appear some time after. By early anagen, a new hair bulb and growing hair shaft begin to develop. The new hair often follows the same path as the old hair follicle.

The follicle population determines the quantity and quality of wool production. As a general rule, a high number of hair follicles leads to production of fibers with a lower diameter, but the opposite is true with low follicle density, that is, fibers that are thicker and more coarse (Hocking Edwards et al., 1996). It is also apparent that hair growth is cyclic, but that this basic rhythmic pattern can be modified by external cues— for example, the seasonal pelage cycles in mammals. Recent studies have focused on the role of the pitu-

itary hormone prolactin in wool growth, for example. The secretion of prolactin is well known to be altered by changes in photoperiod, specifically decreased secretion during short days, also typically cooler temperatures in regions well above or below the equator, but increased secretion during long days and warmer temperatures. Reduced photoperiod and correspondingly reduced prolactin concentrations in the blood are associated with the stimulation of hair growth and generation of the winter pelage. Nixon et al. (2002)

reported changes in expression of prolactin receptor within the dermal papilla and the outer root sheath of wool follicles of sheep. Moreover, changes in receptor expression were altered in sheep subjected to photo-period-induced changes in circulating prolactin. This suggests that changes in expression of prolactin receptor within specific regions of the follicle are involved with seasonal changes in hair growth.

Biochemical properties of skin

In this section we consider some of the important physiological attributes of the integumentary system. Included here are aspects related to vitamin D synthesis and homeostasis. We also discuss factors that control skin and coat color.

Skin and coat color

In the human, three primary pigments give color to skin. Melanin is especially important and can produce various shades of yellow, brown, or black. The rate of melanin synthesis is largely genetically determined. For example, if you have very fair skin, melanin production is low and it is a very light shade. If you have very dark skin, on the other hand, melanin production is higher and the pigment inherently darker. It is believed that the average density of melanocytes is relatively constant between people but rates of cellular activity vary. The yellow-orange pigment carotene also impacts skin color. It tends to collect in the stratum corneum and in the adipose tissue of the hypodermis. Hemoglobin, the oxygen-carrying protein of red blood cells also impacts skin color. For example, a blush, especially in a fair-skinned person is a result of a quick flush of oxygenated blood through the capillaries of the dermis of the cheek. In fact, clinically the appearance of a bluish cast to the skin or nail beds is an indication of inadequate oxygenation of blood, perhaps as a consequence of anemia or some other problem, i.e., respiratory or cardiac problem. Other items related to skin color include 1) jaundice—caused by deposition of bile pigments in certain liver diseases, 2) hematoma—the blue-black color produced by bruising when blood vessels in the skin rupture, and 3) erythema—the reddish cast produced by blushing, fever, or strenuous exercise.

What about skin or hair color in animals? In reality there are two subtypes of melanin: eumelanin (brown-black) and pheomelanin (yellow-red). The making and processing of melanin, melanogenesis, is complex because of interactions of multiple cell types in the skin. In mice, for example, nearly 100 genes are known to affect coat color. However, these genes can be clas-

sified into two primary groups: 1) those that act on the melanocyte and 2) those that directly impact the biochemistry of pigmentation. The melanocytes residing in the stratum basale and within hair bulbs synthesize and package melanin into secretory vesicles called melanosomes. The melanosomes are then distributed to surrounding cells. It is easy to imagine sources of variation in these steps and how this might affect skin or hair color. For example, which type of melanin is made, how much, where is it distributed, how quickly degraded, and so forth. Tyrosinase is the essential regulatory enzyme in melanin synthesis. With high rates of enzyme activity the formation of eumelanin is enhanced; lower rates favor formation of pheomelanin. In addition to synthesis variation, melanocortin receptors are critical in initiation of melanin synthesis. Hormone control of pigmentation is evident in many situations—for example, changes in fur color in arctic mammals and increased skin pigmentation that is a symptom of primary adrenal gland dysfunction. Melanocortin refers to a large family of structurally related hormones derived from the precursor protein proopiomelanocortin (POMC). This protein is abundant in the intermediate lobe of the pituitary gland. Depending on processing, at least four melanocortin peptides can be generated. These are proteins that can interact with the melanocortin 1 receptor (MC1R). These include adrenocorticotrophic hormone (ACTH), as well as α-, β-, and γ-melanocyte stimulating hormone (MSH). Excess production of ACTH explains the excess skin pigmentation that occurs with adrenal insufficiency disease, since ACTH readily binds to the MC1-R receptor on the melanocytes. MC1-R is a G-protein (see Chapter 12) linked receptor with 7 transmembrane spanning domains. However variants of the receptor (MC 2, 3, or 4-R) are expressed in other tissues. This suggests that the melanocortin ligands have a variety of physiological effects in addition to pigmentation of skin or hair.

Mouse coat color genes were some of the first mutations discovered that have been related to regulation of coat color. Resource animals for many of the classic mammalian genetic studies, have their foundations in the very large numbers of coat color variations (brown, silver, and yellow) that were described by fanciers of unusual mice in Europe and Asia in the 18th and 19th centuries. During this time, animals with unusual or striking variations in their pelage were prized and consequently saved as breeding stock. These fancy mice provided many of the initial resources to generate strains of mice that are used extensively in research today. Of course understanding of the molecular basis for variations in these traits has mushroomed in recent years. Table 5.2 summarizes some selected mutations and corresponding phenotypes related to pigmentation in mice.

Table 5.2.   Mutations, gene products, and phenotypes related to pigmentation genes in mice.

Mutation	Gene Product	Phenotype
Albino	Tyrosinase; required to melanin synthesis	Complete absence of pigmentation (snow white hair and red eyes)
Agouti	Secreted ASP; antagonist of MC1-R	Loss of function = black hair Gain of function = yellow hair
Brown	Tyrosinase-related protein 1	Loss of function = brown instead of black hair
Lethal spotting	Endothelin 3—peptide related to angiogenesis	Piebald spotting, deafness, death
Piebald spotting	Endothelin receptor type β	Same as for lethal spotting
Pink-eyed dilution	Integral membrane protein in the melanosomes (eumelanosomes)	Loss of function = pink eyes, yellow-gray hair
Recessive yellow	Melanocortin 1 receptor	Loss of function = yellow hair Gain of function = black hair
Slaty	Tyrosinase-related protein 2	Partial loss of function = dilution of black pigment
Steel	Mast cell growth factor	White hair, black eyes, sterility
White spotting	Receptor tyrosine kinase (encoded by the proto-oncogene kit)	Partial loss of function = piebald spotting

It is now recognized that most of these mouse genes have counterparts in other animals. For example, black horses are homozygous for a deletion in the Agouti locus. The mutation producing the chestnut allele is a single base substitution on the MC1-R gene (Rieder et al., 2001). In domestic pigs, the predominant white phenotype is linked with two mutations in the KIT proto-oncogene, which encodes for mast (stem) cell growth factor receptor. The many millions of white pigs around the world are assumed to be heterozygous or homozygous for these two mutations (Marklund et al., 1999). In the bovine, three alleles of the MSH receptor gene (localized to chromosome 18) have been reported. A point mutation in the dominant allele ED results in black coat color. However, a frameshift mutation, which causes a synthesis of a shortened receptor protein in homozygous e/e animals, leads to a red coat color. The wild type allele E$^+$ allows production of a variety of colors. This likely reflects the great variety in regulation of the normal receptor (Klungland et al., 1995).

In mice, the switch between production of eumelanin and pheomelanin production is tied not only to the binding of the melanocortin ligands to MC1-R, but also to signaling from the agouti signaling protein (ASP). ASP is a soluble paracrine protein made by dermal papilla cells within the hair follicles. Binding of ASP to MC1-R prevents normal binding of α-MSH and thereby promotes production of pheomelanin rather than eumelanin. In mice with the agouti phenotype, the promoter of the ASP gene is transiently activated during the midphase of the hair growth cycle. This causes a band of yellow pigment (accumulation of pheomelanin) in hair that is otherwise black (eumelanin accumulation). Strains of mice with entirely yellow hair coats have mutations that involve this ASP gene. For example, in one case, a prevailing mutation in the agouti locus (A^y/A) results in excessive production of ASP throughout the body. This causes the complete yellow hair coat as well as obesity. The obesity results from ASP antagonism of the MC4-R receptor in the hypothalamus. In another strain the complete yellow coat is produced in a recessive allele (e/e), in the gene for MC1-R. In these animals the receptor protein is synthesized with extra amino acids (extension locus), which causes a failure of signaling. This leads to the exclusive production of pheomelanin and the total yellow hair color. Interestingly, yellow mouse hair is thought to be the murine equivalent of red hair in humans (Shaffer and Bolognia, 2001).

Vitamin D metabolism

Vitamin D has three major effects: 1) promotes absorption of calcium from the intestine, 2) activates resorption of calcium from bones, and 3) increases excretion of phosphate via the kidneys. In conjunction with increased concentrations of parathyroid hormone, increased amounts of biologically active vitamin D act to increase blood calcium. Thus, overall health and homeostasis requires this vitamin. This story begins in the skin. Vitamin D$_2$ is a plant product generated by ultraviolet irradiation of ergosterol. This material

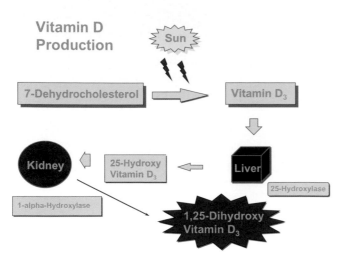

Fig. 5.8.   Metabolism of vitamin D.

can appear in the diet. However, vitamin D_3 or cholecalciferol is also synthesized in the skin. This is induced by the UV irradiation of 7-dehydrocholesterol. However, before the vitamin D_3 is fully active it must be modified. This first step occurs in the liver with the conversion of vitamin D_3 into 25-hydroxycholecalciferol by the addition of a hydroxy group by the action of the enzyme 25-hydroxylase. This material again enters the blood stream and is taken up by the kidney cells. A second hydroxy group is added to create the most potent form of vitamin, 1, 25-dihydroxycholecalciferol. This requires the actions of the 1α-hydroxylase. This form of the molecule acts on the intestinal epithelial cells to stimulate the synthesis of calcium transporter molecules that increase the absorption of calcium.

Deficiencies of vitamin D can lead to malfunctions in calcium homeostasis so that bone growth and development is impaired in growing animals. This produces rickets, a syndrome characterized by bowlegs or knock-knees. In human medicine, as the importance of vitamin D was realized, the practice began of fortifying milk with vitamin D to help ensure that children received adequate amounts of the vitamin to minimize the appearance of rickets. Interconversions of vitamin D are illustrated in Figure 5.8.

Nails, claws, hoofs, and feathers

Let's begin by first considering the nails of humans and other primates. Nails are hard plates of tightly packed keratinized cells. They are clear and cover the dorsal surface of the last phalanges of fingers and toes. Each nail is made of three regions: 1) the nail body, 2) the free edge, and 3) the nail root. The body of the nail is the visible portion. It rests on the nail bed, essen-

tially a combination of the stratum basale and the stratum spinosum. The free edge is that part that extends past the end of the digit. The nail root is hidden from view and is embedded in a fold of skin (or nail fold). The cuticle, for example, is the stratum corneum of the nail fold that gets pushed outward over the surface of the nail body.

Nail growth depends on the nail matrix located under the nail root. As you might guess from your review of the epidermis, the nail matrix consists of the two deepest layers of the epidermis (stratum basale and stratum spinosum). The keratinization of the cells of the nail matrix develops directly from the spinosum, so the stratum granulosum and lucidum are absent. The result is the creation of a hard, durable plate. As the nail matrix thus proliferates and the cells are keratinized, this hard plate is pushed forward onto the nail bed and the nail lengthens. If you consider your own nails, you can see a small white crescent. This is called the lunule and it corresponds with the presence of the thick matrix underneath. So how does this differ from claws and hoofs?

We'll use the horse as an example of the remarkable development of hooves. Let's begin with the lower leg and foot. The foot includes the hoof (epidermis) and the underlying dermis and associated structures. Specifically, these include the corium or dermis, digital cushion, terminal phalanx or coffin bone, distal end of the second phalanx (short pastern bone), navicular bone, and a variety of muscles, tendons, ligaments, and nerves. Some of these major features are illustrated in Figure 5.9.

The hoof is largely an insensitive cornified layer derived from the epidermis. Strictly speaking the terms *epidermal* and *dermis* are more accurate than the common terms *insensitive* and *sensitive*, respectively. The structure of the hoof is produced in two fashions. In some regions the dermis is very highly papillated; this mirrors the general appearance of dermal papillae in other regions of the body, but they are more abundant and highly interlinked with corresponding epidermal pegs. This organization increases strength and assists interchange between the dermal blood vessels and the avascular epidermis. In other areas the papillae and epidermal pegs are so confluent that the adjacent epidermal and dermal tissues create distinct layers or lamina.

The hoof is essentially an extension of the skin of the lower limbs. This boundary area that circles the leg just above the hoof is called the coronet. In this region the dermis of the skin is continuous with the dermis or corium of the hoof. The subdivisions of the corium correspond with the adjacent epidermal regions of the hoof. As you move from the anterior surface of the hoof in a caudal direction you pass through the following epidermal layers: stratum

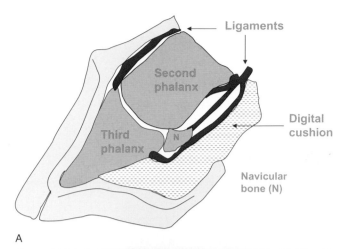

A

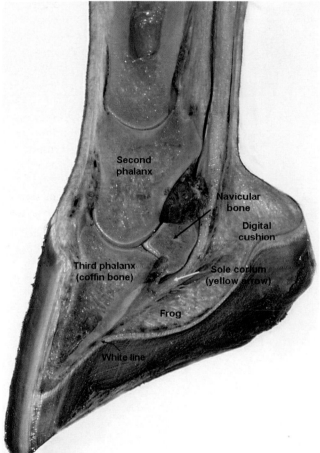

B

Fig. 5.9. Equine foot and hoof. Diagram (A) and corresponding photograph of cross section (B) of the equine foot.

tectorium, stratum medium, and stratum internum. The stratum tectorium extends from the periople layer of the skin epidermis in the area of the coronet. Most of the wall is made up of the stratum medium and is organized in a tubular arrangement of cells. This is similar in appearance to compact bone if cut in cross

section. These tubular structures are sometimes noticeable as lines oriented from the coronet toward the ground in the wall of the hoof. The boundary between the outer "insensitive" epidermis and the "sensitive" dermis occurs in the stratum internum. Here, there is a complex interaction between the outer epidermis and underlying laminar corium. Specifically, papillae from the dermis extend into the epidermis in a regular repeating array. Beyond the dermis (depending on the angle) you would penetrate the bone of the distal phalanx. This is illustrated in Figure 5.10. If you penetrated from the bottom of the hoof near the center, you would pass through similar (but thinner) layers of epidermis and the tubular and intertubular horn of the sole, the solar corium (dermis), the periosteum, and the compact bone of the distal phalanx.

In addition to these complex histological structures, there are also a number of well-defined structures associated with the hoof. These include the frog (so named because of its shape), bulbs, and the sole. The anterior edge is the toe and the caudal margin the heel. The white line, most apparent when the hoof is trimmed, is created by the epidermal laminae and represents the boundary between the dermis and epidermis. The frog is a wedge-shaped mass of mostly keratinized tissue that is softer than in other areas because of higher water content. The tubules of the sole are arranged vertically in correspondence with the papillae of the dermis or corium of the sole. The corium itself has a good supply of nerve and blood vessels. Figure 5.10 illustrates the gross anatomy of an equine hoof. The photograph is of the bottom or ventral surface of a freeze-dried hoof. It is easy to imagine the structure like a shoe that surrounds the dermis bones, blood vessels, and nerves of the lower foot.

Horns

The horns of cattle, goats, and sheep are generated in the region over the horn process, a germinal center that projects from the surface of the frontal bone of the skull. The dermis or corium envelops the horn core so that it is fused with the outer covering of the bone tissue or periosteum. As the horn develops the corium at its base is especially thick where it links to the skin via abundant long, slender papillae. The papillae become shorter and less abundant toward the apex of the horn. The bulk of the horn tissue consists of tubules that extend from the base of the horn toward the apex. Softer tissue covers the surface of the horn near the base and extends a variable distance toward the apex. This is similar to the outer covering of the hoof, the periople. Growth of the horn varies with nutrition.

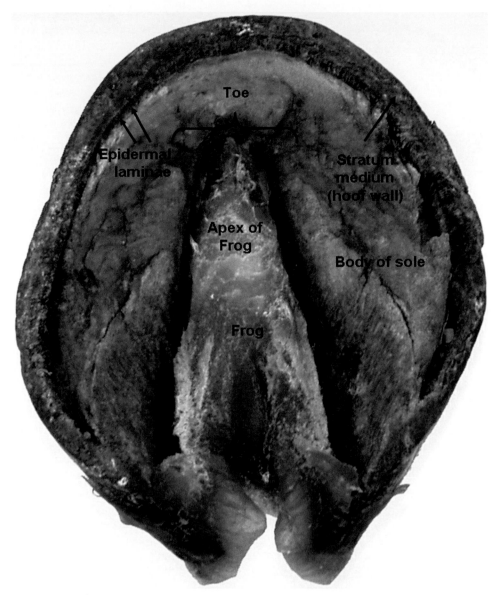

Fig. 5.10. View of the plantar (bottom) of the equine hoof.

This can be especially evident in wild animals with seasonal variation in available nutrients. This variation is reflected in the appearance of rings in the horn that can be used to estimate age.

In many commercial situations, especially dairy, polled cattle are often dehorned. This is usually accomplished by destroying the corium when only the horn buttons are present. This is typically accomplished by either surgical removal or destruction with a hot iron or application of caustic paste. Once the horn has begun to develop, both the corium and entire horn must be removed to prevent the horn from redeveloping. Even a small amount of corium can produce a crooked stubbed horn.

Feathers

As you might guess, a feather is likely the most complex structure that is derived from the integument among vertebrates. It is also clear that there are dramatic differences between avian species as well as marked differences depending on location and purpose. For example, the tail feathers of a rooster are more than a 1,000 times larger than the smallest feathers on his body. First let's consider what feathers actually do. Protection from the elements and maintenance of body temperature are clearly critical in all birds, but in addition they allow the bird to fly. Other aspects include protection from predators and the ability to attract the members of the opposite sex. Feathers are also plentiful. For example, a mature chicken has about 5,000 feathers.

Feathers come in several forms, but they are all made up of the same basic parts. These parts may be absent or rearranged from type to type. The predominant feather type on a bird's body is called the pennae or contour feather. Other feathers vary from this common type to large stiff feathers of the wings, small fluffy down feathers, hairlike filoplumes, and small bristlelike structures. Major features of a contour feather include the shaft, the vanes on either side, and often an after-feather underneath. The shaft, familiar as the writing end of a quill pin, is the longitudinal axis of the feather. It in turn has two parts: the calamus and the rachis. The calamus is the portion that penetrates into the skin and the feather follicle. The distal end tapers and has an opening called the inferior umbilicus. This entrance allows the development of the pulp of the shaft as the feather develops. The nib of the quill pin is anchored in this opening. The rachis is the long slender portion of the center of the feather that protrudes above the skin. On either side of the rachis there are fine branches. Each branch is called a barb, but each branch also has smaller branches called barbicels. The barbicels are typically hooked so that the structure of the feather is maintained. You can distinguish this yourself by stroking a feather in the "wrong direction." You'll notice that that there is a particular direction that the branches prefer. These parts are collectively called the vane and are responsible for the distinctive shape of the feather.

In fact, the barbicels can hold the feather vane together so closely that water is excluded. Have you heard the expression, "like water off a duck's back"? This elegant structural arrangement is responsible for this effect. It is also true that birds use secretions from their oil or uropygial glands to keep their feathers clean and in good condition, but contrary to popular belief the secretions do not provide a waterproof coating.

Leather

Leather is made from animal skins or hides that are chemically treated, or tanned. When properly done the resulting product is strong, flexible leather that is able to resist decay and spoilage. Most leather made is produced from tanned cattle hides, but a variety of skins can be used, including those from sheep, goats, calves, horses, pigs, ostrich, seals, and various reptiles.

The skins are typically cured, a process that involves either salting or drying the hide as soon as it is removed. In the so-called "wet" salting process, the skins are rubbed with salt, stacked, and bundled together. After about a month, most of the salt is absorbed into the skin. An alternative is to pack the skins in vats with a mixture of salt and disinfectants. This process can be completed in less than 24 h and is called brine curing. After curing, the hides are allowed to soak in water to remove excess salt and debris. In the next step the preserved flesh is usually stripped away mechanically.

Skins are usually then moved to large vats and again soaked up to 2 weeks in a mixture of lime and water. This process loosens the hair and makes subsequent removal easier. Bits of hair and fat that are missed by machinery are removed by scraping the skins by hand with a plastic scraper or dull knife. This process is called scudding. Once the skins are cleaned they pass to a vat containing acid. This acts to remove excess lime. The hides are then typically treated with enzymes to smooth the grain of the leather and to make the skin softer and more flexible. The tanning process follows.

Hides can be subjected to a variety of steps at this point, depending on the desired product. For example, vegetable tanning produces leathers that are flexible but stiff. This material would be used in belts, luggage or furniture. In these cases, the hides are often stretched onto frames and suspended in vats containing various tannins. These are agents found in bark, wood, and leaves. Tannins from oak, chestnut, or hemlock trees are frequently used. The hides are often transferred to multiple vats containing progressively stronger concentrations of tannins. Mineral or chrome tanning is an alternative process that is used to produce leathers for use in shoes, gloves, and clothing. After curing, scudding, and lime removal, the hides are soaked in a chromium-sulfate solution. Depending on the desired product, the hides can then be dyed. This not only adds color as desired; it also adds moisture to increase softness and flexibility. Vegetable-tanned hides are usually bleached and then soaked with oils and soaps to increase flexibility.

References

Bitman, J., D.L. Wood, S.A. Bright, R.H. Miller, A.V. Capuco, A. Roche, and J.W. Pankey. 1991. Lipid composition of teat canal keratin collected before and after milking from Holstein and Jersey cows. J. Dairy Sci. 74: 414–420.

Capuco, A.V., D.L. Wood, S.A. Bright, R.H. Miller, and J. Bitman. 1990. Regeneration of teat canal keratin in lactating dairy cows. J. Dairy Sci. 73: 1745–1750.

Hocking Edwards, J.E., M.J. Birtles, G.A. Wickham, P.M. Harris, and S.N. McCutcheon. 1996. Pre- and post-natal wool follicle development and density in sheep of five genotypes. J. Agric. Sci. 126: 363–370.

Klungland, H., D.I. Vage, L. Gomez-Raya, S. Adalsteinsson, and S. Lein. 1995. The role of melanocyte-stimulating hormone (MSH) receptor in bovine coat color determination. Mammalian Genome 6: 636–639.

Marklund, S., J. Kijas, H. Rodriguez-Martinez, L. Ronnstand, K. Funa, M. Moller, D. Lange, I. Edfors-Lilja, and L. Andersson. 1999. Molecular basis for the dominant white phenotype in the domestic pig. Genome Res. 8: 826–833.

Nixon, A.J., C.A. Ford, J.E. Wildermoth, A.J. Craven, M.G. Ashby, and A.J. Pearson. 2002. Regulation of prolactin receptor expression in ovine skin in relation to circulating prolactin and wool follicle growth status. J. Endocrinol. 172: 605–614.

Rieder, S., S. Taourit, D. Mariat, B. Langlois, and G. Guerin. 2001. Mutations in the agouti (ASIP), the extension (MC1R), and the brown (TYRP!) loci and their association to coat color phenotypes in horses (Equus caballus). Mammalian Genome 12: 450–455.

Schaffer, J.V. and J.L. Bolognia. 2001. The melanocortin-1 receptor. Arch Dermatol. 137: 1477–1485.

Schroder, J.M. and J. Harder. 1999. Human beta-defensin-2. International J. Biochem. Cell. Biol. 31: 645–651.

6 Bones and skeletal system

Contents

Bones

Introduction

Osteology is the study of bones. The skeleton provides the basic scaffolding for the body. The skeletal system includes the bones, and the cartilage, ligaments, and connective tissues that hold everything together.

Classification of bones

The human skeleton contains 206 major bones whereas the number of bones in different animals varies. The bones can be classified into five categories including long bones, short bones, flat bones, irregular bones, and sesamoid bones (Fig. 6.1).

- Long bones. These are bones that are longer than they are wide. Some of the bones of the limbs are

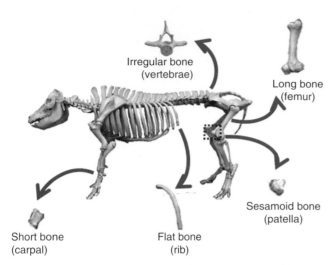

Fig. 6.1.   Types of bones. Examples of the various types of bones as found in the pig skeleton.

long bones. Long bones are characterized by an elongated shaft and somewhat enlarged extremities that bear articular surfaces. Examples of long bones include the humerus, radius, femur, tibia, metacarpals, and metatarsals.

- Short bones. Short bones are generally cube-shaped, and examples include the carpal and tarsal bones.
- Flat bones. Flat bones, as the name implies, are thin and flattened. They include two plates of compact bone separated by cancellous or spongy bone. Examples include the sternum, ribs, scapula, and certain skull bones.
- Irregular bones. These are complex and irregularly shaped bones. Examples include the vertebrae and certain facial bones.
- Sesamoid bones. Sesamoid bones are small bones embedded in a tendon and resemble the shape of a sesame seed. Examples include the patella, and proximal and distal sesamoid bones of the digits.

Bone structure

Gross anatomy

Each bone consists of compact bone and cancellous bone. Compact bone, also called dense or cortical bone, is a term describing solid-looking bone. Compact bone is found on the surface of bones forming a protective outer coating; cancellous bone is found on the interior.

Cancellous bone, also called spongy bone, consists of a network of pieces of bone called trabeculae or spicules, interspersed with spaces filled with red or

yellow bone marrow. Spongy bone predominates in short, flat, and irregular bones, as well as in the epiphyses of long bones. It is also found as a narrow lining of the medullary cavity of the diaphysis of long bones. The epiphyses consist mostly of cancellous bone with a thin outer coat of compact bone.

In developing long bones, the shaft is called the diaphysis and each extremity is called an epiphysis (pl. = epiphyses) (Fig. 6.2). The epiphysis consists mostly of cancellous bone with a thin outer coat of compact bone. It is generally enlarged relative to the diaphysis. The metaphysis is the joining point of the diaphysis and epiphysis. Between the diaphysis and epiphysis of growing bones is a flat plate of hyaline cartilage called the epiphyseal plate. After growth is complete, the plate is replaced by the epiphyseal line. The medullary cavity (*medulla*, "innermost part") is the space in the diaphysis containing bone marrow. At the joint surface on the bone is an articular surface consisting of a smooth layer of hyaline cartilage that covers the epiphysis where one bone forms a joint with another bone.

The fibrous covering surrounding that part of the bone not covered with articular cartilage is called the periosteum. It consists of dense irregular connective tissue. Its innermost layer consists of an osteogenic layer containing osteoblasts (bone germinators) that make new bone, and osteoclasts that break down bone. The periosteum contains nerve fibers, lymphatic vessels, and blood vessels that supply the bone. The periosteum is attached to the underlying bone by Sharpey's fibers extending from the fibrous layer into the bone matrix. There is a high density of Sharpey's fibers where tendons and ligaments attach to the periosteum.

The internal surfaces of the bone are covered with the endosteum. The endosteum lines the medullary cavity in long bones and covers the trabeculae of spongy bone.

Short, irregular and flat bones vary in the proportion of compact and cancellous (Fig. 6.3). Furthermore, these bones also do not have a shaft or epiphyses. They contain bone marrow between their trabeculae, but there is no bone marrow cavity. The internal spongy layer in flat bones is called the diploë (folded).

Microscopic anatomy of bone

There are four major cell types found in bone (Fig. 6.4). Osteocytes are the mature cells within bone that account for most of the population of bone cells. They are found within a lacuna (see next section, "Compact Bone"). Osteoblasts are cells that secrete the extracellular matrix on bone. They secrete collagen and ground

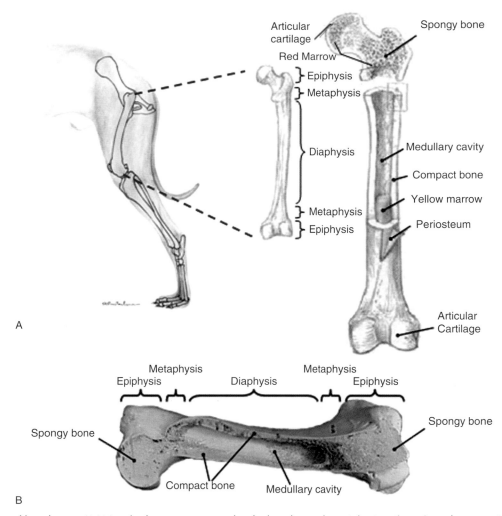

Fig. 6.2. Anatomy of long bones. A) Using the femur as an example of a long bone, the epiphysis is the enlarged area at either end of the bone while the diaphysis is the long shaft in the middle portion of the bone. The metaphysis is the joining point between the epiphysis and diaphysis. The periosteum is the fibrous covering around the outside of the bone not covered with articular cartilage. The endosteum is the fibrous and cellular tissue lining the medullary cavity of the bone. B) Cross section of an equine humerus showing exterior and interior anatomy.

substance that makes up unmineralized bone, called osteoid. Once these cells get embedded within the matrix, they become osteocytes. Osteoclasts are cells involved in resorption of bone, and are therefore present in areas where bone is being removed. Osteoclasts are giant multinucleated cells. Bone also contains a small number of mesenchymal cells known as osteoprogenitor cells. These are stem cells that can produce osteoblasts, and are therefore important in fracture repair. They are located in the inner, cellular layer of the periosteum, the endosteum that lines the marrow cavity, and the lining of vascular passageways in the matrix.

Compact bone

Although compact bone appears solid to the unaided eye, microscopically it contains considerable detail.

The structural unit of compact bone is the osteon, or Haversian system (Fig. 6.5). Each osteon appears as a cylindrical unit consisting of 3–20 concentric lamellae of bone matrix surrounding the central osteonal canal (Haversian canal, or central canal) that runs parallel to the long axis of the bone. The lamellae are like paper towels wrapped around a cardboard roll (i.e., osteonal canal). The osteonal canal contains the vascular and nerve supply of the osteon. The osteonal canals run parallel to the long axis of the bone, and they carry small arteries and veins.

A second group of canals, called perforating or Volkmann's, or lateral, canals, run at right angles to the long axis of the bone. These canals connect the blood vessel and nerve supply of the periosteum with that in the osteonal canal. These canals are lined with endosteum.

During bone formation, osteoblasts secrete the bone matrix. However, osteoblasts maintain contact with one another via connections containing gap junctions. As the matrix hardens, the osteoblasts become trapped within it, thus forming the lacunae and canaliculi. The osteoblasts become osteocytes, or mature bone cells.

Osteocytes, the spider-shaped mature bone cells, are found in lacunae, the small cavities at the junctions of the lamellae. Only one osteocyte is found per lacunae,

and these cells cannot divide. Numerous processes extend from each osteocyte into little tunnels running through the mineralized matrix called canaliculi, which connect adjacent lacunae. Therefore, there is a continuous network of canaliculi and lacunae containing osteocytes and their processes running throughout the mineralized bone. Canaliculi are important because they provide a route by which processes from one osteocyte can contact those of adjacent osteocytes. Therefore, via the canalicular system, all osteocytes are potentially in communication with one another. They pass information, nutrients, and/or wastes from one place to another.

Osteocytes can synthesize or absorb bone matrix. If the osteocyte dies, bone matrix resorption occurs due to osteoclast activity, which is later followed by repair or remodeling by osteoblast activity.

While mature compact bone has a lamellar structure in which the fibers run parallel, immature bone, also called woven bone, has a nonlamellar structure. Woven bone is put down rapidly during growth or repair, and its fibers are aligned at random resulting in lower strength. Woven bone is generally replaced by lamellar bone as growth continues.

Cancellous or spongy bone

Unlike compact bone, spongy bone does not contain osteons. As mentioned earlier, it consists of an irregular lattice network of bone called trabeculae. Red bone

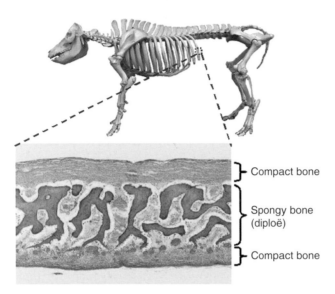

Fig. 6.3.   Internal anatomy of flat bone. Flat bones consist of an outer layer of compact bone that sandwiches an inner layer of spongy, or trabecular, bone (diploë).

Compact bone

Spongy bone (diploë)

Compact bone

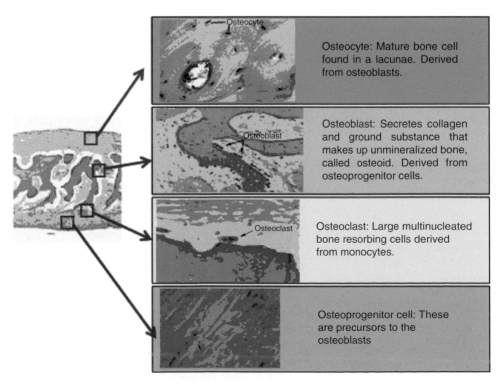

Osteocyte

Osteocyte: Mature bone cell found in a lacunae. Derived from osteoblasts.

Osteoblast

Osteoblast: Secretes collagen and ground substance that makes up unmineralized bone, called osteoid. Derived from osteoprogenitor cells.

Osteoclast

Osteoclast: Large multinucleated bone resorbing cells derived from monocytes.

Osteoprogenitor cell: These are precursors to the osteoblasts

Fig. 6.4.   Bone cells. The four types of bone cells, and their locations, are shown.

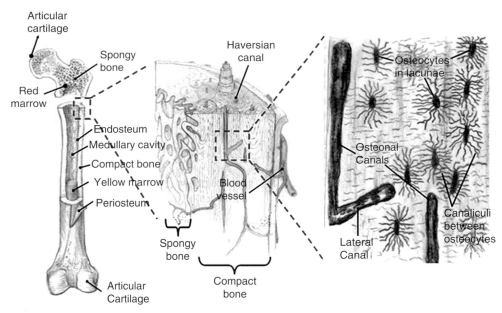

Fig. 6.5. Microscopic structure of compact bone. These figures represent longitudinal sections of the bone shown in increasing magnification from left to right. The osteon, or Haversian system, consists of a central osteonal canal surrounded by concentric lamellae of bone matrix. These canals are all interconnected by lateral canals that run horizontal, or at right angles, to the osteonal canals. Osteocytes, or mature bone cells, are found in cavities called lacunae that lie between the lamellar layers. The osteocytes have processes that project into canaliculi, which are narrow canals interconnecting the lacunae. The osteocytes pick up nutrients and oxygen from the blood and pass it via the canalicular system. (Figure modified from Marieb, 2003.)

marrow can be found in the space between the trabeculae. Osteocytes are found in lacunae within the trabeculae, and canaliculi radiate from the lacunae.

Chemical composition of bone

Bone consists of both organic and inorganic components. The major inorganic component is calcium phosphate, $Ca_3(PO_4)_2$, accounting for two-thirds of the weight of bone. Calcium phosphate interacts with calcium hydroxide, $Ca(OH)_2$, to form hydroxyapatite, $Ca_{10}(PO_4)_6(OH)_2$. As the crystals of hydroxyapatite form, they also incorporate other inorganic materials including calcium carbonate, sodium, magnesium, and fluoride.

The remaining organic portion of the bone is made up of cells (osteoblasts, osteocytes, and osteoclasts) and osteoid, which includes collagen fibers and ground substance (proteoglycans and glycoproteins). The osteoid is secreted by osteoblasts.

Hematopoietic tissue in bones

Red bone marrow, which is hematopoietic (i.e., blood forming), is found in the spongy bone of long bones and the diploë of flat bones. Red bone marrow consists of mature and immature red blood cells, white blood

cells, and stem cells that produce them. In newborns, the medullary cavities of spongy bones contain red bone marrow. In adult long bones, the medullary cavities of spongy bone become large fat-filled medullary cavities containing yellow bone marrow and extending into the epiphysis. Yellow marrow functions in fat storage, and contains mostly fat cells. Therefore, blood cell production in adult long bones is restricted to the head of the femur and humerus. However, if an animal is anemic, the yellow marrow can revert to red marrow to supplement red blood cell production. In contrast, the spongy bone found in flat bones, such as those in the hips, remains hematopoietic and therefore a good source when needing to sample bone marrow.

The osteonal and lateral canals are also the way in which blood cells formed in the marrow enter circulation. The sinuses of the bone marrow connect with the venous vessels running through these channels, and newly formed blood cells are released into them. From there they can leave the confines of the bone and enter the general circulation.

Bone development

Osteogenesis, or ossification, is the process of bone formation. Calcification, the process of calcium salt deposition, occurs during ossification. While calcification is

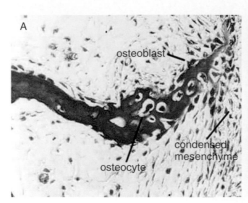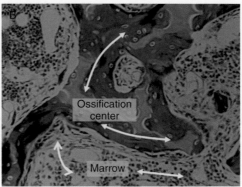

Fig. 6.6. Intramembranous ossification. A) Mesenchymal cells within the mesenchyme migrate and condense in specific areas forming a membrane that will become ossified. This condensed mesenchyme becomes more vascularized, and the cells become larger and rounded. The cells differentiate into osteoblasts secreting collagen and proteoglycans (osteoid). As the matrix becomes more dense and calcified, the osteoblasts become osteocytes contained within canaliculi. Some of the surrounding cells become osteoprogenitor cells. As osteoprogenitor cells come into apposition with the initial bone spicules, they become osteoblasts and continue appositional growth. B) Ossification begins in a relatively confined region called the ossification center.

associated with bone formation, it can occur in other tissues.

There are two general classes of bone formation. Intramembranous ossification occurs when bone develops from a fibrous membrane. The flat bones of the skull and face, the mandible, and the clavicle if present, are formed by this method. Intramembranous ossification can also result in the formation of bones in abnormal locations such as testes or whites of the eyes. Such bones are called heterotopic bones (*hetero* = different; *topos* = place). If cartilage serves as the precursor for the bone, formation is called endochondral ossification. Because of remodeling that occurs later, the initial bone laid down by either method is eventually replaced.

Intramembranous ossification

Early in embryonic development, elongate mesenchymal cells migrate and aggregate in specific regions of the body. Remember, mesenchyme is tissue from which all connective tissue develops. As these cells condense, they form the membrane from which the bone will develop (Fig. 6.6). This presumptive bone site becomes more vascularized with time, and the mesenchymal cells enlarge and become rounder. As the mesenchymal cells change from eosinophilic (i.e., stained with eosin dyes) to basophilic (affinity for basic dyes), they differentiate into osteoblasts. These cells secrete the collagen and proteoglycans (osteoid) of the bone matrix. As the osteoid is deposited, the osteoblasts become increasingly separated from one another, although they remain connected by thin cytoplasmic processes.

The site where the matrix begins to calcify is called the ossification center. Eventually, as the matrix becomes calcified, the osteoblasts become osteocytes. The osteocytes are contained in canaliculi. Some of the surrounding primitive cells in the membrane proliferate and give rise to osteoprogenitor cells. These cells come in opposition to the spicules, and become osteoblasts, thus adding more matrix. This results in appositional growth in which the spicules (areas of calcification extending from the ossification center) enlarge and become joined into a trabecular network having the shape of bone.

Endochondral ossification

Endochondral ossification begins similar to intramembranous ossification, with mesenchymal cells migrating and aggregating (Fig. 6.7). However, these cells now become chondroblasts, instead of osteoblasts, and begin making a cartilage matrix. Once made, the cartilage matrix grows by both interstitial and appositional growth. Interstitial growth is responsible for most of the increase in length of the bone, whereas the increase in width is produced by new chondrocytes that differentiate from the chondrogenic layer of the perichondrium surrounding the cartilage mass.

Bone formation begins when perichondrial cells in the midregion give rise to osteoblasts rather than chondrocytes. At this point, the connective tissue surrounding the middle of the cartilage changes from perichondrium to periosteum. A thin layer of bone begins forming around the cartilage model. This bone can be called either periosteal bone because of its location, or endochondral bone because of its method of

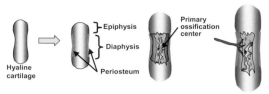

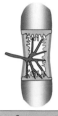

Step 1:	Step 2:	Step 3:	Step 4:
A hyaline cartilage model is produced by chondrocytes. It increases in length by interstitial growth, but also grows by appositional growth	The connective tissue around the middle of the cartilage changes to periosteum, which is osteogenic and contains osteoblasts	Chondrocytes in midregion hypertrophy forming irregular cartilage plates; cells synthesize alkaline phosphatase; surrounding matrix calcifies	Chondrocytes die, matrix begins breaking down. Blood vessels grow into this region. Fibroblasts migrate with blood vessels, differentiate into osteoblasts; they lay down osteoid on remaining spicules

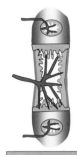

Step 5:	Step 6:
Chondrocytes die; calcified matrix begins breaking down. Other primitive cells enter via new vasculature and give rise to marrow. Endochondral bone forms on remaining spicules	A secondary ossification center is established in the upper epiphysis.

Fig. 6.7. Endochondral ossification.

development. This periosteal bone is sometimes termed the bony collar.

As the chondrocytes in the midregion become hypertrophic, the matrix becomes compressed. These cells begin to synthesize alkaline phosphatase, and the surrounding matrix begins to calcify. As the chondrocytes die, the matrix breaks down and the neighboring lacunae become interconnected. At the same time, blood vessels begin to enter this diaphyseal area vascularizing the developing cavity.

Cells from the periosteum migrate inward with the blood vessels and become osteoprogenitor cells. Other cells also enter to give rise to the marrow. The breakdown of the matrix leaves spicules that become lined with osteoprogenitor cells that then differentiate into osteoblasts. Osteoblasts then begin to produce the osteoid on the spicule framework. Bone formed in this manner is called endochondral bone, and this region becomes the primary ossification center. As the cartilage is resorbed (i.e., broken down), the bone deposited on the calcified spicules becomes spongy bone.

Eventually, a secondary ossification center develops in each epiphysis. Bone develops in these regions similarly to that in the primary ossification center. As the secondary ossification develops, the only cartilage remaining is that at the ends of the bones, and a transverse region known as the epiphyseal plate separating the diaphyseal and epiphyseal cavities.

As the cavity in the diaphyseal marrow enlarges, there is a distinct zonation that develops in the cartilage at either end of the diaphysis (Fig. 6.8). The following five regions develop beginning most distal from the diaphysis:

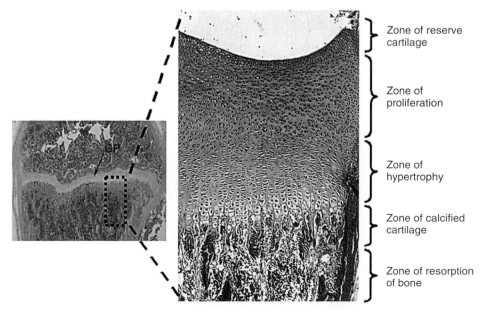

Zone of reserve cartilage

Zone of proliferation

Zone of hypertrophy

Zone of calcified cartilage

Zone of resorption of bone

Fig. 6.8. Epiphyseal plate. The area between the diaphysis and epiphysis is the growth plate (GP), and it is characterized by distinct zonation as shown in this longitudinal section.

1. Zone of reserve cartilage. This region contains no cellular proliferation or matrix production. It contains small, scattered chondrocytes.
2. Zone of proliferation. The cartilage cells are dividing and organized in distinct columns in this area. The cells are larger than in the reserve zone, and are producing matrix.
3. Zone of hypertrophy. The cartilage cells are large with a clear cytoplasm containing glycogen in this region. The matrix is found in columns between the cells.
4. Zone of calcified cartilage. This area contains enlarged cells that are degenerating. The matrix is calcified.
5. Zone of resorption: Nearest the diaphysis, the cartilage in this region is in direct contact with connective tissue in the marrow cavity.

Bone growth, remodeling, and repair

Bone growth

As the bone grows, there is constant internal and external remodeling in the epiphyseal plate. While the epiphyseal plate remains constant in size, new cartilage is produced in the zone of proliferation while a similar amount of cartilage is resorbed in the zone of resorption due to the action of osteocytes. The resorbed cartilage is replaced by spongy bone produced by osteoblasts found between the zone of resorption and the diaphysis. As the cells in the proliferative region divide, an increase in length of the bone occurs as the epiphysis is moved away from the diaphysis.

The width of bone is increased by appositional growth of bone that occurs between the cortical lamellae and the periosteum as bone resorption occurs on the endosteal surface of the outermost region of the bone. As bones elongate, they are constantly remodeling, which involves resorption of bone in some areas concomitant with deposition in other areas.

Eventually, new cartilage production ceases. The cartilage that is present in the epiphyseal plate is converted to bone until no more cartilage exists. This is termed epiphyseal closure, and growth of the bone is complete. The only remaining cartilage is at the articular (i.e., regions where bones form joints) surfaces on the bone. The epiphyseal plate now becomes the epiphyseal line.

The major hormone controlling bone growth in young animals is growth hormone that is released from the anterior pituitary. Excessive secretion of growth hormone can cause gigantism, whereas hyposecretion can cause dwarfism. Thyroid hormones also play an important role in bone development. The action of these hormones is discussed in Chapter 12.

Bone remodeling and repair

While bone may appear to be dormant after animals reach adulthood, this is not true. In fact, bone remains very active, and is constantly being broken down (resorbed) and replaced in response to various physical or hormonal changes. This constant breakdown by osteoclasts and formation by osteoblasts is termed remodeling, and occurs at both the periosteal and endosteal surfaces.

The breakdown of bone by osteoclasts is called bone resorption. Osteoclasts bind tightly to either the endosteum or periosteum forming a leakproof seal. The osteoclasts release lysosomal enzymes and acids into this sealed region, which then digests the collagen fibers and organic matrix while the acid digests the minerals. The digested components are engulfed by the osteoclasts by endocytosis, packaged into vesicles, translocated across the osteoclast by the process of transcytosis, and released by exocytosis into the interstitial space where the material is absorbed into the capillaries. The canal that is formed establishes the future Haversian system. Eventually, the osteoclasts are replaced by osteoblasts that rebuild the bone.

Hormonal control

The control of bone homeostasis is poorly understood. Since bones are a major calcium storage site, calcium homeostasis plays a major role in bone mineralization (Fig. 6.9). The two hormones involved in calcium homeostasis are parathyroid hormone (PTH), produced by the parathyroid glands, and calcitonin, from the parafollicular cells (C cells) of the thyroid gland). PTH is released in response to low plasma ionic calcium levels, while calcitonin is released when plasma ionic calcium levels rise.

If resorption predominates, bones get weak such as in osteoporosis. If deposition predominates, bone spurs can develop. Estrogens are known to reduce bone resorption whereas parathyroid hormone promotes bone resorption. The decrease in estrogen level associated with menopause is linked with a weakening of the bones.

Repair of fractures

Fractures can be classified several ways:

- Bone end alignment. If the bone ends remained aligned following a fracture, it is called a nondisplaced fracture. Displaced fractures occur when the bone ends are out of alignment.
- Degree of break. If the break is all the way through the bone, it is termed a complete fracture; if not all the way through, it is an incomplete break.

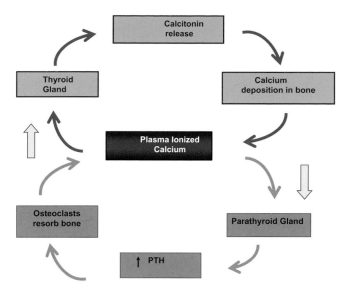

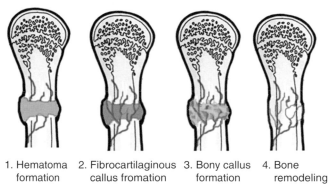

1. Hematoma formation   2. Fibrocartilaginous callus fromation   3. Bony callus formation   4. Bone remodeling

Fig. 6.10.   Steps in fracture repair.

Fig. 6.9.   Hormonal control of plasma ionic calcium concentration. An increase in plasma ionic calcium concentration results in the release of calcitonin from the thyroid gland. Calcitonin stimulates calcium deposition in bone. In contrast, a decrease in plasma ionic calcium concentration stimulates the release of parathyroid hormone (PTH) from the parathyroid glands, which promotes osteoclast activity resulting in an increase in plasma ionic calcium levels.

- Orientation of the break. If the break is parallel to the long axis, it is a linear fracture; if it is perpendicular to the long axis, it is a transverse fracture.
- Skin penetration. If bone protrudes through the skin, it is an open, or compound, fracture. A nonprotruding break is called a closed, or simple fracture.

The repair process for a fractured bone involves four steps (Fig. 6.10):

1. Hematoma formation. As a result of a fracture, the blood vessels tear causing the formation of a hematoma, a mass of clotted blood, at the fracture site. Bone cells begin to die and the site shows the classic signs of inflammation, i.e., pain, swelling, redness, and loss of function.
2. Fibrocartilaginous callus formation. Capillaries grow into the hematoma from which phagocytic cells invade and remove the debris. Fibroblasts and osteoblasts migrate into the fractured area from the periosteum and endosteum. The fibroblasts form collagen fibers, which serve to span the space in the break, thus connecting the two ends. As the fibroblasts differentiate into chondroblasts, they secrete cartilage matrix. Finally, osteoblasts close to the capillaries begin forming spongy bone; those found further away, secrete a bulging cartilaginous matrix. This entire mass,

called a fibrocartilaginous callus, spans the fractured area.
3. Bony callus formation. Bone trabeculae begin to appear as a result of the actions of the osteoblasts converting the fibrocartilaginous callus into a bony callus made of spongy (or woven) bone. Bony callus formation continues until the two ends of the bone are firmly attached.
4. Bone remodeling. Remodeling begins during bony callus formation and continues until the bony callus is remodeled. The excess material is removed from both the periosteal and endosteal area, and compact bone is formed along the shaft.

Response to mechanical stress

Although bone deposition occurs in response to a bone injury, it can also occur when additional strength is needed. This can occur in response to new physical pressures placed on the bone as would occur if the bone is bearing weight at a different angle. Wolff's law states that a bone grows or remodels in response to forces placed on the bone. Such forces include weight bearing on the bone or muscles pulling on the bone. Since such forces are generally off-center, they tend to bend the bone. In response, the compact bone thickens on one side while thinning on the other side through the remodeling process. Spongy bone forms in the middle since mechanical forces acting on the bone sum to zero in this region (Fig. 6.11).

Nutrients necessary for bone deposition

Bone deposition requires vitamin C for collagen synthesis, vitamin D for calcium absorption in the gut, and vitamin A for bone deposition and removal, in addition to calcium, phosphorus, magnesium, and manganese.

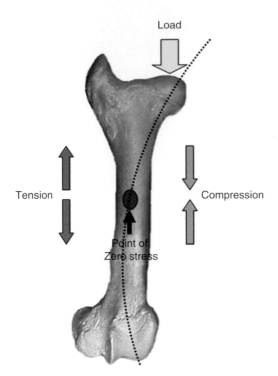

Fig. 6.11. Mechanical stress on bone. Using the femur as an example, the bone is acted upon by the load of the body weight. This load is transmitted through the bone as indicated by the dashed arc. This causes compression on one side of the bone while stretching the other side. These two forces sum to zero in the middle of the bone, creating the point of zero stress.

Homeostatic imbalances of bone

Osteomalacia and rickets

Osteomalacia is a condition in which the bones are insufficiently mineralized. Rickets is a name for the same condition when it is present in prepubertal animals. While osteoid is produced, calcium salts are not deposited; thus the bones remain soft. This is caused by inadequate calcium or vitamin D in the diet. Vitamin D is necessary for intestinal absorption of Ca^{2+}. When blood calcium levels decrease due to inadequate intestinal absorption, parathyroid hormone maintains plasma Ca^{2+} by stimulating the release of Ca^{2+} from the bone.

Parturient paresis (milk fever)

As dairy cattle begin milk production, the first milk produced (called colostrum) contains high concentrations of Ca^{2+}. Colostrum requires approximately 3 g of calcium per hour to produce. When the cow cannot mobilize this amount of calcium, she can develop milk

fever within 72 hrs following parturition. Symptoms include loss of appetite, followed by muscle weakness, decreased body temperature, labored breathing, and paralysis of hind legs. If left untreated, the cow can collapse into a coma and die.

To prevent milk fever, cows should be given sufficient vitamin D in the diet prior to parturition. If milk fever develops, cows are given an oral bolus of calcium carbonate.

Egg-laying fatigue in birds

Similar to milk fever in cows, high-producing egg-laying hens can develop weak and brittle bones. A hen must deposit as much as 8–10% of her total calcium into the eggshell each day. Since the eggshell is deposited during the night, the hen must draw upon the calcium reserves located in a specialized type of bone called medullary bone. Under the influence of estrogens and androgens secreted from the developing follicles, medullary bone is produced in hens 2 weeks prior to commencement of egg laying. As blood calcium levels decrease during eggshell formation, the hen releases parathyroid hormone, which mobilizes bone calcium. If there are insufficient stores of calcium in the bones, the bones become weaker as they become demineralized.

Bones and skeleton

Markings on bones

The surface of bone is seldom smooth. Instead, it contains various depressions, bumps, and ridges that serve as sites where muscles and tendons originate or attach, and blood vessels and nerves travel. These various markings are shown in Table 6.1 and Figure 6.12. Learning them is helpful when studying the origins and insertions of muscles.

Skeleton

The skeleton includes all the bones of the body. These bones, and their articulations, have been altered during evolution to accommodate various functions. Therefore, the skeleton is an excellent example of the complementary nature of form and function. The skeletons of various species are shown in Figure 6.13. Since most of the remainder of the chapter is concerned with mammals, a brief discussion of features unique to avian species will be included at the end of the section on the skeleton.

Table 6.1. Bone markings.

Term	Description	Example
Projections Where Muscles and Ligaments Attach		
Crest	Narrow ridge of bone; usually prominent	Iliac crest
Epicondyle	Raised area on or above a condyle	Lateral epicondyle of the humerus
Fossa	Shallow depression, often serving as an articular surface	Olecranon and radial fossae of the humerus
Line	Narrow ridge of bone; less prominent than a crest	Gluteal line on wing of ilium
Process	Generally any bony prominence; sometimes used to name specific prominences	Crest, spine, trochanter, tubercle, tuberosity, etc.; olecranon process
Ramus	Armlike bar of bone	Ramus of the mandible
Spine	Sharp, slender, often pointed projection	Spine of the scapula
Tuberosity	Large rounded projection	Deltoid tuberosity of the humerus
Trochanter	Very large, blunt, irregular-shaped process; found only on the femur	Trochanter of the femur
Tubercle	Small rounded projection or process	Greater tubercle of the humerus
Projections That Help Form Joints		
Condyle	Rounded articular projection	Occipital condyle of the skull
Cotyloid	A deep articular depression	Acetabulum of the hip joint
Facet	Smooth, nearly flat articular surface	Superior costal facet of the vertebrae
Head	Bony expansion carried on a narrow neck	Head of the femur
Trochlea	A pulley-shaped, articular structure	Trochlea of the femur
Depressions and Openings Allowing Blood Vessels and Nerves to Pass		
Fissure	Narrow, slitlike opening	Palatine fissure
Foramen	Round or oval opening through a bone	Foramen magnum
Fovea	A shallow, nonarticular depression	Fovea capitis on the head of the femur
Incisure	A notch-shaped depression at the edge of a bone	Semilunar notch of the ulna
Meatus	Canal-like passageway	External auditory meatus
Sinus	Cavity within a bone, filled with air and lined with mucous membrane	Nasal sinuses
Sulcus	Furrowlike groove	Brachial groove of the humerus

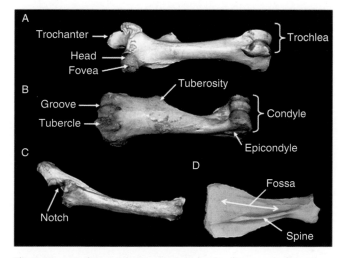

Fig. 6.12. Marking on bones. Various bovine bones are shown, including the femur (A), humerus (B), radius-ulna (C), and scapula (D), which are labeled to illustrate bone markings.

Functions of the skeletal system

The skeleton has five primary functions:

1. Support. The skeletal system provides the structure to which the bones attach, as well as the structural support for the entire body.
2. Storage of minerals and lipids. The bones provide a major storage for various minerals, particularly calcium. In addition, the bones contain a substantial amount of lipid.
3. Blood cell production. The bone marrow is a site of formation for all types of blood cells.
4. Protection. The vital organs of the body are protected by the skeletal system. The ribs surround the visceral organs, whereas the central nervous system is encased within the skull and spinal cord.
5. Leverage. Many of the joints of the body act as levers therefore assisting with movement.

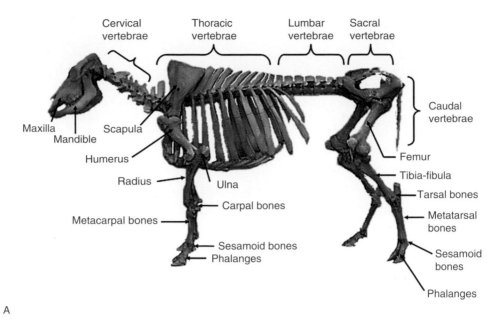

A

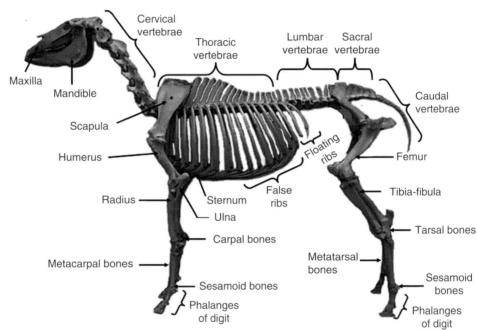

B

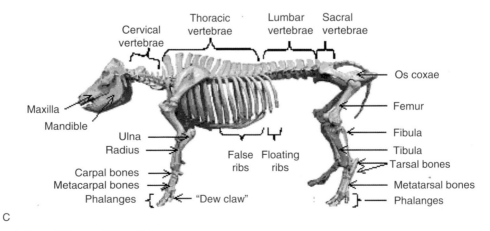

C

Fig. 6.13. Skeletons. A) Cow. B) Horse. C) Pig. D) Dog.

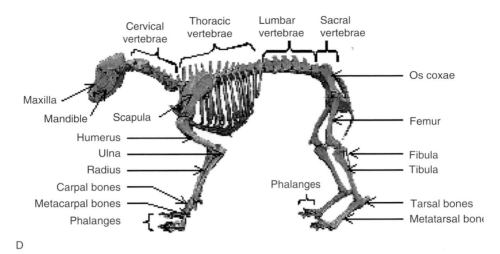

Cervical vertebrae · Thoracic vertebrae · Lumbar vertebrae · Sacral vertebrae · Os coxae · Femur · Fibula · Tibula · Maxilla · Mandible · Scapula · Humerus · Ulna · Radius · Carpal bones · Metacarpal bones · Phalanges · Phalanges · Tarsal bones · Metatarsal bone

D

Fig. 6.13. *Continued*

Skeletal cartilage

Types of cartilage

The skeleton begins as cartilage and fibrous membranes, but then is replaced with ossified tissue as the animal develops through gestation. Cartilage contains no nerves or blood vessels and is surrounded by a layer of dense irregular connective tissue called the perichondrium. Blood vessels found within the perichondrium provide nutrients for the chondrocytes within the cartilage.

There are three types of cartilage found in the skeleton. Hyaline cartilage is the most abundant and provides support and flexibility for the skeleton. The matrix contains only fine collagen fibers. Hyaline cartilage is found 1) on articular surfaces, 2) within costal cartilage connecting the ribs to the sternum, 3) in the respiratory cartilages forming the skeleton of the larynx and reinforcing passageways of the respiratory system, and 4) in nasal cartilages supporting the external nose.

Elastic cartilage contains more elastic fibers than hyaline cartilage. It, therefore, is better able to withstand bending. It is found in only two places in the skeleton: 1) the external ear, and 2) the epiglottis, which is the flap of tissue that covers the opening of the larynx during swallowing.

Fibrocartilage is highly compressible, possessing great tensile strength. It contains approximately parallel rows of chondrocytes with intervening thick collagen fibers. It is found in the menisci within the knee and intervertebral discs.

Growth of cartilage

Cartilage can continue to grow by two processes. Appositional growth occurs when new cartilage forms

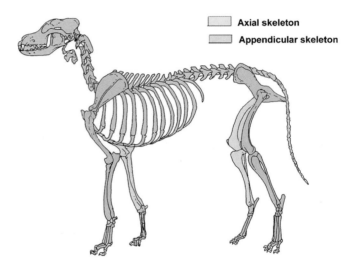

☐ **Axial skeleton**
☐ **Appendicular skeleton**

Fig. 6.14. Axial and appendicular skeleton. As shown with this dog skeleton. The axial skeleton includes the bones and cartilage protecting the soft structures in the head, neck, and trunk, and consists of the skull, hyoid apparatus, vertebral column, and thorax. The appendicular skeleton includes the limbs and bones connecting the limbs to the axial skeleton.

on the surface of preexisting cartilage. Interstitial growth occurs from inside of the cartilage mass in which lacunae-bound chondrocytes inside the cartilage divide and secrete new matrix, thereby expanding the cartilage from within.

Skeleton classification

The skeleton is divided into the appendicular skeleton and the axial skeleton (Fig. 6.14). The axial skeleton includes the skull, hyoid apparatus, vertebral column, ribs, and sternum. The appendicular skeleton includes the bones of the limbs and limb girdles. The thoracic limb or pectoral limb includes the scapula, humerus, radius, ulna, carpal bones, metacarpal bones, phalanges, and their sesamoid bones. The thoracic girdle or shoulder girdle includes the two scapulae, and the clavicle in man, which holds the shoulder laterally, but which is only vestigial in domestic animals.

Axial skeleton

The skull

The skull is a very complex structure made mostly of flat bones. Except for the mandible that is attached via a movable joint, the bones of the skull are connected by interlocking joints called sutures. The suture joints are characterized by a saw-toothed or serrated appearance that keeps the bones attached, but allows the cranium to expand and contract while remaining intact.

Suture lines are visible between the bones of the skull (Fig. 6.15). The internasal suture is between the two nasal bones while the frontonasal suture separates the frontal bones from the nasal bones. The frontoparietal suture separates the frontal bones from the parietal bones. The nasomaxillary suture separates the nasal bones from the maxillary bones.

The skull contains both cranial and facial bones (Table 6.2). The cranium includes those bones that surround the brain. The cranium consists of the cranial vault, also called the calvaria, forming the superior, lateral, and posterior aspects of the skull, and the cranial base or floor that forms the inferior aspect of the cranium. The cranial base is divided by bony ridges into three distinct fossae: the anterior, middle, and posterior cranial fossa. The cranial bones form the cranial cavity that houses the brain, and also provide the site for attachment of head and neck muscles.

The skull contains approximately 85 named openings, including foramina, canals, fissures, and orbits. These provide passageways for the spinal cord, blood vessels, and the 12 cranial nerves to enter and leave the brain.

Cranium

The roof of the cranium is formed by the paired frontal and parietal bones (Fig. 6.16). The caudal aspect of the skull is formed by the unpaired occipital bone. The floor of the cranium is formed by the unpaired sphenoid bone. Finally, the rostral wall of the cranium is formed by the ethmoid bone.

The facial bones include those bones enclosing the nasal and oral cavities. These bones form the structure of the face; contain cavities for special senses, including sight, taste, and smell; provide openings for air and food; secure teeth; and provide attachment sites

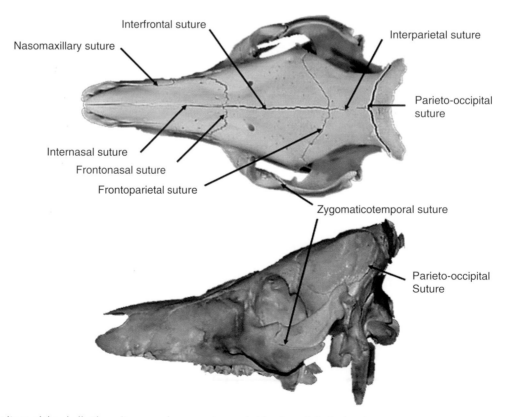

Fig. 6.15.   Suture lines of the skull. These lines are shown on top and side view of skull of a pig.

Table 6.2. Bones of the skull.

Term	Description	Major Markings
Cranial Bones (Number)		
Frontal (2)	The rostral portion of the roof of the cranial cavity in most domestic species; in the ox, it forms the entire roof of the cranial cavity	Supraorbital foramina—allows the supraorbital arteries and nerves to pass
Parietal (2)	Along with frontal, forms the roof of the cranial cavity in most domestic animals except ox	
Occipital (1)	Forms caudal aspect of the cranial cavity, as well as the skull	Foramen magnum—allows spinal cord to enter the vertebral canal Hypoglossal canal—passageway for hypoglossal nerve (XII) Occipital condyles—articulate with the atlas (first cervical vertebra) External occipital protuberance—site of muscle attachments; site of attachment of ligamentum nuchae in horse and ruminants
Temporal (2)	Forms caudolateral wall of the cranial cavity	Zygomatic process—forms part of zygomatic arch, which forms bulge in cheek Mandibular fossa—articulation site for mandibular condyle External auditory meatus—canal leading from external ear to the eardrum Styloid process—attachment site for hyoid bone and some neck muscles Mastoid process—attachment site for some neck and tongue muscles Stylomastoid foramen—passageway for facial nerve (VII) Jugular foramen—passageway for internal jugular vein and cranial nerves IX, X, and XI Internal acoustic meatus—passageway for cranial nerves VII and VIII Carotid canal—passageway for internal carotid artery
Sphenoid (1)	Unpaired bone forming floor of cranial cavity; it has several parts, including the body, greater wings, lesser wings, and pterygoid processes	Sella turcica—helps form cavity for pituitary Optic canals—passageway for optic nerve (II) and ophthalmic arteries Superior orbital tissures—passageway for cranial nerves III, IV, VI, part of V, and ophthalmic vein Foramen rotundum—passageway for mandibular division of cranial nerve V Foramen ovale—passageway for cranial nerve V Foramen spinosum—passageway for middle meningeal artery
Ethmoid (1)	Unpaired bone forming rostral wall of cranial cavity; forms part of the nasal septum, caudal wall of nasal cavity, and part of medial wall of the orbit	Crista galli—attachment for the falx cerebri portion of dura mater Cribriform plate—passageway for the olfactory nerves (I) Dorsal and middle nasal conchae—forms part of lateral walls of nasal cavity
Facial Bones (Number)		
Mandible (1)	The lower jaw	Coronoid processes—insertion site of temporalis muscles Mandibular condyles—articulate with the temporal bones forming the temporomandibular joint in the jaw Mandibular symphysis—medial fusion site of mandibular bones Alveoli—sockets for teeth Mandibular foramina—passageway for alveolar nerves Mental foramina—passageway for blood vessels and nerves going to the chin and lower lip

Table 6.2. *Continued*

Term	Description	Major Markings
Maxilla (2)	Forms the upper jaw, and parts of the hard palate, orbits, and nasal cavity	Alveoli—sockets for teeth Zygomatic processes—forms caudal part of zygomatic arches Palatine processes—forms much of the bony hard palate Incisive—passageway for blood vessels and nerves going through hard palate (fused palatine processes) Orbital fissures—passageway for maxillary branch of cranial nerve V, the zygomatic nerve and blood vessels Infraorbital foramen—passageway of infraorbital nerve to skin of face
Zygomatic (2)	Cranial portion of zygomatic arch; forms part of cheek and orbit	Temporal process—forms cranial part of zygomatic arch
Nasal (2)	Along with cranial portion of frontal bone, forms osseous roof of nasal cavity	
Lacrimal (2)	Forms medial surface of orbit	Lacrimal fossa—houses the lacrimal sac
Palatine (2)	Forms part of hard palate along with maxillary and incisive bones	
Vomer (1)	Unpaired bone forming part of osseous nasal septum	
Ventral nasal concha (2)	A fragile scroll of bone that increases nasal surface area	
Pterygoid (2)	Small bones in caudal part of nasopharynx	
Incisive or premaxillary (1)	Holds upper incisors	

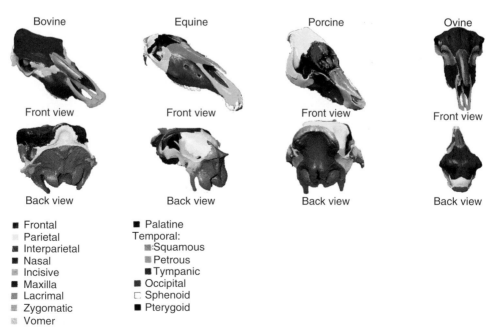

Fig. 6.16. Skulls of various species. The skulls of different species showing main bones.

- ■ Frontal
- ▢ Parietal
- ▨ Interparietal
- ■ Nasal
- ▨ Incisive
- ■ Maxilla
- ▨ Lacrimal
- ▨ Zygomatic
- ▨ Vomer
- ■ Palatine
- Temporal:
  - ▨ Squamous
  - ▨ Petrous
  - ■ Tympanic
- ■ Occipital
- ▢ Sphenoid
- ■ Pterygoid

A

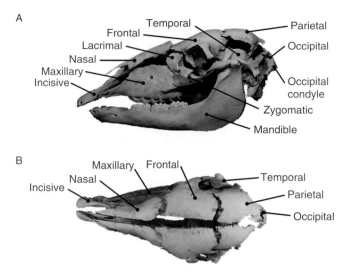

B

Fig. 6.17. Exploded equine skull. The various bones of the equine skull have been separated, showing side (A) and top (B) view.

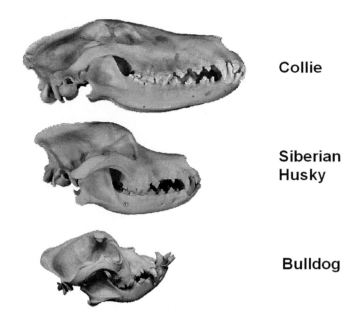

Collie

Siberian Husky

Bulldog

Fig. 6.18. Examples of dog skulls. The three general types of dog skulls are represented. The collie, Siberian husky, and bulldog represent the dolichephalic, mesaticephalic, and brachiocephalic types of skulls, respectively. Note the relatively long facial component on the collie and the short facial component on the bulldog.

for facial muscles. The facial region is divided into the oral, nasal, and orbital regions.

The oral region includes the incisive, maxillary, and palatine bones, as well as the mandible surrounding the oral cavity. The nasal region includes the nasal, maxillary, palatine, and incisive bones surrounding the nasal cavity. The orbital region includes the bony socket holding the eye, formed by portions of the frontal, lacrimal, palatine, sphenoid, and zygomatic bones. The zygomatic arch, which forms the ventral wall of the orbit, consists of the zygomatic bone and the zygomatic process of the temporal bones. An exploded view of the equine skull is shown in Figure 6.17.

Species differences

Unique to the horse and cat, the interparietal bone is found between the two parietal bones. In other species, this bone is present in the fetus, but fuses with surrounding bones during gestation. In the ox, the frontal bone forms the entire roof of the cranium, whereas the parietal bones help form the roof in other species.

In the dog, there are three types of skulls based on the proportions of the facial bones and cranial cavity (Fig. 6.18).

1. Mesaticephalic. Average conformation. Example, Siberian husky.
2. Dolichephalic. Has an elongated facial component. Example, collie.
3. Brachiocephalic. Has a shorter facial component. Example, bulldog.

The vertebral column

The vertebral column, also called the spine, protects the spinal cord, supports the head and serves as an attachment site for muscles affecting body movements. It consists of irregular bones connected by slightly movable joints.

The vertebrae (sing. = vertebra) are the irregularly shaped bones making up the spinal column. They are grouped into the cervical (neck), thoracic (back), lumbar (loin), sacral (croup), and caudal (tail) vertebrae. Each is named by the first letter of the group followed by the number within the group, e.g., C1, T3, L5, S3, and Ca20. The number of vertebrae by species is shown in Table 6.3.

Typical vertebrae are shown in Figure 6.19. The common features of a vertebra include the body, vertebral arch, vertebral foramen, and processes. The body is the thick, spool-shaped ventral portion of the vertebra. It is convex at the cranial end and concave at the caudal end, allowing articulation with the adjacent vertebrae. The vertebral arch is the dorsal portion of the vertebra consisting of two upright pedicles that form the wall of the vertebral foramen. Two half- (or hemi-) laminae project from the pedicles, and, meeting in the midline to complete the lamina, form the roof of the vertebral foramen. The vertebral foramen of each vertebra connects to form the vertebral canal.

Table 6.3. Number of vertebrae.

Species	Cervical	Thoracic	Lumbar	Sacral	Caudal
Carnivore	C7	T13	L7	S3	Ca20–24
Pig	C7	T11–15	L6–7	S4	Ca20–23
Horse	C7	T18	L6	S5	Ca15–21
Ox	C7	T13	L6	S5	Ca18–20
Sheep	C7	T13	L6–7	S4	Ca16–18
Chicken	C7	T7	L14 (lumbarsacral)		

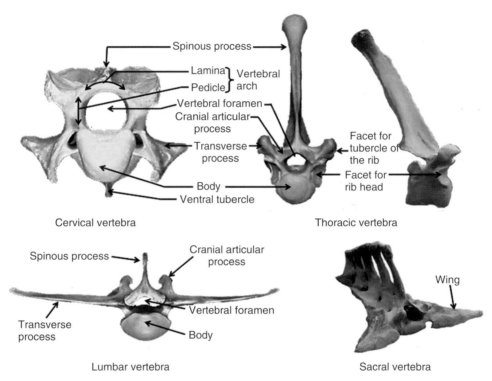

Fig. 6.19. Examples of various vertebrae. Examples of cervical, thoracic, lumbar, and sacral vertebrae are shown. Note that the cervical vertebrae have a reduced spinous process. Thoracic vertebrae have an exaggerated spinous process, and lumbar vertebrae have an exaggerated transverse process. Sacral vertebrae are generally fused, with the processes also tending to fuse.

There are seven processes coming from each vertebra. These include a midsaggital dorsal projection called the spinous process, two lateral extensions called the transverse processes, and four articular processes. The articular processes include two cranial and two caudal articular processes.

The first and second cervical vertebrae are called the atlas and axis, respectively (Fig. 6.20). The atlas supports the head, hence its name. It articulates with the occipital condyles (see Fig 6.17) forming the atlanto-occipital joint, which allows the head to make a "yes" motion, i.e., flexion and extension. The atlas is unique in that it lacks a body or a spinal process. The axis contains a large ridgelike spinous process and the dens, a peglike cranial process forming a pivot articulation with the atlas, and allowing a "no" motion.

The thoracic vertebrae have articular facets for each pair of ribs to which they attach. The anticlinal vertebra is the one with the most upright-oriented dorsal process. Cranial to this vertebra, the dorsal processes are inclined cranially while those caudal to this vertebra are inclined caudally. This is an important landmark when reading radiographs.

Lumbar vertebrae are characterized by their large size and long, flatlike transverse processes. These vertebrae also lack costal facets since ribs do not articulate with them.

The sacral vertebrae fuse to form the sacrum. The wings of the sacrum (Fig. 6.19) articulate with the ilium forming the sacroiliac joint. This is the one site of connection between the axial skeleton and pelvic limb. Each sacral vertebra has dorsal and ventral foramina allowing the passage of spinal nerves.

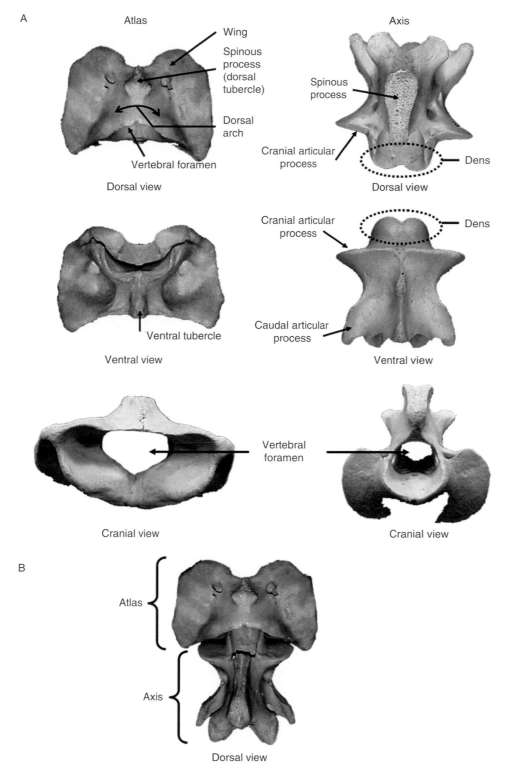

Fig. 6.20. Atlas and axis. The atlas and axis are the first and second cervical vertebrae, respectively. A) The dorsal, ventral and cranial views of the atlas and axis of a cow. B) The articulation between the atlas and axis.

Thorax

The thorax is the bony cavity formed by the sternum, ribs, costal cartilages, and bodies of the thoracic vertebrae (Fig. 6.21). The sternum, or breastbone, is composed of the unpaired bones (sternebrae) forming the floor of the thorax. The number of sternebrae is eight in carnivores; six in pigs, horses, and humans; and seven in ruminants. The manubrium is the enlarged first sternebra while the xiphoid process is the last

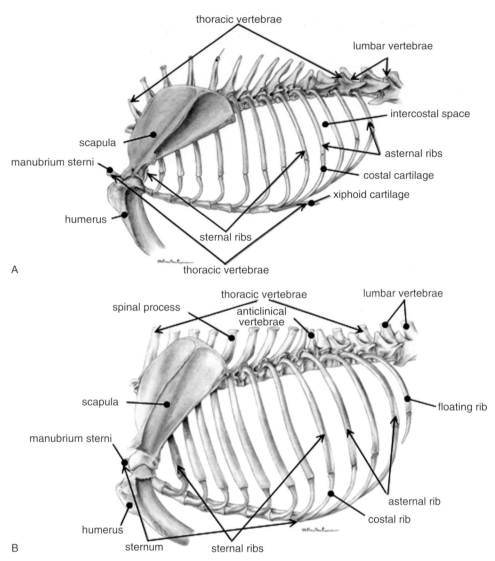

Fig. 6.21.   Thorax of different species. A) Lateral aspect of cat. B) Lateral aspect of dog. (Reprinted from Constantinescu, 2002. Used by permission of the publisher.)

sternebra capped by the xiphoid cartilage. The thoracic inlet is a region formed by the last cervical vertebra, the first pair of ribs, and the sternum.

The ribs consist of long, curved bones that form the lateral wall of the thorax. The ribs can be grouped as follows:

1. True ribs. They articulate directly to the sternum via their costal cartilage.
2. False ribs. They include all ribs that are not true ribs. Their costal cartilages merge to form the costal arch, which indirectly joins them to the sternum in all domestic species except the dog. Costal cartilage consists of hyaline cartilage.
3. Floating ribs. They include the last false ribs in the dog and man. There is one pair in dogs and two pairs in man. They end in costal cartilage that does not join to the sternum or the costal arch.

As shown in Figure 6.22, each rib consists of a head and a tubercle. The head articulates with the caudal and cranial costal fovea of adjacent thoracic vertebrae in the intervertebral disc found in between. The tubercle of the rib articulates with the transverse process of the same numbered vertebra. Between each rib is the intercostal space.

Appendicular skeleton

Thoracic limb

While humans have the clavicle to keep the shoulder in a lateral position, domestic animals lack this bone since their thoracic limb is maintained under their body. The top of the thoracic limb begins at the scapula.

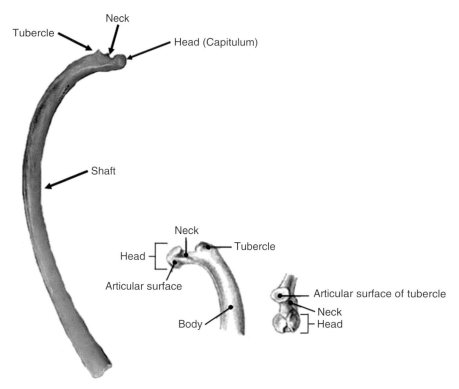

Fig. 6.22. Typical rib. A picture of a rib is shown. (The inserted rib drawing is from Constantinescu and Constantinescu, 2004.)

This is a flat, triangular bone in the shoulder (Fig. 6.23). The two scapulae constitute the thoracic girdle.

The lateral surface of the scapula contains the spine of the scapula that ends in the acromion, the expanded distal end of the spine of the scapula. The acromion is absent in the horse and pig. The area cranial to the spine is the supraspinous fossa; the area caudal to it is the infraspinous fossa. The medial surface of the scapula is called the subscapular fossa. On the dorsal border of the scapula is the scapular cartilage. The cavity in which the humerus articulates is the glenoid cavity. The supraglenoid tubercle, located near the cranial aspect of the glenoid cavity, is the site of attachment of the biceps brachii muscle. The coracoid process (Greek for "crowlike") is a small process on the medial side of the supraglenoid tubercle where the coracobrachialis muscle attaches. Found only in cats, the suprahamate process is a caudal projection from the acromion.

The humerus, sometimes called the brachial bone, is the largest bone in the thoracic limb (Fig. 6.24). It articulates proximally with the scapula in the glenoid cavity forming the shoulder joint, and distally with the radius and ulna forming the elbow joint.

The head of the humerus is a rounded process articulating with the glenoid cavity. The greater (lateral, major) tubercle is the large process craniolateral to the head, and can be palpated as the point of the shoulder. The lesser (medial, minor) tubercle is located on the medial side of the head. The bicipital, or intertubercular, groove is a sulcus between the greater and lesser tubercles through which the tendon of the biceps brachii muscle passes. The body of the humerus connects the two epiphyses of the bone. The deltoid tuberosity, to which the deltoid muscles attach, is the largest tuberosity on the bone. The distal end of the bone is called the humeral condyle and includes the humeral capitulum and humeral trochlea that are the two articulating surfaces, two fossae (three in cats), and the medial and lateral epicondyles. The olecranon fossa is a groove on the caudal surface of the distal end of the humerus in which the olecranon process of the ulna rests. The radial fossa, opposite the olecranon fossa, receives the proximal end of the radius while the elbow is flexed. The dog, and sometimes the pig, also has a supratrochlear foramen, which is a hole between the olecranon and radial fossa through which nothing passes.

The radius is the main weight-bearing bone of the forearm (Fig. 6.25). It articulates with the humerus and ulna in the elbow, and with the carpal bones and ulna at the distal end forming the antebrachiocarpal joint. The head of the radius articulates with the capitulum of the humerus, as well as the ulna. The styloid process is on the distal end of the radius.

The ulna functions mainly as a site for muscle attachments and formation of the elbow. It articulates proximately with the humerus and radius, and dis-

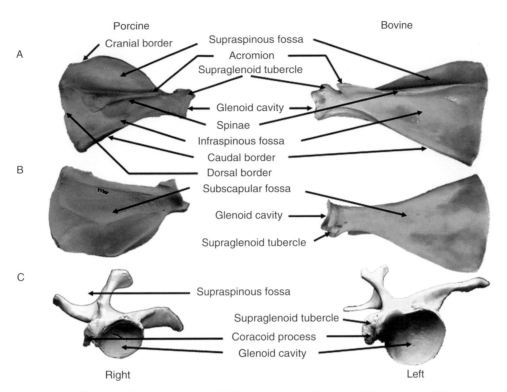

Fig. 6.23. Scapula of porcine and bovine. The lateral (A), medial (B), and caudal (C) views of the porcine and bovine scapula.

tally with the radius and carpal bones. The proximal end of the ulna is called the olecranon process, the point of the elbow, where the extensor muscles of the elbow attach. The trochlear notch is where the humerus articulates with the ulna. The distal end of the ulna also ends in the styloid process.

The radius and ulna fuse in the horse and ruminants. Because they are fused, these animals cannot supinate; therefore, the hand (mannus) is committed to permanent pronation. In contrast, these bones are not fused in carnivores; therefore, these animals can at least partially supinate their hands (paws).

Premature closing of the growth plates in the radius or ulna can cause deviations in these bones resulting in valgus or vargus deviations. Valgus is a lateral deviation distal to a joint; vargus is a medial deviation distal to a joint. For example, carpus valgus or carpus vargus are lateral and medial deviations distal to the carpus. Carpal valgus, a lateral deviation of the joints distal to the carpus, is also called "knock-knee"; carpal vargus, a medial deviation of the bones distal to the carpus, is called "bowlegged."

The distal portion of the thoracic limb is technically the manus (hand), commonly called the forepaw in carnivores (Fig. 6.26). It consists of the carpus, metacarpus, and digits, the latter with their individual phalanges, and their associated sesamoid bones.

The carpus, the wrist of man, consists of two transverse rows of carpal bones. The number of carpal bones varies between species. The pig and horse have eight carpal bones, although the first carpal bone in the distal row is sometimes missing in the horse. Dogs and cats have seven carpal bones due to the fusion of two carpal bones. Ruminants have six carpal bones since the first carpal bone is missing, the second and third are fused.

The metacarpal (MC) bones are located between the carpus and digits. In general, they are numbered I–V from medial to lateral. Species differ in the number of metacarpal bones due to absence or fusion of these bones. For example, the pig has four metacarpal bones since the MC I is missing, and the III and IV metacarpals are the weight-bearing bones; the II and V are reduced in size. Sesamoid bones (i.e., proximal and distal sesamoid bones) are associated with each weight-bearing metacarpal.

The horse has three metacarpals, with MC I and V missing. The II and IV metacarpals are commonly called splint bones because they are greatly reduced in size. The distal end of the splint bones is called the buttons of the splints. The III metacarpal is called the cannon bone.

Carnivores have five metacarpals, but MC I is reduced in size and bears no weight. It is part of the dewclaw, a digit that is not weight-bearing. Ruminants have two metacarpal bones since the MC I and II are missing and MC III and IV are fused into the so-called large metacarpal bone.

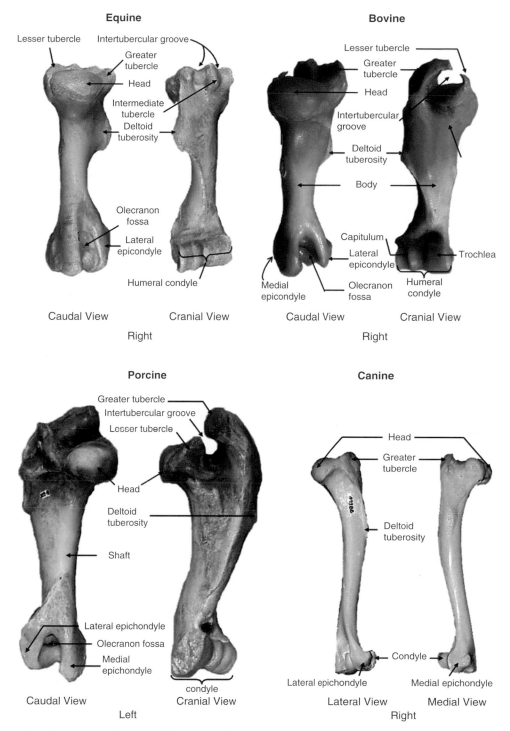

Fig. 6.24. Humerus of various species. The parts of the equine, bovine, porcine, and canine humerus.

The digits correspond with the fingers and toes of man. In general, there are five digits numbered from medial to lateral. However, the number varies by species. Digits generally consist of three phalanges, sesamoid bones, tendons, ligaments, vessels, nerves, and skin. The three phalanges are named the proximal phalanx, middle phalanx, and distal phalanx.

In carnivores, there are four main weight-bearing digits. The dewclaw consists of digit I and MC I. The first digit is reduced in size, and has only two phalanges and one proximal sesamoid bone. Horses have one digit per limb that corresponds with the MC III metacarpal bone; pigs have four digits, with the first missing.

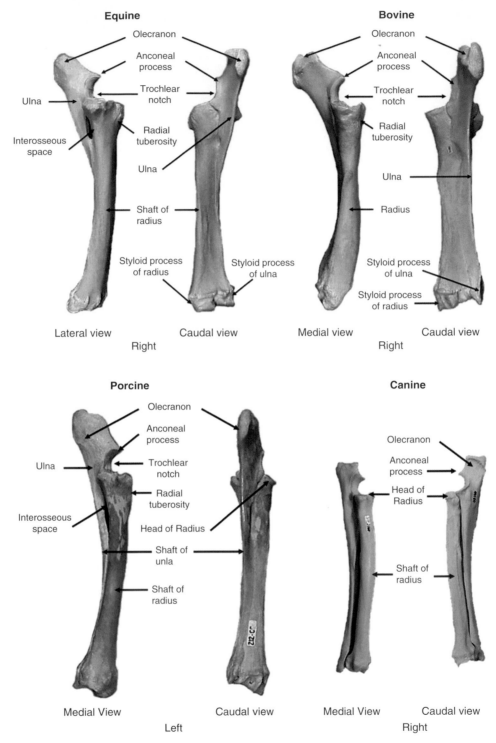

Fig. 6.25. Radius and ulna. The radius and ulna of various species.

Pelvic limb

The pelvic girdle, or bony pelvis, consists of the two hip bones (ossa coxarum), sacrum, and the first few caudal vertebrae (Fig. 6.27). It encases the pelvic cavity. The hip bone (os coxae) consists of the fused ilium, ischium, pubic, and acetabular bones. The acetabular bone is found in the center of the acetabulum, where it has fused with the other bones. The two hip bones are fused at the pelvic symphysis. This fusion includes the two pubic and two ischial bones.

The ilium is the largest and most cranial of the os coxae, consisting of a wing and body. It forms the cranial part of the acetabulum and articulates with the

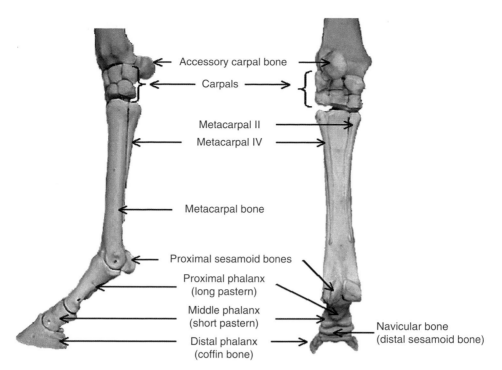

Accessory carpal bone

Carpals

Metacarpal II
Metacarpal IV

Metacarpal bone

Proximal sesamoid bones

Proximal phalanx
(long pastern)

Middle phalanx
(short pastern)

Distal phalanx
(coffin bone)

Navicular bone
(distal sesamoid bone)

Fig. 6.26. Lower leg, including the mannus, of the horse.

sacrum at the sacroiliac joint. The tuber coxae are the prominences of the lateral wings, sometimes called the "hook" in the ox. The tuber sacrale is the medial process of the wing next to the sacrum. The ischium is the caudal-most portion of the os coxae forming the horizontal portion of the obturator foramen, the large opening in the floor of the ox coxae. The ischiatic tuberosity ("pin bone" in the ox) is the caudal part of the ischium, and is referred to as the "sit bones" in man. The pubis forms the cranioventral part of the os coxae. It consists of a central body and two branches.

The acetabulum is the site where the head of the femur articulates. It is formed by the fusion of the ilium, ischium, pubic, and acetabular bones.

The femur, or thigh bone, articulates proximately with the hip bone forming the hip joint, and distally with the tibia forming the stifle joint (Fig. 6.28). Proximally, the head of the femur articulates with the acetabulum. There is a small depression, the fovea, in the head of the femur that allows for passage of the round ligament of the femur. The head of the femur is joined to the body of the femur by the neck. The greater trochanter is the large prominence found lateral to the head of the femur; the lesser trochanter is the smaller prominence found distal to the head on the medial side. Also found on the lateral side, distal to the greater trochanter, is the third trochanter, which is absent in dogs and ruminants. Note that trochanters are unique to the femur. The medial and lateral condyles are the two large prominences found at the distal end of

the femur, and articulate with the tibia. Also on the distal end of the femur is the patellar surface, a groove bordered by two ridges that articulates with the patella. The patella, or kneecap, is the largest sesamoid bone.

The tibia and fibula are located between the femur and metatarsal bones (Fig. 6.29). The tibia, or shin bone, is located medially, and is the major weight-bearing bone of the two bones. Located at the proximal end of the tibia are the medial and lateral condyles, separated by the intercondylar eminence. The condyles articulate with the corresponding condyles of the femur. The fibula is located more laterally and bears little weight. Distally, the fibula articulates with the tibia and the fibular tarsal bone. The distal fibula in the cow is represented by the separate malleolar bone.

The tarsus, or hock, consists of the three rows of bones between the tibia/fibula and metatarsal region (Fig. 6.30). Carnivores and pigs have seven tarsal bones, ruminants have five tarsal bones since four of them fuse, and horses have six.

The largest bone of the tarsus is the talus, or tibial tarsal bone. It is located on the dorsomedial side, and articulates with the tibia, or tibia and fibula in the dog, via its trochlea. The calcaneus is the second bone on the proximal row, just lateral to the talus. The calcanean tuberosity is a large process of the fibular tarsal bone acting as a lever for the common calcanean tendon, and is commonly called the point of the hock.

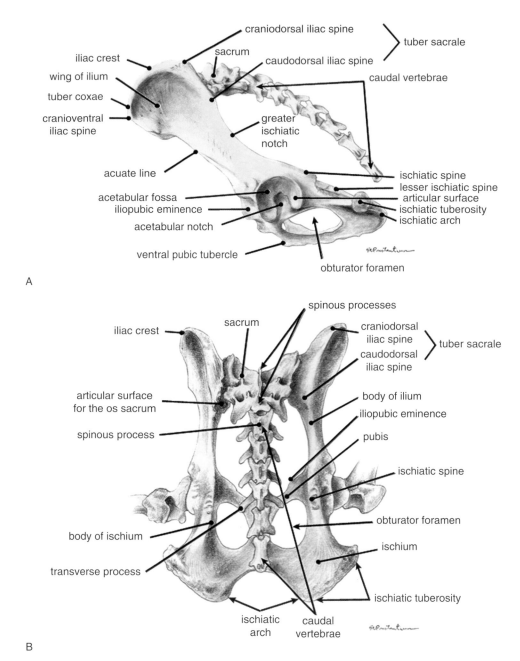

Fig. 6.27. Dog, pelvic girdle. A) Lateral view. B) Dorsal view. (Reprinted from Constantinescu, 2002. Used by permission of the publisher.)

Metatarsal bones and digits are located distal of the tarsus. In the horse and pig, they follow the same pattern as the thoracic limb. In carnivores, the first metatarsal bone is more reduced than in the front limb, and the digit is often absent. In ruminants, the first and fifth metatarsal bone is absent, and the second is reduced to a tiny element.

Avian skeleton

The skeleton of birds has been adapted for flight (Fig. 6.31). This has resulted in many significant differences compared to mammals. The neck consists of varying numbers of cervical vertebrae, with the joint between the vertebrae being synovial. The atlas articulates with a single occipital condyle, thus allowing great mobility. The extensive mobility in the atlanto-occipital joint and the neck allows the beak to be used in many motions.

The last cervical vertebra and first three thoracic vertebrae form the notarium. This fused structure, along with the synsacrum, provides rigidity to the spine in order to help with flight. The synsacrum consists of fused thoracic, lumbar, sacral, and caudal vertebrae. The synsacrum is also fused to the ilium. The

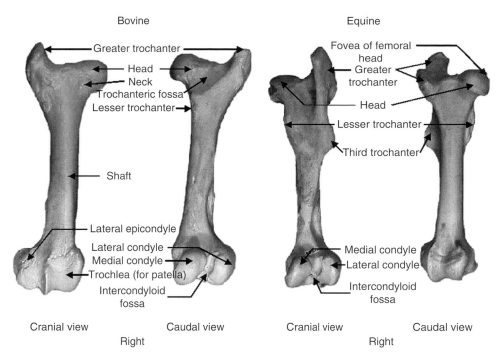

Fig. 6.28. Femur of bovine and equine.

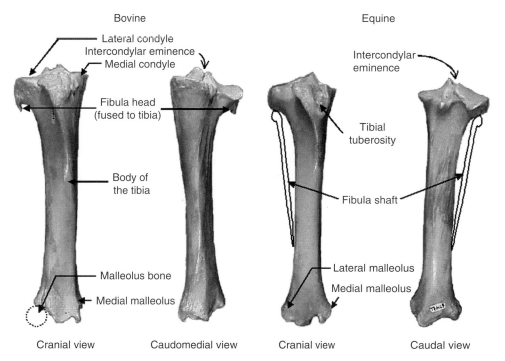

Fig. 6.29. Tibia and fibula of various species. The fibula for the equine was drawn to show where these bones would be if they were present on these specimens.

chicken has six free caudal vertebrae allowing flexibility of the tail. The caudal end of the spinal column, called the pygostyle, consists of four to six fused caudal vertebrae, and provides the site of attachment of some of the tail feathers.

The pectoral girdle has evolved for flight. It consists of the scapula, coracoid bone, and clavicle (wishbone). The latter two bones are either missing or rudimentary in most mammals. The coracoid serves as a brace to essentially immobilize the shoulder joint from the

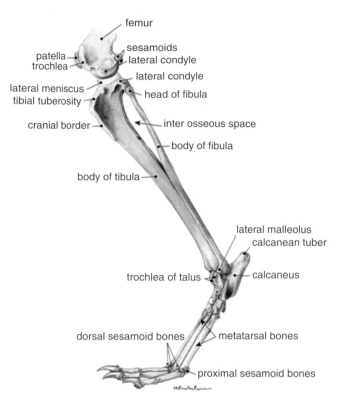

Fig. 6.30. Pelvic limb of the dog. The lateral aspect of the pelvic limb of the dog. (Reprinted from Constantinescu, 2002. Used by permission of the publisher.)

sternum. The sternum has ligamentous attachments directly to the ribs to further brace the shoulder from the sternum. Thus, the shoulder is not pulled toward the sternum as the pectoralis muscles pull the wings downward during flight.

The ulna is larger than the radius and the two are separated by a relatively large space; together they form a unit with a slight mediolateral convex configuration. The increased distance between these two bones adds strength that resists bending of these two bones during flight. The distal row of carpal bones fuses with the metacarpus forming the carpometacarpus. The carpometacarpus articulates with the radial and ulnar carpal bones at the wrist. Finally, there are three digits, including the alular digit having two phalanges, the major digit with two phalanges, and a minor digit with one phalanx.

The avian pelvic girdle consists of a partly fused ilium, ischium, and pubis. The ilium is joined to the synsacral portion of the vertebral column. The pelvic girdle has no pubis symphysis.

There are two articulations between the femur and the pelvis. The head of the femur articulates with the acetabulum formed by the pelvis similar to that in mammals. In addition, the femoral trochanter articulates with the antitrochanter of the ilium. The tarsal

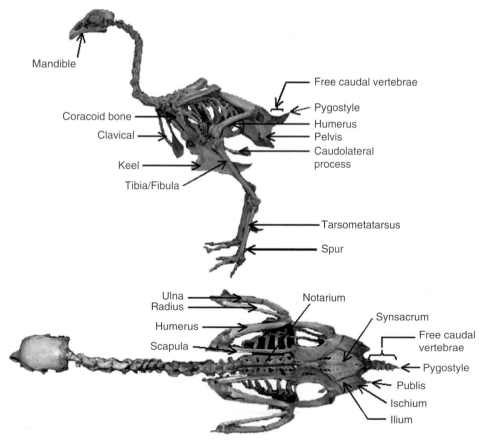

Fig. 6.31. Chicken skeleton.

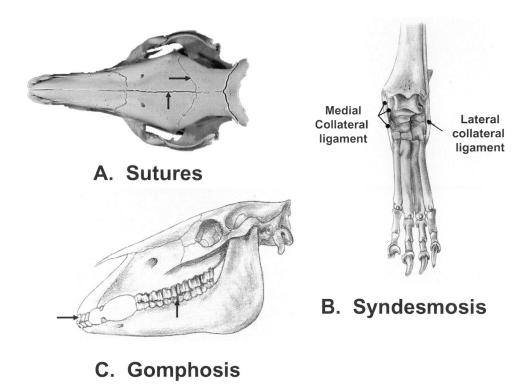

A. Sutures

B. Syndesmosis

Medial Collateral ligament

Lateral collateral ligament

C. Gomphosis

Fig. 6.32. Fibrous joints. Examples of fibrous joints include the following: A) Sutures as found between the bones in the skull. B) Syndesmosis joints in which ligaments connect the bones. C) Gomphosis joints exemplified by the teeth located in alveolar sockets.

bones are fused with other bones, giving the tibiotarsus and tarsometatarsus. Four digits are present and an accessory structure, the metatarsal spur, develops in males.

Laying hens have a special type of bone, called medullary bone, which allows hens to store calcium necessary for eggshell production. Medullary bone is found in bones possessing a good blood supply. It is absent in the humerus, metatarsus, and toes, with small amounts found in the skull and cervical vertebrae and larger amounts found in the femur and tibia. Found only when the birds are producing eggs, medullary bone grows from the inner endosteal surface of the shaft of long bones forming interlacing spicules that fill the marrow space.

Eggshell formation occurs largely at night, a time when laying hens are not eating and therefore are not absorbing dietary calcium. During the time of eggshell deposition, osteoclasts surround the trabeculae and actively reabsorb this bone in order to supply the calcium necessary for eggshell formation, which lasts approximately 20 hours. During the last 15 hours of eggshell formation, the shell gland of the hen secretes calcium at the rate of 100–150 mg/hr, a rate that would deplete blood calcium in 8–18 min. Thus, medullary bone provides an essential source of blood calcium necessary for shell deposition. The deposition of medullary bone is induced by estrogen.

Joints

Types of joints

Arthrology is the study of joints. Joints are vital to allow for the movement of the skeleton. Joints can be classified several ways including 1) the number of articulating bones, 2) structural classification, and 3) functional classification:

1. Number of articulating bones. A simple joint has two articulating joints, whereas a compound joint has more than two articulating bones.
2. Structural classification. Joints can be classified by the medium holding the joint together (Table 6.4):
    a. Fibrous joint has fibrous tissue between bones allowing little or no movement, and has no joint capsule (Fig. 6.32). These joints usually ossify later. There are three types of fibrous joints: sutures, syndesmoses, and gomphoses.
    b. Cartilaginous joints are held together by fibrocartilage, hyaline cartilage, or both (Fig. 6.33). These joints have slight movement, and like fibrous joints, they lack a joint capsule. There are two types of cartilaginous joints: synchondroses and symphyses. The best examples of

Table 6.4.   Structural classification of joints.

Structural Class	Characteristics	Type	Mobility	Example
Fibrous	Ends of bones united by fibrous tissue	1. Sutures	Immobile (synarthrosis)	Bones of the cranium
		2. Syndesmosis	Slightly mobile (amphiarthrosis) and immobile	Distal tibiofibular joint
		3. Gomphosis	Immobile	The only example is the articulation of a tooth with its socket
Cartilaginous	Ends of bones united by cartilage	1. Synchondrosis (hyaline cartilage)	Immobile	Epiphyseal plates
		2. Symphysis (fibrocartilage)	Slightly movable	Pubic symphysis
Synovial	Ends of bones covered with articular cartilage, and a joint cavity enclosed with a joint capsule	1. Ball-and-socket	Freely movable	Coxofemoral (hip) joint and glenohumeral (shoulder) joint
		2. Pivot	Rounded end of one bone projected into sleeve or ring on another bone; freely movable but allows only uniaxial rotation	Between atlas and dens of axis; Proximal radioulnar joint in animals where pronation and supination possible
		3. Ellipsoidal	Both articulating surfaces are oval. Freely movable allowing flexion, extension, abduction, adduction, and circumduction	Radiocarpal joints
		4. Saddle	Each articulating surface has both concave and convex areas, resembling a saddle; freely movable	Carpometacarpal joint of thumb in man
		5. Plane (or gliding)	Articulating surfaces essentially flat; freely movable, but only slipping or gliding motions	Intercarpal and intertarsal joints; articulating surfaces of vertebral processes
		6. Hinge	Cylindrical projection of one bone fits into troughlike depression of other bone; freely movable but restricted to flexion and extension	Knee, elbow and interphalangeal joints.

synchondroses are the epiphyseal plates in long bones, which eventually close, and the joint between the first rib and the manubrium. An example of a symphysis is the pubic symphysis.

c. Synovial joints have a joint cavity bounded by the articular surfaces joined by a synovial joint capsule, and are freely movable. The structure and types of synovial joints are discussed below.

3. The functional classification of joints indicates the degree of mobility in the joint:
a. Synarthrotic. Movements in these joints are absent or extremely limited. Examples of these joints include the sutures in the cranium.
b. Amphiarthrotic. There is slight movement in these joints. Examples include the intervertebral joints of sternoclavicular joints.
c. Diarthrotic. Also called synovial joints, these joints have considerable movement. They

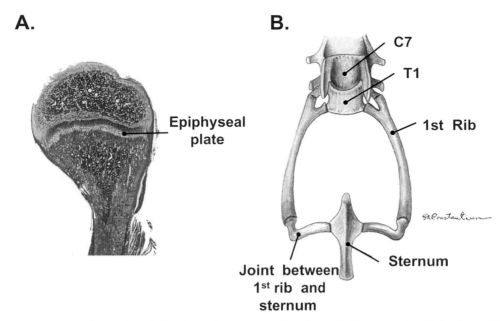

A.

Epiphyseal plate

B.

C7

T1

1st Rib

Sternum

Joint between 1st rib and sternum

Fig. 6.33. Cartilaginous joints. A) The epiphyseal plate located in a growing long bone. B) The sternoclostal joint located between the 1st rib and sternum.

allow for one-, two-, or three-dimensional movement, and contain articular cartilage and synovial membranes. Many such joints also contain bursae sacs. Examples include shoulder, knee, wrist, and elbow.

Synovial joints

Anatomy of synovial joints

The synovial joint is a complicated joint, involving many parts. It is movable, and consists of a joint cavity, articular cartilage, and joint capsule with an inner synovial membrane, and an outer fibrous layer (Fig. 6.34). The fibrous layer attaches to the periosteum on or near the articular cartilage. The synovial membrane is highly vascular, well innervated, and produces synovial fluid. Synovial fluid is viscous and acts to lubricate the joint, provide nutrients, and remove waste from the hyaline articular cartilage.

The articular cartilage is a translucent, bluish-tinged cartilage, usually hyaline, that covers the articulating surfaces of the bone. The joint cavity is unique to synovial joints and contains a trace amount of synovial fluid. Outside the fibrous layer of the joint capsule may be ligaments that hold together the bones of the joints. The ligaments consist of bands of white fibrous connective tissue holding the joints together.

The meniscus or articular menisci is fibrocartilage that partially or completely divides a joint cavity. Menisci are found only in the stifle and temporoman-

dibular joints. They serve to make the joint more stable by improving the fit between two articulating bones.

A bursa is a saclike structure between different tissues that acts as a ball bearing reducing the friction between the bones. The bursa is a flattened sac lined with a synovial membrane and containing a small amount of synovial fluid. While technically not part of the synovial joint, bursae are associated with such joints where ligaments, muscles, skin, tendons, or bones rub together. A bunion is an enlarged bursa at the base of the big toe in humans.

A tendon synovial sheath wraps completely around a tendon. It acts similar to a bursa, reducing friction between the tendons and bones.

Classification of synovial joints

The types of synovial joints can be classified as follows:

1. Ball-and-socket. Also called a spheroid or triaxial, this joint allows all movements, thus allowing the greatest range of motion. Examples include the iliofemoral (hip) joint and glenohumeral (shoulder) joint.
2. Hinge. Also called a ginglymus or monaxial joint, movement is limited to flexion and extension. Examples include the knee, elbow, and interphalangeal joints.
3. Pivot. Also called a trochoid or monaxial joint, it allows movement limited to rotation. Examples include the atlantoaxial or proximal radioulnar joint.

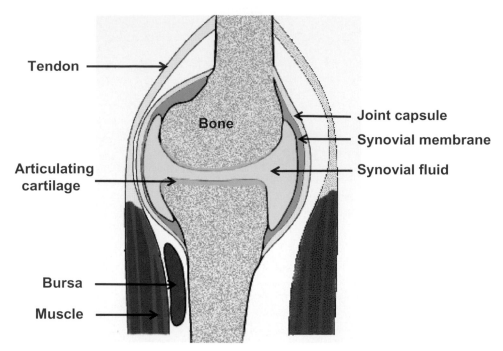

Fig. 6.34. General structure of a synovial joint. Modified from http://www.arthritis.ca/images/user/%7B9078931D-CA9E-4682-B65C-70F8782D168D%7D.gif

4. Ellipsoidal or condyloid. Also called a condyloid or biaxial joint, it is essentially a reduced ball-and-socket joint. Allows all angular motions, including flexion, extension, abduction, and adduction, but not rotation. Examples include the radiocarpal joints.
5. Saddle. Also known as sellar or biaxial, allows all movements except rotation. An example includes the carpometacarpal joint of thumb.
6. Plane. Also called an arthrodia, gliding, or biaxial joint, allows gliding in flexion, extension, abduction, and adduction. Such joints are present in intercarpal and intertarsal joints.

Movements of synovial joints

Synovial joints can make various types of movements and display different ranges of motion. The range of motion of synovial joints varies from nonaxial movement, which includes slipping motions only; to uniaxial movement involving motion in one plane; to biaxial movement, (movement in two planes); and to multiaxial movement involving movement in three planes.

There are three general types of movements possible in synovial joints: rotation, gliding, and angular. These are listed in Table 6.5.

In addition, there are special movements unique to synovial joints. The manus (hand) can undergo supination, palm-up position, and pronation, palm-down or back position. Supination involves the lateral rotation of the radius; pronation involves the medial rotation of the radius relative to the ulna. During pronation, the distal end of the radius crosses over the ulna so that the bones form an "X."

Inversion and eversion are terms describing the movement of the foot. During inversion, the sole of the foot turns medially; during eversion, the sole faces laterally.

Protraction and retraction involve nonangular anterior or posterior movement along a transverse plane. When the mandible is pushed outward from the jaw, this is protraction; pulling the mandible back is called retraction.

Elevation and depression are terms used to describe shoulders or jaw movement. When the shoulders are moved dorsally, it is called elevation; lowering the shoulders is called depression. The mandible is elevated or depressed during chewing.

Specific joints

Intervertebral articulations

The intervertebral articulations consist of cartilaginous and synovial joints. The cartilaginous joints are formed by the intervertebral discs joining the bodies of the vertebrae. The synovial joints are formed by

Table 6.5. Types of movements within synovial joints.

Movement	Description	Example
Rotation		
Rotation	Turning a bone around its own long axis	Femur can rotate away from median plane (lateral rotation) or toward median plane (medial rotation)
Nonangular Movements		
Gliding	One flat or nearly flat bone surface slips over another similar surface	Intercarpal and intertarsal joint movements
Angular Movements		
Flexion	Decreasing the angle of the joint	The elbow joint (humerus-radius/ulna)
Extension	Increasing the angle of the joint	The elbow joint (humerus-radius/ulna)
Dorsal and ventral flexion	Bending the spinal column dorsally or ventrally	The spine
Abduction	Moving a part away from the median plane	The shoulder joint (humerus-glenoid fossa)
Adduction	Moving a part toward the median plane	The shoulder joint (humerus-glenoid fossa)
Circumduction	Movement that traces a cone shape, thus combining flexion, abduction, extension, and adduction	Movement of a limb in a circular motion with the shoulder or hip remaining essentially stationary
Rotation	Movement around the long axis of a part	Radio-ulnar joint
Universal	All of the above movement	The shoulder joint

caudal and cranial articular processes of the adjacent vertebrae.

The first two joints within the vertebral column are atypical. The first, the atlanto-occipital joint, is a modified hinge type of synovial joint between the occipital condyles and the cranial articular surfaces of the atlas (i.e., first vertebral vertebra). This joint has a spacious joint capsule, and is specialized to allow a "yes" motion. The atlanto-axial joint is a pivot type of synovial joint. It is between the dens of the axis and the cranial articulation surfaces on the atlas.

Costovertebral joints

There are two types of articulations between the ribs and the vertebral column. The head of each rib forms a ball-and-socket type of synovial joint, with the causal and ostal facets of adjacent vertebrae. The tubercle of each rib forms a plane type of synovial joint with the transverse process of the corresponding rib.

Sternocostal joints

There is a pivot type of synovial joint between the first eight costal cartilages and the sternum. Each joint has a joint capsule and ligaments.

Costochondral joints

There is a fibrous joint between the ribs and costal cartilage. These have no synovial cavities or joint capsule.

Box 6.1 Rupture of an intervertebral disc

The rupture or degeneration of a disc between the vertebrae allows the pulpy nucleus to bulge or leak out of the disc. This usually occurs dorsally, or dorsolaterally. This can result in pressure being placed on the spinal cord or spinal nerves. It most commonly occurs at the thoracolumbar junction or neck region.

Thoracic limb

Shoulder joint

Also called the glenohumeral or scapulohumeral joint, the shoulder joint is a ball-and-socket type of synovial joint. The head of the humerus articulates with the glenoid cavity of the scapula. It contains a loose joint capsule with no true collateral ligaments. Instead, the muscles crossing the joint provide the support to minimize shoulder luxation (i.e., separation). Functionally, this is a freely movable joint (Fig. 6.35).

The intertubercular, or bicipital, sulcus is a groove between the greater and lesser tubercles. This site holds the biceps brachii tendon. There is a synovial sheath around this tendon as it passes through the intertubercular groove in carnivores, pigs, and sheep. In horses, oxen, and goats, there is an intertubercular bursa found between the intertubercular groove and the bicipital tendon. The transverse humeral ligament attaches between the greater and lesser tubercles

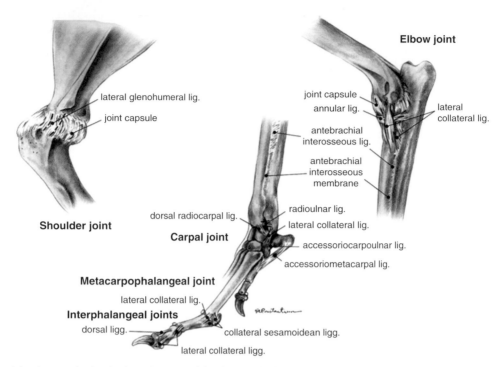

Fig. 6.35. Joints of the thoracic limb. The lateral aspect of the thoracic limb of the dog. (Reprinted from Constantinescu, 2002. Used by permission of the publisher.)

holding the biceps tendon in the intertubercular groove.

Elbow joint

The humeroradioulnar articulation is a hinged type of synovial joint allowing flexion and extension. It is a compound joint since it consists of three bones. There is a joint capsule encasing all three bones.

The humeral condyle consisting of the capitulum and trochlea articulates with the head of the radius, and the anconeal process of the ulna fits into the olecranon fossa of the humerus. The medial and lateral collateral ligaments located on the sides of the joint restrict the movement to flexion and extension.

In horses and ruminants the proximal and distal joint between the radius and ulna is fused. In carnivores, these joints are not fused. This allows some rotation of the radius and, hence, some degree of supination of the forepaw, as well as return to pronation.

Carpal joint

The carpal joint consists of three main joints including the antebrachiocarpal, middle carpal, and carpometacarpal joint. The carpal joint is a hinged type of synovial joint. The antebrachiocarpal joint consists of an articulation between the distal radius and ulna and the proximal row of carpal bones. The distal row of carpal bones articulate with the metacarpal bones con-

stituting the carpometacarpal joint. The middle carpal joint is between the two rows of carpal bones. There are plane joints between individual carpal bones.

Pelvis

Pelvic symphysis

This is a slightly movable fibrocartilaginous joint between the hip bones (os coxae). The front portion of this joint is formed by the pubic symphysis between the two pubic bones; the caudal portion is formed by the ischial symphysis between the two ischial bones.

Sacroiliac joint

The sacroiliac joint is a relatively immobile joint between the wings of the sacrum and the ilium. It is a combination of a cartilaginous and synovial joint. Fibrocartilage unites the ilium with the wing of the sacrum.

The sacrotuberous ligament connects the sacrum and first caudal vertebrae with the ischiatic tuberosity. This ligament stabilizes the caudad end of the sacrum between the os coxae. It is absent in cats.

Hip joint

Also called the coxal or coxofemoral articulation, this is a ball-and-socket synovial joint between the head of the femur and the acetabulum of the hip bone. It is a freely movable (diarthrodial) joint allowing universal movement (i.e., flexion, extension, abduction, adduction, lateral rotation, and circumduction). It has no collateral ligaments; instead, its stability depends on the ligament of the head of the femur, a strong joint capsule, and a large muscle mass surrounding it. The ligament of the head of the femur connects from the acetabular cavity to the notch on the fovea capitis, a notch on the head of the femur. Found only in horses, the accessory ligament of the head of the femur extends from the prepubic tendon through the acetabular notch under the transverse acetabular ligament to the fovea capitis of the head of the femur. This ligament makes it harder for the horse to kick to the side, i.e., cow kick, although it doesn't totally prevent it.

Box 6.2   Hip dysplasia

Hip dysplasia involves a malformed hip joint resulting in a progressive degenerative disease. This disease has a high incidence in some breeds of dogs. Diagnosed radiographically, the condition causes pain. Treatments include cutting the pectineous muscle, removing the neck and head of the femur (head and neck osteotomy), or remodeling the acetabulum by cutting the hip bones and repositioning them.

Pelvic limb

Knee (stifle joint)

The knee, also known as the stifle joint, is a compound joint involving the femur, patella, and tibia. It is a hinge type of synovial joint allowing flexion and extension with little rotation (Fig. 6.36).

The joint between the patella and femur is called the femoropatellar joint, and contains a large joint capsule. The patellar ligament runs between the patella and the tibial tuberosity. Remember that the patella is a sesamoid bone, meaning that it is found within a tendon. Carnivores, pigs, and small ruminants have one patellar ligament; horses and oxen have three, including the lateral, middle, and medial.

The femorotibial joint is the articulation between the femur condyles and the tibia, and has an interposed menisci. These menisci include the medial and lateral menisci that sit between the tibial and femoral condyles.

The medial collateral ligament fuses with the joint capsule and medial meniscus and stabilizes the medial side of the stifle. The lateral collateral ligaments connect the lateral epicondyle and head of the fibula. It is separated from the lateral meniscus by the tendon of the popliteus muscle.

The cranial cruciate ligament originates on the caudolateral femur and inserts cranially on the tibia. It

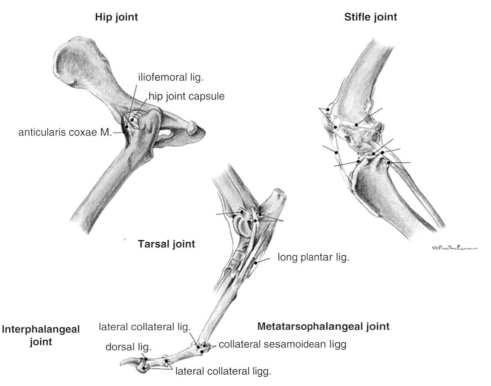

Fig. 6.36. Joints of the pelvic limb. The lateral aspect of the pelvic limb of the dog. (Reprinted from Constantinescu, 2002. Used by permission of the publisher.)

prevents cranial movement of the tibia relative to the femur. The caudal cruciate ligament arises from the craniomedial distal femur and inserts on the tibia. It prevents caudal movement of the tibia relative to the femur.

Tarsus

The tarsus, or hock, is a compound hinge type of synovial joint. It allows only flexion and extension. The tibiotarsal portion of the tarsus is the most movable joint, and is an articulation between the proximal row of tarsal bones (i.e., the talus and calcaneus), and the fibula and tibia. The cochlea of the tibia receives the trochlear ridges of the talus. The proximal intertarsal joint is the articulation between the proximal row of tarsal bones and the central and fourth tarsal bones. The distal intertarsal joint includes the articulation between the central tarsal and tarsal bones I, II, and III.

References

Constantinescu, G.M. 2002. Clinical Anatomy for Small Animal Practitioners. Iowa State Press, Ames, Iowa.

Constantinescu, G.M. and I.A. Constantinescu. 2004. Clinical Dissection Guide for Large Animals. Iowa State Press, Ames, Iowa.

Marieb, E.N. 2003. Human Anatomy & Physiology. Pearson Benjamin Cummings, San Francisco.

7 Muscular tissue

Contents

Muscle tissue overview

Introduction

Muscle tissue is specialized for contraction and is responsible for body movements and changes in size and shape of internal organs. Muscle cells are usually elongated and arranged in parallel arrays.

Muscle is classified based on the appearance of its cells. The two principle types of muscle include striated and smooth muscle. Striated muscle appears to have cross striations when viewed under the light microscope, whereas smooth muscle lacks such striations. Striated muscle can be further subdivided into two types: skeletal muscle that is attached to bone and responsible for the movements of the axial and appendicular skeleton, and cardiac muscle that makes up the majority of the heart. Skeletal muscle and cardiac muscle are sometimes referred to as voluntary striated and involuntary striated muscle, respectively.

The prefixes *myo* and *sarco* refer to muscle. Therefore, terms such as *myofibril* or *myofilament* reference structures within a muscle. For example, the plasma membrane of a muscle cell is called the sarcolemma, the cytoplasm the sarcoplasm, and the endoplasmic reticulum the sarcoplasmic reticulum. In addition, a single skeletal muscle cell is also called a muscle fiber.

Properties of muscles

Four properties of muscles enable them to perform their functions. These properties include

- Excitability. Sometimes called irritability. Muscle cells maintain a membrane potential and are able to respond to a stimulus such as a neurotransmitter by developing an electrical impulse. The stimulus is usually neurochemical, but can also be mechanical or chemical. The electrical impulse can migrate across the sarcolemma.
- Contractility. When stimulated, the electrical impulse spreading across a muscle cell can cause the cell to contract.
- Extensibility. In addition to contraction, muscle cells can lengthen in response to stretch. This is more evident in smooth muscle compared to skeletal muscle.
- Elasticity. Once stretched, muscle fibers can recoil to their original resting length due to the elastic elements within the muscle.

Functions of muscles

Muscles serve four major functions including production of movement, maintenance of posture, stabilization of joints, and generation of heat:

- Production of movement. One feature unique to animals compared to plants is their ability to move. The action of skeletal muscle is responsible for moving joints and thus allowing locomotion. However, movement can be viewed more broadly than locomotion. An animal can change its posture or facial features as a result of muscle contraction. In addition, generally as a result of smooth or cardiac muscle contraction, materials can be relocated within the body. For example, contraction of the heart helps propel blood through the vessels; contraction of the bladder or gastrointestinal tract can also move materials.
- Maintaining posture. Maintaining a position is generally an active, rather than a passive, process. Through the actions of signals generated from sensors located in joints, tendons, and muscles, minute adjustments are automatically made to maintain the position of joints.
- Stabilizing joints. In addition to moving joints, muscles also stabilize the joints, thus minimizing dislocations.
- Generating heat. Endotherms maintain a relatively constant body temperature over a range of environmental temperature. Skeletal muscles are an important organ in heat production, such as through the process of shivering.

Skeletal muscle

Skeletal muscle accounts for approximately 40% of body weight. Each skeletal muscle is considered an organ, and is made up of muscle fibers as well as connective tissue, blood vessels, and nerve fibers.

Connective tissues

As with neurons, each muscle has three connective tissue layers (Fig. 7.1).

1. Epimysium. The entire muscle is surrounded by a dense irregular connective tissue layer called the epimysium containing a dense concentration of collagen fibers. This layer separates the muscle from surrounding tissue.
2. Perimysium. In cross section, a muscle consists of multiple groupings of muscle fibers called fascicles (bundles). Each fascicle is surrounded by the perimysium (*peri* = around) containing collagen

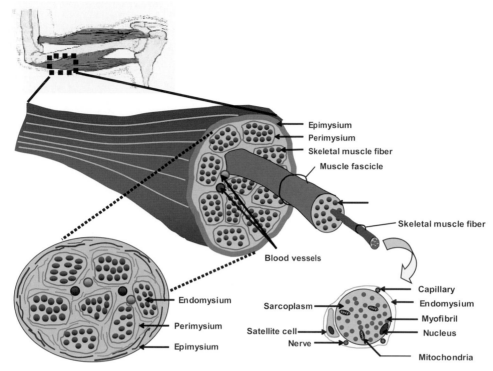

Fig. 7.1. Connective tissue sheaths in skeletal muscle. Each skeletal muscle represents skeletal muscle fibers grouped into a muscle surrounded by a thin connective tissue sheath called the epimysium. Within the muscle are groupings of muscle fibers called fascicles, which are surrounded by the perimysium. Within each fascicle are individual muscle fibers surrounded by the endomysium.

and elastic fibers. This layer contains blood vessels and nerves supplying the fascicles.

3. Endomysium. Within each fascicle are individual skeletal muscle cells, called muscle fibers, each surrounded by the endomysium (*endo* = within). Within this connective tissue layer are capillaries supplying each muscle fiber, nerve fibers controlling the muscle, and satellite cells. These latter cells serve as stem cells that can help repair damaged muscle.

Near the ends of the muscle, the epimysium, perimysium, and endomysium blend together forming either a bundle called a tendon or a broad sheet called an aponeurosis. Tendons and aponeuroses attach muscle to bones blending with the periosteum of the bone. These attachments allow contraction of the muscles to move the bones.

Blood vessels and nerves

The two innermost layers of connective tissue within the muscle each contain blood vessels and nerves. Skeletal muscle is generally under voluntary nervous control, and therefore requires stimulation for nerve fibers to initiate contraction. Therefore, individual nerve fibers must innervate each muscle fiber to control contraction. While the diaphragm consists of skeletal muscle, it usually is under involuntary control but can be under voluntary control as well.

Skeletal muscle fibers

Skeletal muscle tissue consists of large, multinucleated cells commonly referred to as muscle fibers (Fig. 7.2). Muscle fibers can be 100 μm in diameter and run the entire length of a muscle, and can contain hundreds of nuclei. These cells form from the fusion of small, individual muscle cells called myoblasts during development (Fig. 7.2). Instead, some remain unfused and become satellite cells. While skeletal muscle fibers are incapable of dividing, new muscle fibers are produced from satellite cells located in the adult muscle. Not all myoblasts fuse to form muscle fibers. The satellite cells can later enlarge, divide, and then fuse with damaged muscle cells, thus regenerating the muscle.

The nuclei are located immediately under the plasma membrane, which, in skeletal muscle is called the sarcolemma. There is a resting membrane potential present due to the unequal distribution of ions

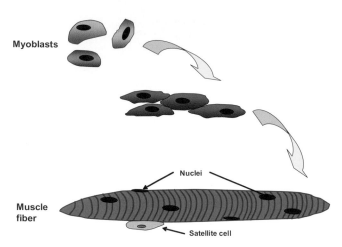

Fig. 7.2. Formation of skeletal muscle cell. During embryonic development, myoblasts begin to fuse forming a large, multinucleated skeletal muscle cell called a muscle fiber. Nonfused myoblasts remain as satellite cells that function as muscle stem cells.

across the sarcolemma similar to that found in neurons. The cytoplasm of skeletal muscle is called sarcoplasm. Within the sarcoplasm are glycosomes, storage granules of glycogen, and myoglobin, a red pigmented protein that stores oxygen.

Although skeletal muscle fibers are large, an electrical signal must be able to propagate throughout the cell quickly to cause contraction. Transverse, or T, tubules are small diameter tubes running perpendicular to the sarcolemma and traveling into the sarcoplasm. These tubes are continuous with the extracellular space, and thus they contain extracellular fluid. They can be thought of as extensions of the sarcolemma. As we will see later, the action potential can travel along the sarcolemma and down the T tubules.

Myofibrils

Muscle fibers are composed of functional subunits called myofibrils. Each muscle fiber contains hundreds to thousands of myofibrils that run longitudinally the length of the fiber. The myofibrils consist of bundles of myofilaments that are protein filaments composed primarily of actin and myosin, the two contractile proteins in muscle. Actin forms the bulk of the thin filaments and myosin forms the bulk of the thick filaments. The myofibrils are packed tightly into the muscle fiber forcing the mitochondria, nuclei, and other organelles to be squeezed toward the outer edge of the cell.

The myofibrils contain three types of proteins that will be discussed in more detail when describing the structure of thin and thick filaments below:

1. Contractile proteins. Contractile proteins generate the force during contraction. These proteins include myosin and actin.
2. Regulatory protein. Regulatory proteins help initiate and terminate the contraction process and include tropomyosin and troponin found on the thin filaments.
3. Structural proteins. Structural proteins help maintain the alignment of the thin and thick filaments, provide elasticity and extensibility, and attach the myofibrils to the sarcolemma. These proteins include titin, myomesin, and dystrophin.

The myofibrils are attached to the inner surface of the sarcolemma. The outer surface of the muscle fibers is attached to collagen fibers that help connect the cells to the tendon or aponeuroses. Therefore, as the muscle fibers contract, they exert force on the bones causing them to move.

Sarcoplasmic reticulum

Similar to the endoplasmic reticulum in nonmuscle cells, the sarcoplasmic reticulum (SR) forms a tubular network surrounding each myofibril (Fig. 7.3). The terminal cisternae (end sacs) of the sarcoplasmic reticulum are always found in pairs, with an intervening T tubule. The combination of a terminal cisterna, a T tubule, and the adjacent terminal cisterna form a triad. Note that the T tubule communicates with the extracellular space while the SR is intracellular.

The terminal cisternae have an active calcium pump that pumps calcium from the sarcoplasm into the SR. This maintains a low concentration of free calcium within the sarcoplasm, whereas the free calcium concentration inside the SR may be 1,000 times greater. Also found within the terminal cisternae is the protein calsequestrin that reversibly binds Ca^{2+}. The free and calsequestrin-bound calcium concentrations can be 40,000 times that in the sarcoplasm. As we will discuss later, the terminal cisternae of the SR are the source of calcium for skeletal muscle contraction.

Sarcomeres

The functional unit of skeletal muscle is the sarcomere. A myofibril consists of thousands of sarcomeres (Fig. 7.4). In stained cross sections of skeletal muscle, alternating light and dark bands are evident, which are called the I band and A band, respectively. These bands give skeletal muscle its striated appearance. The dark bands alter the plane of the polarized light and are therefore anisotropic (i.e., not having the same properties in all directions), whereas the light bands

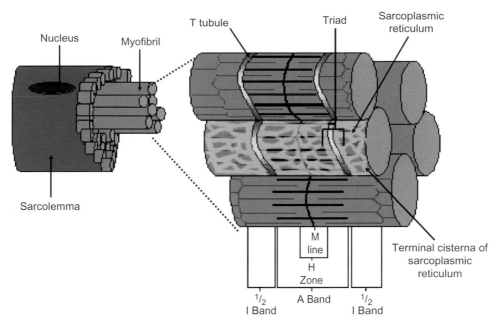

Fig. 7.3. T tubule and sarcoplasmic reticulum. The transverse, or T, tubules are inwardly directed invaginations of the sarcolemma found near the junction of the A and I bands. The sarcoplasmic reticulum is a network of tubules found inside the cell and which have terminal cisternae near the T tubules. Two terminal cisterna and the intervening T tubule make a triad.

do not alter the plane of polarized light and are therefore isotropic (i.e., appear the same in all directons), thus the names A band and I band, respectively.

The sarcomere is composed of thick and thin filaments, proteins that stabilize those filaments, and proteins that regulate the interactions between thick and thin filaments. As shown in Figure 7.4, a sarcomere is the region between two adjacent Z discs (or Z lines). It consists of one-half an I band, an A band, and one-half an I band. The A band is the length of the thick filament, and can contain both thick and thin filaments. In a muscle at rest, a lighter region can be found in the center of the A band called the H zone (from *helle*, meaning bright), which contains only myosin. This region disappears as skeletal muscle contracts and the actin filaments overlap, thus entering this area. The M line, named for being in the middle of the sarcomere, transects the H zone and is composed of proteins that stabilize the position of the thick filaments. Near the ends of the A band are zones of overlap where thin and thick filaments are found side by side.

The I band, located between each intervening A band, contains thin filaments. The I band is bisected by the Z line that consists of proteins called actinins, which interconnect adjacent thin filaments.

There are several structural proteins associated with the myofibrils making the sarcomere. Titin (from *titan*, meaning gigantic) is a large protein, and the third most abundant protein in the sarcomere behind myosin and actin. Each titin molecule extends from the Z line to the M line and helps anchor a thick filament to both the Z line and M line. This provides stabilization for the position of the thick filaments. As shown in Figure 7.4, the portion of the titin molecule located between the Z line and the end of the thick filament is very elastic and can stretch up to four times its resting length. Therefore, titin probably assists in returning the muscle to its resting length following stretching.

The Z line is composed of the protein nebulin. Nebulin anchors thin filaments and connects myofibrils to each other throughout the muscle cell. The M line is composed of the protein myomesin. The M line binds to titin, thus helping to connect adjacent thick filaments. Dystophin is another structural protein that links thin filaments to integral membrane proteins in the sarcolemma. Other proteins in the sarcolemma then attach to the connective tissue sheath surrounding the muscle. Thus, the contractive forces generated in the sarcomere are transferred throughout the muscle.

Thin filaments

Thin filaments are 5–6 nm in diameter and 1 μm in length (Fig. 7.5). Each thin filament is composed of four proteins:

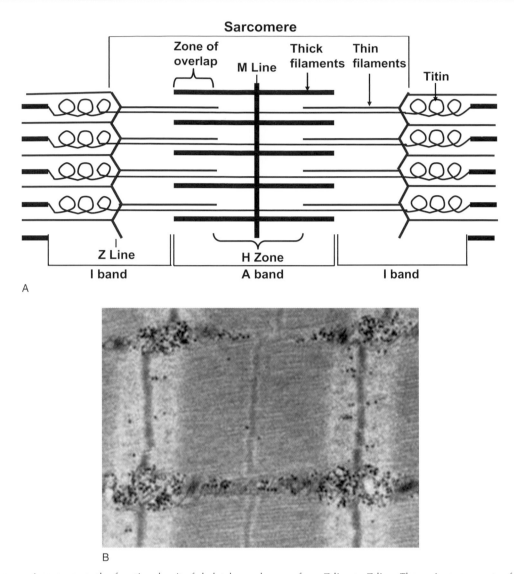

Fig. 7.4. Sarcomere. A sarcomere, the functional unit of skeletal muscle, runs from Z line to Z line. The various segments of the sarcomere are identified in the top portion of the figure, and a photomicrograph of a sarcomere is shown below.

1. F actin. Thin filaments are composed of two strands of F actin, also called filamentous actin, arranged in a double-stranded helix. Each strand of F actin is composed of polymers of G actin, or globular actin. Therefore, the F actin appears as two twisted strands of pearls, with each pearl being analogous to a molecule of G actin.
2. Tropomyosin. Strands of tropomyosin (*trope* = turning), wrap around the length of the F actin. Each tropomyosin molecule is a double-stranded protein, which, at rest, covers seven myosin-binding sites on the actin filament.
3. Troponin. A globular protein, troponin consists of three subunits. One binds to tropomyosin (TnT), one to G actin (TnI), and the other to calcium ions (TnC). Therefore, troponin controls the structural

relationship between tropomyosin and F actin. At rest, troponin allows tropomyosin to be positioned such that it covers the myosin-binding sites. When a muscle is stimulated, and intracellular calcium levels increase, calcium binds to troponin causing a conformational change that allows the tropomyosin to slide into the grooves of the double helix of actin and thus uncover the myosin binding sites.

Thick filaments

Thick filaments are 10–12 nm in diameter and 1.6 μm in length (Fig. 7.6). Thick filaments consist of approximately 500 myosin molecules, each composed of two myosin subunits wrapped around each other. The

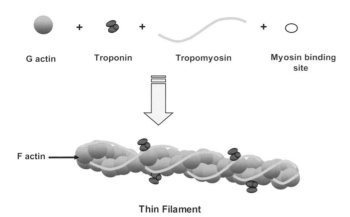

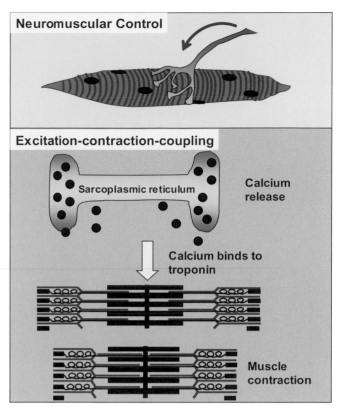

Fig. 7.5. Thin filament. The thin filaments in skeletal muscle consist of G-actin, troponin, and tropomyosin. G actin polymerizes into F actin, or filamentous actin. Troponin is made of three globular proteins binding G actin, tropomyosin, and calcium ions, respectively. Two strands of tropomyosin, a rod-shaped protein, intertwine around the F actin covering the myosin binding sites while the muscle is at rest.

Fig. 7.7. Summary of skeletal muscle contraction. Stimulation of α-motor neurons going to skeletal muscle causes the release of acetylcholine at the neuromuscular junction. This causes the production of an action potential in the muscle fiber that spreads along the sarcolemma and down the T tubules where it causes the release of calcium ions from the sarcoplasmic reticulum. Calcium then diffuses to the thin filaments where it binds to troponin to initiate contraction.

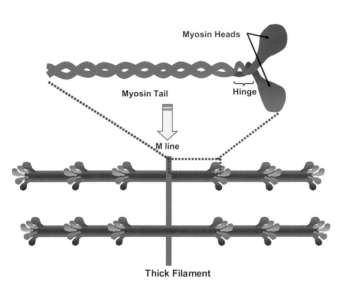

Fig. 7.6. Thick filament. A single myosin molecule is shown at the top. It contains a pair of intertwined subunits each consisting of a tail, a hinge region, and a globular head. The thick filaments contain approximately 500 myosin molecules in which the tails are lined up so that the heads project away from the M line.

long tails of the myosin molecules line up forming the thick filament, and the heads of the myosin molecules project off the filament toward the adjacent thin filaments. The head of the myosin molecule consists of two globular proteins, has ATPase activity, and is able to bind to the actin filament. A cross bridge is formed when the head of the myosin binds to the actin filament. There is a hinge between the head and the tail

of the myosin molecule that allows the head to pivot toward or away from the M line.

The myosin molecules are arranged so that their tails point toward the M line. In the H zone, there are no myosin heads, only tails. Also within each thick filament is a molecule of titin extending from the M line to the Z line.

Contraction of skeletal muscle

As summarized in Figure 7.7, the control of skeletal muscle contraction involves the voluntary stimulation of motor neurons innervating the muscle. The release of the neurotransmitter from these motor neurons initiates excitation-coupling-contraction in which an action potential is generated within the skeletal muscle fiber. The action potential causes the release of calcium from the SR, which then causes muscle contraction.

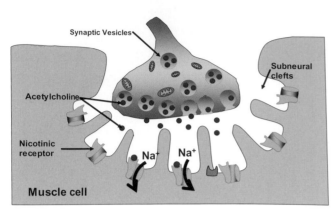

Fig. 7.8. Neuromuscular junction. The neuromuscular junction is a specialized synapse between an α-motor neuron and skeletal muscle fibers. The synaptic bouton is imbedded in the sarcolemma. At this site are subneural clefts that increase the surface area surrounding the synapse. Synaptic vesicles containing acetylcholine (ACh) are located in the nerve ending. Upon stimulation, the α-motor neuron releases ACh that can diffuse across the synaptic cleft and bind to nicotinic receptors on the skeletal muscle fiber. Upon binding to the receptor, ACh causes Na+ ions to enter the skeletal muscle fiber, causing a postsynaptic potential. The postsynaptic potential is always large enough to induce an action potential in the skeletal muscle fiber.

Neuromuscular junction

Skeletal muscle is controlled by the somatic nervous system. The cell bodies of the α-motor neurons, i.e., somatic motor neurons, that innervate skeletal muscle reside in the central nervous system. The axons of these neurons leave the CNS and innervate skeletal muscle fibers at a specialized junction called the neuromuscular junction, or myoneural junction (Fig. 7.8).

Each muscle fiber is innervated by a neuron, although a single neuron may innervate multiple muscle fibers. The neuron branches as it enters the perimysium, and each branch ends in a synaptic terminal, sometimes called a synaptic bouton. The synapse is the region of contact between a neuron and its target cell, which in this case is a skeletal muscle fiber. The space between the neuron and the muscle fiber is the synaptic cleft. The sarcolemma in the region of the neuromuscular junction is called the motor end plate.

Since an electrical signal cannot traverse the synaptic cleft, the signal from the motor neuron is communicated via the release of a neurotransmitter. The neurotransmitter released from α-motor neurons is acetylcholine (ACh). Acetylcholine is contained in synaptic vesicles located in the synaptic bouton. When the action potential arrives at the synaptic bouton, it causes the release of ACh that then diffuses across the

synapse and binds to a specialized cholinergic receptor located on the muscle fiber. This receptor is called a nicotinic receptor. This is a transmembrane protein that binds ACh, and can also be stimulated by the agonist nicotine.

When ACh binds to the nicotinic receptor, it causes the opening of a ligand-gated ion channel that allows sodium ions to enter the muscle fiber. This causes the production of a postsynaptic potential that results in the production of an action potential in the muscle fiber.

Pharmacology of the neuromuscular junction

Since the neuromuscular junction (NMJ) is a chemical synapse, it is prone to pharmacological manipulation. Curare, produced by certain frogs, is a compound used by South American Indians to make poisonous arrows and darts. Curare blocks nicotinic receptors and thereby prevents ACh from inducing skeletal muscle contraction. Derivatives of curare are sometimes given prior to surgery in order to relax the skeletal muscles.

Clostridium botulinum is a bacteria often found in contaminated canned foods. The toxin from this organism prevents the release of ACh from somatic motor neurons. Botulinum toxin prevents skeletal muscle contraction. A very tiny amount of this toxin can cause death by paralyzing the diaphragm and other respiratory muscles. Recently, this toxin has been increasingly used in human medicine (Botox) to reduce wrinkles, control strabismus (crossed eyes), blepharospasm (uncontrolled blinking), or cervical dystonia (also known as spasmodic torticollis), which is characterized by involuntary tonic contractions or intermittent spasms of the neck muscles.

ACh is normally inactivated by the enzyme acetylcholinesterase (AChE). Agents known as AChE inhibitors can be used to strengthen weak skeletal muscle contractions. An autoimmune disease called myasthenia gravis, in which there is reduced nicotinic receptor function, is treated with the AchE inhibitor neostigmine. This drug can also be used to reverse the effects of curare.

Excitation-contraction coupling

The process by which an action potential in skeletal muscle fibers induces contraction is called excitation-contraction coupling (Fig. 7.9). The action potential migrates along the sarcolemma and down the T tubules. At the triad, the action potential triggers the release of Ca^{2+} from the terminal cisterns of the SR.

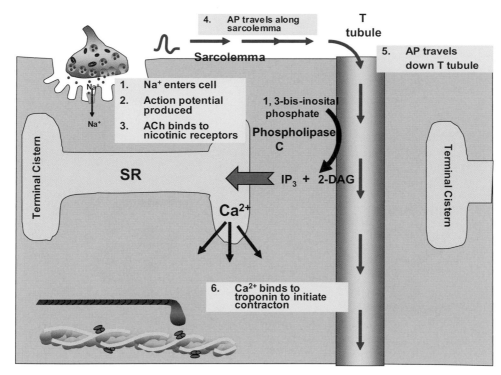

Fig. 7.9. Increasing sarcoplasmic calcium concentration. The action potential (AP) migrates along the sarcolemma and down the T tubule. When reaching the triad, the AP activates the enzyme phospholipase C, resulting in the production of 2-diacylglycerol (2-DAG) and inosital triphosphate (IP_3). The 2-DAG remains membrane bound while IP_3 diffuses through the sarcoplasm to the terminal cistern of the SR. This opens Ca^{2+} release channels, causing the release of Ca^{2+} from the SR into the sarcoplasm. Ca^{2+} then binds to troponin, which initiates contraction.

The release of Ca^{2+} from the terminal cisterns involves the production of inosital triphosphate (IP_3). Upon arrival at the triad, the action potential causes the stimulation of phospholipase C. This enzyme causes the production of IP_3 and diacyl-glycerol. IP_3 diffuses in the cytosol and interacts with the calcium release channels on the terminal cisterns of the SR causing the release of Ca^{2+}.

Cytosolic calcium levels increase at least tenfold. As cytosolic calcium levels increase, Ca^{2+} binds to troponin, causing a conformational change in the shape of this globular protein. This change in shape allows tropomyosin to slide into the grooves of the double helix formed by F-actin (Fig. 7.10). As tropomyosin slides into the groove, it uncovers the myosin binding sites on G actin. Once uncovered, the heads of the myosin filament binds to the myosin-binding sites, and contraction begins.

When stimulation from the motor neurons ends, the action potential is no longer propagated down the T tubules. At this point, a calcium active transport pump called calsequestrin actively pumps Ca^{2+} back into the terminal cisterns of the SR. This process requires ATP, and allows for the concentration of Ca^{2+} in the SR to be 10,000 times higher than in the sarcoplasm. As the

Ca^{2+} levels in the sarcoplasm decrease, troponin returns to its resting configuration and tropomyosin again covers the myosin-binding sites on the G actin.

Sliding filament theory

During skeletal muscle contraction, the length of the thin and thick filaments does not change. Instead, the thin filaments slide between the thick filaments as the myosin heads "grab" the actin filaments and pull them toward the M line (Fig. 7.11). Hence, as the thin filaments move toward the M line, the Z lines get closer, thus decreasing the length of the sarcomere and the myofibril. As the sarcomere width decreases, the muscle shortens.

Contraction of skeletal muscle involves four steps:

1. Hydrolysis of ATP. In the resting position, the myosin head is perpendicular to the thin filament, and ATP has been hydrolyzed to ADP and inorganic phosphate (P_i), creating a charged intermediate. The myosin head is "waiting" for a binding site to become available on the thin filament.

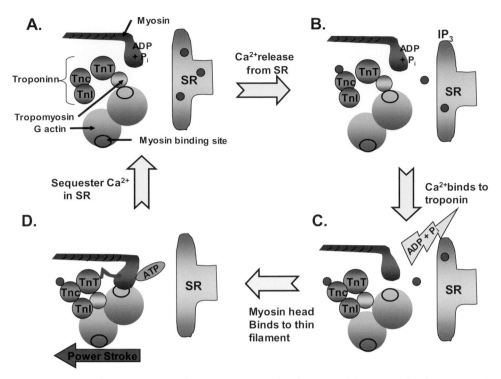

Fig. 7.10. Excitation-contraction coupling. A) At rest, calcium is sequestered in the SR, and the myosin head sits perpendicular to the thin filament. The myosin head is a charged intermediate with ADP and inorganic phosphate (P$_i$) attached. B) Calcium released from the SR binds to the TnC component of troponin. C) The conformational change in troponin results in the tropomyosin filament sliding into the groove of the double helix formed by F actin, thus uncovering the myosin-binding site located on the actin filament. The myosin head binds to actin, releasing ADP and P$_i$. D) The power stroke occurs when the myosin head tilts toward the M line.

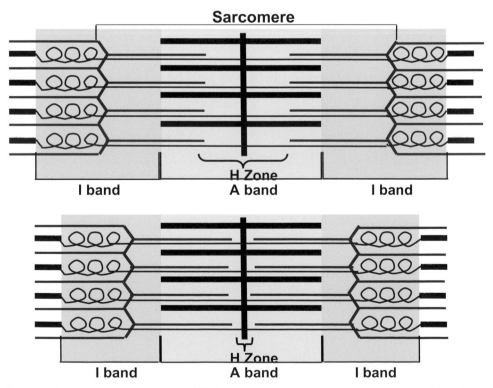

Fig. 7.11. Sliding filaments. The top sarcomere is at rest while the bottom sarcomere is in a contracted state. Note that in the contracted state, the Z lines move closer together and the I bands and H zone shorten while the A band remains the same width.

2. Formation of cross bridges. When tropomyosin uncovers the myosin-binding sites on the thin filament, the myosin head binds to one of these sites liberating ADP and P_i.
3. Power stroke. Release of P_i initiates the power stroke in which the myosin head tilts toward the M line, and ADP is released. The myosin head thus pulls the thin filament toward the M line so that there is greater overlap between the thick and thin filaments. Hence the name, the sliding filament theory.
4. Detachment of the myosin head. At the end of the power stroke, the myosin head remains attached to actin until a molecule of ATP attaches to the myosin head, thus breaking the bond between myosin and actin. The myosin head returns to its perpendicular position as it hydrolyzes ATP, thus returning to step 1.

This cycle then repeats itself as long as the myosin binding sites on the actin remain uncovered and sufficient ATP is present. Each thick filament possesses about 600 myosin heads. As contraction occurs, these heads are attaching and detaching throughout the cycle such that at any given time, there are many myosin heads attached. Therefore, contraction force is always being generated during this time. The myosin heads are sequentially "walking" the thin filament toward the M line throughout the contraction cycle, and therefore pulling the Z lines closer together.

The elastic components in muscle include titin, tendons, and the connective tissue sheaths (endomysium, perimysium, and epimysium). As the muscle fibers contracts, the elastic components are stretched. This stretch is relayed out to the tendons, which then pull on the bones causing them to move.

As calcium is sequestered in the SR, tropomyosin again covers the myosin binding sites. Hence, the myosin head, with its hydrolyzed molecule of ATP attached, assumes its resting position poised to attach to actin when a binding site becomes available. As contraction ceases, the elastic components of the muscle help return the muscle to its resting position.

Rigor mortis

After death, the supply of energy within the cells diminishes as metabolism ceases. As such, the cells can no longer synthesize ATP. ATP is needed to actively remove sequestered Ca^{2+} into the terminal cisterns of the SR. In addition, since the cross bridges can be broken only in the presence of ATP, myosin and actin remain attached following death. This occurs in all the skeletal muscles creating a state called rigor mortis (rigidity of death) in which the animal appears rigid. Rigor mortis ceases only as proteolytic lysosomal enzymes released by autolysis digest the cross bridges.

Summary of skeletal muscle contraction

The following steps summarize the contraction of skeletal muscles:

1. Release of acetylcholine. Stimulation of the α-motor neuron to skeletal muscle causes release of ACh at the neuromuscular junction.
2. Activation of nicotinic receptors. ACh binds to nicotinic receptors causing an influx of Na^+ into the muscle fiber resulting in the generation of an end plate potential.
3. Generation of an action potential. Generation of an end plate potential results in an AP developing in the muscle fiber.
4. Release of Ca^{2+} from the SR. The AP is propagated along the sarcolemma and down the T tubules where it causes the production of IP_3 at the triad. IP_3 then diffuses to the SR where it causes the release of Ca^{2+} into the sarcoplasm.
5. Uncovering myosin binding sites. Ca^{2+} binds to troponin causing a conformational change resulting in the movement of tropomyosin into the grooves of the thin filament, thus uncovering the myosin binding sites on the thin filament.
6. Power stroke. Once uncovered, the heads of the myosin filaments bind to their binding sites on the actin filament. Once bound, the myosin head tilts toward the M line, dragging the thin filaments in the same direction.
7. Breaking the myosin-thin filament bond. If present, ATP binds to the myosin head, which breaks the bond between myosin and the thin filament.
8. Termination of ACh activity. At the conclusion of motor neuron stimulation, ACh is broken down in the synaptic cleft by the enzyme acetylcholinesterase.
9. Sequester calcium. At the conclusion of motor neuron stimulation, calcium is actively sequestered back into the terminal cisterns of the SR by the protein calsequestrin.
10. Myosin head returns to resting position. After detaching from the thin filament, the myosin head hydrolyzes ATP and returns to a position perpendicular to the thin filament. ADP and P_i remain bound to the myosin head until it attaches to another myosin binding site on a thin filament.

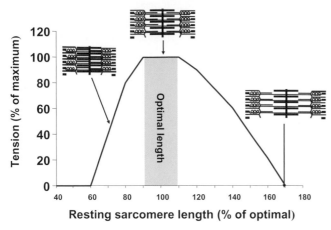

Fig. 7.12. Length-tension relationship. At the optimal resting sarcomere length, the maximum number of cross bridges can be formed between myosin and the thin filament resulting in the maximum tension. As the length of the sarcomere is stretched or compressed, the number of cross bridges is reduced, resulting in less tension.

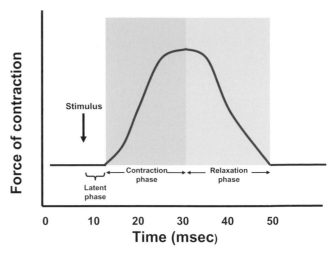

Fig. 7.13. Muscle twitch. A myogram showing the three stages of an isometric muscle twitch. The stimulus is followed by a latent period during which calcium is released from the sarcoplasmic reticulum (SR) and then binds to troponin. The contraction period is when the myosin head actively binds and pulls on the thin filaments, and the relaxation period occurs when calcium is sequestered in the SR.

Length-tension relationships

The tension developed by a muscle fiber during contraction is dependent on the length of the sarcomere prior to contraction. At a sarcomere length of approximately 2.0–2.4 μm, or 90–110% of the resting sarcomere length, the overlap between the actin and myosin filaments is optimal, and the muscle can generate the maximum tension (Fig. 7.12). At these lengths, the maximum number of cross bridges can be formed between the myosin head and thin filament. As the muscle is either contracted or stretched, the number of cross bridges that can form decreases, and less tension is generated during contraction.

As the muscle fiber is stretched to approximately 170% of its resting length, the thick and thin filaments no longer overlap, and therefore, no tension can be generated. Conversely, as the length of the sarcomere gets too short, the thick filaments are compressed against the Z line, decreasing the number of cross bridges that can be produced.

A muscle twitch

A single stimulation of a motor neuron results in a single contraction, or twitch (Fig. 7.13). Although twitches can produce heat during shivering, they are not generally observed during normal muscle contraction. Instead, prolonged stimulation results in more tension being produced than caused by a single twitch.

A recording of a single muscle twitch is called a myogram. A single twitch can last from 20 to 200 msec. depending on the type of muscle, temperature, stretch of the muscle, etc. A muscle twitch consists of three phases:

1. Latent phase. Following stimulation by the motor neuron, the action potential moves along the sarcolemma and down the T tubules to the triad where it induces the release of Ca^{2+} from the terminal cisterns of the SR. The calcium then diffuses to troponin where it binds. This process generally lasts about 2 msec.
2. Contraction Phase. After a conformational change in troponin allows tropomyosin to move, thus uncovering the myosin binding sites on the actin filament, the myosin head binds to the actin filament and the power stroke pulls the thin filament toward the M line, which produces tension. This lasts about 10–100 msec.
3. Relaxation phase. Calcium is sequestered into the SR, the tropomyosin covers the myosin binding sites on the actin filament, and ATP causes the myosin head to detach from the actin filament, decreasing the number of cross bridges and tension. This phase can also last 10–100 msec.

Treppe

If skeletal muscle is stimulated a second time, shortly after the relaxation phase of the first twitch, the second

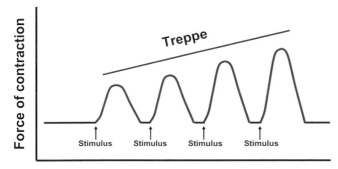

Fig. 7.14. Treppe. If the muscle is stimulated shortly after the relaxation phase, the subsequent muscle twitches generate greater tension, producing a steplike increase in magnitude called treppe. The increase in tension in subsequent twitches results from the increase in sarcoplasmic calcium due to the inability of the SR to recapture all the calcium between twitches.

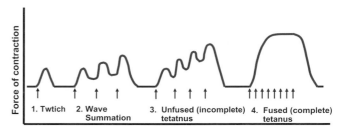

Fig. 7.15. Wave summation and tetanus. 1. A single twitch. 2. The muscle is stimulated (↑) before the relaxation phase is complete, causing wave summation and increased contraction force. 3. Frequency of stimulation is more rapid, resulting in unfused tetanus in which the individual twitches can still be discerned. 4. Frequency of stimulation is so rapid that individual twitches cannot be distinguished, resulting in fused tetanus.

twitch will generate greater tension (Fig. 7.14). This increase in tension is known as treppe, German for "stairs." The increase in tension caused by subsequent stimulations results from the gradual increase in sarcoplasmic calcium since the calcium pumps located in the SR are unable to sequester all the calcium between twitches.

Summation

While a muscle twitch is an all-or-none response, muscle contraction is graded, meaning that it displays varying length and strength of contraction. There are two mechanisms leading to graded responses: 1) changing the frequency of stimulation, and 2) changing the strength of the stimulus.

Wave summation

While muscle twitches can be observed in the laboratory, muscle contraction generally involves smooth sustained contraction resulting from frequent stimulation. If a second stimulation occurs before the muscle completes its relaxation phase, the second twitch will create greater tension than the original twitch. This process is called wave summation (Fig. 7.15). This generally occurs at stimulation rates of about 50 per second. Stimulation occurs rapidly enough that the SR is no longer able to sequester Ca^{2+} between twitches. In addition to prolonging contraction, the second contraction causes greater shortening than the first contraction because it is superimposed on an already contracted muscle, thus increasing tension.

As the frequency of stimulation increases, the tension developed also increases. Incomplete tetanus (*tetan* = rigid or tense) occurs when the individual twitches are still distinguishable. When the frequency of stimulation is rapid enough to eliminate the relaxation phase, and the individual twitches are no longer distinguishable, the contraction is termed complete tetanus. Complete tetanus is the normal state observed during muscle contraction. Wave summation results in smooth, continuous muscle contraction. Note that the frequency of nerve stimulation cannot be faster than the absolute refractory period of the neurons.

Multiple motor unit summation

A second type of summation that increases the force of muscle contraction is called multiple motor unit summation, or recruitment. Skeletal muscles have thousands of muscle fibers. All of the muscle fibers innervated by a single motor neuron constitute a motor unit (Fig. 7.16). The size of a motor unit can vary with a single motor neuron innervating as few as 4–6 muscle fibers, or as many as several thousand. Where fine, delicate movements are necessary, such as in the lips, motor units are small, whereas in areas where precise movements are not necessary, such as in the hindquarter of a beef cow, the motor units are much larger. Motor units are intermingled within a muscle so that they always deliver force on the tendon attaching to a bone.

As an animal begins a task, it generally stimulates the smallest motor units. However, if more force is required, more and larger motor units are recruited in order to increase the tension produced by the muscle.

Muscle tone

Skeletal muscle is seldom flaccid, but instead maintains a degree of tension called muscle tone. Since skeletal muscle contraction is controlled by motor neurons releasing ACh, muscle tone is established by the central nervous system. If these motor neurons are cut, skeletal muscle becomes flaccid. Muscle tone is due to the alternating stimulation of motor units by the central nervous system. Such tone helps keep an animal upright, keep the head held up, stabilize joints, and maintain posture.

Muscle tone is not unique to skeletal muscle, but it is also found in smooth muscle. For example, blood vessels generally maintain a vascular tone as does the gastrointestinal tract.

Isometric versus isotonic contraction

There are two major categories of muscle contraction: isotonic and isometric (Fig. 7.17). During isotonic (*iso* = same; *tonos* = tension), the length of the muscle changes as force is generated, resulting in movement. There are two types of isotonic contractions, concentric and eccentric. In a concentric contraction, the muscle gets shorter as it works. In other words, the muscle forms cross bridges and the thin filaments interdigitate within the thick filaments overcoming the resistance of the load on the muscle. During eccentric contraction, the tension developed by the muscle is less than the load on the muscle. As a result, the muscle lengthens. As an animal walks down a steep incline, the animal controls the rate of elongation of muscles as the legs stretch to the next location.

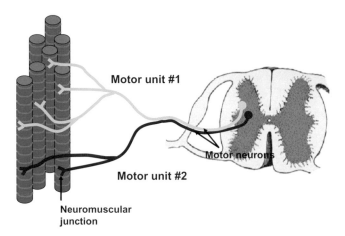

Fig. 7.16. Motor units. All of the muscle fibers innervated by a single motor neuron constitute a motor unit. Motor unit #1 is larger than motor unit #2 because it innervates more muscle fibers. Motor unit #2 would be involved in more precise motor movement than motor unit #1.

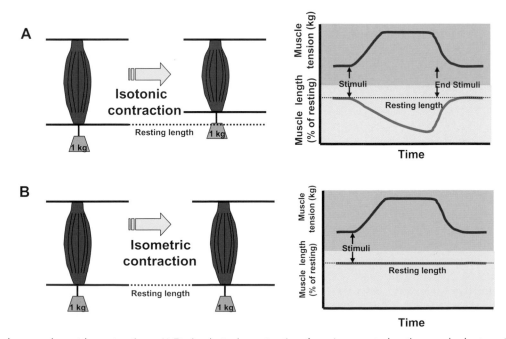

Fig. 7.17. Isotonic versus isometric contractions. A) During isotonic contraction, force is generated as the muscle shortens. B) In isometric contraction, force is generated, but there is minimal shortening of the muscle.

During isometric (*metric* = measure) contraction, the length of the muscle does not change because the tension produced does not exceed the resistance. Isometric contraction is commonly observed in postural muscles that maintain a constant body position while opposing gravity.

When performing various movements, animals use all these types of contractions. Consider the motions as a dog sits and then stands back up. The quadriceps are involved in controlling this motion. As a dog begins to sit, the knees begin to bend, or flex (eccentric). As the dog holds a position part way through the sitting motion, an isometric condition exists. As the dog stands, thus extending the knee, isometric and concentric contractions occur.

Muscle relaxation or return to resting length

While muscle contraction is an active process requiring energy, the relaxation of muscle is a passive process. Elastic forces, opposing muscles, and gravity act to return the muscle to its resting length. Such elastic fibers include connective tissue and many of the muscle proteins such as titin.

Contraction of the opposing muscle will also help return a muscle to its resting length. For example, as the triceps brachii muscle in the back of the front leg contracts, it causes the biceps brachii on the anterior portion of the leg to extend.

Similarly, gravity can cause muscles to extend. The neck of a horse is extended in order to look upward, and then when the muscles are relaxed, the head will move toward the ground, thus stretching the neck muscles that originally were involved in extension.

Metabolism of skeletal muscle

The major energy source for muscle metabolism is ATP. It is used for cross bridge formation, to actively pump calcium into the SR, and to pump Na^+ out and K^+ into the muscle fiber. The endogenous stores of ATP are able to last only about 4–6 seconds. Therefore, there must be mechanisms to replenish this limited store.

While at rest, skeletal muscle makes sufficient ATP to meet its metabolic needs, and to store surplus energy in the form of creatine phosphate and glycogen. Resting muscle can use fatty acids that are broken down in the mitochondria and the ATP used to make creatine phosphate. The glucose that is delivered through the blood stream can be converted to glycogen. When the demands for ATP become greater, there

are three pathways for generating ATP. 1) aerobic respiration, 2) ADP interacting with creatine phosphate, and 3) from stored glycogen through the anaerobic process of glycolysis (Fig. 7.18).

Aerobic mechanism

When O_2 is present, pyruvate enters the mitochondria where aerobic respiration occurs. This process produces 36 moles of ATP for every 1 mole of glucose. During aerobic respiration, the following reaction occurs:

$$Glucose + O_2 \rightarrow CO_2 + water + ATP$$

Since muscle is able to store glycogen, the breakdown of glycogen can yield glucose for aerobic metabolism. In addition, muscle can get energy from blood-borne glucose, pyruvic acid, free fatty acids, and some amino acids. During moderate exercise, aerobic metabolism is able to meet the energy of the muscle

Creatine phosphate

While at rest, muscles are able to produce more ATP than is utilized. This surplus energy is used to synthesize creatine phosphate, an energy storage form found exclusively in muscle. The enzyme creatine kinase catalyzes the transfer of a high-energy phosphate group from ATP to creatine. When ADP is present in the muscle, creatine kinase catylyzes the transfer of a high-energy phosphate group from creatine phosphate to ADP forming ATP. Creatine phosphate is 3–6 times more plentiful in muscle than ATP. These two compounds together can provide enough energy for muscles to contract for approximately 10–15 seconds. When energy is plentiful, creatine phosphate is replenished.

Anaerobic mechanism

Although ATP and creatine phosphate can provide energy for short periods of time, other mechanisms are needed to produce ATP. Glucose can be metabolized through glycolysis, the initial phase of glucose respiration. Glycolysis does not require oxygen, and therefore is termed an anaerobic (without oxygen) process, anaerobic glycolyis. Therefore, this process is utilized when there is insufficient O_2 available for aerobic metabolism to sustain the energy needs of the muscle.

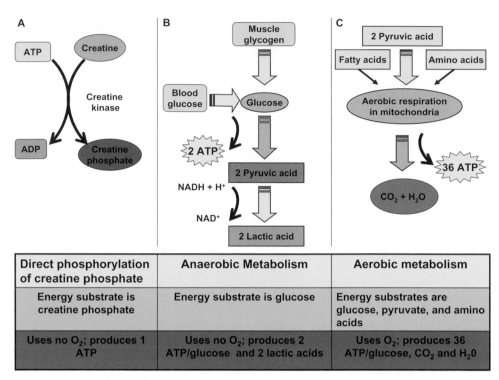

Fig. 7.18. ATP production in muscle. There are three mechanisms for generating ATP in muscle fibers. A) During the direct phosphorylation of creatine phosphate, a phosphate group is moved from ATP to creatine producing creatine phosphate, an energy storage form in muscle. When ADP is plentiful, this reaction is reversed to produce ATP. B) During glycolysis, glucose is anerobically broken down to two molecules of pyruvate, which are then converted to lactic acid in order to regenerate NAD^+. C) In the presence of O_2, pyruvate is further metabolized to CO_2 and H_2O, plus ATP.

During glycolysis, one molecule of glucose is metabolized to 2 molecules of pyruvic acid. During this process, 2 ATPs are produced per molecule of glucose. Therefore, anaerobic glycolysis can produce only 5% of the amount of ATP from glucose as aerobic respiration whereas aerobic respiration produces 95% of the ATP.

In the process of breaking down glucose, NAD^+ is reduced to $NADH+H^+$. In order to continue glycolysis, the cell must be able to oxidize NADH back to NAD^+. When oxygen is not present, the cell can do this only by converting pyruvate to lactic acid, during which NAD^+ is regenerated. Lactic acid then diffuses out of the cells and goes to the liver, heart, or kidney. In the liver, it can be converted back to glycogen.

Muscle fatigue and oxygen consumption

Muscle fatigue is the inability of muscle to contract after prolonged activity. This effect is due to conditions within the muscle fiber, since it occurs even in the presence of sustained neural input. Muscle fatigue differs from central fatigue, in which the muscle is still able to function but the mind is unwilling.

While the exact mechanism of muscle fatigue is unknown, several factors probably play a role. These include inadequate release of Ca^{2+} from the SR, depletion of creatine phosphate, insufficient O_2, depletion of glycogen, buildup of lactic acid (decrease in pH) and ADP, or depletion of ACh from motor neurons. Furthermore, the lack of ATP in fatigued muscle may compromise the action of the Na^+–K^+ pump on the sarcolemma, causing a loss of intracellular K^+.

During prolonged exercise, muscles accumulate lactic acid. This lactic acid must be reconverted to pyruvic acid. In addition, the animal must replenish glycogen stores and replace creatine phosphate and ATP, and the liver must convert blood lactic acid to glycogen. These processes all require O_2, leading to what was termed the "oxygen debt," or the amount of extra O_2 that an animal must inspire to restore homeostasis. Since body temperature and enzymatic reaction rates are elevated for a period of time after exercise, a better term for the increased oxygen needed following exercise is recovery oxygen uptake. During the recovery period, the muscle fibers return to their preexertion conditions.

Heat production

Since metabolism is not 100% efficient, the by-product of metabolism is heat. While a resting muscle fiber is approximately 42% efficient, an active fiber is only about 30% efficient. The remainder of the energy appears as heat that is used to warm the tissues and fluids and help maintain normal body temperature. The excess heat produced when muscles are active is the reason body temperature climbs during exercise.

Types of muscle fibers

There are three functional ways to classify skeletal muscle fibers: 1) Speed of contraction, 2) metabolic pathways forming ATP, and 3) myoglobin content:

1. Speed of contraction. Based on rate of contraction, fibers can be classified as fast or slow. Speed is based on the rate at which the myosin ATPase splits ATP.
2. Metabolic pathways forming ATP. Fibers that rely on oxygen-requiring pathways for generating ATP are called oxidative, whereas those that rely on anaerobic glycolysis are called glycolytic.
3. Myoglobin content. Some muscle fibers have a large amount of myoglobin, the red-colored protein that binds oxygen in muscle fibers. These

fibers are termed red muscle fibers. In contrast, some fibers have low myoglobin content, and are called white muscle fibers.

Based on these criteria, there are now three major categories of muscle fibers, including slow oxidative fibers, fast oxidative-glycolytic fibers, and fast glycolytic fibers—sometimes called slow, intermediate, and fast fibers, respectively. To further complicate matters, these fibers are also called Type I, Type II-A or Type II-B fibers, respectively. While there are many more types of fibers, these are three such classifications that allow for the discussion of general characteristics (Table 7.1). For example, slow fibers allow for prolonged, sustained activities that are powered by aerobic metabolism and which fatigue slowly. Such fibers have a good blood supply, a high myoglobin content and many mitochondria. Conversely, fast glycolytic fibers are better suited for quick, powerful movements that occur over a short period of time and which fatigue quickly. Since these latter fibers contract quickly, they rely on endogenous glycogen stores rather than glucose delivered via the blood stream, and they have fewer mitochondria and little myoglobin.

Table 7.1. Characteristics of skeletal muscle fibers.

	Slow Oxidative Fibers (Type I fibers)	Fast Oxidative-Glycolytic Fibers (Type II-A)	Fast Glycolytic Fibers (Type II-B)
Structural Characteristics			
Fiber diameter	Smallest	Intermediate	Largest
Myoglobin content	Large	Large	Small
Capillaries	Many	Many	Few
Mitochondria	Many	Many	Few
Color	Red	Red-pink	White
Functional Characteristics			
Capacity to generate ATP	High	Intermediate	Low
Method to generate ATP	Aerobic respiration	Both aerobic respiration and glycolysis	Glycolysis
Rate of ATP hydrolysis	Slow	Fast	Fast
Contraction velocity	Slow	Fast	Fast
Fatigue resistance	High	Intermediate	Low
Creatine kinase content	Low	Intermediate	High
Glycogen stores	Low	Intermediate	High
Order of recruitment	First	Second	Third
Primary function of fibers	Postural, endurance-type activities	Sprinting, walking	Short-term activities

Effects of exercise on muscles

Exercise results in changes in the muscle. With endurance exercise, there is a prolongation of the time to fatigue. This resistance to fatigue appears associated with increases in aerobic power and anaerobic capacity. Such changes include increases in muscle buffering capacity and citrate synthase activity, and reduced glycogen utilization. There is also an increase in the capillary-to-muscle fiber ratio, the number of mitochondria, and the amount of myoglobin.

With sustained but relatively weak muscle activity, the muscle does not display significant hypertrophy. However, high-intensity anaerobic activity is associated with muscle hypertrophy. This is because this type of exercise is associated with strength more than with endurance. Such hypertrophy is due to increased muscle fiber size rather than hyperplasia (i.e., increase in cell number).

Cardiac muscle

Cardiac muscle, composed of cardiac muscle cells called cardiocytes or cardiac myocytes, is found exclusively in the heart. It is considered involuntary, striated muscle.

Cardiac versus skeletal muscle cells

Cardiac muscle has several structural differences from skeletal muscle fibers:

1. Cardiocytes are smaller in diameter and length than skeletal muscle fibers.
2. Cardiocytes generally have a single, centrally located, nucleus, although occasionally a cell may have two or more nuclei. In comparison, skeletal muscle fibers are multinucleated.
3. T tubules are shorter and broader, and they lack a triad. The T tubules encircle the sarcomere at the Z line rather than at the overlap between thin and thick filaments.
4. The SR lacks terminal cisternae.
5. The sarcoplasm of cardiocytes contains a large number of mitochondria since cardiac muscle is almost exclusively dependent on aerobic metabolism.
6. Cardiocytes connect with each other at specialized junctions called intercalated (*intercal* = to insert between) discs.

At the intercalated discs, the sarcolemma of the adjacent cardiocytes have irregular thickenings that connect the cells to one another. Within these regions are desmosomes that hold the cells together, as well as gap junctions. The gap junctions allow ions, small molecules, and an action potential to move between adjacent cells. Since the cardiocytes are mechanically and functionally connected, they are said to act as a functional syncytium, meaning that they act as a fused mass of cells.

Functional characteristics

Unlike skeletal muscle, cardiac muscle can contract without neural stimulation. Therefore, cardiac muscle is said to be autorhythmic. Such contraction is generally controlled by a specialized group of cardiac cells that act as the pacemaker cells.

As will be discussed in Chapter 13, contraction of cardiac muscle cells lasts approximately 10 times longer than that of skeletal muscle. This is due to the differing mechanism of the action potential. In addition, cardiac muscle cells cannot display wave summation, nor can they produce titanic contractions. These features are important for the pumping function of the heart.

Smooth muscle

Smooth muscle, also called nonstriated, involuntary muscle, can be found surrounding the blood vessels, digestive tract, urinary system, reproductive system, and respiratory system. It can be found in the form of bundles or sheets around other tissues.

Structure

Smooth muscle cells are long and slender, varying from 5 to 10 μm in diameter and 30–200 μm in length,

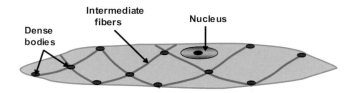

Relaxed Smooth Muscle Cell

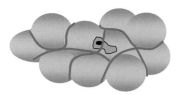

Contracted Smooth Muscle Cell

Fig. 7.19.   Smooth muscle cell. A smooth muscle cell is long and slender, with a single nucleus. Unlike the skeletal muscle fibers, the smooth muscle fibers lack cross striations. However, smooth muscle fibers have intermediate fibers attached to dense bodies. Many of the dense bodies are attached directly to the sarcolemma. Since the intermediate fibers crisscross the cell, when stimulated, a smooth muscle fiber contracts in multiple directions.

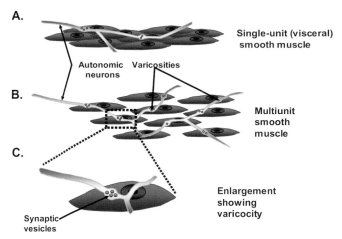

Fig. 7.20.   Types of smooth muscle, and their innervations. A) In single-unit, or visceral, smooth muscle, there are gap junctions between the individual muscle cells. Therefore, when one cell is stimulated by an autonomic neuron, the action potential can spread among cells so that single-unit smooth muscle can contract as a unit. B) In multiunit smooth muscle, individual muscle cells are separated from one another; therefore, each fiber needs its own innervation. C) The autonomic fibers that innervate smooth muscle have varicosities along their length that make diffuse synaptic connections with muscle cells releasing neurotransmitters at these locations.

with a single, centrally located nucleus. There are no T tubules, and the sarcoplasmic reticulum is not as well organized as in skeletal and cardiac muscle. As discussed below, the source of Ca^{2+} for smooth muscle contraction is mostly the extracellular space. To facilitate the entry of Ca^{2+}, the sarcolemma of smooth muscle has in-foldings called caveoli that increase the surface area.

Smooth muscle also lacks the well-organized connective tissue sheaths found in skeletal muscle. There is an endomysium found between smooth muscle cells that is secreted by the smooth muscle cells and which contains blood vessels and nerves.

While smooth muscle contains actin and myosin, it lacks myofibrils and sarcomeres that cardiac and skeletal muscles possess. As a result, smooth muscle lacks striations, hence the name smooth or nonstriated muscle.

Thick filaments are found throughout the smooth muscle cell. Cross bridges are more numerous in smooth muscle since they are found along the entire length of the myosin filament, which is also longer than in skeletal muscle. In addition, scattered throughout the sarcoplasm is a network of intermediate filaments composed of the protein desmin (Fig. 7.19).

Attached to the intermediate fibers are structures called dense bodies. Some dense bodies attach directly to the sarcolemma, and the thin filaments are attached to dense bodies. Therefore, dense bodies act similarly to the Z discs in striated muscle. The ratio of thin to thick filaments is much lower in smooth muscle (1 : 13) than in skeletal muscle (1 : 2). However, the thick and thin filaments do interdigitate.

Due to the network of attachments between the thin filaments and the sarcolemma, when the thick filaments pull on the thin filaments, this causes the cell to shorten, with the areas between the dense bodies bulging outward creating an irregular cell surface (Fig. 7.19). Since the network of intermediate fibers cross throughout the cell, during contraction the cell does not simply shorten in one plane, but rather shortens in multiple directions.

Types of smooth muscle

There are two types of smooth muscle: single-unit smooth muscle and multiunit smooth muscle (Fig. 7.20).

1. Single-unit smooth muscle. Single-unit smooth muscle, also called visceral smooth muscle, is widely distributed throughout the body. The cells

are electrically coupled by gap junctions allowing an electrical impulse to move between cells. Since the cells are electrically connected, they function as a unit in which an entire sheet of cells are interconnected. Such muscle is found along the wall of the digestive tract, the gall bladder, the urinary bladder, and most other internal organs.

This type of muscle is often found as two layers, a longitudinal layer running parallel to the long-axis of the organ, and a circular layer in which the fibers encircle the organ. When the longitudinal layer contracts, this dilates and shortens the organ, whereas contraction of the circular layer constricts the lumen of the organ. Such muscle generally displays rhythmic contractions that are controlled by pacesetter cells that can spontaneously depolarize and trigger contraction of the remainder of the muscle.

2. Multiunit smooth muscle. In contrast to single-unit smooth muscle, individual cells are separated from one another in multiunit smooth muscle. Such cells generally lack gap junctions. This necessitates that each cell must be innervated by a nerve ending. Therefore, such muscle has a richer nerve supply than single-unit smooth muscle. There is seldom synchronous contraction of the entire muscle. This type of muscle is found in the iris of the eye, along portions of the male reproductive tract, surrounding the walls of large arteries, and in the arrector pili muscle of the skin.

Neural innervation of smooth muscle

Smooth muscle is innervated by the autonomic nervous system, whereas skeletal muscle is innervated by the somatic nervous system. Unlike skeletal muscle that has a well-defined neuromuscular junction, autonomic fibers run over the surface of smooth muscle cells and have many bulbous swellings called varicosities. The neurotransmitter is released from these varicosities and diffuses into a wide synaptic cleft, forming a diffuse junction.

Contraction of smooth muscle

Contraction of smooth muscle takes longer to develop, but lasts longer, than skeletal muscle. Smooth muscle can also shorten and stretch further than skeletal muscle. This is due to the differences in the structure between the two muscle types. While tropomyosin is found in smooth muscle associated with the thin filaments, troponin is lacking. There is less SR in smooth muscle, and smooth muscle lacks T tubules. As a result, the action potential must spread only along the surface of the cell, and the greatest source of calcium for muscle contraction is the interstitial space. The sequences of events for smooth muscle contraction are as follows:

1. The muscle is stimulated by autonomic fibers releasing either norepinephrine or acetylcholine.
2. An action potential spreads along the sarcolemma.
3. Cytosolic Ca^{2+} levels increase, with calcium coming mostly from the interstitial space, but some from the SR.
4. Ca^{2+} binds to the calmodulin, a second messenger, causing its activation.
5. The activated calmodulin then activates myosin light-chain kinase.
6. The activated protein kinase phosphorylates the myosin head.
7. Phosphorylation allows cross bridges to form between myosin and actin.
8. The muscle contracts as Ca^{2+} is pumped out of the cell.

Note that in smooth muscle, calmodulin is serving a role similar to that of troponin in skeletal muscle in that it binds calcium. Once activated, calmodulin activates a myosin light chain kinase that uses ATP to phosphorylate the myosin head, thus allowing the myosin head to attach to actin. The pumping of calcium out of the cell is a slow process partially explaining the delay in smooth muscle relaxation.

In addition to responding to the autonomic nervous system, smooth muscle can contract and relax in response to stretching; hormones; or changes in local factors, including pH, O_2, CO_2, temperature, and ion concentrations. For example, stretching of the bladder can cause contractions. Hence, the bladder can continue to function in an animal with a spinal cord injury. Epinephrine, released from the adrenal medulla during a stress response can cause the bronchioles to dilate. For a comparison of skeletal, smooth, and cardiac muscle, (discussed in Chapter 13), see Table 7.2.

Muscle system

Naming muscles

The muscle system includes all the skeletal muscle and is therefore responsible for voluntary movement. It is not the intent of this book to cover all the muscles, but rather to give an overview of many of the major muscles involved in movement. The muscles will be covered by functional area.

Table 7.2. Comparison of skeletal, cardiac, and smooth muscle tissues.

Properties	Skeletal Muscle	Cardiac Muscle	Smooth Muscle
Location	Attached to bones, or occasionally to skin in the case of some facial muscle	Wall of the heart	Single-unit found in walls of hollow organs, multiunit found in intrinsic eye muscles
Size	Single, long, cylindrical; striated; 100 μm–30 cm	Branching, striated, 10–20 μm × 50–100 μm	Fusiform, nonstriated, 5–10 μm × 30–200 μm
Number of nuclei	Multinucleated	Uni- or binucleated	Uninucleated
Connective tissue components	Epimysium, perimysium, and endomysium	Endomysium attached to fibrous skeleton	Endomysium
Presence of sarcomere	Yes	Yes	No; actin and myosin scattered throughout sarcoplasm; actin attached to dense bodies
Presence and location of T tubules	Yes; located at junction of A and I bands	Yes; located at Z disc	No; caveoli instead
Presence of gap junctions	No	Yes; located at intercalated discs	Present in single-unit, but not multiunit, smooth muscle
Fibers contain individual neuromuscular junctions	Yes	No	Present in multiunit, but not single-unit, smooth muscle
Source of calcium for contraction	Sarcoplasmic reticulum	Sarcoplasmic reticulum and extracellular fluid	Mostly extracellular fluid, but also sarcoplasmic reticulum
Site of calcium binding and regulation	Troponin located on thin filaments	Troponin located on thin filaments	Calmodulin located in sarcoplasm
Contraction	Rapid onset, can tetanize; depending on fiber type, can fatigue rapidly	Develops slowly; cannot tetanize	Slow onset; may tetanize, but generally fatigues slowly
Effect of nervous system input	Excitation at nicotinic receptors	Excitation at β_1 receptors; inhibition at muscarinic receptors	Excitation or inhibition at muscarinic receptors; excitation at α or β receptors
Respiration	Aerobic and anaerobic	Aerobic	Primarily aerobic

Generally, the name of the muscle gives considerable information about its location or role. Muscles are named by several criteria:

1. Location. Sometimes, a bone or body region is included in the name giving an indication of its location (e.g., temporalis is located over the temporal bone and the intercostal muscles are found between the ribs). The word *deep* (e.g., deep digital flexor) indicates that the muscle is not found at a superficial level.
2. Action. The action performed by the muscle may be included in the name. For example, the extensor digitorum extends a digit while the pronator teres pronates a limb.
3. Size. Whether the muscle is large or small may be indicated in the name (e.g., pectoralis major, adductor longus). The name may include such terms as longus (long), brevis (short), maximus (largest), minimus (smallest).
4. Shape. Sometimes muscles are named according to their shape (e.g., deltoid or trapezius muscles).

5. Direction of the fibers. Terms, such as rectus, indicate that the muscle fibers run parallel or straight relative to the body axis, whereas transverse runs at right angles to the same axis. Oblique fibers run at some other angle relative to that axis.
6. Number of origins/bellies. The name may include the number of heads (e.g., biceps brachii) or bellies (digastricus).
7. Attachment. Many times, the origin or attachment site is included in the name of the muscle (e.g., cleidomastoid is attached to the clavical, or its remnant, and mastoid process).

Muscles can have several types of attachments. They may attach to a bone via either 1) a tendon, which is a dense cord of regular connective tissue, 2) an aponeurosis, which is a tendinous sheet, or 3) fascia, which is common for superficial muscles, or 4) they may attach directly to the periosteum of the bone. Examples of each include the biceps brachii, which attaches via a tendon, the latissimus dorsi, which attaches via the thoracolumbar aponeurosis, the

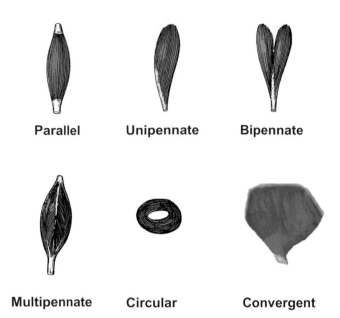

Fig. 7.21. Fascicle arrangement. Muscle fascicles can have varying arrangements allowing for different functions.

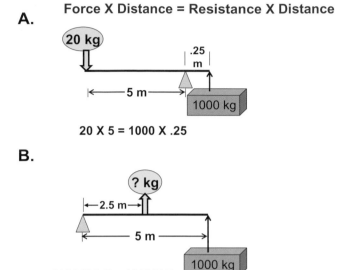

Fig. 7.22. Mechanical advantage versus disadvantage. A lever system can provide a mechanical advantage or a mechanical disadvantage. The equation shown at the top explains the relationship between force and distance. A) With this lever system, a mechanical advantage is provided because of the position of the fulcrum relative to the force and load. Twenty kg of force is able to lift 1,000 kg of load. B) With the fulcrum and load placed at opposite ends of the lever, and a force provided in the middle, it requires 100 times the amount of force needed in the example shown in A to move the same load. This is a mechanical disadvantage.

platysma attaches via the fascia, and the masseter, which attaches to the mandible.

Arrangements of fascicles

As stated previously, skeletal muscles are arranged in fascicles (Fig. 7.1). The fascicle arrangement can vary (Fig. 7.21). Fascicles are sometimes found to be arranged in a straight line and are referred to as parallel muscles (an example is the abductor digiti minimi). If the arrangement is circular, the fascicles appear as concentric rings. Such an arrangement is typically found around an orifice such as the orbicularis oris muscle that surrounds the mouth. In a convergent muscle, the fascicles converge to the tendon for insertion. Therefore, the muscle begins wide similar to the shape of a fan, and then narrows such as seen in the pectoralis major muscle. In the pennate muscle, such as the gastrocnemius muscle, the fascicles are short and attach obliquely (*penna* = feather) to the tendon. In a unipennate muscle, the tendon runs along one side of the tendon, whereas in multipennate, the tendon branches within the muscle and looks like many feathers laying side by side.

Muscles as levers

The muscular and skeletal system work together to function as a lever system. A lever consists of a rigid structure (i.e., bone) that moves around a fixed point called the fulcrum. Muscle contraction acts as the force

to move a load, or bone. Levers provide a mechanical advantage allowing a force to move a heavier load either further or faster (Fig. 7.22).

Three different classes of levers exist, depending on the relationship of the force, fulcrum, and load (Fig. 7.23). In a first-class lever, the fulcrum is between the force and load, which are at either end of the lever. This is similar to a playground seesaw, and it provides a mechanical advantage. The act of an animal lifting its head functions as a first-class lever.

A second-class lever exists when the force is applied at one end and the fulcrum is found at the other end, while the load is placed in between. Such levers create a mechanical disadvantage, and are thus rarely found in the body. A wheelbarrow acts as such a lever. The calf muscles act as a second-class lever when causing plantar flexion.

In a third-class lever, the fulcrum and load are at either end of the lever, and the force is applied between the two. Tweezers work in this manner, as do most skeletal muscles. When the biceps brachii flexes the elbow, the insertion is located on the radius-ulna while the origin is located in the shoulder region. Contraction of the muscle causes the leg to flex at the elbow. In a third-class lever, the speed and distance traveled by the load are increased at the expense of effective force.

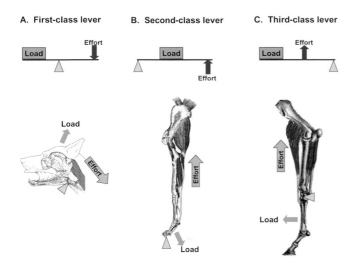

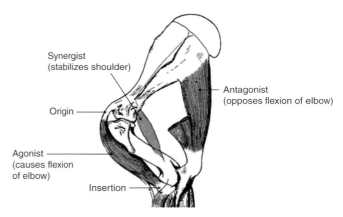

Fig. 7.24. Muscle functions and attachments. Using the thoracic limb of the horse, this figure demonstrates the origin and insertion of muscles, as well as the agonist and antagonist functions with regards to the elbow. (Figure modified from Getty, 1964.)

Fig. 7.23. Anatomical examples of lever systems. A) In a first-class lever, the force and load are on opposite sides of the fulcrum. B) In a second-class lever, the load is between the force and the fulcrum. 3) In a third-class lever, the force is between the load and the fulcrum.

Muscle terminology

Origins and insertions

Muscles are always attached to other structures at either end. Generally, one end is in a fixed position while the other end moves toward it when the muscle is contracted. The fixed attachment site is called the origin, and the movable end is called the insertion (Fig. 7.24). While the origin is normally proximal or superior to the insertion, this is not always the case. The sternocleidomastoid muscle originates at the sternum, and inserts at the mastoid process of the temporal bone.

Actions

The movements of the skeleton caused by muscle contraction involve flexion or extension, adduction or abduction, protraction or retraction, elevation or depression, rotation, circumduction, pronation or supination, inversion or eversion. These actions are defined in Table 7.3.

Muscles typically work in groups rather than individually. For example, the biceps branchii and brachialis cause flexion of the elbow, and the triceps brachii, tensor fasciae anterbrachii, and anconeus cause exten-

sion of the elbow. The agonist is the muscle primarily responsible for producing a certain movement and the antagonist is the muscle whose action opposes that movement. In the case of the elbow, the biceps brachii is the agonist for flexion of the elbow and the triceps branchii is the antagonist. A synergist is a muscle that helps the agonist work more efficiently. Synergists may either provide additional force to move the joint, or they may help stabilize the joint.

Muscle attachments

Muscles can make three types of attachments. In a fleshy attachment, there is an apparent direct attachment of the muscle to the bone, as in the case of muscle attachments to the scapula. In actuality, the muscles are attached to the bones by very short tendons. In a tendinous attachment, the muscle is attached to the bone via dense connective tissue. In an aponeurotic attachment, there is a flat, tendinous sheet attaching the muscle, as is seen in the abdominal wall.

Major skeletal muscles

There are over 600 skeletal muscles in the body. We will only cover the principle muscles, presenting them as groups controlling various parts of the body (see Tables 7.4–7.6 and Figs. 7.25–7.29).

Table 7.3. Muscle terminology.

Term	Description
Abduction	Movement of the limb or structure away from the median plane of the body. Example: spreading the toes.
Adduction	Movement of the limb or structure toward the median plane of the body. Example: bringing the toes together or moving a limb toward the center of the body.
Antagonist	Opposing the movement of the prime mover. Example: the triceps brachii muscle, which causes extension of the elbow joint is the antagonist of the biceps brachii during flexion of the elbow.
Circumduction	Movement of an extremity that describes the surface of a cone. Involves successive flexion, abduction, extension, and adduction. Example: moving a limb in a circular motion.
Depression	Moving a structure in an inferior direction. Example: dropping the shoulders.
Elevation	Moving a structure in a superior direction. Example: shrugging the shoulders upward.
Eversion	Twisting to face the sole outward.
Extension	Increasing the angle between bones. Example: bending the head back, which is hyperextension of the neck, or pushing the arm backward, which extends the shoulder.
Flexion	Decreasing the angle between bones. In the limbs, it is usually the more distal attachment. Example: bending the elbow toward a 90° angle.
Trunk lateral flexion	Bending to the side.
Trunk flexion	Bending forward.
Shoulder flexion	Swinging the limb forward.
Plantar flexion	Movement of the ankle joint to push the sole of the foot downward.
Dorsiflexion	Flexion of the ankle joint in order to raise the top of the foot upward.
Insertion	The more movable of the two attachments. In the limbs, this is normally the more distal attachment.
Inversion	Twisting to face the sole inward.
Origin	The less movable of the two attachments. In the limbs, it is usually the more proximal attachment.
Pronation	Movement of the palmar side of the paw or foot downward or backward.
Protraction	Moving a part of the body anteriorly in the horizontal plane. Example: pushing the shoulders forward.
Retraction	Moving a part of the body posteriorly. Example: pulling the shoulders back.
Rotation	Movement around the long axis.
Lateral rotation	Turning the anterior surface of a limb away from the long axis of the trunk.
Medial rotation	Turning the anterior surface of a limb toward the long axis of the trunk.
Supination	Movement of the forearm (radius and ulna) so the palmar side is rotated upward or forward as when a cat laps milk off its paw.
Synergist	A muscle that indirectly aids the action of the prime mover. Example: teres major muscle is a synergist to the latissimus dorsi muscle.

Muscles of the head and neck

Table 7.4. Muscles of the head and neck.

Muscle	Description	Origin (O)/Insertion (I)	Action
Muscles of Facial Expression and Mastication			
Buccinator			
Masseter	Most powerful muscle for closing jaw	O—Zygomatic arch I—Masseteric fossa of mandible	Elevates mandible
Mentalis	Major muscle making bulk of muscle mass of chin	O—Rostral end of mandible I—Skin of chin	Elevates and protrudes lower lip
Orbicularis oris	Multilayered muscle of the lips	O—Lips I—Lips	Compresses lips
Pterygoid			
Medial	Two-headed muscle running along internal surface of mandible	O—Sphenoid bone and pterygoid bones I—Medial surface of mandible	Acts with temporalis and masseter muscle to elevate mandible
Lateral	Two-headed muscle lying superior to medial pterygoid muscle	O—Sphenoid bone I—Neck of condyle of mandible	Protrudes mandible; in herbivores, cross-jaw action
Platysma		O—Skin of neck I—Angle of lips	Retracts lips
Temporalis	Fan-shaped muscle covering part of temporal, frontal, and parietal bones	O—Temporal fossa I—Coronoid process of mandible	Closes jaw, elevates and retracts mandible
Zygomaticus	Muscle running diagonally from cheek bones to corner of mouth	O—Zygomatic bone near zygomaticomaxillary suture I—Angle of the mouth	Retracts and elevates corners of mouth
Muscles of the Neck			
Brachiocephalicus	Wide muscle extending from head to thoracic limb	O—Clavicle I—Skull and humerus	Pulls limb forward or flexes neck laterally
Sternocephalicus	In carnivores, consists of sternomastoid and sternoocipitalis; in ox and goats, the sternoocipitalis is replaced by the sternomandibularis	O—Cranial part of the sternum I—Mastoid process	Flexes the head and neck and inclines them to one side

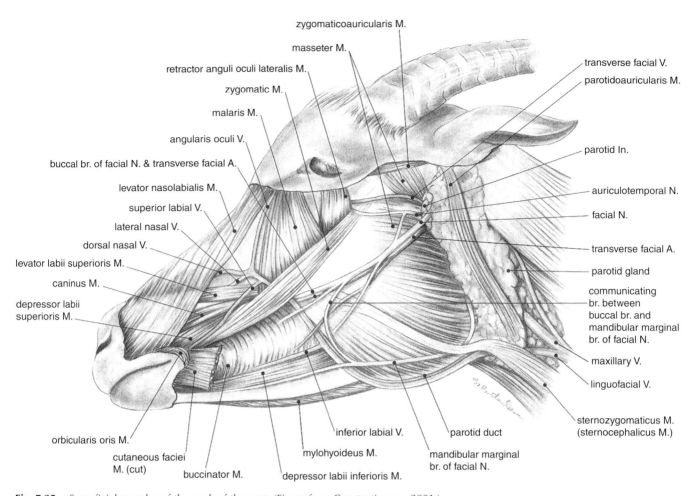

zygomaticoauricularis M.

masseter M.

retractor anguli oculi lateralis M.

zygomatic M.

malaris M.

angularis oculi V.

buccal br. of facial N. & transverse facial A.

levator nasolabialis M.

superior labial V.

lateral nasal V.

dorsal nasal V.

levator labii superioris M.

caninus M.

depressor labii superioris M.

transverse facial V.

parotidoauricularis M.

parotid ln.

auriculotemporal N.

facial N.

transverse facial A.

parotid gland

communicating br. between buccal br. and mandibular marginal br. of facial N.

maxillary V.

linguofacial V.

sternozygomaticus M. (sternocephalicus M.)

orbicularis oris M.

cutaneous faciei M. (cut)

buccinator M.

inferior labial V.

mylohyoideus M.

depressor labii inferioris M.

parotid duct

mandibular marginal br. of facial N.

Fig. 7.25. Superficial muscles of the neck of the goat. (Figure from Constantinescu, 2001.)

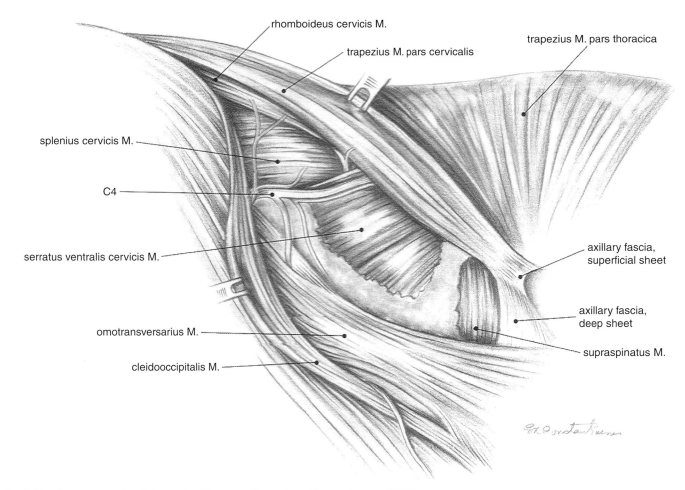

Fig. 7.26. Deeper muscles of the neck of the goat. (Figure from Constantinescu, 2001.)

Muscles of the pectoral limb and lateral thorax

Table 7.5. Muscles of the pectoral limb.

Muscle	Description	Origin (O)/Insertion (I)	Action
Extrinsic Muscles of Thoracic Limb[1]			
Brachiocephalicus	A wide muscle running from the head and neck to the front limb; the clavicular intersection divides the muscle into the cleidocephalicus (clavotrapezius) and cleidobrachialis (clavodeltoid)	O—Clavicle I—Skull and humerus	Draws the lifted forelimb forward or draws the head to the side
Cleidocephalicus		O—Occiput and dorsal midline of neck I—Clavicle	Pulls humerus forward
Clavodeltoid		O—Clavicle I—Cranial border of humerus	Pulls humerus forward
Pectoralis	A broad flat muscle extending from the sternum to the humerus		
Pectoralis superficialis		O—Sternum I—Humerus (greater and lesser tubercles)	Adducts and retracts limb (flexes shoulder)

Table 7.5. *Continued*

Muscle	Description	Origin (O)/Insertion (I)	Action
Pectoralis profundus		O—Sternum I—Cranial surface of the humerus	Depresses, protracts, and laterally rotates the scapula
Rhomboid	Extrinsic muscle lying deep to the trapezius	O—Dorsal neck and thorax; nuchal crest of skull I—Dorsal border of scapula and scapular cartilage	Draws scapula dorsocranially
Trapezius	Triangular-shaped muscle extending from the dorsomedial neck and thorax to the spine of the scapula	O—Median fibrous raphe of neck; Spines of T_3–T_8 or T_9 I—Spine of scapula	Elevates shoulder and draws it forward or backward
Latissimus dorsi	Broad, flat, fan–shaped muscle extending from dorsal thoracolumbar region to medial side of humerus	O—Thoracolumbar fascia of thorax and some posterior ribs I—Teres tuberosity of humerus	Pulls humerus backward; medially rotates, adducts the shoulder
Intrinsic Muscles of Shoulder[2]			
Biceps brachii	Two-headed fusiform muscle	O—Tubercule of scapula I—Bicipital tuberosity of radius	Extends shoulder and, with brachialis muscle, flexes elbow joint
Coroacobrachialis	Small muscle extending from the coracoid process to the humerus, on medial side of axilla	O—Coracoid process of scapula I—Proximal shaft of humerus	Flexes shoulder joint
Deltoid	Extends from scapular spine over shoulder joint to the deltoid tuberosity of the humerus	O—Spine of scapula; acromion process of scapula I—Deltoid tuberocity of humerus	Flexes shoulder joint
Supraspinatus	Originates from and fills the supraspinous fossa of the scapula	O—Supraspinous fossa of scapula I—Greater and lesser tubercule of humerus	Extends shoulder joint
Infraspinatus	Originates in and fills the infraspinatous fossa of the scapula	O—Infraspinous fossa of scapula I—Greater tubercule of humerus	Abducts and rotates humerus
Teres major	Extends from caudal border of scapula and inserts on latissimus dorsi muscle on medial side of humerus	O—Inferior half of lateral border of scapula I—Teres tuberocity of humerus	Flexes shoulder joint
Teres minor	Small muscle ventral to the tendon of the infraspinatus muscle	O—Caudal border of scapula I—Teres minor tuberocity of humerus	Flexes shoulder
Subscapularis	Large muscle originating from subscapular fossa and inserting on humerus	O—Subscapular fossa of scapula I—Lesser tubercle of humerus	Adducts and extends shoulder joint
Intrinsic Flexor Muscles of Leg[2]			
Biceps brachii	Extends from supraglenoid tubercles to radius	O—Supraglenoid tubercle of scapula I—Radial tuberosity	Flexes elbow and extends shoulder
Brachialis	Extends from caudal part of humerus to the radius	O—Brachial groove of humerus I—Radius	Flexes elbow

Table 7.5. *Continued*

Muscle	Description	Origin (O)/Insertion (I)	Action
Intrinsic Extensor Muscles of Leg[2]			
Triceps brachii	Consists of long head, lateral head, and medial head		
Long Head		O—Caudal border of scapula I—Olecranon process	Extends elbow joint
Lateral Head		O—Lateral surface of humerus I—Olecranon process	Extends elbow joint
Medial Head		O—Medial surface of humerus I—Olecranon process	Extends elbow joint
Tensor fasciae anterbrachii	Thin, insignificant muscle arising from the latissimus muscle	O—Latissimus dorsi I—Olecranon process of tibia and antebrachial fascia	Extends elbow
Anconeus	Crosses lateral aspect of elbow under triceps brachii muscle	O—Epicondyles of humerus I—Olecranon process of ulna	Extends elbow

[1] Muscles that attach to the thoracic limb and some other part of the body.
[2] Muscles having both attachments on the thoracic limb bones.

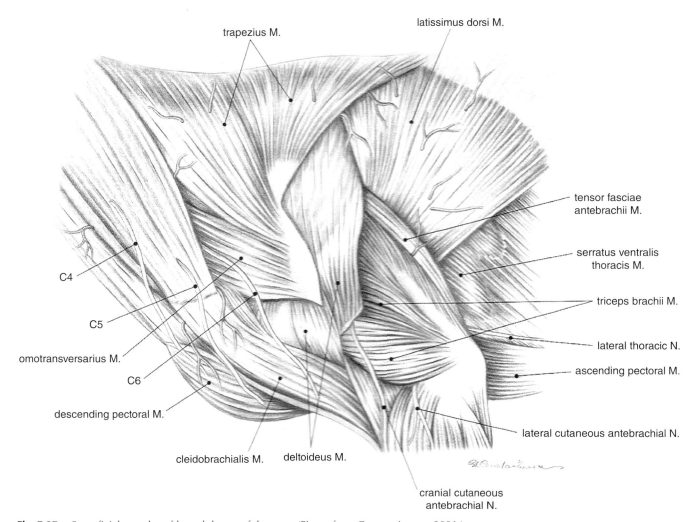

Fig. 7.27. Superficial muscles of lateral thorax of the goat. (Figure from Constantinescu, 2001.)

Muscles of the pelvic limb and body wall

Table 7.6. Muscles of the pelvic limb and body wall.

Muscle	Description	Origin (O)/Insertion (I)	Action
Sublumbar Muscles[1]			
Psoas minor	A long, thin muscle extending from lumbar vertebral bodies to ilium	O—Vertebrae T_{13}–L_5 I—Body of ilium	Stabilizes back
Iliopsoas (psoas major and iliacus)	Fused psoas major and iliacus muscle; is chief flexor of hip	O—Lumbar vertebrae I—Lesser trochanter of femur	Flexes hip and outwardly rotates thigh
Quadratus lumborum	Lies along underside of transverse processes of lumbar vertebrae	O—Transverse processes of lumbar vertebrae I—Wing of sacrum and ilium	Stabilizes lumbar vertebrae
Rump Muscles[2] *Gluteal Muscle*			
Superficial	Arises from sacral vertebrae and inserts on 3rd trochanter	O—Sacral vertebrae I—Third trochanter	Abducts limb of femur
Medial	Largest gluteal muscle; runs over deep gluteal muscle	O—Wing of ilium I—Greater trochanter of femur	Extends hip, abducts limb
Deep	Extends from shaft of ilium over hip joint and inserts on greater trochanter	O—Body of ilium I—On or near greater trochanter	Extends hip, abducts limb
Tensor fasciae latae	Triangular-shaped; inserts on lateral femoral fascia, thus the patella	O—Tuber coxae I—Lateral femoral fascia, patella	Tenses lateral femoral fascia and thus flexes hip joint and extends stifle
Pelvic-Associated Muscles[3] *Obturators*			
External	Fan-shaped; arises from ventral surface of os coxae and covers obturator foramen externally	O—Ventral surface of pubis and ischium I—Trochanteric fossa of femur	Adducts thigh
Internal	Fan-shaped; arises from pelvis floor covering obturator foramen	O—Interior (floor) of pelvis I—Trochanteric fossa of femur	Rotates femur laterally
Gemelli	Fairly insignificant hip rotator	O—Ischium I—Trochanteric fossa of femur	Rotates femur laterally
Body Wall Abdominal Obliques	Four muscles forming ventrolateral abdominal wall		
External	Sheetlike muscle extending from ribs and thoracolumbar facia	O—Lumbar last thoracic I—Midventral	Support/balance
Internal	Sheetlike muscle deep to the external abdominal oblique	O—Lumbar fascia I—Midventral	Support/balance
Gracilis	Broad, superficial muscle extending from pelvic symphysis to medial thigh and inserting on the tibia	O—Pubis and ischium I—Medial surface of knee/leg	Adducts thigh
Rectus abdominis	Two long, straight muscles running from sternum to prepubic tendon	O—Sternum I—Prepubic tendon	Support/balance

Table 7.6. *Continued*

Muscle	Description	Origin (O)/Insertion (I)	Action
Thigh Muscles[4]			
Hamstrings			
Biceps femoris	Largest and most lateral of caudal thigh muscles	O—Ischial tuberocity I—Lateral surface of knee/leg	Extends thigh, flexes leg
Semimembranosus	Arises with semitendinosis muscle form ischiatic tuberosity; splits into two bellies	O—Ischial tuberocity I—Posterior surface of femur and tibia	Extends hip, flexes or extends stifle
Semitendinosus	The longest hamstring; forms caudal border of thigh	O—Ischial tuberocity I—Tibia and calcanean tuberosity	Extends hip and tarsus, flexes stifle
Pectinius	Long, spindle-shaped muscle on medial thigh	O—Pubic tendon I—Femoral shaft	Adducts limb and flexes hip
Quadraceps femoris	Large muscle covering lateral, medial, and cranial surfaces of femur		Main stifle (knee) joint extensor
Vastus lateralis		O—Cranial and inferior to greater trochanter of femur and along linea aspera I—Tibial tuberosity via patellar ligament	Extends knee (stifle)
Vastus intermedius		O—Craniolateral surface of femur and linea aspera of femur I—Tibial tuberosity via patellar ligament	Extends knee (stifle)
Vastus medialis		O—Entire length of linea aspera of femur I—Tibial tuberosity via patellar ligament	Extends knee (stifle)
Rectus femoris		O—Rectus femoris area of ilium I—Tibial tuberosity via patellar ligament	Extends knee (stifle), flexes hip
Sartorius	A straplike muscle; the "tailor's" muscle on medial thigh	O—Ilium I—Knee	Flexes hip joint and extends knee

[1] Originates from ventral surface of caudal thoracic and lumbar vertebrae and inserts on the os coxae and femur.

[2] Originates from the ilium and inserts on the femur.

[3] Originates caudomedial to the hip joint and inserts in or near trochanteric fossa.

[4] Includes extensors of the stifle that are innervated by the femoral nerve, adductors, and hamstring muscles.

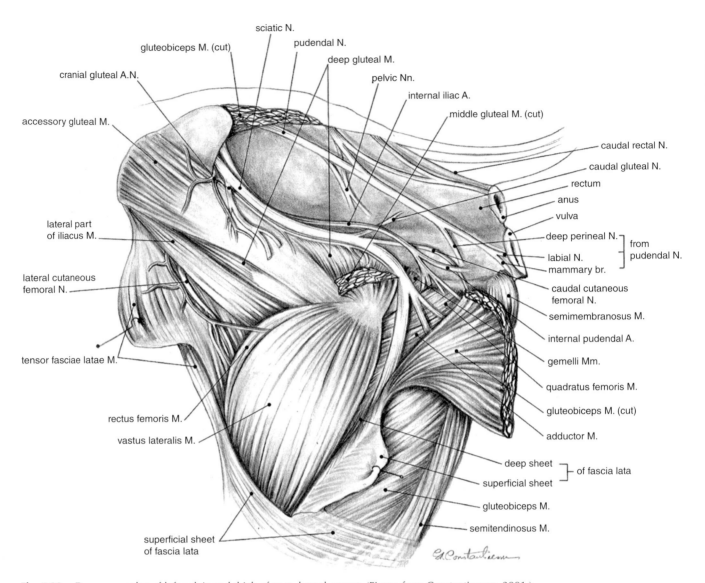

Fig. 7.28. Deeper muscles of left pelvis and thigh of goat, lateral aspect. (Figure from Constantinescu, 2001.)

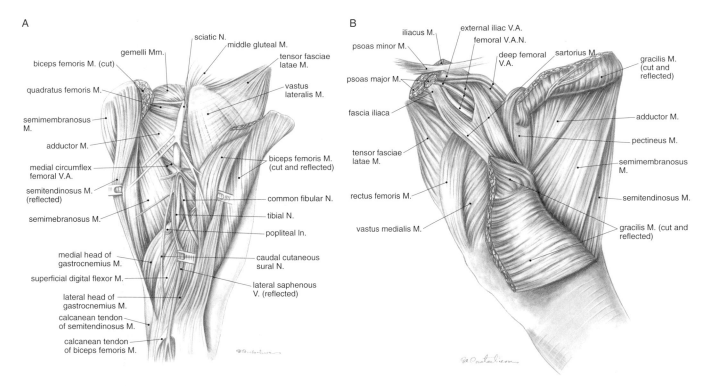

Fig. 7.29. Superficial and deep muscles in right thigh of goat. A) Lateral aspect. B) Medial aspect. (Figure from Constantinescu, 2001.)

Stay apparatus of a horse

The stay apparatus allows a horse to rest while standing, using little muscular activity or fatigue. The stay apparatus uses a system of tendons and ligaments to "lock" the lower portion of the leg, thus requiring minimal muscular effort to stand (Fig. 7.30). The stay apparatus of the thoracic limb consists of the tendinous tissue of the serratus ventralis muscles, biceps brachii, lacertus fibrosus, radial carpal extensor, common digital extensor, long head of the triceps, suspensory ligament and its branches, collateral ligaments, superficial and deep digital flexor tendons, and their accessory ligaments. The stay apparatus works as follows:

1. Shoulder flexion. Prevented by the tendon of the biceps brachii.
   a. Serratus ventralis. When the horse is at rest, the body is suspended from the scapulae by fibrous tissue in the serratus ventralis that causes the shoulder to flex.
   b. Biceps brachii. The tendon of the biceps brachii runs the length of the muscle. Stretching this tendon prevents flexion of the shoulder.
2. Elbow flexion. The elbow tends to flex because of the weight of the animal. This is prevented by

placement of collateral ligaments behind the axis of the joint.
3. Carpus flexion. The carpus would tend to flex, but this is prevented by the tendon of the biceps brachii, the lacertus fibrosus, and the tendon of the extensor carpi radialis acting cranially, and the flexor tendons and accessory ligaments acting caudally.
   a. The lacertus fibrosus is a tendinous band that connects the tendon of the biceps brachii muscle to the tendon of the extensor carpi radialis muscle, thus forming an unbroken line of force from the shoulder to the metacarpus.
   b. Tendon of the extensor carpi radialis. Tension is transmitted through the tendon of the biceps brachii and pulls the lacertus fibrosus, which directs tension down to the tendon of the extensor carpi radialis and then down to the metacarpus.
4. Carpus hyperextension. This is prevented by the cube shape of the carpal bones and the palmar carpal ligament.
5. Fetlock hyperextension. This is prevented by the suspensory apparatus, the extensor branches of the suspensory ligament, and the flexor tendons and their accessory ligaments.

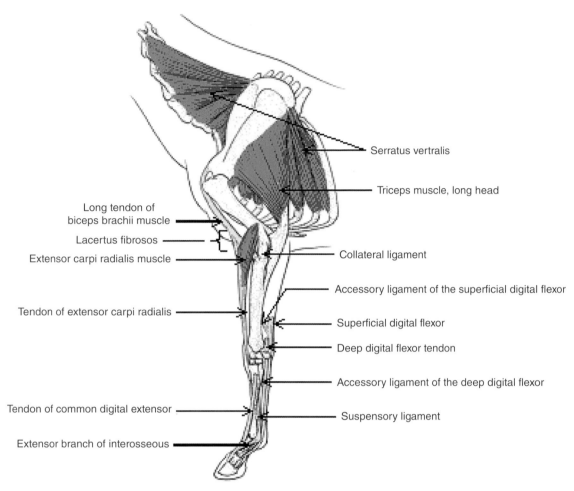

Serratus vertralis

Triceps muscle, long head

Long tendon of
biceps brachii muscle

Lacertus fibrosos

Extensor carpi radialis muscle

Collateral ligament

Accessory ligament of the superficial digital flexor

Tendon of extensor carpi radialis

Superficial digital flexor

Deep digital flexor tendon

Accessory ligament of the deep digital flexor

Tendon of common digital extensor

Suspensory ligament

Extensor branch of interosseous

Fig. 7.30. Stay apparatus of the thoracic limb of the horse. (Modified from Pasquini et al., 1995.)

References

Constantinescu, G.M. 2001. Guide to Regional Ruminant Anatomy Based on the Dissection of the Goat. Iowa State Press, Ames, Iowa.

Getty, R. 1964. Atlas for Applied Veterinary Anatomy. Iowa State Press, Ames, Iowa.

Pasquini, C., T. Spurgeon, and S. Pasquini. 1995. Anatomy of Domestic Animals, 8th Edition. SUDZ Publishing, Pilot Point, Texas.

8 Introduction to the nervous system

Contents

The body must be in constant communication with both the internal and external environment. To maintain homeostasis, the body must receive information about the environment, and then must be able to respond to that information. These responses must be rapid and coordinated. The nervous system carries out these functions.

The nervous system is responsible for collecting information about what is happening inside (internal environment), as well as outside (external environment), the body. It communicates with all parts of the body via electrical signals. This communication occurs in a highly coordinated and specific manner much like our older phone system in which signals were carried to and from various locations via wire that had to pass through a central switching station.

The nervous system can be viewed as having three components: sensory input, integration, and motor output (Fig. 8.1):

1. Sensory information about both the internal and external environment must be gathered. Any change in the environment can act as stimuli. Such sensory, or afferent information, is collected by specialized neurons called sensory neurons and transmitted as sensory input.
2. The processing and interpreting of sensory input is called integration.

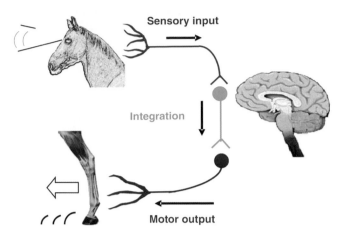

Fig. 8.1. Components of the nervous system. The nervous system has a sensory component responsible for detecting stimuli and transmitting that information to the integration center. There, the information is processed and the appropriate response is conveyed to an effector organ via the motor output.

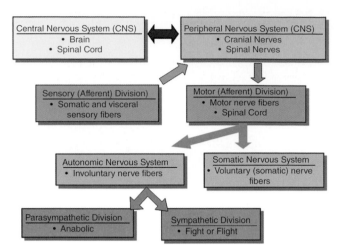

Fig. 8.2. Organization of the nervous system. The two main divisions of the nervous system include the central and peripheral nervous system. The peripheral nervous system has a sensory division that carries signals toward, and a motor division that carries signals away from, the central nervous system, respectively. The motor division is further divided into the autonomic component that controls involuntary functions, such as gastrointestinal tract motility and heart rate, and a somatic component that controls skeletal muscle. The autonomic nervous system is made of the parasympathetic and sympathetic divisions.

3. Once the information has been processed, the appropriate response is elicited by sending a motor, or efferent, signal to an effector organ. As an example of this process, when an animal sees feed being placed in a feeder, the visual information is gathered by the eyes, which sends that information to the brain (sensory input). The brain processes that information (integration) and then sends a signal to the legs to enable the animal to walk to the feeder (motor output).

Organization of the nervous system

For the purpose of presentation, the nervous system is generally divided into two major divisions: the central and the peripheral nervous system (Fig. 8.2). The central nervous system (CNS) includes the brain and spinal cord. These are located in the dorsal body cavity and are encased in the skull and vertebrae. The central nervous system includes not only neurons, but also blood vessels, connective tissue, and supportive cells. The central nervous system is responsible for the integrative function in which sensory information from both inside and outside the body is processed and the appropriate response is generated.

The peripheral nervous system (PNS) includes all the neurons outside the CNS. These include the spinal nerves that carry impulses to and from the spinal cord and the cranial nerves that carry impulses to and from the brain. Peripheral nerves consist of the neurons and associated blood vessels and connective tissue that lie outside of the CNS.

The PNS is further divided into the sensory, or afferent (*ad* = to + *ferre* = to carry), and motor, or efferent

(*ex* = from), division. The sensory division consists of sensory neurons located throughout the body that project to the brain and spinal cord. This sensory input is carried in the sensory division of the PNS. Sensory input originates from receptors, which are specialized structures that detect changes in either the internal or external environment. These receptors can be as simple as the dendrite of a neuron, or they can consist of an organ adapted to detect a specialized type of information such as the Golgi tendon organ, which detects the stretch of the tendons. The motor response generated via the integrative function of the CNS is carried to either a muscle or endocrine gland by the motor division of the PNS.

The motor division of the PNS is further divided into two parts: somatic nervous system and autonomic nervous system. The somatic nervous system controls skeletal muscle contractions, and is under voluntary control. Therefore, an animal can consciously control the somatic nervous system.

The autonomic nervous system, also called the visceral motor system, controls smooth muscle, cardiac muscle, and glandular secretions. In contrast to the somatic nervous system, the autonomic nervous system is under involuntary control, meaning that its regulation generally occurs at the subconscious level. An animal does not have to consciously control the dilation or constriction of a blood vessel in the skin in response to heat. Instead, this happens automatically—hence the name autonomic nervous system. The autonomic nervous system includes the sympathetic and parasympathetic divisions. These two divisions generally have an antagonistic effect on various functions. For example, stimulation of the sympathetic nervous system will increase heart rate, whereas stimulation of the parasympathetic nervous system will decrease heart rate.

The neuron

The nervous system consists of neurons and supportive cells. Neurons are excitable cells that are able to transmit an electrical impulse along their length. Supportive cells are responsible for making the myelin sheath surrounding many neurons, providing nutrients, as well as performing a phagocytic role.

Neurons are highly specialized cells that can respond to stimuli, and produce an impulse, and transmit that information to a distant site (Fig. 8.3). Neurons come in many sizes and shapes. They have a long life span and are generally considered amitotic, meaning that they no longer divide. However, recent evidence has revealed that within certain sites in the brain, neurons do reproduce. It has been demonstrated in songbirds that the number of neurons in regions of the brain associated with the production of songs increases in the spring as the birds increase their repertoire in preparation for mating. Similarly, the number of neurons in sites within the human brain, such as the hippocampus, has been shown to increase under

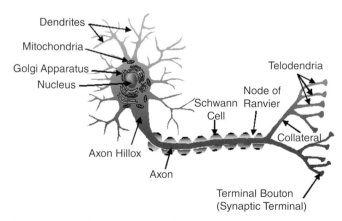

Fig. 8.3. A typical neuron. A typical neuron has a cell body (soma) that contains various organelles. The dendrites act as afferent fibers carrying signals to the soma. A neuron typically has a single axon that is the efferent fiber carrying signals away from the cell body. Many times the axon is surrounded by a myelin sheath that acts to insulate the process. In the periphery, Schwann cells make the myelin, whereas in the central nervous system, it is made by oligodendrocytes. The space between adjacent Schwann cells is called the node of Ranvier.

certain conditions. It is assumed this happens in other species.

Cell body

The cell body, or soma, consists of a large, round, nucleus 5–10 μm in diameter surrounded by cytoplasm, also called perikaryon (karyon = nucleus). Within the cytoplasma are the normal cell organelles except for the lack of centrioles that are responsible for formation of the mitotic spindle associated with cell division.

The cytoplasma contains free ribosomes, smooth and rough endoplasmic reticulum (ER), mitochondria, and Golgi apparatus. The rough endoplasmic reticulum is also known as nissl substance that stains darkly in the presence of basic dyes called nissl stains. The rough ER is the major site of protein synthesis destined for insertion into the membrane of the cell or an organelle. Free ribosomes are responsible for the synthesis of proteins destined for the cytosol. Smooth ER can be continuous with rough ER and act as a site where newly synthesized proteins are folded into their three-dimensional structure. Smooth ER can also regulate cytosolic concentrations of ions such as calcium.

Also within the cytosol is internal scaffolding called the cytoskeleton. The cytoskeleton consists of several components. The largest are the microtubules measuring about 20 nm in diameter and running longitudinally down the neurites (axons and dendrites). They are formed through polymerization of molecules of the protein tubulin. Associated with the microtubules are another class of proteins called microtubule-associated proteins, or MAPs. These proteins help anchor microtubles to other parts of the neuron, and to each other. The second component of the cytoskeleton is neurofilaments, which are called intermediate fibers in other cell types, measuring 10 nm in diameter. They consist of multiple subunits connected end to end. Each subunit consists of three proteins interwoven together. A third component are the microfilaments measuring 5 nm in diameter. They consist of two braided strands, each of which is made of polymers of the protein actin. Microfilaments not only run longitudinally down the neurites, but are also anchored to the inside of the cell membrane.

Dendrites

The term *dendrite* is derived from the Greek word for "tree," and as such they look like the branches of a tree originating from the cell body. All of the dendrites collectively make up the dendritic tree. The dendrites on some neurons also have on their surface dendritic spines. Dendrites act as the receptive region of the neuron. The combination of the dendritic tree and dendritic spines makes for a large surface area that facilitates this function. The cytoplasm of the dendrites resembles that of the soma. As discussed below, neurons can be classified based on dendrites.

Axon

While the structures discussed above are common to most cells, the axon is unique to neurons. The axon is specialized to allow an impulse to be transmitted along its length and thus carried from one location to another. A long axon is sometimes called a nerve fiber. A bundle of axons within the central nervous system is called a tract; it is called a nerve in the periphery.

A neuron has a single axon that originates from the soma in a region called the axon hillox. This is where the nerve impulse originates, and therefore is sometimes called the trigger zone. The axon is unique in that it contains no rough ER; it contains few, if any, free ribosomes; and its membrane has a different protein composition from that of the soma.

While the axoplasm (cytoplasm inside the axon) contains neurofibrils, neurotubules, lysosomes, mitochondria, and small vesicles, it lacks rough ER and ribosomes. Therefore, protein synthesis does not occur in the axon. Instead, proteins must be synthesized in the soma and transported along the axon.

Axons may extend less than a millimeter or over a meter in length. Axons typically branch, forming collaterals that enable one neuron to communicate with several other sites. Occasionally, an axon collateral may communicate with the same neuron from which it originated, thus forming a recurrent collateral. The diameter of an axon can range from less than 1 μm to as large as one mm. The thicker the axon, the faster the speed of conduction of the nerve impulse down its length.

The nerve fibers of many nerves are covered with a whitish, fatty sheath called myelin. Myelin acts to protect and insulate the axon and increases the speed of conduction of the impulse. Whereas the speed of conduction may be 1 m/sec in unmyelinated fibers, it can be 150 m/sec in myelinated fibers. The dendrites are always unmyelinated.

In the peripheral nervous system, the myelin is produced by the Schwann cells. The Schwann cell spirals around the axon producing many concentric circles enclosing the axon and forming the myelin sheath. During the spiraling process, the nucleus and cytoplasm of the Schwann cell gets squeezed to the outer layer of the cell and appears as a bulge on the outer surface. The outer layer is the neurilemma. Occasionally, the Schwann cell does not spiral around the axon, but instead encloses many axons at one time in what look like indentations on its surface. Such axons are said to be unmyelinated. Adjacent Schwann cells do not touch one another, but instead form a space called the node of Ranvier, or neurofibral nodes, in which the axonal membrane is exposed.

In the central nervous system, myelin is produced by another type of cell called an oligodendrocyte. Oligodendrocytes are a type of glial, or supportive, cell in the central nervous system. Instead of spiraling around the axon, the oligodendrocytes form end feet that surround the axon and form the myelin sheath. One oligodendrocyte can thereby myelinate many axons, whereas a Schwann cell myelinates only a single axon. In the central nervous system, areas containing myelinated fibers are referred to as white matter and generally consist of fiber tracts. Areas containing cell bodies are referred to as gray matter; collections of cell bodies are called nuclei.

The collaterals off the main axon trunk end in a series of fine extensions called telodendria. A collection of telodendria is called a terminal arbor. The telodendria end in a knoblike structure called the axon terminal, terminal bouton, or synaptic knob. Microtubules do not extend into the terminal, but the terminal will typically contain synaptic vesicles. Synaptic vesicles are small membrane-bound spheres measuring 50 nm in diameter and containing quanta of neurotransmitters. The axon terminal will end at another neuron or cell such as an endocrine gland or muscle cell.

Synapse

Where the axon terminal meets another cell is called the synapse. It consists of a presynaptic membrane, a synaptic cleft, and a postsynaptic membrane. The axon terminal will typically contain synaptic vesicles. The average neuron forms approximately 1,000 synaptic junctions.

The synaptic terminal of one neuron can synapse on any part of an adjacent neuron. Therefore, this can create synapses such as axo-axonic, axo-dendritic, axo-somatic. When a neuron synapses on a skeletal muscle cell, it creates a specialized junction called a neuromuscular junction. If the neuron synapses with a gland, it creates a neuroglandular synapse.

There are two types of synapses, electrical and chemical, which have different functional properties (Table 8.1). While chemical synapses are much more common between neurons in the mammalian and avian brain, electrical synapses are common between nonneural cells such as glial cells, epithelial cells,

Table 8.1. Electrical versus chemical synapses.

Type of Synapse	Distance Within Synaptic Cleft	Components of Synapse	Agent of Transmission	Synaptic Delay	Direction of Transmission
Chemical	20–40 nm	Synaptic vesicles, active zone, postsynaptic receptors	Chemical	1–5 ms	Unidirectional
Electrical	3.5 nm	Gap-junction channels	Electrical	Virtually absent	Bidirectional

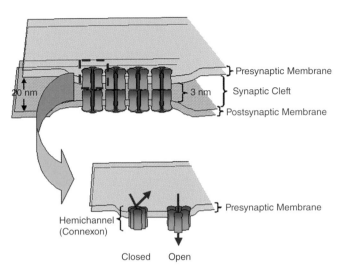

Fig. 8.4. An electrical synapse. An electrical synapse consists of a gap junction between two adjacent cells. The space between the presynaptic and postsynaptic cells contains channels called connexons, each composed of six protein subunits called connexins. The connexon forms a cytoplasmic connection between adjacent cells allowing ions and small molecules to pass between both cells. The connexins can tilt toward each other, closing the channel.

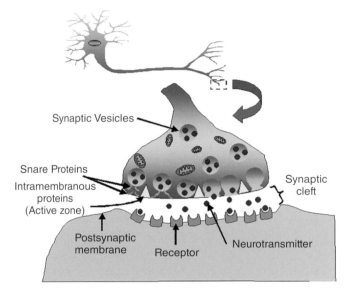

Fig. 8.5. A chemical synapse. A chemical synapse consists of synaptic membrane, synaptic cleft, and a postsynaptic membrane. Since the nerve impulse cannot jump across the synaptic cleft, a neurotransmitter is released, which carries the signal to the postsynaptic cell. The active zone of the presynaptic cell contains intramembranous proteins, thought to be calcium channels. When the neuron is depolarized, calcium enters through the calcium channels and causes the synaptic vesicles to bind to the presynaptic membrane and release their contents through a process of exocytosis. SNARE (soluble N-ethylmaleimide-sensitive proteins) attaches synaptic vesicles to the presynaptic membrane.

smooth and cardiac muscle cells, liver cells, and some glandular cells.

In electrical synapses, the pre- and postsynaptic cells communicate through special channels called gap junctions (Fig. 8.4). These junctions provide a channel between the cytoplasm of the adjacent cells. Gap junctions consist of a pair of hemichannels, with one associated with the presynaptic membrane and the other the postsynaptic membrane. Each hemichannel consists of specialized proteins called connexins. Six connexins combine to form a channel called a connexon through which ions can pass from the cytoplasm of one cell to the cytoplasm of another cell. The pore formed within the connexon is about 2 nm in diameter, making it one of the largest known, and is of sufficient size to allow small organic molecules to pass. It appears that the connexins can tilt toward one another to close the channel.

The electrical synapse allows an action potential to pass from one cell to another with virtually no delay. This is beneficial when it is necessary for a signal to pass rapidly to another cell, and for that signal to not be modified.

The chemical synapse is characterized by a synaptic cleft 20–50 nm wide (Fig. 8.5). Within the synaptic cleft is a fibrous protein matrix to help the two cells adhere to one another. An electrical signal cannot cross the synaptic cleft, so a chemical substance called a neurotransmitter carries the signal to the postsynaptic cell. The neurotransmitter is stored in the synaptic vesicles. The concentration of neurotransmitter can be 10,000 times higher than in the cytosol. This is accomplished by a countertransport system in which a molecule of transmitter enters the vesicle in exchange for a H^+ ion (Fig. 8.6).

Also found on the presynaptic membrane are pyramid-shaped proteins projecting into the cyto-

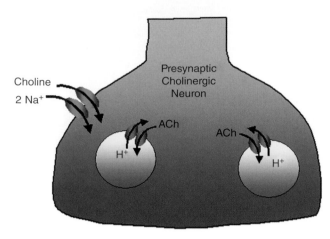

Fig. 8.6. Pumping neurotransmitters. Neurotransmitters are actively concentrated into the synaptic vesicles, using a countertransport system. The vesicle membrane has an H⁺-ATP pump that loads the vesicle with H⁺. The neurotransmitter then enters the vesicle in exchange for a molecule of H⁺. In addition, there is a transport system on the presynaptic neuron membrane that transports either the neurotransmitter, or its precursor, into the cell. In this example, choline, the precursor of acetylcholine (ACh) is actively cotransported into the cell with Na⁺.

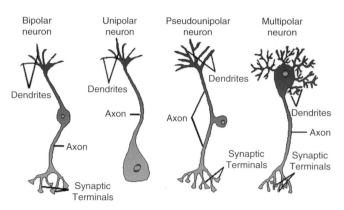

Fig. 8.7. Classification of neurons. Anaxonic neurons lack an axon. Bipolar neurons have one dendrite and one axon originating from the cell body. In unipolar neurons, the dendrite and axon merge into a single process having a dendritic and axonic component. Pseudounipolar have a small process coming off at the cell body and leading to the axon. In multipolar neurons, there are many dendrites but a single axon originating from the cell body.

plasm. These proteins, and the associated cell membrane, make the active zone. The active zone is the site of neurotransmitter release. The pyramid-shaped proteins associated with the active zone are believed to be calcium channels.

Classification of neurons

Neurons can be classified based on several characteristics. These include the structural classifications based on the number of neurites that extend from the soma or the length of the axon, the function, or the neurotransmitter they contain.

Classification based on neurite number

Based on neurite number, neurons can be classified as unipolar, bipolar, pseudounipolar, or multipolar (Fig. 8.7). Unipolar neurons are the simplest nerve cells, and they have a single process. They are found in the autonomic nervous system. Bipolar neurons have an oval-shaped soma from which two processes emerge: the dendrite and the axon. Many sensory neurons are bipolar, such as those in the retina of the eye and olfactory epithelium of the nose. Pseudounipolar cells serve as mechanoreceptors that sense touch, pressure, and pain. The pseudounipolar develops embryologically as a bipolar neuron with two processes, but eventually these two processes fuse into a single axon that emerges from the soma. The axon then divides into two segments, with one going to the

periphery and one going to the spinal cord. The predominate type of neuron is the multipolar neuron that has a single axon and generally has many dendrites.

Classification based on axon length

Classifications based on axon length include Golgi type I and Golgi type II neurons. Golgi type I neurons have long axons and are considered projection neurons since they carry signals to other sites. An example would be pyramidal cells with the cell bodies located in the cerebral cortex and whose axons extend to the spinal cord. Golgi type II neurons have short axons and are involved in local circuits. Examples include stellate or basket neurons in the cerebellum.

Classification based on function

Based on function, neurons are classified the following ways: 1) sensory, or afferent neurons; 2) motor, or efferent neurons; 3) interneurons, or association neurons. Sensory neurons respond to sensory stimuli, and transmit that information to the nervous system, with most information being carried to the CNS. Most sensory neurons are pseudounipolar, and their cell bodies are located in the dorsal root ganglion of the spinal nerves. Motor neurons transmit signals from the brain or spinal cord to the muscles or glands. Their cell bodies are located in the CNS. Interneurons are the largest class of neurons—constituting 99% of all neurons, including all those neurons that are not sensory or motor—and are generally multipolar. This class can be divided into two groups. Relay or projection interneurons have long axons and transmit signals over considerable distances, such as the dorsal columns

A. Convergence

B. Divergence

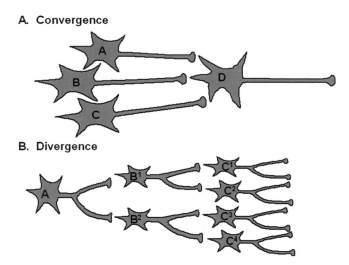

Fig. 8.8. Diverging and converging neuronal pools. Interneurons are involved in making neuronal pools. A) Convergence occurs when several interneurons synapse on a single neuron. B) Divergence occurs when a single interneuron synapses on more than one interneuron.

located in the spinal cord. Local interneurons have short axons and are involved in processing information in localized circuits, such as the horizontal cells in the retina or stellate cells that inhibit Purkinje cells in the cerebellum.

Interneurons, sometimes called association neurons, are the most numerous of all neuronal types. Mostly located in the brain and spinal cord, some are found in autonomic ganglia. They function to distribute sensory information and coordinate motor activity. Interneurons produce patterns of connections such as divergence and convergence (Fig. 8.8). Information coming from a single source and spreading to multiple neurons is known as divergence, whereas input from multiple neurons synapsing on a single interneuron is called convergence.

Classification based on neurotransmitter

Finally, neurons can be classified according to the neurotransmitter they release. In the case of motor neurons, which innervate skeletal muscle, they all release acetylcholine and are called cholinergic neurons. Neurons that release serotonin, such as 5-hydroxytryptamine (5-HT), are called serotonergic neurons. An example would be those neurons in the raphe nucleus of the brain stem.

Supportive cells

Although neurons are the fundamental cell of the nervous system and are responsible for transmitting a

signal, they make up only 10% of nervous tissue. The remaining 90% is made of several cell types collectively called neuroglia, or glia, that support, protect, and nourish neighboring neurons both in the central and peripheral nervous system. The neuroglia of the CNS include 1) ependymal cells, 2) astrocytes, 3) oligodendrocytes, and 4) microglia. The neuroglia of the peripheral nervous system include 1) satellite cells and 2) Schwann cells.

Ependymal cells

The brain has four fluid-filled cavities within its borders called cerebroventricles; the spinal cord has a central canal. These cavities are lined with ependymal cells that range in shape from squamous to columnar, and may be ciliated. These cells generally form a permeable barrier between the cerebrospinal fluid and tissue. The exception is ependymal cells covering the choroid plexus (capillary tuft in each cerebroventricle responsible for forming cerebrospinal fluid). These ependymal cells form tight junctions creating a barrier between the blood and brain. The cilia located on ependymal cells help "circulate" or move the cerebrospinal fluid within the ventricular system.

Astrocytes

Astrocytes are star-shaped, and are the most abundant glial cells. They have radiating processes that expand at the end and form end feet that wrap around capillaries. The astrocytes secrete some chemical that causes the endothelial cells lining the brain capillaries to form tight junctions. These tight junctions form the blood-brain barrier that greatly restricts the movement of compounds into the brain. Astrocytes also help guide the migration and connections of new neurons, control the chemical environment around neurons and help inactivate neurotransmitters that are released into the synapse. Since astrocytes are also connected via gap junctions, they also signal one another, although the function is unclear.

Oligodendrocytes

Oligodendrocytes have fewer processes than astrocytes and smaller cell bodies. As already discussed, these cells are responsible for producing the myelin sheath found around axons in the CNS. This sheath is formed by the process of the oligodendrocyte that wraps around an axon forming concentric layers or circles, much like wrapping layers of gauze around a cut finger.

Microglia

These are small ovoid cells that have narrow cytoplasmic processes with many branches. These cells originate from mesodermal stem cells related to those that produce monocytes and macrophages. They can migrate within the CNS where they phagocytize microorganisms and dead neurons. Although cells in the peripheral immune system cannot enter the CNS, the microglia seem to partially fill this role.

Satellite cells and Schwann cells

Also called amphicytes, satellite cells surround neuronal cell bodies in peripheral ganglia. Their function is unknown. As previously discussed, Schwann cells form the myelin sheath around peripheral axons. Therefore, they are analogous to oligodendrocytes.

Neurophysiology

The neuron is a highly excitable cell that is able to respond to and transduce a stimulus into an electrical potential. Like an electrical wire, an axon carries a signal along its length. Whereas in an electrical wire, the signal involves the flow of electrons along the length of the wire, nerve cells are poor conductors of electricity over a long length. Instead of the movement of electrons, neurons rely on the flow of charged ions to propagate the signal. The nerve impulse, or action potential, can travel over long distances without diminishing.

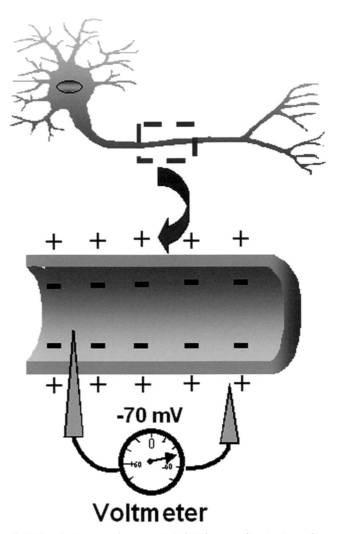

Fig. 8.9. Resting membrane potential. When a voltmeter is used to compare the voltage difference between the inside and outside of a neuron membrane, a membrane potential of approximately −70 mV is typically measured.

The resting membrane potential

Nerve cells and muscle cells have an excitable membrane. When such a cell is not generating an impulse, it is said to be at rest. When at rest, the cytosol has a negative electrical charge relative to the outside of the cell (Fig. 8.9). The potential energy generated by the separation of charge across the membrane is called voltage, and is measured in volts or millivolts (1 V = 1,000 mV). By placing an electrode both inside and outside the cell, a voltage can be measured between these two sites. That voltage is called the potential difference, or potential. The difference in electrical charge across the membrane of a cell at rest is called the resting membrane potential, and it is typically about −60 to −70 mV.

The inside and outside of the cell is separated by a membrane that acts as a semipermeable membrane. The membrane potential is caused by the unequal distribution of ions across the membrane. For the four most important ions with regard to membrane potential, the concentration of Na^+ and Cl^- is higher outside the cell, whereas the concentration of K^+ and organic anions is higher inside the cell. The organic anions consist mostly of proteins and amino acids. These differences in ion concentrations establish chemical gradients.

The lipid bilayer of the cell membrane acts as an insulator between the interior and exterior of the cell. Ions cannot cross the membrane except by way of ion channels. Within the membrane there are passive ion channels, sometimes called leak channels, which remain open. These passive channels are most permeable to K^+ and chloride ions, relatively less permeable to Na^+, and impermeable to proteins. Since K^+ is in higher concentrations inside the cell, it tends to diffuse outwardly, down its concentration gradient. The movement of ions to eliminate the potential difference is called a current. How much the membrane restricts the movement of ions is a measure of its resistance. As K^+ moves outward, an excess of negatively charged anions remain inside the cell, thus establishing an electrochemical gradient. Eventually, the movement of K^+ outward reaches equilibrium because the outwardly directed chemical gradient is opposed by the inwardly directed electrical gradient. This point is called the ionic equilibrium potential, or equilibrium potential, and is represented by the symbol E_{ion}.

The equilibrium potential of an ion can be calculated using the Nernst equation:

$$E_{ion} = 2.303 \frac{RT}{zF} \log \frac{[ion]_{outside}}{[ion]_{inside}}$$

where E_{ion} equals ionic equilibrium potential, R equals the gas constant, T equals absolute temperature, z equals charge on the ion, F equals Faraday's constant, and [ion] is the concentration of the ion either inside or outside the cell. At body temperature, the Nernst equation for the monovalent ions K^+, Na^+, and Cl^- can be simplified to

$$E_{ion} = 61.54 \, mV \log \frac{[ion]_{outside}}{[ion]_{inside}}$$

whereas for Ca^{++}, a divalent cation, the equation would be

$$E_{ca} = 30.77 \, mV \log \frac{[Ca^{++}]_{outside}}{[Ca^{++}]_{inside}}$$

E_{ion} is very important for understanding the effect an ion has on the membrane potential (Table 8.2).

If the membrane were permeable only to K^+, the membrane potential would be approximately −80 mV. At this point, the chemical gradient for K^+ would equal the electrochemical gradient. However, the membrane is permeable to ions other than K^+. The Nernst equation does not take into consideration the permeability of multiple ions, or that the relative permeability of the various ions is different. If the permeabilities of the ions are known, the membrane potential can be calculated using the Goldman equation:

$$V_m = \frac{RT}{F} \ln \frac{P_K[K^{++}]_{outside} + P_{Na}[Na^+]_{outside} + P_{Cl}[Cl^-]_{inside}}{P_K[K^+]_{inside} + P_{Na}[Na^+]_{inside} + P_{Cl}[Cl^-]_{outside}}$$

where V_m is the membrane potential, and P is the permeability of the respective ion. The relative permeability of the ions is $P_K:P_{Na}:P_{Cl} = 1.0 : 0.04 : 0.45$. Note that in the Goldman equation, the concentrations of Cl^- inside and outside the membrane are reversed compared to Na^+ and K^+ since Cl^- is an anion.

At rest, the flow of ions is not static, but is in equilibrium such that Na^+ is moving into the cell while K^+ is moving out (Fig. 8.10). This movement is countered by an active Na^+–K^+ATPase. This active transport system pumps 3 molecules of Na^+ out of the cell for every 2 molecules of K^+ pumped back in. The helps maintain the unequal distribution of ions across the cell membrane.

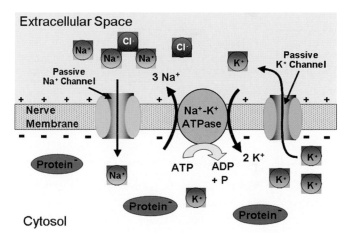

Fig. 8.10. The basis of the resting membrane potential. In a nerve at rest, there is an unequal distribution of ions across the cell membrane. The concentration of Na^+ and Cl^- is higher outside the cell, while that of K^+ and anions is higher inside the cell. Moving down their concentration gradient, Na^+ passively moves into the cell while K^+ moves out of the cell. A Na^+–K^+ ATPase then actively pumps three molecules of Na^+ out of the cell for every two molecules of K^+ pumped in while cleaving ATP to ADP plus inorganic phosphate (P).

Table 8.2. Ion concentrations and equilibrium potentials in neurons.

Ion	Concentration Outside (mM)	Concentration Inside (mM)	Ratio Outside : Inside	E_{ion} (mV)
K^+	5	100	1 : 20	−80
Na^+	150	15	10 : 1	62
Ca^{++}	2	.0002	10,000 : 1	123
Cl^-	150	13	11.5 : 1	−65

Membrane channels

The neuron is excitable, and thus able to generate and transmit an impulse. A nerve impulse is a change in the resting membrane potential. It is generated in a rather complex process. We have already discussed passive membrane channels that allow ions to move through the membrane of a resting neuron. In addition, there are also active channels, sometimes called gated channels, in the cell membrane. The gated channels open or close in response to stimuli. There are three classes of gated channels: 1) chemically gated; 2) voltage-gated; 3) mechanically gated.

Chemically gated channels

Chemically gated channels, sometimes called neurotransmitter-gated channels, are located on the post-synaptic membrane. These channels are found most abundantly on the dendrites and cell body, and they respond to a neurotransmitter binding to its receptor. The binding of a neurotransmitter will generally cause these channels to either open or close. However, a high concentration of neurotransmitter can cause these channels to become inactivated.

Chemically gated channels can be either directly gated or indirectly gated (Fig. 8.11). Directly gated channels consist of a single macromolecule in which part of the molecule serves as an extracellular domain forming a receptor for a neurotransmitter while the second part of the molecule consists of a membrane-spanning domain, which forms an ion channel. Such receptors are sometimes called ionotropic receptors. Binding of the neurotransmitter to the receptor portion of the molecule causes a conformational change that results in opening the channel.

Ionotropic receptors are relatively large and contain multisubunits that form an ion channel through the cell membrane. Binding of a neurotransmitter to such

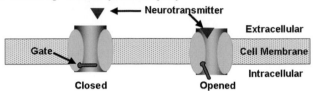

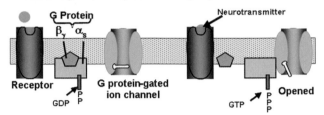

Fig. 8.11. Indirectly and directly gated channel. Neurotransmitters can activate either directly or indirectly gated channels. 1. In directly gated, or ionotropic, channels the neurotransmitter receptor and ion channel are the same protein. When the neurotransmitter binds to the receptor, it causes a conformation change that results in either an opening or closing of the ion channel. 2. In indirectly gated, or metabotropic, channels the neurotransmitter binds to a receptor that is distinct from the ion channel. Binding of the neurotransmitter to the receptor activates a G protein. The G protein can act either act directly on a G protein–gated ion channel, or affect the action of an enzyme that makes a second messenger.

a receptor causes a conformational change that opens the channel permitting ions to flow down their electrochemical gradients. Ionotropic receptors act in submilliseconds.

Indirectly gated channels, often called metabotropic receptors, consist of macromolecules that are distinct from the ion channels they affect. Binding of the neurotransmitter to these channels stimulates or inhibits the production of second messengers such as cAMP, inositol triphosphate, or diacylglycerol. The second messengers then activate protein kinases that are enzymes that phosphorylate other proteins such as ion channels. This can result in opening or closing of ion channels, thus altering the membrane potential.

Metabotropic receptors are composed of a single polypeptide. In contrast to ionotropic receptors, instead of opening an ion channel in response to binding of a neurotransmitter, metabotropic receptors instead normally activate GTP-binding proteins (G proteins). Such receptors generally display slower onset and longer duration than ionotropic receptors.

Voltage-gated channels

Voltage-gated channels are found on those membranes that generate an action potential, including axons and the sarcolemma of skeletal and cardiac muscle. These channels open or close in response to changes

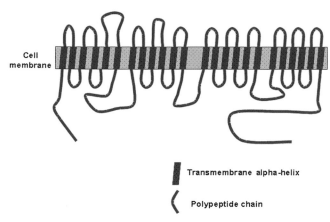

Transmembrane alpha-helix

Polypeptide chain

Fig. 8.12. Voltage-gated sodium channel. The voltage-gated sodium channel consists of four groups of homologous domains of similar sequences of amino acids, with each domain being comprised of six transmembrane segments. Each transmembrane segment consists of nonpolar amino acids coiled into an alpha-helix. The peptide chains connecting the transmembrane domains consist of polar amino acids.

in membrane potential. More precisely, when the membrane potential reaches a critical level called the threshold, voltage-gated channels open. The threshold is normally between −55 and −50 mV.

For our discussion, the most important such channels are those for sodium, potassium, and calcium. The voltage-gated sodium channel is created by a long polypeptide having four distinct domains, each consisting of six transmembrane segments (Fig. 8.12). As the membrane potential becomes more positive due to stimulation, positively charged amino acids lining the pore formed by the channel move away from the center, thus opening the channel. The voltage-gated sodium channel is unique in that it operates in three stages. When stimulated by depolarization, the channel opens rapidly. It remains open for about 1 msec and then becomes inactivated. It cannot be opened again until the membrane potential returns to a negative value below or near the value that originally caused the channel to open. These channels can be blocked by the neurotoxin tetrodotoxin that is found in the ovaries of the puffer fish (see Box 8.2).

Voltage-gated potassium channels do not open immediately upon stimulation. In addition to having a delayed opening, they also do not become inactivated after stimulation. The voltage-gated calcium channels are similar to the other voltage-gated channels, and will be discussed below with regards to neurotransmitter release.

Mechanically gated channels

These channels open and close in response to physical distortion of the cell membrane. They are found in

Box 8.2 Voltage-gated channels: neurotoxins and anesthetics

The puffer fish is considered a delicacy in Japan. When prepared properly, its consumption results in numbness around the mouth. It is prepared by chefs who are licensed by the government for preparation of this fish. Yet each year, dozens of people die from eating this fish. The ovaries of the puffer fish contain a tetrodotoxin, a compound that specifically blocks voltage-gated sodium channels. Blockage of these channels results in the inability of neurons to generate an action potential.

Dinoflagellates of the genus *Gonyaulax* produce a neurotoxin called saxitoxin that similarly blocks voltage-gated sodium channels. Dinoflagellates can contaminate shellfish such as clams and mussels. Occasionally, there is a sudden increase in the level of dinoflagellates resulting in a "red tide" that causes contamination resulting in occasional human deaths from consumption of these seafoods.

Local anesthetics such as lidocaine also work by blocking voltage-gated sodium channels. Lidocaine binds to the S6 alpha helix of domain IV of the channel, thus blocking the flow of Na+ into the neuron. These anesthetics affect smaller axons before affecting larger axons. Fortunately, it is the smaller axons that carry pain signals.

sensory neurons such as those that respond to touch, pressure, or vibration.

Postsynaptic potentials

At rest, only the passive channels are open while the neurotransmitter-gated channels are closed. When a neurotransmitter binds to a postsynaptic receptor, it activates a neurotransmitter-gated, or chemically gated, channel that causes a change in the membrane potential. This change in potential is called a postsynaptic potential since it occurs in the postsynaptic cell. Postsynaptic potentials are also graded because their magnitude depends on both the amount and the duration of action of the neurotransmitter.

If the neurotransmitter is excitatory, it generates an excitatory postsynaptic potential (EPSP). During an EPSP, the membrane potential moves toward 0 mV, or becomes depolarized. If the neurotransmitter is inhibitory, it generates an inhibitory postsynaptic potential (IPSP). An IPSP results in the membrane potential becoming more negative, or hyperpolarized. The activation of mechanically gated channels can also cause the generation of an EPSP or IPSP.

Excitatory postsynaptic potentials

The binding of an excitatory neurotransmitter to a postsynaptic receptor causes channels to open that allow both sodium and potassium to simultaneously move down their concentration gradient. However, sodium moves inward more rapidly than potassium moves outward due to the electrochemical gradient that exists. Remember that the inside of the cell is negatively charged and thus attracts positively charged molecules. The net result of this ion movement is an increase in intracellular sodium, resulting in depolarization.

The EPSPs are generated in the dendrites and cell bodies. Dendrites and cell bodies do not have voltage-gated channels, which are necessary for the generation of an action potential. An EPSP is not the same as an action potential, but instead is graded.

Inhibitory postsynaptic potential

The binding of an inhibitory neurotransmitter to its receptor causes the cell membrane to become hyperpolarized. Inhibitory neurotransmitters generally cause the opening of transmitter-gated potassium channels, chloride channels, or both. Opening potassium channels allows potassium to move out of the cell, thus making the interior of the cell more negative. Conversely, opening chloride channels allows chloride to move into the cell that also makes the cell more negative.

Generation of an action potential

Neurons are able to generate and propagate an electrical impulse, called an action potential, along their length. The action potential is a stereotypic depolarization and repolarization of the membrane. It is an all-or-none response that means that within a given cell, the response always looks identical both in amplitude and duration, independent of the stimulus. The action potential is generated at one site in the neuron, the axon hillox, and is then propagated down the length of the axon;

Step 1—Resting state. At rest, the voltage-gated channels are closed, and there is only passive movement of ions across the cell membrane.

Step 2—Depolarization. When a neuron receives stimuli, the chemically or mechanically gated channels respond. This results in the production of postsynaptic potentials. These are graded potentials, and they can summate (Fig. 8.13). For example, if a neuron generates a volley of EPSPs in rapid succession, they will summate, or add up algebraically, over time, which is called temporal

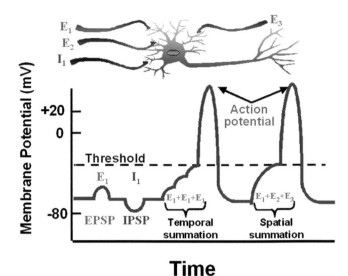

Fig. 8.13. Summation. In response to activation of chemically or mechanically gated channel, neurons can develop postsynaptic potentials, which can be either excitatory (EPSP) or inhibitory (IPSP). These postsynaptic potentials summate algebraically. EPSPs result in depolarization whereas IPSPs cause hyperpolarization. If a neuron receives stimuli from a single neuron in rapid succession, the postsynaptic potentials can cause temporal summation, whereas if a neuron receives input from multiple locations at the same time, it causes spatial summation.

summation. If a neuron receives many stimuli simultaneously from various neurons synapsing on its surface, the postsynaptic potentials summate via spatial summation, meaning that it is occurring across space rather than time. A neuron typically receives both inhibitory and excitatory input that is summated. The postsynaptic potentials are generated in the dendrites and cell's body, and they travel to the axon hillox.

Step 3—Generation of the action potential. If summation brings the membrane to threshold, the voltage-gated channels are activated (Fig. 8.14). Upon reaching threshold, the voltage-gated Na^+ channels open, increasing the permeability to Na^+ a thousandfold, and allowing Na^+ to rapidly move inward. This causes the membrane potential to move toward the equilibrium potential for Na+ ($E_{Na} = +62$ mV). This results in the upstroke, or rising phase, of the action potential. At the peak of the action potential, the voltage-gated Na^+ channels become inactivated. Therefore, Na^+ can no longer move inward. However, at this time, the voltage-gated potassium channels are opening, thus allowing K^+ to move outward. The outward movement of K+ causes the repolarization phase, also called the downstroke or falling phase, of the action potential in which the membrane potential moves back toward its resting membrane potential.

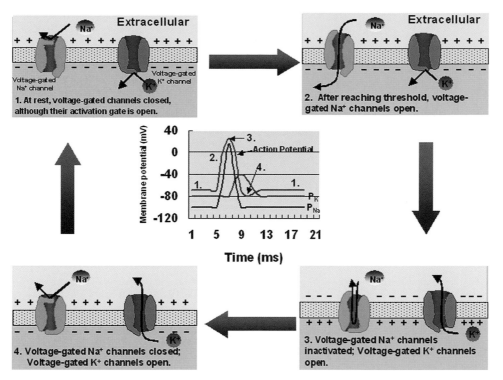

Fig. 8.14. Generation of an action potential. 1. At rest, the voltage-gated Na$^+$ and K$^+$ channels are closed. 2. When the neuron is depolarized to threshold by the summation of postsynaptic potentials, the voltage-gated Na$^+$ channels open. The movement of Na+ into the cell results in the upstroke of the action potential as the membrane potential moves toward the equilibrium potential for Na$^+$. 3. At the peak of the action potential, the voltage-gated Na$^+$ channels become inactivated, while the voltage-gated K$^+$ channels are opening. This results in the downstroke of the action potential as the membrane potential moves toward the equilibrium potential for K$^+$. 4. If the voltage-gated K$^+$ channels remain open for an extended period of time, a hyperpolarizing after-potential can develop. Finally, the voltage-gated K$^+$ channels close, and the membrane potential returns to rest.

At the end of the repolarization phase, if the voltage-gated potassium channels are slow to close, K$^+$ continues to move outward. This results in a hyperpolarizing afterpotential, or undershoot, in which the membrane potential becomes hyperpolarized relative to the original resting membrane potential before returning to normal.

At the peak of the action potential, the voltage-gated sodium channels become inactivated. This creates a brief time period called the absolute refractory period during which no stimuli, no matter how large, can generate an action potential. This is followed by another brief period of time, called the relative refractory period, during which only a greater than normal stimuli can initiate an action potential. A summary of the generation of the action potential is shown in Figure 8.15.

Propagation of the action potential

Once the action potential is generated, it must be carried along the length of the axon. During the generation of the action potential, there is a reversal in membrane potential induced by the movement of Na$^+$ inward, causing the interior of the membrane to temporarily become positive while the outside becomes negative. After this happens, the positively charged ions now inside the membrane move laterally since they are attracted by the negatively charged ions lining the inside of the membrane. Conversely, the positively charged ions found on the outside of the membrane migrate toward the new sink of negatively charged ions created by the reversal in membrane potential, thus completing the circuit.

The local flow of current caused by the opening of the voltage-gated Na$^+$ channels results in a series of electrotonic changes (Fig. 8.16). As the positive ions on the inside of the membrane flow to an area of negative ions, this depolarizes that area and thus causes the voltage-gated Na$^+$ channels in that area to open. A positive feedback system is initiated that allows the action potential to be propagated down the length of the axon without diminishing in amplitude. The process is self-propagating. As the action potential migrates down the axon, the voltage-gated Na$^+$ channels in the area it just moved from are absolutely refractory. Therefore, the action potential cannot go backward through that area since the voltage-gated Na$^+$ channels cannot open. Since the action potential

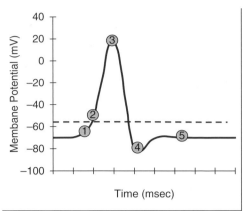

Step 1: Depolarization to threshold – Postsynaptic potentials summate temporally or spatially to reach threshold.

Step 2: Opening voltage-gated Na⁺ channels - Voltage-gated sodium channels open allowing Na⁺ to rush inward and membrane potential to move towards E_{Na^+}

Step 3: Inactivation of voltage-gated Na⁺ channels, activation of voltage-gated K⁺ channels - At the peak of the action potential, the voltage-gated sodium channels become inactivated. This results in the absolute refractory period during which time another action potential can not be generated. This is immediately followed by the relative refractory period when a greater than normal stimuli can again open the voltage-gated Na⁺ channels. At the peak of the action potential, the volatge-gated K⁺ channels are opening allowing K⁺ to flow outward and the membrane potential to move towards E_K.

Step 4: After potential – If the voltage-gated K⁺ channels are sluggish in dosing, then the membrane potential will move closer to the E_{K^+} and will drop below the original resting membrane potential.

Step 5: Resting Membrane potential – The cell returns to the original resting membrane potential

Fig. 8.15. Summary of an action potential.

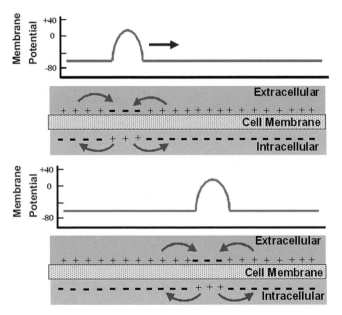

Fig. 8.16. Propagation of an action potential. Local current flows between the site of the action potential and the adjacent inactive areas. This flow of current triggers an action potential in the adjacent area while returning the original site to its resting membrane potential. In this manner, the action potential is able to propagate down the axon.

originates in the axon hillox, in vivo the action potential moves only from the axon hillox toward the nerve bouton. If the nerve is removed and placed in vitro, and the axon is stimulated in the middle, the action potential can travel in either direction.

Conduction velocity

Conduction velocity refers to the speed with which an action potential is propagated down the length of the axon. Two factors control the conduction velocity: axon diameter and myelin sheath:

- Axon diameter. The larger the axon diameter, the faster the conduction velocity. During an action potential, the cations that enter the cell can either move through the cytoplasm, or back through the cell membrane. Both the membrane and the cytoplasm offer resistance. While the cytoplasm offers resistance, the larger the diameter of the axon, the resistance in the cytoplasm becomes less, relative to that of the axon membrane. The farther the current can flow down the axon due to less resistance in the larger diameter axons, the farther the wave of depolarization moves, and thus the faster the speed of conduction.
- Myelin and saltatory conduction. While increasing the diameter of an axon is one strategy to increase conduction velocity, another strategy found in nature is to myelinate the axon. The myelin acts as an insulative sheath enwrapping an axon. There are 0.2–2.0 mm breaks in the myelin sheath called node of Ranvier. Voltage-gated channels are concentrated in the nodes. An action potential is propagated down a myelinated axon by a process called saltatory conduction (from Latin, "to leap"). In essence, the action potential skips along the axon from node to node (Fig. 8.17).

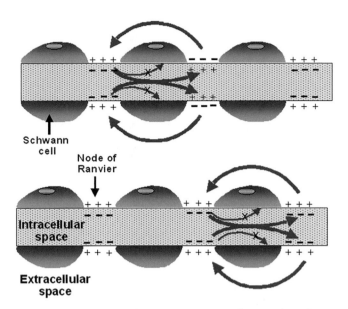

Schwann
cell

Node of
Ranvier

**Intracellular
space**

**Extracellular
space**

Fig. 8.17. Saltatory conduction. On myelinated axons, the voltage-gated channels are clustered at the node of Ranvier. An action potential propagates along the axon by "jumping" from node to node. Since there are no voltage-gated channels in the internode area, there is no movement of ions nor reversal of membrane potential in these regions.

Myelinating a neuron also decreases the amount of energy needed for neural transmission. This is because Na$^+$ and K$^+$ move across the axon membrane only at the nodes; therefore, less energy is expended via the Na$^+$-K$^+$ ATPase to restore the Na$^+$ and K$^+$ concentration gradients.

Box 8.3 Demyelinating diseases

Problems with myelin can result in several disease states. Multiple sclerosis (MS) is a disease involving the myelin sheath of axons in the brain, spinal cord, and optic nerve. Sclerosis is derived from the Greek word for "hardening." In this disease, the myelin sheath in many areas (i.e., multiple) becomes hardened, resulting in a multitude of symptoms such as weakness, lack of coordination, and impaired vision and speech. In Guillain-Barré syndrome, the myelin of peripheral nerves innervating muscle and skin is affected.

Coding of stimulus intensity

If the action potential is an all-or-none response, how does the CNS determine the intensity of a stimulus? How does the brain know whether the animal just touched something warm versus something very hot?

The answer lies in the frequency of the action potentials. As a stimulus increases in intensity, a neuron will produce more frequent action potentials. For example, as an area of the skin gets warmer, the frequency of the firing rate of warm receptors will increase. Conversely, as the site gets cooler, the frequency of the firing rate of the warm receptors will decrease, while those of cold receptors will increase.

Synaptic transmission

Electrical transmission

As discussed above, electrical synapses are relatively rare. They allow the electrical signal to be propagated from one cell to another with virtually no delay. Cells are connected via a connexon, and ions can flow from one cell to the other. The electrical signal can be propagated bidirectionally, without modification, across the electrical synapse.

Chemical transmission

Far more numerous, chemical synapses are responsible for most communication between neurons and adjacent cells. As shown in Figure 8.5, a chemical synapse is much more complicated. An action potential arriving at the synaptic bouton initiates a series of events:

Step 1—Depolarization of the synaptic bouton. The arrival of the action potential at the nerve ending causes depolarization of this region.

Step 2—Opening voltage-gated calcium channels. Depolarization of the nerve ending allows the voltage-gated calcium channels to open. This allows the influx of calcium from the extracellular space into the synaptic bouton. Calcium causes the synaptic vesicles to bind to the presynaptic membrane. Calcium is then sequestered by the mitochondria or endoplasmic reticulum, or is actively pumped out of the cell.

Step 3—Exocytosis. Once bound to the presynaptic membrane, the synaptic vesicles release their contents into the synaptic cleft through a process of exocytosis. The vesicles contain quanta, or packages, of neurotransmitter molecules. The neurotransmitter diffuses throughout the synaptic cleft. The amount of neurotransmitter released is dependent on the frequency of impulses reaching the synaptic bouton. The higher the frequency of impulses, the more synaptic vesicles that bind to the presynaptic membrane, and the more neurotransmitter released.

Step 4—Binding of neurotransmitter to postsynaptic membrane. If the neurotransmitter binds to a postsynaptic receptor, it activates the transmitter-gated channels. This will result in either an IPSP or EPSP in the postsynaptic cell, depending on whether the neurotransmitter is inhibitory or excitatory.

Step 5—Inactivation of the neurotransmitter. The neurotransmitter can continue to cause an effect on the postsynaptic cell until it is inactivated. The action of neurotransmitters is short-lived due to rapid methods of inactivation. The methods of inactivation include 1) enzymatic breakdown, 2) reuptake into the neurons that released the neurotransmitter, 3) uptake by glial cells, or 4) diffusion from the site.

During chemical transmission, there is a synaptic delay of 0.2–0.5 msec between the time an impulse reaches the nerve bouton, and the initiation of a postsynaptic potential in an adjacent cell. This delay is due to the time it takes for all the events associated with chemical transmission, including 1) opening voltage-gated calcium channels, 2) entry of calcium, 3) binding of synaptic vesicles to the presynaptic membrane, 4) exocytosis, 5) diffusion of the neurotransmitter to postsynaptic membrane, and 6) activation of transmitter-gated channels.

Modulation of the synaptic signal

The transmission of a signal across the chemical synapse can be modified both over the short or long term. This is known as synaptic plasticity. It can be controlled by either internal processes within a neuron or by extrinsic processes.

For short-term regulation, the amount of transmitter released at the synapse is dependent on the concentration of presynaptic calcium. Calcium enters the presynaptic terminal through L-type voltage-gated Ca^{2+} channels. Hyperpolarizing or depolarizing the resting membrane potential can decrease or increase the entry of Ca^{++} through these channels, thus affecting neurotransmitter release. In addition, another neuron can synapse on the axon terminal of the neuron, and also control the amount of neurotransmitter released by that cell. This can cause either presynaptic inhibition or facilitation depending on whether the amount of neurotransmitter released is decreased or increased, respectively (Fig. 8.18).

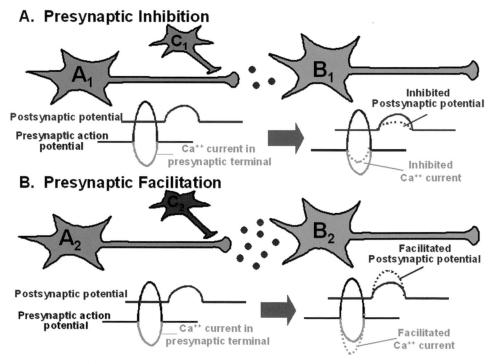

Fig. 8.18. Presynaptic inhibition and facilitation. A) An inhibitory neuron (C_1) can synapse on the axon terminal of a presynaptic neuron (A_1). Release of a neurotransmitter from C_1 can hyperpolarize A_1 reducing the influx of Ca^{++} into the presynaptic terminal and thereby decreasing the amount of neurotransmitter released from A_1, which acts on neuron B_1. B) An excitatory neuron (C_2) can synapse on a presynaptic neuron (A_2). Release of the excitatory neurotransmitter can enhance the entry of Ca^{++} into neuron A_2 and thereby increase the release of a neurotransmitter from A_2, which acts on neuron B_2.

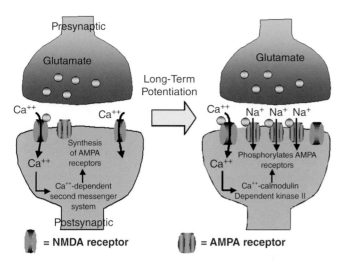

= NMDA receptor   = AMPA receptor

Fig. 8.19. Long-term potentiation. Stimulation of presynaptic glutaminergic neurons causes the release of glutamate. Glutamate binds to postsynaptic glutamate NMDA receptors leading to the entry of Ca^{++} into the postsynaptic cell. Ca^{++} stimulates a Ca^{++}-dependent second messenger system, resulting in the formation of new AMPA glutamate receptors. Thereafter, stimulation of NMDA receptors allows the entry of Ca^{++}, which stimulates Ca^{++}-calmodulin dependent kinase II to phosphorylate AMPA receptors. The AMPA receptors then allow the entry of Na$^+$, which results in enhanced depolarization of the postsynaptic cell, and thus long-term potentiation.

The neurotransmitter GABA has been shown to cause presynaptic inhibition by increasing the presynaptic influx of Cl$^-$ through GABA-gated Cl$^-$ channels. This causes hyperpolarization of the presynaptic neuron that results in less influx of Ca^{++} into the presynaptic terminal in response to an action potential in that cell. In contrast, serotonin has been shown to activate a cAMP-dependent protein kinase causing phosphorylation and closure of K$^+$ channels. This results in depolarizing the presynaptic terminal, allowing the entry of Ca^{++} to persist longer, and thus enhancing the release of the neurotransmitter from the presynaptic neuron.

Calcium also appears involved in another type of synaptic plasticity that lasts for a longer period of time called long-term potentiation (Fig. 8.19). Stimulation of the glutamate NMDA receptor, named after the chemical N-methyl D-aspartate, results in an influx of Ca^{++} into the postsynaptic nerve terminal. Although this does not cause an EPSP, it does cause activation of a Ca^{++}-dependent second messenger pathway, which results in an increase in the number of another type of glutamate receptors called AMPA (α-amino-3-hydroxy 5-methylisoaxzole-4-propionic acid) receptors at the same site. Now, when glutamate stimulates NMDA receptors, thus allowing Ca^{++} to enter, Ca^{++} stimulates calcium-calmodulin-dependent protein kinase II, which phosphorylates AMPA receptors. The AMPA receptors then open and allow Na$^+$ to enter, resulting in enhanced formation of EPSPs. Because of the increased number of AMPA receptors, the cell now displays an enhanced sensitivity to glutamate resulting in long-term potentiation.

Neurotransmitters

Neurotransmitters are the means by which signals are carried across the chemical synapse. To be considered a neurotransmitter, a compound must satisfy the following four criteria:

1. It must be synthesized in the neuron.
2. It must be present in the presynaptic terminal and released in amounts sufficient to exert a defined action on the postsynaptic cell.
3. When administered exogenously, it must exactly mimic the action of the endogenously released neurotransmitter.
4. There must be a specific mechanism of inactivation.

It was originally believed that neurons released a single neurotransmitter. This is known as Dale's principle. Although some neurons make and release a single neurotransmitter, it is now known that some neurons release more than one neurotransmitter. It is not uncommon for a peptide-containing neuron to also release an amino acid or amine type neurotransmitter. If a cell releases more than one neurotransmitter, it can either be coreleased or released separately in response to various stimulation frequencies.

Neurotransmitters are generally grouped into four chemical categories: 1) amino acids, 2) amines, 3) peptides, or 4) dissolved gases (Table 8.3). The term *biogenic amines* has classically been used to include the catecholamines and serotonin. Occasionally, histamine is also considered a biogenic amine. The term *classical neurotransmitters* refer to acetylcholine, biogenic amines, and the amino acid neurotransmitters.

Amines

Acetylcholine

Acetylcholine (ACh) was the first neurotransmitter discovered. It is the transmitter at the neuromuscular junction. It is therefore synthesized in all motor neurons whose cell bodies are in the spinal cord and brain stem. It is also used in other cholinergic neurons both in the CNS and peripheral nervous system.

Table 8.3. Major neurotransmitters.

Amines	Amino Acids	Peptides	Dissolved Gases
Acetylcholine (ACh)	Aspartic acid	Cholecystokinin (CCK)	Nitric oxide (NO)
Dopamine (DA)	Gamma-amino butyric acid (GABA)	Dynorphin	Carbon monoxide (CO)
Epinephrine (E)	Glutamic acid	Enkephalins	
Histamine	Glycine	Neuropeptide Y	
Norepinephrine (NE)		Somatostatin	
Serotonin (5-HT)		Substance P	
ATP		Thyrotropin-releasing hormone	
Adenosine		Vasoactive intestinal peptide	

Box 8.4   Acetylcholinesterase

Many pharmacological agents have been developed in order to manipulate the synaptic levels of acetylcholine (ACh). Acetylcholinesterase inhibitors increase the synaptic levels of ACh. Examples of such inhibitors include various nerve gases, such as sarin, that were developed for chemical warfare and organophosphates, such as parathion, that are used as insecticides. Succinylcholine, which is a competitive neuromuscular blocking agent, is used as an adjunct with anesthetics to increase muscle relaxation during surgery.

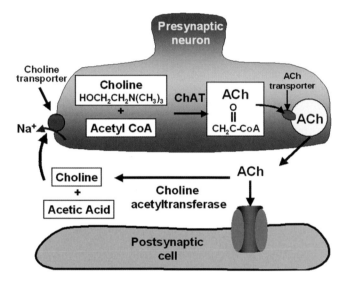

Fig. 8.20. Cholinergic neuron. Choline plus acetyl CoA, acted upon by choline acetyltransferase, combine to form acetylcholine (ACh). ACh is actively pumped into the synaptic vesicles by an ACh transporter. When released from the presynaptic cell ACh can either bind to a presynaptic receptor or be broken down by choline acetyltransferase into choline and acetic acid. Choline is then actively pumped back into the presynaptic cell by a choline transporter where it can be used to make more ACh.

Synthesized in a one-step enzymatic process within the nerve ending, choline acetyltransferase transfers an acetyl group from acetyl CoA to choline to form ACh (Fig. 8.20). Once synthesized in the cytosol of the cell, ACh is concentrated into the synaptic vesicles by an ACh transporter. Upon stimulation of the cell, ACh is released into the synaptic cleft where it can bind to a cholinergic receptor or be enzymatically degraded by acetylcholinesterase (AChE). AChE is secreted into the synaptic cleft, and its action represents the major route of inactivation for ACh. The action of AChE yields choline and acetic acid. Choline is taken back into the cholinergic axon terminals by a specific choline transporter. Since the availability of choline limits how much ACh can be synthesized, the transport of choline into the presynaptic terminal is the rate-limiting step.

Catecholamines

The amino acid tyrosine is the precursor to a group of neurotransmitters that all contain the chemical structure called a catechol. Collectively, this group of neurotransmitters are called catecholamines and include dopamine, norepinephrine, and epinephrine. Catecholamines are compounds that contain both a cate-

chol and an amine group (Fig. 8.21). Since norepinephrine (NE) and epinephrine (E) are found in the adrenal medulla, they are sometimes called noradrenaline and adrenaline, respectively. Catecholaminergic neurons are found throughout the peripheral and central nervous system. The role of epinephrine within the CNS is limited since it is found in only two medullary sites, known as the C1 and C2 cell groups.

The first step in the synthesis of catecholamines is catalyzed by tyrosine hydroxylase that converts tyrosine to L-dopa (L-dihydroxyphylalanine). This step is under end-product inhibition so that if the levels of catecholamines in the synapse rise, they can inhibit the activity of this enzyme. Furthermore, when catecholaminergic neurons are stimulated, enzymatic activity of this enzyme increases in response to depletion of

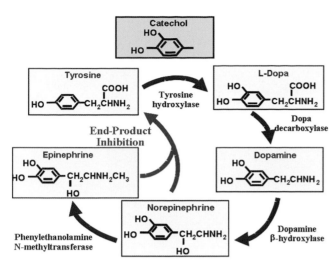

Fig. 8.21. Catecholamine synthesis. Catecholamines are a group of compounds that contain both a catechol and an amine group. Synthesized from tyrosine, the catecholamines include dopamine, norepinephrine, and epinephrine. The rate-limiting enzyme, tyrosine hydroxylase, is under end-product inhibition. If a neuron releases only dopamine, it will lack those enzymes and compounds found further along in the biosynthetic pathway.

the catecholamines. The remainder of the biosynthetic pathway is shown in Figure 8.21.

Catecholamines are inactivated at the synapse by selective reuptake into the presynaptic terminal. This reuptake system involves Na^+-dependent active transporters. These transporters are subject to pharmacological manipulation. For example, amphetamine and cocaine can block these transporters, thus prolonging the action of the neurotransmitter in the synapse. After reuptake, the neurotransmitters can be enzymatically degraded by monoamine oxidase (MAO), or they can be reloaded into the synaptic vesicles. Another enzyme, catechol-O-methyltransferase is also found in the synapse and can break down catecholamines.

Indoleamine

The neurotransmitter serotonin, also called 5-hydroxytryptamine (5-HT), is an indoleamine. It is synthesized from the amino acid tryptophan (Fig. 8.22). While in relatively low concentrations in the CNS, 5-HT is involved in mood, emotional behavior, and sleep. Because the synthesis of 5-HT is not under end-product inhibition, the endogenous levels of 5-HT can be increased by dietary supplementation with tryptophan.

Once in the synapse, 5-HT is inactivated by a specific serotonergic reuptake transporter. Like the transporter for catecholamines, this transporter is subject to pharmacological manipulation. One very

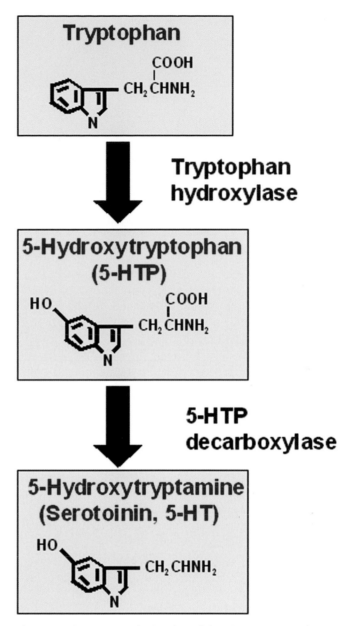

Fig. 8.22. Serotonin synthesis. The indoleamine serotonin, also called 5-hydroxytryptamine, is synthesized from the amino acid tryptophan. The synthesis of serotonin is not under end-product inhibition.

successful class of antidepressants is known as specific serotonergic reuptake inhibitors (SSRI), which include Prozac®. Once inside the cell, 5-HT is degraded by MAO.

Adenosine

There is growing evidence that ATP, and its derivatives such as adenine, can act as neurotransmitters. Adenine and guanine, and their derivatives, are called purines. These compounds act as purinergic receptors. Adenosine acts to dampen sympathetic function

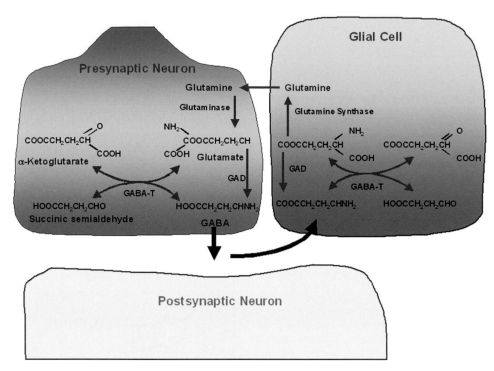

Fig. 8.23. Gamma amino butyric acid synthesis (GABA). GABA is ultimately synthesized from glucose metabolism in which α-ketoglutarate formed in the Krebs cycle is transaminated to glutamate catalyzed by the enzyme α-oxo-glutarate transaminase (GABA-T). The amino acid glutamate is decarboxylated by the enzyme glutamic acid decarboxylase (GAD). Upon release, GABA is taken back into the presynaptic neurons or glial cells. Once inside the glial cells, glutamate is formed. Glutamate must be converted to the noncharged glutamine by glutamine synthetase in order to be transported back to the presynaptic neuron where it is deaminated by glutaminase.

following intense sympathetic activity, thus reducing further release of norepinephrine and ATP, which are coreleased from sympathetic fibers.

Amino acids

Amino acids are ubiquitous within the body, and some appear to act as neurotransmitters. The amino acids glutamate and aspartate act as excitatory neurotransmitters, whereas glycine acts as an inhibitory neurotransmitter in the interneurons of the spinal cord. Although these amino acids are found in all cells, the concentrations are about two to three times higher (~20 mM) in those cells in which they are neurotransmitters. Furthermore, there are transporters within those cells that load the amino acids into vesicles, thus further increasing their concentrations (50 mM). These transporters are found only in neurons in which the amino acid is a neurotransmitter.

The neurotransmitter gamma-aminobutyric acid (GABA) is synthesized from the amino acid glutamate (Fig. 8.23). However, unlike other amino acids that are found ubiquitously throughout the body, GABA is found only in neurons that use it as a neurotransmitter. GABA serves as the neurotransmitter at most CNS synapses where it acts as an inhibitory neurotransmitter. It is also found in other tissues, including the islet

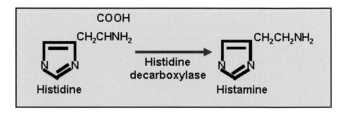

Fig. 8.24. Histamine synthesis. Histamine is synthesized from histidine by the action of histamine decarboxylase.

cells of the pancreas and adrenal gland. GABA is inactivated by uptake into the presynaptic terminals and glia by Na^+-dependent transporters.

Histamine, in addition to serving a role in the immune system where it is found in mast cells, also acts as a neurotransmitter. It is localized in the hypothalamus. It is synthesized from the amino acid histidine by decarboxylation (Fig. 8.24).

Peptides

Peptides consist of strings of amino acids connected in amide linkages. Unlike the classical neurotransmitters discussed above, which are synthesized in the nerve ending, peptides are synthesized in the cell body and transported to the nerve ending (Fig. 8.25).

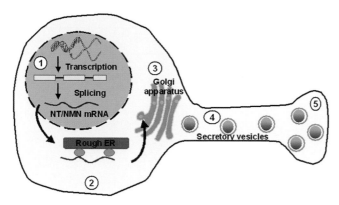

Fig. 8.25. Peptide neurotransmitter synthesis. Peptide neurotransmitters are generally synthesized by transcription in a prohormone form. 1. For example, the 170 amino acid prohormone precursor of neurotensin (NT) is encoded by a single gene. 2. The mRNA is translated by the rough endoplasmic reticulum. The prohormone that is made also contains one copy each of neurotensin and neuromedin N (NMN). 3. The prohormone is targeted to the Golgi apparatus where it is packaged into secretory vesicles. 4. The secretory vesicles are transported anterogradally toward the nerve bouton. 5) The peptide transmitter is ready for release by the process of exocytosis.

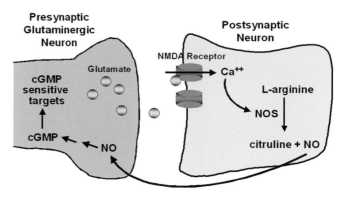

Fig. 8.26. Nitric oxide (NO) containing neuron. Nitric oxide is synthesized from arginine by the action of nitric oxide synthase (NOS) that forms citrulline and NO. Glutamate, acting on NMDA receptors, causes an influx of Ca^{++} into the postsynaptic cell. Calcium then induces NOS. Nitric oxide, which is small and membrane-permeable, acts as a retrograde messenger causing the synthesis of cGMP in the presynaptic cell.

Peptides are generally synthesized as a prohormone in the rough endoplasmic reticulum. This prohormone is packaged in secretory vesicles that bud off from the Golgi apparatus. Peptidases then act on the prohormone to produce the active transmitter. In addition to being synthesized differently from classical neurotransmitters, peptides are inactivated by enzymes rather than by reuptake processes.

Whereas the amounts of classical neurotransmitters can be enhanced through increased local synthesis, peptide transmitters require activation of gene expression that takes hours or days. The classical neurotransmitters are generally stored in relatively small vesicles (~50 nm), whereas peptides are stored in larger vesicles 100 nm in diameter. In addition, peptide neurotransmitters are typically released at higher neuronal firing rates than are necessary to release the classical neurotransmitters.

Unconventional neurotransmitters

Nitric oxide

Although its mechanism was unknown, for decades, nitroglycerine was used to treat cardiovascular disorder. In the 1980s, it was known that a factor called endothelial-derived relaxation factor was produced by the cells lining blood vessels and caused vasodilation. This factor was shown to be nitric oxide (NO). Nitric oxide is an unconventional neurotransmitter for several reasons: 1) it is a gas, 2) it is not stored, 3) it is not released in an exocytotic manner, and 4) there is

no active process that terminates the action of NO. Instead, since NO is small and uncharged, it readily crosses membranes, and due to its short half-life of less than 30 sec, it decays spontaneously to nitrite.

The synthesis of NO is very simple, involving one enzymatic step in which L-arginine is converted to citrulline and NO (Fig. 8.26). The enzyme that catalyzes this reaction is nitric oxide synthase (NOS). There are three known isoforms of NOS, including macrophage-inducible NOS present in microglia, endothelial NOS found in endothelial cells lining blood vessels, and neuronal NOS.

NO can act as a retrograde messenger, meaning that it is produced in a postsynaptic cell and acts on the presynaptic cell where it activates guanlylyl cyclase resulting in the production of cGMP, which then enhances the release of the neurotransmitter from the presynaptic cell. As such, NO is believed to facilitate long-term potentiation in which the release of a neurotransmitter from a presynaptic cell is increased upon increased firing rate at the synapse.

Carbon Monoxide

Carbon monoxide (CO) is a gas that forms in the body by the enzyme heme oxygenase-2, the same enzyme responsible for degrading heme in aging red blood cells. This enzyme is localized in discrete neuronal populations suggesting that CO, like NO, may act as a neurotransmitter. In fact, from using knock-out mice (i.e., mice that have a gene removed or inactivated), it appears that CO and NO both function in the relaxation of smooth muscle associated with peristalsis in the gastrointestinal tract. Like NO, CO activates guanlylyl cyclase.

Table 8.4. Neurotransmitters and their receptors.

Neurotransmitter	Receptors	Mechanism of Signal Transduction*	Functions
Acetylcholine (ACh)	Nicotinic	$\uparrow gCa^{2+}$, gK^+, and gNa^+	Contract skeletal muscle and excite postganglionic neurons
	Muscarinic		
	M_1, M_3, M_5	$\uparrow IP_3$ and DAG	M_3: contract smooth muscle
	M_2, M_4	$\downarrow cAMP$; $\uparrow gK^+$	M_2: $\uparrow$heart rate M_4: modulate neurotransmission
Dopamine (DA)	D_1, D_5	$\uparrow cAMP$	Inhibitory
	D2, D3, D4	$\downarrow cAMP$	Inhibitory
Epinephrine (E) and norepinephrine (NE)	α_1	$\uparrow IP_3$ and DAG	Excitatory
	α_2	$\downarrow cAMP$	Inhibitory
	β_1	$\uparrow cAMP$	Excitatory
	β_2	$\uparrow cAMP$	Inhibitory
Histamine	H_1	$\uparrow IP_3$ and DAG	Excitatory
	H_2	$\uparrow cAMP$	Excitatory
	H_3	Unknown	?
Serotonin (5-HT)	$5\text{-}HT_1$	$\downarrow cAMP$; $\uparrow gK^+$	Inhibitory
	$5\text{-}HT_2$	$\uparrow IP_3$ and DAG	Inhibitory
	$5\text{-}HT_3$	$\uparrow gK^+$ and gNa^+	Excitatory
	$5\text{-}HT_4$	$\uparrow cAMP$	Excitatory
	$5\text{-}HT_5$	$\downarrow cAMP$	Inhibitory
	$5\text{-}HT_6$	$\uparrow cAMP$	Excitatory
	$5\text{-}HT_7$	$\uparrow cAMP$	Excitatory
Opioid peptides	δ, κ, and μ	$\downarrow cAMP$ and gCa^{++}; $\uparrow gK^+$	Inhibitory
ATP	P1 purinoceptors		
Adenosine	P2 purinoceptors	$\downarrow cAMP$	Inhibitory
		$\uparrow cAMP$	Excitatory

* DAG, diacyl glycerol; g, conductance; $\uparrow$, increased; $\downarrow$, decreased.

Neurotransmitter receptors

The action of neurotransmitters is dependent on the receptor to which they bind. Neurotransmitters can generally act at multiple receptors, resulting in differential responses. Each of the receptors to which a neurotransmitter binds is called a receptor subtype.

For example, acetylcholine can bind to both nicotinic and muscarinic receptors. Although acetylcholine can bind to both receptor subtypes, the subtypes mediate different responses. Nicotinic receptors are found in skeletal muscle where their stimulation results in contraction of skeletal muscle. In contrast, muscarinic receptors are found on postsynaptic cells of the parasympathetic nervous system and their stimulation can cause contraction of smooth muscle or decreased heart rate.

The same neurotransmitter can cause opposite effects depending on which receptors it stimulates. When norepinephrine binds to β_2-adrenergic receptors, it causes vasodilation, whereas binding to α_1-adrenergic receptors causes vasoconstriction. Examples of receptors and their effects are shown in Table 8.4

Neuropharmacology deals with the action of various neurotransmitters and explores drugs that either

Table 8.5. Neurotransmitters: Agonists and antagonists.

Neurotransmitter	Receptors	Agonists	Antagonists
Acetylcholine (ACh)	Nicotinic	Nicotine	Curare
	Muscarinic	Muscarine	Atropine
Dopamine (DA)	Dopaminergic	Apomorphine	Haloperidol
Epinephrine (E) and norepinephrine (NE)	α	Phenylephrine	Phenoxybenzamine
	β	Isoproterenol	Propranolol
GABA	$GABA_A$	Muscimol	Bicuculline
	$GABA_B$	Baclofen	Phaclofen
Serotonin (5-HT)	Serotonergic	Quipazine	Methysergide

mimic or block the action of neurotransmitters. A drug that mimics the action of a neurotransmitter at its receptor is called an agonist; a drug that blocks the neurotransmitter is called an antagonist (Table 8.5).

Agonists and antagonists are routinely used in animal and human medicine. They have been developed because they generally have fewer side effects because of their specificity, and have longer half-lives than neurotransmitters. Treatments typically involve either stimulating or inhibiting the action of a neurotransmitter. Since atropine can block the action of the parasympathetic nervous system, it is commonly given prior to surgery in order to reduce the production of saliva and thereby reduce the chances of suffocation during surgery. In glaucoma, it is necessary to increase smooth muscle tone in order to increase outflow of aqueous humor. The administration of acetylcholine would be ineffective because of its rapid hydrolysis by acetylcholinesterases. Instead, a muscarinic agonist, such as pilocarpine, is given.

9 Central nervous system

Contents

The central nervous system includes the brain and spinal cord. One of the major factors distinguishing animals into different classes is the degree of development of the brain that has occurred during evolution. This process, called cephalization, has resulted in an increase in size and complexity of the rostral, or front, portion of the brain.

Embryonic development

The central nervous system is derived from the ectoderm, the outermost layer of the embryo. During gastrulation, the notochord develops from the chorda-mesodermal tissue. The notochord, in a process called primary induction, sends a signal to the overlying ectoderm to begin to thicken, thus forming the neural plate (Fig. 9.1). The inducing signal is a protein called noggin.

Shortly after formation of the neural plate, its lateral edges become elevated forming the neural folds, which flank the neural groove. As the neural plate begins to invaginate, the neural folds surround it. The lateral edges of the neural folds eventually migrate toward the longitudinal midline of the embryo, thus forming the neural tube. The neural tube then separates from the overlying cutaneous ectoderm. The cavity inside the neural tube is called the neurocoele. Closure of the tube first occurs in the upper spinal

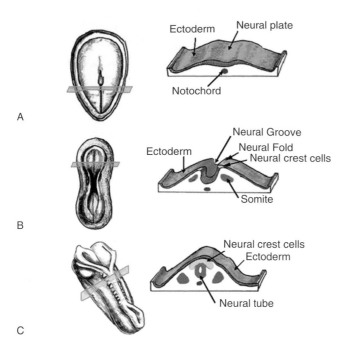

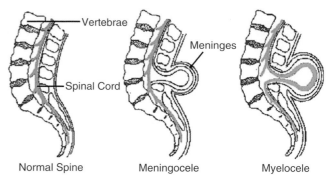

Fig. 9.2. Spina bifida. Spina bifida aperta produces a noticeable sac in the back. A meningocele, in which a portion of the meninges protrudes, produces little or no muscle paralysis or incontinence once it is repaired. However, in 90% of all spina bifida cases, a portion of the undeveloped spinal cord itself protrudes through the spine and forms a sac called a myelocele. Any portion of the spinal cord outside the vertebrae is undeveloped or damaged, causing paralysis and incontinence.

Fig. 9.1. Neurulation. A) During early development, shortly after formation of the primitive streak, the notochord sends a signal to the overlying ectoderm to begin to flatten and the cells elongate, thus forming the neural plate. B) After induction from the notochord, the overlying ectoderm begins to involute, and a neural groove is formed in the midline while the sides of the area involuting form the neural folds. C) Later in embryonic development, the neural tube forms and is covered by the overlying ectoderm.

cord and progresses both cephalad (toward the head) and caudad (toward the tail).

In the chick, neurulation occurs in the cephalic region while gastrulation is still occurring in the caudal region. The opened ends of the tube are called the anterior and posterior neuropore, respectively.

In mammals, neural tube closure is initiated at several sites along the tube. Failure of the tube to close at different sites results in various birth defects. Spina bifida occurs if the posterior neural tube does not close, whereas anencephaly is a lethal condition that results when the anterior neural tube fails to close. Craniorachischisis is a failure of the entire tube to close. There are different forms of spina bifida. In spina bifida occulta, often called hidden spina bifida, the spinal cord and the nerves are usually normal and there is no visible opening on the back (Fig 9.2). Usually harmless, there is a small defect or gap in a few of the vertebrae. When the meninges protrude from the spine, it is called a myelocele (or meningo-myelocele). The sac is filled with cerebrospinal fluid, but there is generally no nerve damage. In a myelo-meningocele, the meninges and spinal nerves push through an opening in the vertebrae.

Box 9.1   Folic acid and birth defects in humans

Neural tube defects (NTD) are among the most common birth defects in humans. Folic acid appears very important in neural tube development. In 1992, it was recommended by the Public Health Service, and endorsed by the American Academy of Pediatrics, that women who might become pregnant should take 400 micrograms of folic acid daily. For women at higher risk for giving birth to a child with spinal bifida, it is recommended that they take 4,000 micrograms of folic acid/day by prescription. Studies have shown that 50% or more of NTD can be prevented if women consume adequate folic acid before and during the early weeks of pregnancy.

Folic acid is a synthetic compound used in fortified foods and dietary supplements. Folate is a term describing all compounds having the same vitamin activity.

As the neural tube is closing, a group of ectodermal cells separates from the neural tube and locates on the dorsal lateral edge of the tube. These cells become the neural crest cells, which eventually migrate throughout the body producing all neurons that have cell bodies in the peripheral nervous system, including 1) neurons and glial cells of the sensory, sympathetic, and parasympathetic nervous system; 2) norepinephrine and epinephrine producing cells of the adrenal gland; 3) pigment-containing cells of the epidermis; and 4) skeletal and connective tissues of the head.

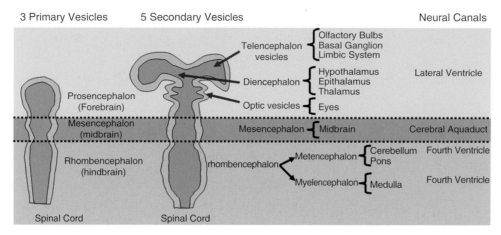

Fig. 9.3. Brain development. During embryonic development, the brain begins as three vesicles. The most rostral is the prosencephalon which gives rise to the telencephalon and diencephalon vesicles. The most caudal, the rhombencephalon, gives rise to the metencephalon and myelencephalon.

The neural crest cells develop in conjunction with the underlying mesoderm. The mesoderm on either side of the neural tube forms the somites. The somites produce the vertebrae and the associated skeletal muscle. The nerves that innervate the skeletal muscle are called somatic motor neurons since they are derived from somites.

Three brain vesicles

As the brain develops from the neural tube, three swellings form at its rostral end. These three vesicles include the prosencephalon; the mesencephalon, or midbrain; and the rhombencephalon, or hindbrain. The rhombencephalon connects the brain with the spinal cord (Fig. 9.3).

During the next stage of development, two secondary vesicles called the optic vesicles and telencephalic vesicles form from the prosencephalon. The remaining unpaired vesicle in the middle is called the diencephalon, or "between brain." The telencephalon vesicles grow to become the two cerebral hemispheres, collectively called the cerebrum. Finally, another pair of vesicles forms on the ventral surface of the telencephalic vesicles and eventually become the olfactory bulbs. The olfactory bulbs participate in the sense of smell. The mesencephalon does not divide, but instead remains the midbrain while the rhombencephalon divides into the metencephalon and myelencephalon. The metencephalon includes the pons (*pons* = bridge) and cerebellum, and the myelencephalon includes the medulla oblongata. Collectively, the midbrain, pons, and medulla oblongata constitute the brain stem.

Organization of the brain

The cerebral hemispheres

The telencephalic vesicles form the telencephalon, which consists of two cerebral hemispheres. As the brain develops, the telencephalic vesicles grow posteriorly and laterally until they encase the diencephalon. There is a proliferation of neurons resulting in the formation of three major white matter systems, including the cortical white matter, the corpus callosum, and the internal capsule. The cortical white matter includes neurons that run to and from the cerebral cortex. The corpus callosum includes neurons that connect the two cerebral hemispheres and the internal capsule connects the cortex with the brain stem.

The surface of the brain is marked by many convolutions. The grooves are called sulci (sing. = sulcus); the ridges are called gyri (sing. = gyrus). The outer six layers of neurons constitute the cerebral cortex. The convolutions greatly increase the surface area, thus increasing the amount of cortex. Whereas the brain of a chicken has a relatively flat surface, the brain of most domestic animals is considerably convoluted (Fig. 9.4).

The larger grooves that separate brain regions are called fissures. The longitudinal fissure separates the two cerebral hemispheres, whereas the cerebral hemispheres are separated from the cerebellum by the transverse fissure which runs perpendicular to the longitudinal fissure.

When viewing an intact brain, four lobes—frontal, parietal, temporal, and occipital—are visible in the cerebral hemispheres. In most animals, the lobes are

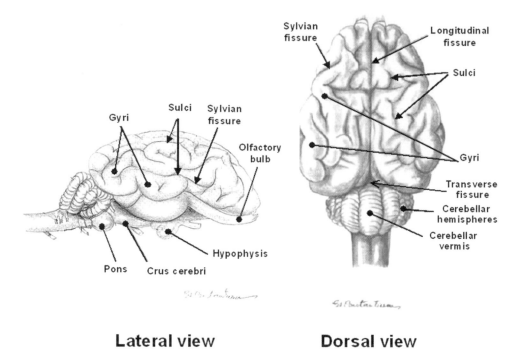

Lateral view   **Dorsal view**

Fig. 9.4.   Cytoarchitecture of the goat brain surface. Cephalization has resulted in the formation of ridges, called gyri, and valleys, called sulci. Fissures are larger grooves separating major brain areas, such as the longitudinal fissure that separates the two cerebral hemispheres. (Reprinted from Constantinescu, 2001. Used by permission of the publisher.)

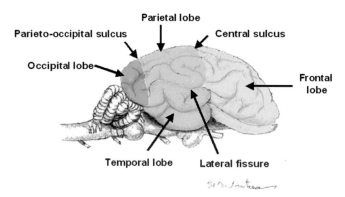

Fig. 9.5.   Lobes of the brain. Four lobes are visible on the surface of the brain. The frontal lobe is most rostral. Caudad to the frontal lobe is the parietal lobe. Below the lateral fissure is the temporal lobe. The most caudal lobe is the occipital lobe. (Modified from Constantinescu, 2001.)

not delineated by sulci, but are named for the cranial bones under which they lie (Fig. 9.5). In the human brain, various sulci separate the lobes, as will be described below. The frontal lobe lies just under the frontal bone making up the most rostral lobe of the cerebral hemispheres. Immediately caudal to the frontal lobe is the parietal lobe, which is separated from the frontal lobe by the central sulcus.

Two important gyri are also bordered by the central sulcus: the precentral gyrus anterior and the postcentral gyrus posterior to the central sulcus.

Below the parietal lobe is the temporal lobe that is found under the temporal bone. The temporal lobe is separated from the frontal and parietal lobes by the lateral sulcus (lateral fissure, Sylvian fissure). Finally, at the back surface of the cerebral hemispheres is the occipital lobe, which is separated from the parietal lobe by the parieto-occipital sulcus.

Although not visible on the surface, there is a fifth lobe called the insula that is found by spreading the brain apart at the lateral fissure. It is covered by parts of the temporal, parietal, and frontal lobes.

Ventricles of the brain

As development progresses, the neurocoel expands to produce four chambers, called cerebroventricles. Ependymal cells line the cerebroventricles. Each cerebral hemisphere contains a lateral ventricle, also called the first and second ventricle. A thin layer of tissue called the septum pellucidum separates the two lateral ventricles from each other. The third ventricle is found in the diencephalon, and the fourth ventricle extends from the posterior surface of the pons and the anterior surface of the cerebellum to the superior portion of the medulla oblongata (Fig. 9.6). The fourth ventricle is continuous with the central canal of the spinal cord.

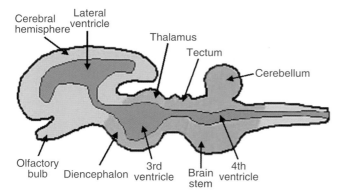

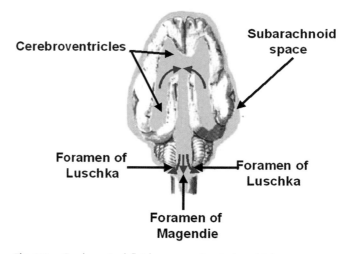

Fig. 9.6. Cerebroventricles. The neurocoele, or central cavity, in the neural tube eventually enlarges into four cerebroventricles filled with cerebrospinal fluid. Two lateral ventricles, one in each cerebral hemisphere, empty into the medially located third ventricle located in the diencephalon. This empties into the fourth ventricle located between the cerebellum and brain stem.

Fig. 9.8. Cerebrospinal fluid movement out of ventricles. Cerebrospinal fluid (CSF) travels from the fourth ventricle to the subarachnoid space via the medially located foramen of Magendie and the two lateral foramina of Luschka.

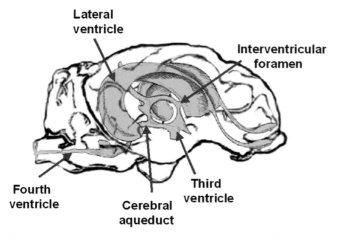

Fig. 9.7. Cerebroventricles of the sheep. Cerebrospinal fluid (CSF) is formed in the choroid plexus located in each lateral ventricle. Via bulk flow, the CSF flows from the lateral ventricles through the interventricular foramen of Monroe to the third ventricle. It then flows through the cerebral aqueduct to the fourth ventricle.

The lateral ventricles are connected to the third ventricle via the interventricular foramen of Monroe (Fig. 9.7). The third ventricle connects to the fourth ventricle via the mesencephalic aqueduct, also called the aqueduct of Sylvius or cerebral aquaduct. Cerebrospinal fluid flows by bulk flow from the lateral ventricles, to the third ventricle, to the fourth ventricle.

Cerebrospinal fluid can leave the fourth ventricle through the medial aperture called the foramen of Magendie and the two lateral apertures called the foramina of Luschka and enter the subarachnoid space (Fig. 9.8). This space is found between the arachnoid and pia mater, which, along with the dura mater, form the three meningeal layers covering the brain. The fluid in the subarachnoid space bathes the surface of

the brain and spinal cord. Should the cerebrospinal fluid not be able to flow through the ventricular system, it will back up in the ventricles causing hydrocephalus, or swelling of the ventricles. Since the skull cannot expand, increased pressure in the ventricles causes the soft tissue of the brain to be compressed that leads to impaired brain function, and death if untreated.

The adult human contains about 150 ml of CSF, and it is estimated that 430 to 450 ml are produced daily. Therefore, CSF is turned over every 6 to 7 hours. After entering the subarachnoid space, cerebrospinal fluid moves through one-way valves called arachnoid villi that project into the superior sagittal sinus formed by the dura mater located in the longitudinal fissure. The superior sagittal sinus is filled with venous blood. Therefore, once the cerebrospinal fluid enters the superior sagittal sinus, it returns to the circulatory system.

Cerebral cortex

The cerebral cortex is arranged as layers of cells that lie parallel to the surface of the brain. The layer closest to the surface of the brain is separated from the pia mater by a zone, called the molecular layer or layer I, that lacks neurons. Furthermore, at least one layer contains pyramidal cells that project large dendrites, called apical dendrites, that project to layer I where they form multiple synapses.

The neocortex, which is found only in mammals and is associated with higher brain functions such as conscious behavior, is found over most of the surface

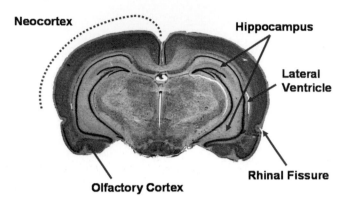

Fig. 9.9. Three types of mammalian cortex. The neocortex is found on the outer surface of the cerebral hemispheres. Medial to the lateral ventricles is a second type of cortex called the hippocampus, part of the limbic system. The third type of cortical tissue is the olfactory cortex, located ventrally and laterally to the hippocampus.

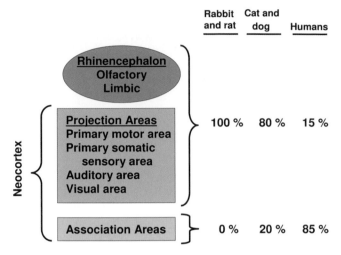

Fig. 9.10. Evolutionary changes in cerebrocortex. Through evolutionary development, the ability to display higher-order thinking is associated with enhanced development of the association areas. (Modified from King, 1987.)

of the cerebral hemisphere and consists of six layers of cells (Fig. 9.9). Medial to the lateral ventricles is an area of cortex named for its unique shape called the hippocampus (Greek for "seahorse"). It is only a single cell layer. Ventral and lateral to the hippocampus is the third area of cortex called the olfactory cortex (piriform, or pyriform cortex) that consists of two cell layers. The olfactory cortex connects with the olfactory bulbs. The olfactory cortex is separated from the neocortex by the rhinal fissure.

In humans, the neocortex was extensively mapped by Korbinian Brodmann in 1906 in which he numbered 52 different cortical areas each having a common cytoarchitecture. Such an extensive mapping has not been done in other animals. The cortex can be designated into three areas: 1) motor areas responsible for the control of voluntary motor functions, 2) sensory areas responsible for perception of various sensations, and 3) Association areas that integrate the motor and sensory signals.

The motor and sensory areas can be grouped together into projection areas, thus allowing the cortex to be subdivided into three components including the projection areas, rhinencephalon (olfactory and limbic) areas, and association areas. The projection and association areas comprise the neocortex. Association areas receive sensory information, process that information, develop a response, and predict its consequences. As animals became more evolutionarily advanced, the association areas became more developed (Fig. 9.10).

The white matter, or fibers, in the cerebral cortex form three types of fibers:

1. Association fibers. Association areas allow complex problem solving and creative thinking. There are association areas found in the frontal, temporal, parietal, and occipital lobes. These fibers course within a cerebral hemisphere, thus connecting various areas of the cortex. The parietal and occipital lobe association areas are involved with cognitive functions, whereas the frontal association areas are involved with general alertness, intelligence, and temperament. The temporal association area is involved with learning and memory. Although these areas are not well developed in cats and dogs, lesions to the frontal association area result in changes in behavior and personality.

2. Projection fibers. Neurons that leave the cerebrum and enter the brain stem via the internal capsule are called projection fibers. They therefore connect the cortex with subcortical structures, as well as the remainder of the nervous system.

3. Commissural fibers. Each cerebral hemisphere generally controls the contralateral side of the body, therefore, fibers need to cross between hemispheres. When crossing from one side of the cerebral cortex to the other, they do so as commissural fibers.

Motor areas

These are cortical areas responsible for motor functions. The primary motor cortex is the final site for cortical processing of motor commands before messages are then sent to the somatic muscles. While in humans, the primary motor area lies in the posterior part of the frontal lobes just anterior to the central sulcus, in mammals this area lays in the rostral region of the frontal lobes (Fig. 9.11). Unlike birds, reptiles,

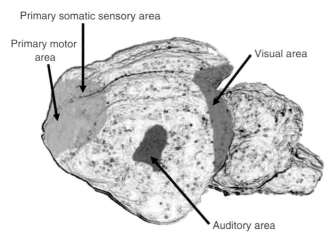

Fig. 9.11. Primary projection areas of the cat. The primary motor and somatic sensory areas spread over the medial surface of the frontal lobes. The visual area is located in the occipital lobe; the auditory area is located in the temporal lobe.

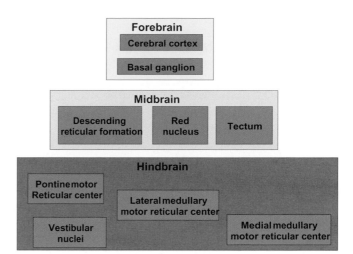

Fig. 9.12. Extrapyramidal system. The extrapyramidal system is a multisynaptic motor pathway that includes all those motor neurons not part of the pyramidal system. It consists of nine motor centers scattered throughout the brain.

amphibians, and fish, mammals possess a pyramidal system. The pyramidal system consists of corticospinal fibers that travel from the primary motor area, through the medullary pyramids located at the base of the medulla oblongata, to the somatic motor neurons found in the spinal cord. It also includes the corticonuclear fibers that project to the nuclei of those cranial nerves that innervate striated muscles in the head. The pyramidal fibers decussate, or cross over, in the pyramids of the medulla.

The extrapyramidal system includes all the descending somatic motor pathways excluding those described above that constitute the pyramidal system. The extrapyramidal system is phylogenetically old, and found in all but the lowest vertebrates. It consists of nine main motor areas located in the forebrain, midbrain, and hindbrain (Fig. 9.12). These will be discussed in depth later in the chapter.

Sensory areas

Unlike the motor areas that are located in the frontal lobe, sensory areas are located throughout the cortex. The primary somatosensory cortex receives information from sensory receptors located in the skin and proprioceptors in skeletal muscles.

Cerebral white matter

Basal ganglion

In addition to the cerebral cortex discussed above, and its commissures, and association and projection fibers,

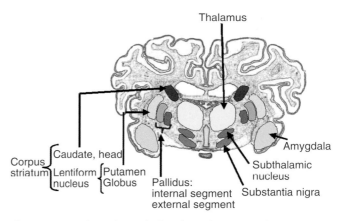

Fig. 9.13. Basal ganglion. The basal ganglion, or nucleus, is a collection of brain nuclei that function in motor movement as part of the extrapyramidal system. The basal ganglion includes the globus pallidus and putamen, which together constitute the lentiform nucleus. Also included is the caudate, which, combined with the lentiform nucleus, forms the corpus striatum. Finally, also included in the basal ganglion are the amygdala, subthalamic nucleus, and substantia nigra.

there are some deep subcortical nuclei called the basal ganglia or nuclei (Fig. 9.13). Although the definition of the structures included in the basal ganglion varies, it generally includes the caudate nucleus, putamen, globus pallidus, substantia nigra (consisting of the pars reticulata and pars compacts), and subthalamic nucleus. The putamen and globus pallidus (or pallidum) together form the lentiform nucleus that laterally borders the internal capsule. The lentiform nucleus and caudate are collectively called the corpus striatum because the fibers of the internal capsule, a collection of fibers that runs between the neocortex and thalamus, pass through them giving them a striated appearance.

The corpus striatum receives most of the inputs to the basal ganglion from the cerebral cortex, thalamus, and brain stem. The corpus striatum sends projections to the globus pallidus and substantia nigra that provide the major output projections from the basal ganglion. These projection fibers travel through the thalamus to the premotor and prefrontal cortex, and therefore affect motor movement.

Limbic system

The limbic system consists of a group of structures located in the medial region of each cerebral hemisphere (Fig. 9.14). These structures encircle (*limbus* = ring or border) the brainstem. The limbic lobe of the cerebral hemisphere includes gyri surrounding the diencephalon, as well as other underlying structures. Specifically, it consists of three gyri. The cingulate gyrus is dorsal to the corpus callosum. The dentate gyrus and parahippocampal gyrus form the inferior and posterior portions of the limbic lobe. These later two gyri conceal the hippocampus, which is a nucleus lying inferior to the lateral ventricle. The fornix is a fiber tract running inferior to the corpus callosum and connecting the hippocampus with the hypothalamus where it ends in the mammillary bodies. Also included in the limbic system is the anterior nucleus of the thalamus, which relays information from the mammil-

lary bodies to the cingulate gyrus. The amygdaloid body (nucleus) serves as the interface between the limbic system, cerebrum, and various sensory systems.

The limbic system is involved in emotional and behavioral patterns. The functions of the limbic system include 1) establishment of emotional states, 2) linking of conscious functions with unconscious, autonomic functions, 3) long-term memory storage and retrieval. The rabies virus generally attacks the hippocampus and results in emotional changes including bouts of terror and rage. The amygdala is believed to be the major component of the limbic system involved in emotion since electrical stimulation of this region produces feelings of fear and apprehension whereas damage to this region causes tameness. Removal of the amygdala will allow a cat to wander through a colony of monkeys ignoring the monkey's hoots and threats.

It is believed that the hippocampal formation processes information from the cingulated gyrus. This information is sent to the mammillary bodies of the hypothalamus via the fornix (Fig. 9.14). The hypothalamus gives feedback to the cingulate gyrus by a pathway from the mammillary bodies to the anterior thalamus via the mammillothalamic tract, and then to the cingulate gyrus.

Diencephalon

The telencephalon and diencephalons make up the forebrain and are derived from the rostral-most vesicle called the prosencephalon. Surrounded by the cerebral hemispheres, the diencephalons consist of three paired structures—the thalamus, hypothalamus, and epithalamus.

Thalamus

The thalamus lies dorsal to the hypothalamus, and is bordered by the caudate nucleus dorsally and the internal capsule laterally. Its two halves are separated by the third ventricle. There is a collection of nuclei found in each half of the thalamus (Fig. 9.15). The intermediate mass of the thalamus extends through the third ventricle connecting the two halves.

The thalamus is the major relay station for sensory information generated in the periphery and transferred for processing to the cerebral hemispheres. It also integrates motor information from the cerebellum and basal ganglion and transfers such information to the motor regions of the cortex.

The nuclei of the thalamus are generally classified into four groups—anterior, ventrolateral, medial, and

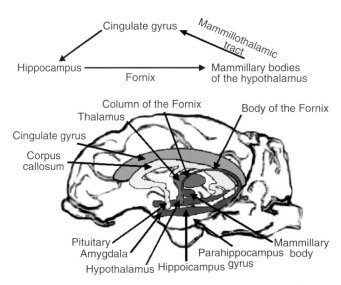

Fig. 9.14. Limbic system. The limbic lobe includes the cingulate gyrus, parahippocampal gyrus, and the hippocampal formation that lies deep in the parahippocampal gyrus. The hippocampal formation includes the hippocampus, dentate gyrus (deep to the parahippocampus gyrus), and subiculum. The limbic system additionally includes parts of the rhinencephalon, amygdala, hypothalamus, and anterior nucleus of the thalamus. The fornix helps connect parts of the limbic system.

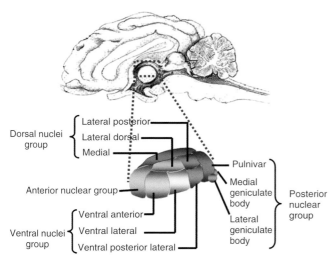

Fig. 9.15. The thalamus. The thalamus consists of four groups of nuclei. The anterior nucleus and pulvinar constitute the anterior and posterior groups, respectively. The medial group consists mainly of the mediodorsal nuclei (not shown).

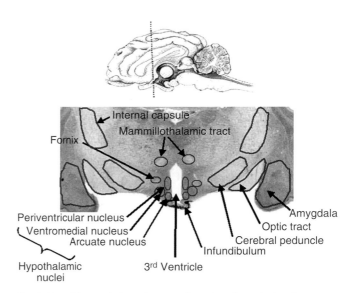

Fig. 9.16. Diencephalon. A coronal section through the sheep brain at the level of the diencephalon is shown. The hypothalamus is that region surrounding the 3rd ventricle.

posterior. The ventrolateral and posterior groups are located lateral to the medullary lamina, a fiber tract that runs the rostrocaudal length of the thalamus. The medial group of nuclei are located medial to the medullary lamina. The medullary lamina splits at the rostral end of the thalamus and encases the anterior group. The posterior nuclear group consists of the pulvinar, whereas the anterior group consists only of the anterior nucleus.

The anterior nucleus receives input from the mammillary nuclei of the hypothalamus, and is thought to participate in memory and emotion. It is also interconnected with the cingulated and frontal cortices, and is therefore part of the limbic system.

The medial group, consisting mostly of the medial nuclei, receives inputs from the basal ganglia, amygdala, and midbrain. It projects to the frontal cortex and has been implicated in memory. The ventrolateral group consists of the remaining nuclei shown in Figure 9.15. The ventral anterior and ventral lateral nuclei carry information from the basal ganglia and cerebellum to the motor cortex. The ventral posterior lateral nucleus carries somatosensory information to the neocortex.

Hypothalamus

The hypothalamus (*hypo* = below) is found ventral to the thalamus and forms the inferolateral walls of the third ventricle (Fig. 9.16). It extends from the optic chiasm, the site where the optic nerves cross to the contralateral sides, to the posterior border of the mammillary bodies. The infundibulum, which connects the

hypothalamus to the pituitary, lies between the optic chiasm and mammillary bodies. It arises from the tuber cinereum, which is an oval protuberance located on the floor of the third ventricle.

The hypothalamus serves an essential role in the control of homeostasis and reproduction. Once termed the "head ganglion" of the autonomic nervous system, the hypothalamus was thought to control the autonomic nervous system. This was due to the observations that electrical stimulation of the hypothalamus altered autonomic functions. However, it is now believed that the hypothalamus plays more of an integrative role in regulating the autonomic nervous system, and that many of the early effects attributed to the hypothalamus were a result of stimulation of fiber pathways that course through the area.

While relatively small, the hypothalamus is a complex structure containing many nuclei (Fig. 9.17). It can be divided into three general areas: anterior, middle, and posterior. The anterior region lies dorsal to the optic chiasm and is called the preoptic region. It contains the suprachiasmatic nucleus, which is involved in circadian rhythms, the anterior hypothalamic nucleus, and the lateral and medial preoptic nuclei. This area also controls blood pressure, body temperature, and reproductive activity.

The middle region lies dorsal to the pituitary and contains various nuclei including the dorsomedial, ventromedial, paraventricular, supraoptic, and arcuate nuclei. The paraventricular nucleus contains magnocellular and parvocellular neuroendocrine regions. The arcuate nucleus and parvocellular region of the paraventricular nucleus produce hormones that

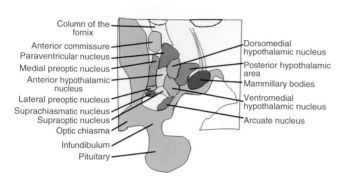

Column of the fornix
Anterior commissure
Paraventricular nucleus
Medial preoptic nucleus
Anterior hypothalamic nucleus
Lateral preoptic nucleus
Suprachiasmatic nucleus
Supraoptic nucleus
Optic chiasma
Infundibulum
Pituitary

Dorsomedial hypothalamic nucleus
Posterior hypothalamic area
Mammillary bodies
Ventromedial hypothalamic nucleus
Arcuate nucleus

Fig. 9.17. Hypothalamus. Saggital view of hypothalamus showing the various hypothalamic nuclei.

control the anterior pituitary. The magnocellular area of the paraventricular nucleus, consisting of large neurons, produces oxytocin that is secreted in the neurohypophysis. The paraventricular nucleus also has connections to both parasympathetic and sympathetic preganglionic neurons in the medulla and spinal cord, and can thus control the autonomic nervous system. The supraoptic nucleus produces antidiuretic hormone also secreted from the neurohypophysis.

The posterior region of the hypothalamus contains the mammillary bodies, tuberomammillary nucleus, and the overlying posterior hypothalamic region. This latter nucleus contains histamine and appears involved in wakefulness and arousal.

The hypothalamus can also be divided longitudinally into the periventricular, medial, and lateral zones that each run the rostral-caudal length of the hypothalamus. The periventricular zone lies immediately adjacent to the third ventricle. There are two major fiber systems running through the hypothalamus. The medial forebrain bundle runs through the lateral hypothalamus connecting the hypothalamus with the brain stem, basal forebrain, amygdala, and cerebral cortex. The second fiber system is located medial to the major hypothalamic nuclei along the wall of the third ventricle, and it links the periaqueductal gray matter in the midbrain with the hypothalamus. This latter fiber system is involved in stereotyped behavioral patterns such as posturing during sexual behavior.

The hypothalamus controls the autonomic nervous system, and thereby controls growth, feeding, drinking, circadian rhythms, and maternal behavior. Specifically, the hypothalamus plays a key role in six physiological areas:

1. It controls blood pressure and electrolyte composition by affecting water consumption and salt appetite as well as controlling blood osmolarity and vasomotor tone. When the blood becomes hyperosmotic, osmoreceptors in the hypothala-

mus are stimulated and result in the release of antidiuretic hormone (vasopressin) from the posterior pituitary that causes the collecting tubules in the kidneys to reabsorb water. This results in a decrease in blood osmolarity.
2. Regulates body temperature by controlling metabolic rate, vasomotor tone, and thermoregulatory behavior.
3. Regulates food and water intake. For example, an increase in white adipose levels in the body causes increased plasma leptin levels. Leptin circulates to the hypothalamus where it decreases the production and release of Neuropeptide Y by neurons in the arcuate nucleus, thus resulting in decreased food intake.
4. Regulates reproduction through the hormonal control of estrus, pregnancy, and lactation. Releasing factors produced in the hypothalamus and released into the hypothalamic-hypophyseal portal system control the release of hormones from the anterior pituitary. Conversely, the hormones released from the posterior pituitary (i.e., oxytocin and antidiuretic hormone) are produced in supraoptic and paraventricular nuclei of the hypothalamus and then travel down the axons and are released from the posterior pituitary.
5. Controls the stress response. This includes the physiological and immunological responses such as increased blood pressure and decreased humoral immunity.
6. Controls circadian rhythms and sleep-wake cycles. The suprachiasmatic nucleus acts as a major internal clock in mammals. This nucleus is entrained by light via the retinohypothalamic tract that runs from the retina to the suprachiasmatic nucleus. Lesioning the suprachiasmatic nucleus attenuates sleep and other circadian rhythms. These rhythms can be restored by transplanting a fetal suprachiasmatic nucleus. Furthermore, stimulation of the posterior hypothalamus produces arousal that is mediated by histaminergic neurons whereas destruction of this area decreases histaminergic output, which causes sleep, much like that caused by antihistamines. In contrast, stimulation of the anterior hypothalamus induces sleep. This appears to be mediated by GABAnergic inhibitory neurons.

Epithalamus

The epithalamus lies superiorly, caudally, and medially relative to the other parts of the diencephalons and thus represents a cephalad extension of the pretectum (just rostral of where the midbrain fuses with the thalamus) of the mesencephalon. The epithalamus

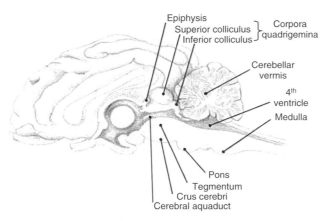

Epiphysis
Superior colliculus } Corpora
Inferior colliculus } quadrigemina
Cerebellar vermis
4th ventricle
Medulla
Pons
Tegmentum
Crus cerebri
Cerebral aquaduct

Fig. 9.18. Mesencephalon. Saggital view of goat brain showing the mesencephalon. (Modified from Constantinescu, 2001.)

includes the pineal body (epiphysis), the habenula, the habenular commissure, and the striae medullares.

The pineal body serves a role in sensing light and thereby controlling the sleep-wake cycle via the production of melatonin. It also has an important role in seasonal breeding animals such as sheep in which a decrease in day length, and therefore a decrease in melatonin levels, results in estrus.

Mesencephalon

The mesencephalon lies between the diencephalons and pons (Fig. 9.18). The tectum (Latin for "roof") forms the roof of the mesencephalon and contains two pairs of prominent bulges known as the corpora quadrigemina. Consisting of the superior and inferior colliculi, these nuclei process visual and auditory stimuli, respectively. The tegmentum forms the floor of the midbrain.

The superior colliculus receives visual input from the lateral geniculate nucleus of the thalamus from the ipsilateral side. The inferior colliculus receives auditory information from the medulla oblongata and pons, and relays that information to the medial geniculate on the same side. The inferior colliculii control orienting movements in response to auditory stimuli. The superior colliculii control orienting movements of the eyes, head, and neck in response to visual stimulation such as bright light.

The cerebral aquaduct connecting the 3rd ventricle with the 4th ventricle runs through the mesencephalon. The tegmentum forms the part of the midbrain lying ventral to the cerebral aqueduct. On the walls and floor of the mesencephalon are found the red nuclei, substantia nigra, reticular formation, and nuclei for the third (occulomotor) and fourth (trochlear) cranial nerves. The red nucleus is named for its red

color caused by the extensive blood supply it receives and the iron pigment found in the cell bodies. It is the largest nucleus of the reticular formation discussed below. It receives information from the cerebrum and cerebellum, and is involved in subconscious motor control of the forelimb positions and background muscle tone. The substantia nigra (*nigra* = black), named for its black pigment, lies lateral of the red nucleus.

Visible on the sides of the mesencephalon are the cerebral peduncles (little feet). They contain descending fibers connecting to the cerebellum via the pons, and descending fibers carrying voluntary motor signals from the cerebral hemispheres.

Metencephalon

The metencephalon consists of the pons and cerebellum. The pons links the spinal cord with the forebrain, as well as the cerebellum with the forebrain and spinal cord. It forms part of the anterior surface of the fourth ventricle.

The pons has four major components:

1. Cranial nerves. Cranial nerves V (trigeminal), VI (abducens), VII (facial) and VIII (vestibulocochlear) are found in the pons.
2. Nuclei controlling respiration. Located bilaterally are two respiratory centers called the apneustic center and the pneumotaxic center.
3. Fiber tracts and nuclei connecting cerebellum to the brain stem, forebrain, and spinal cord.
4. Transverse tracts. Found on the anterior surface of the pons are fiber tracts that link nuclei found in the pons with the contralateral (opposite) cerebral hemisphere.

The cerebellum (Latin for "little brain") is the second largest region of the brain, accounting for 10% of its total mass, but containing half of all neurons in the brain. It is located dorsal to the pons and medulla oblongata, with the fourth ventricle in between, and is separated from the cerebral hemispheres by the transverse fissure.

The cerebellum is important in coordinating muscle movement and maintaining balance. For example, when a horse jumps over an obstacle, it requires the coordinated movement of all the limbs, as well as a good sense of where the horse is in space. The cerebellum compares what movement was intended to what movement happened. The cerebellum can then institute adjustments to the intended movement while they are in progress, or during repetitions.

Resembling a piece of cauliflower, the cerebellum is connected to the brain stem by the inferior, middle, and superior cerebellar peduncles, also called the

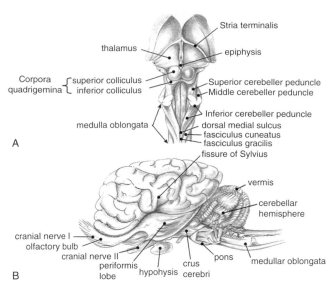

thalamus

Stria terminalis

epiphysis

Corpora quadrigemina { superior colliculus, inferior colliculus

Superior cerebeller peduncle
Middle cerebeller peduncle

Inferior cerebeller peduncle

medulla oblongata

dorsal medial sulcus
fasciculus cuneatus
fasciculus gracilis
fissure of Sylvius

A

vermis

cerebellar hemisphere

cranial nerve I
olfactory bulb
cranial nerve II
periformis lobe
hypohysis
crus cerebri
pons
medullar oblongata

B

Fig. 9.19.   Brain of the horse. A) Dorsal view of brain stem. B) Lateral view of brain. (Reprinted from Constantinescu and Constantinescu, 2004. Used by permission of the publisher.)

restiform body, brachium pontis, and brachium conjuctivum, respectively (Fig. 9.19). The surface of the cerebellum consists of small convolutions similar to small gyri, called folia (leaves), running side to side. The anterior and posterior lobes of the cerebellum are separated by the primary fissure. The anterior and posterior lobes are further subdivided into two and five lobules, respectively. The two lateral cerebellar hemispheres are separated by a narrow ridge of cortex called the vermis (Latin for "worm"). When viewing a saggital cut of the cerebellum, the flocculonodular lobe is seen between the cerebellar hemispheres, vermis, and the roof of the fourth ventricle. This lobe is separated from the body of the cerebellum by the posterolateral fissure (Fig. 9.19).

The surface of the cerebellum is covered with a cortex containing large, highly branched neurons called Purkinje cells. These cells contain an extensive dendritic tree and receive input from up to 200,000 synapses. The importance of this input is evidenced by the fact that 40 times as many axons project to the cerebellum as leave it. Inside the cerebellum, forming the shape of a tree, is white matter called the arbor vitae, or "tree of life." In addition, there are three pairs of deep cerebellar nuclei.

The cerebellum monitors all proprioceptive, visual, tactile, balance, and auditory sensory information. Most of this information is carried to the Purkinje cells, thus bypassing deep cerebellar nuclei. The motor information traveling to the cerebellum from the pyramidal and extrapyramidal system is relayed from nuclei in the pons or cerebellar nuclei found in the arbor vitae.

Information leaves the pons via the cerebellar peduncles. The superior cerebellar peduncle carries signals to the midbrain, diencephalons, and cerebrum while the middle cerebellar peduncle transmits signals to the sensory and motor nuclei in the pons. The inferior cerebellar peduncle relays information between the cerebellum and nuclei in the medulla oblongata and cerebellar tracts from the spinal cord.

Signals generated in the sensorimotor areas of the cortex project to nuclei in the pons, and then to the cerebellum. This is a large pathway containing approximately two times the axons found in the pyramidal tract. The lateral cerebellum then sends signals back to the motor cortex via the ventral lateral nucleus of the thalamus.

Medulla oblongata

Originating from the myelencephalon, the medulla oblongata is continuous with the spinal cord. The rostral portion of the medulla contains part of the fourth ventricle; the caudad portion contains a central canal.

The medulla contains three major groups of nuclei. The first is part of the reticular formation, which extends from the medulla to the mesencephalon, and was described above. The portion of the reticular formation in the medulla is responsible for regulating autonomic functions. The two major reflex centers are the cardiovascular centers and the respiratory rhythmicity center. The cardiovascular centers regulate heart rate, the strength of cardiac contractions, and the flow of blood through peripheral tissues. The cardiovascular centers include the cardiac center and vasomotor center. The respiratory rhythms center regulates the pace of respiratory movements. These are controlled by inputs from the apneustic and pneumotaxic centers in the pons.

The second group of nuclei are for the cranial nerves (see Fig. 9.22, later in chapter). Five cranial nerves originate in the medulla including the VIII (vestibulocochlear), IX (glossopharyngeal), X (vagus), XI (accessory), and XII (hypoglossal) nerves. Note that cranial nerve VIII carries sensory information from the inner ear to both the vestibular and cochlear nuclei that extend from the pons into the medulla.

The third group of nuclei act as relay stations from sensory and motor pathways. They include the nucleus gracilis and nucleus cuneatus that carry somatic sensory information to the thalamus. The solitary nucleus, located bilaterally, receives visceral sensory information coming from the spinal cord and cranial nerves. This information is relayed to the autonomic centers in the medulla and elsewhere. The olivary nuclei, which form olive-shaped bulges along the ventrolateral surface of the medulla, transmit somatic motor commands from higher brain centers to the cerebellar cortex.

Functional systems

The reticular activating system

The reticular formation forms the core of the brain stem tegmentum extending from the medullar oblongata through the pons and midbrain. It consists of loosely clustered neurons, and is homologous to the central gray area of the spinal cord that contains interneurons. It is termed an area since it lacks cell cluster–forming nuclei, and is spanned by long bundles of ascending and descending fibers, giving it a reticulated appearance.

The area can be divided into lateral and medial regions. The lateral region generally consists of parvocellular interneurons found close to motor nuclei of the cranial nerves, and is involved in coordinated reflexes and simple stereotyped behaviors. These are generally related to the vagus nerve and include gastrointestinal responses such as swallowing and vomiting; respiratory activities such as initiation of respiratory rhythm, coughing, hiccupping, and sneezing; and cardiovascular functions including the baroreceptor reflexes. The main descending lateral pathway is the rubrospinal tract originating in the magnocellular portion of the red nucleus and traveling to the lateral column of the spinal cord. The lateral reticulospinal pathway inhibits antigravitational muscles and can lead to atonia.

Neurons in the medial region are larger (magnocellular) and have long ascending and descending axons (e.g., pontine reticulospinal tract) that modulate neurons involved in movement and posture, pain, autonomic functions, and arousal. In particular, this pathway enhances antigravitational reflexes by facilitating extensors and helping standing posture.

Within the reticular formation, certain neurons send continuous impulses via the thalamus to the cerebral cortex. These impulses cause excitation, thus causing arousal. This system is called the ascending reticular activating system (RAS). This system receives input from ascending sensory tracts. It is responsible for filtering out selected sensory signals after they become familiar and weak.

The RAS is inhibited during sleep, and is thus involved in the sleep-wake cycle. Studies in the 1940s and 1950s revealed that electrical stimulation of the midbrain reticular formation (i.e., midline tegmental area) promoted wakefulness, whereas damage to this region caused a state similar to that in non-REM sleep. This area was found to be inhibited by a system in the medulla. Making a cut just caudad to the midbrain (i.e., midpontine-pretrigeminal transection) prevented an animal from sleeping.

Stimulating the RAS increases the firing rate of various neurons including the locus coeruleus in the pons, which contains norepinephrine, the raphe nuclei, which produces serotonin, acetylchonine-containing neurons in the brain stem and forebrain, as well as histamine-containing neurons in the midbrain. These neurons synapse in the thalamus, cerebral cortex, and other brain regions.

Sleep

Sleep can be defined as a readily reversible state of reduced responsiveness to and interaction with the environment. Therefore, behaviorally, sleep has four characteristics: 1) reduced motor activity, 2) decreased responsiveness, 3) stereotypic postures, and 4) ready reversibility. Coma and anesthesia do not qualify as sleep since they are not readily reversible.

Sleep is categorized into two categories. Rapid eye movement, or REM sleep, is noted for the movement of the eyes under the eyelids, and the almost complete inhibition of skeletal muscle tone. This stage of sleep is when most dreaming occurs. Non-REM sleep is characterized by a change in the electroencephalogram (EEG). Non-REM sleep is sometimes called slow-wave sleep because of the large, slow EEG rhythms (Fig. 9.20). All mammals sleep, although the length of sleep varies. Birds also show both REM and non-REM sleep, although their sleep episodes are short, with REM sleep lasting maybe only a few seconds. In addition, muscle atonia during REM sleep is rare in birds.

Non-REM sleep appears designed for rest. Neuronal activity is low, muscle tension is reduced, and movement is minimal, although movement is possible. Body temperature and metabolic rate are at their lowest. Sympathetic outflow decreases while the activity of the parasympathetic nervous system increases. Therefore, heart rate, blood pressure, respiration rate, and kidney function decrease and digestive function increases. The slow, large-amplitude EEG rhythms indicate that the cortex is oscillating in high synchrony while receiving little if any sensory input.

In contrast, the EEG during REM sleep is nearly indistinguishable from that of the awake brain. It displays fast, low-voltage fluctuations and is therefore sometimes called paradoxical sleep. Oxygen consumption of the brain is higher during REM sleep than when an animal is awake and concentrating. While most of the muscles of the body are in atonia, the muscles controlling eye movement and those in the inner ear are active.

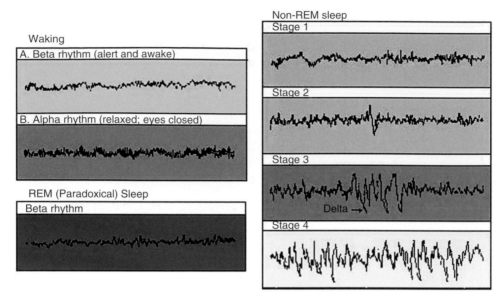

Fig. 9.20.   EEG. Various EEG wave patterns seen during wakefulness and various stages of sleep.

Roughly 75% of the sleep cycle is spent in non-REM sleep and 25% in REM sleep. An animal cycles between these two stages of sleep going from non-REM to REM sleep, and back approximately every 90 min. This is an example of an ultradian rhythms that are shorter than circadian rhythms.

Non-REM sleep is divided into four stages. The lightest stage of sleep, stage 1, is the transition period from wakefulness to onset of sleep and may last 5–10 min. While awake, people show low-voltage EEG activity of 10–30 μV and 16–25 Hz (Fig. 9.20). As they relax, they show alpha activity of 20–40 μV and 10 Hz. During stage 1, the EEG shows a low-voltage mixed frequency pattern known as theta waves. Stage 2 contains theta waves plus K complexes and sleep spindles. Sleep spindles are sudden bursts of electrical activity, 12–14 Hz, lasting 1–2 sec, whereas K complexes are sudden and sharp waves of electrical activity of longer frequency, often triggered by noise. Eye movements almost cease. During stage 3, the EEG contains large-amplitude, slow delta rhythms (.5–2 Hz), and eye and body movements are absent. Delta waves are the slowest and strongest waves produced. Stage 4, the deepest stage of sleep, is characterized by large EEG rhythms of 2 Hz or less (slow wave sleep). Growth hormone, prolactin, and gonadotrophins are released during these last two stages, leading some to speculate that these stages of sleep are restorative. If awakened during stages 3 and 4, an animal will appear confused.

Throughout the night, there is a reduction in the duration of non-REM sleep, particularly stages 3 and 4, while there is an increase in the duration of REM sleep. During REM sleep, brain temperature and metabolic rate rise, although almost all skeletal muscle activity is lost.

During non-REM sleep, GABA-containing neurons in the ventrolateral preoptic (anterior) area of the hypothalamus send a signal to the posterior hypothalamus, particularly the tuberomammillary nucleus, which contains histaminergic neurons. These latter neurons normally project to the thalamus and cortex causing activation. The reticularis nucleus of the thalamus and thalamocortical neurons are reciprocally interconnected, and they shift into a non-REM sleep spindle wave when deactivated by the hypothalamus and brainstem. These cells have a unique property; when they are hyperpolarized, voltage-sensitive calcium channels open, causing a burst of action potentials. Following the calcium spike, the membrane potential returns to the hyperpolarized state. The action potential in the reticularis nucleus leads to the release of GABA that hyperpolarizes thalamic cells projecting to the cortex (thalamocortical neurons), and such hyperpolarization causes a rebound low-threshold calcium spike in these thalamocortical neurons. The firing of the thalamocortical neurons causes synchronized postsynaptic potentials in cortical neurons that cause spindle waves. When the thalamocortical neurons become progressively hyperpolarized, and spindling becomes reduced, cortical neurons spontaneously develop delta waves.

Using brain transection and stimulation experiments, Francois Michel and Michel Jouvet showed that the pons is the source of EEG activation and rapid eye movement during REM sleep. The pons is also the

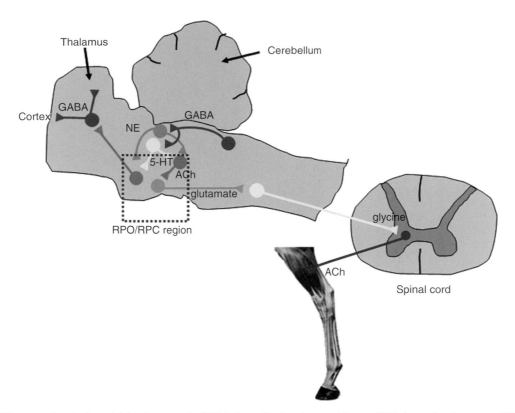

Fig. 9.21. Possible neurochemical model for the control of REM sleep. During the transition to REM sleep, the slow wave EEG associated with stage 4 of non-REM sleep is replaced by a low-voltage EEG. In addition, skeletal muscle tone is reduced. During this transition, GABA containing neurons in the pons become activated. They cause an inhibition of NE- and 5-HT containing neurons found in the locus ceruleus and raphe nucleus, respectively. This causes disinhibition of the cholinergic neurons in the reticularis pontis oralis/caudalis (RPO/RPC) region of the pons. The ascending pontine neurons cause the reduction in EEG voltage associated with REM sleep by blocking the burst firing mode of the GABAergic neurons in the thalamus. The choinergic neurons in the pons also stimulate descending glutamatergic neurons that project to the medulla, synapsing on glycine-containing neurons. These latter neurons project to the central gray area of the spinal cord and synapse on α-motor neurons causing inhibition.

site of inhibitory signals that lead to atonia. Signals, called pontine-geniculate-occipital (PGO) waves are sent from the pons, specifically from the reticularis pontis oralis/caudalis region, to both the forebrain and the spinal cord (Fig. 9.21). These signals cause bursts of firing in cortical neurons while sensory input is suppressed via presynaptic inhibition. The cholinergic PGO-on cells fire in bursts and this leads to the PGO spikes observed in the thalamus during REM sleep. Thus, the brain is blocked from external stimuli. During waking periods, serotonergic neurons from the raphe nucleus called REM-off cells hyperpolarize and block the burst firing of PGO-on cells. Noradrenergic neurons in the locus ceruleus, as well as histaminergic neurons in the posterior hypothalamus, also are involved in inhibition of the PGO cells during waking periods.

Another class of neurons in the nucleus reticularis pontis oralis, the REM-on cells, show little firing during waking and non-REM sleep, but have high activity during REM sleep.

Cranial nerves

Cranial nerves connect directly to the brain rather than the spinal cord (Fig. 9.22). Most are part of the peripheral nervous system, although the first two (olfactory nerve and optic nerve) are considered part of the central nervous system. There are twelve pairs of cranial nerves, and they arise from the ventrolateral surface of the brain. These nerves mostly innervate the head.

The cranial nerves attach to the brain near their associated sensory and/or motor nuclei. As shown in Table 9.1, the cranial nerves can be classified as sensory, special sensory, motor, or mixed. Sensory nerves carry somatic sensory information such as touch, pressure, vibration, temperature, and pain input to the brain. Special sensory nerves carry signals associated with special senses including smell, sight, hearing, taste, or balance. Motor nerves carry somatic motor input to their respective muscles while mixed nerves are both afferent and efferent carrying sensory and motor information.

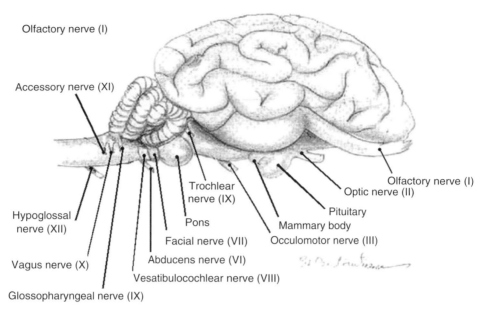

Olfactory nerve (I)

Accessory nerve (XI)

Hypoglossal
nerve (XII)

Vagus nerve (X)

Glossopharyngeal nerve (IX)

Trochlear
nerve (IX)

Pons

Facial nerve (VII)

Abducens nerve (VI)

Vesatibulocochlear nerve (VIII)

Olfactory nerve (I)
Optic nerve (II)

Pituitary
Mammary body
Occulomotor nerve (III)

Fig. 9.22. Cranial nerves. Cranial nerves shown exiting the goat brain. (Reprinted from Constantinescu, 2001. Used by permission of the publisher.)

Table 9.1. Cranial nerves.

Number	Name	Types of Axons	Function
I	Olfactory	Special sensory	Smell
II	Optic	Special sensory	Vision
III	Oculomotor	Somatic motor Visceral motor	Movements of eye and eyelid Parasympathetic control of pupil size
IV	Trochlear	Somatic motor	Movement of the eye
V	Trigenimal	Somatic sensory Somatic motor	Sensation of touch to the face Motor control of mastication
VI	Abducens	Somatic motor	Movement of the eye
VII	Facial	Somatic motor Special sensory	Facial expressions Taste in anterior two-thirds of tongue
VIII	Auditory-vestibular	Special sensory	Hearing and balance
IX	Glossopharyngeal	Somatic motor Special sensory Visceral sensory Visceral motor	Movements in the throat Taste in posterior two-thirds of tongue Detection of BP changes in aorta Parasympathetic control of salivary glands
X	Vagus	Visceral sensory Visceral motor Somatic motor	Sense of pain in viscera Movement in the throat Parasympathetic control of heart, lungs, and abdominal organs
XI	Spinal accessory	Somatic motor	Movement in throat and neck
XII	Hypoglossal	Somatic motor	Movement of the tongue

Cranial nerves III, VII, IX, and X are associated with the parasympathetic nervous system. They carry autonomic signals to preganglionic fibers located in the periphery.

Cranial nerves are involved in cranial reflexes. These are reflexes involving sensory and motor fibers of the cranial nerves. Examples of these reflexes are shown in Table 9.2.

Table 9.2. Cranial reflexes.

Reflex	Stimulus	Afferent Cranial Nerve	Central Synapse	Efferent Cranial Nerves	Response
Somatic Reflexes					
Corneal reflex	Touching corneal surface	Trigeminal	Motor nucleus for facial nerve	VII	Blinking eyelids
Tympanic reflex	Loud noise	Vestibulocochlear	Inferior colliculus	VII	Reduced movement of auditory ossicles
Auditory reflex	Loud noise	Vestibulocochlear	Motor nuclei of brain stem and spinal cord	III, IV, VI, VII, X, and cervical nerves	Eye and/or head movements triggered by sudden sounds
Vestibulo-ocular reflex	Rotation of head	VIII	Motor nuclei controlling eye muscles	III, IV, VI	Opposite movement of eyes to stabilize field of vision
Visceral Reflexes					
Direct light reflex	Light-stimulating photoreceptors	II	Superior colliculus	III	Constriction of ipsilateral pupil
Consensual light reflex	Light- stimulating photoreceptors	II	Superior colliculus	III	Constriction of contralateral pupil

A

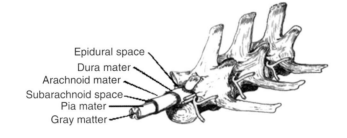

Epidural space
Dura mater
Arachnoid mater
Subarachnoid space
Pia mater
Gray matter

B

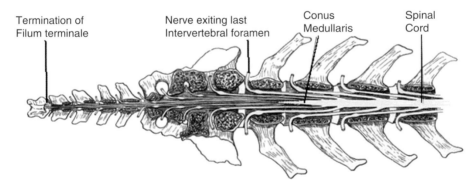

Termination of Filum terminale · Nerve exiting last Intervertebral foramen · Conus Medullaris · Spinal Cord

Fig. 9.23. Spinal cord. A) The spinal cord with its various meningial layers is shown. B) The spinal cord extends only to the level of the first or second lumbar vertebrae in adult animals where it ends in a tapered structure called the conus medullaris. A fibrous extension called the filum terminale anchors the spinal cord to the sacrum. (Modified from Getty, 1964.)

Organization of the spinal cord

The spinal cord is housed in the vertebral column (Fig. 9.23). It extends from the foramen magnum at the base of the skull, to approximately the level of the first or second lumbar vertebra in an adult animal. The spinal cord terminates as a tapered structure called the conus medullaris. It contains ascending and descending pathways to and from the brain, as well as nerve cell bodies which function in motor activity and reflexes.

Continuing as an extension of the medulla oblongata, like the brain, the spinal cord is surrounded by

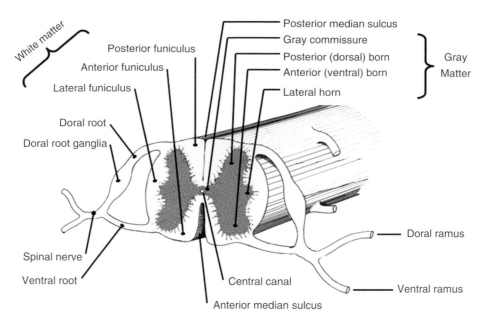

Fig. 9.24. Cross section of the spinal cord. The spinal cord has a central gray area consisting mostly of nerve cell bodies and a surrounding region of white matter consisting of fiber tracts made largely of myelinated fibers. The spinal nerves are shown on either side of the spinal cord. (Modified from Getty, 1964.)

bone, meninges, and cerebrospinal fluid. The dura mater over the spinal cord is a single layer that is not attached to the vertebral column. Instead, between the walls of the vertebral canal and the spinal cord is the epidural space containing loose connective tissue, blood vessels, and a layer of fat. The arachnoid mater and pia mater extend further down the spinal canal than does the spinal cord. This fibrous extension is called the filum terminale, which extends to the second sacral vertebrae and anchors the spinal cord.

In cross section, the spinal cord has a central core of gray matter consisting mostly of cell bodies and an outer region of white matter containing myelinated and unmyelinated nerve fibers (Fig. 9.24). The anterior and posterior surface of the spinal cord each contains a groove called the anterior median fissure and the posterior median sulcus, respectively.

The central gray area approximates the shape of a butterfly. The relative amounts of gray and white matter change at successive levels of the spinal cord. Moving from the inferior end toward the medulla oblongata, the relative amounts of gray matter decreases as white matter increases. Therefore, there are increasing numbers of fibers carrying information to the brain. The central gray area has two posterior (dorsal) horns and two anterior (ventral) horns. In addition, in the thoracic and superior lumbar region of the spinal cord, the central gray area also has lateral horns on either side. The central gray area also has a gray commissure that connects both sides of the central gray area. The posterior horns contain interneurons;

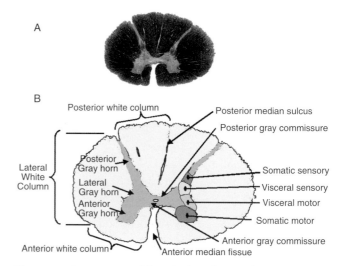

Fig. 9.25. Organization of the spinal cord. A) A photomicrograph of a cross section of the thoracic spinal cord. B) A drawing showing the important landmarks of the same cross section.

the anterior horns contain both interneurons and cell bodies of somatic motor neurons. The lateral horns contain motor neurons of the sympathetic nervous system.

The white matter of the spinal cord is grouped into three white columns, also called funiculi (long ropes). Named according to their location, they include the posterior, lateral, and anterior columns (Fig. 9.25). The fiber tracts within these columns are named according to their origin and destination (Fig. 9.26).

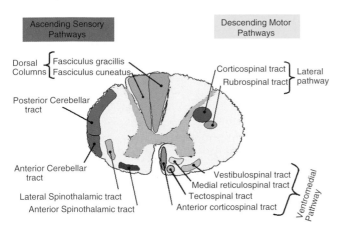

Fig. 9.26. The major ascending (sensory) and descending (motor) pathways of the spinal cord. The left side shows ascending pathways; the right side shows descending pathways within the spinal cord.

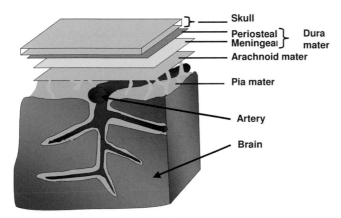

Fig. 9.27. The meninges. There are three connective tissue layers, collectively called the meninges, which cover the brain. The outermost layer, the dura mater, is a tough, fibrous connective tissue consisting of two layers: a periosteal layer attached to the inner surface of the skull and a meningeal layer. The arachnoid mater lies inside the dura mater, and is a loosely knit layer. The deepest layer is the pia mater, which also courses into the brain closely adhering to capillaries as they move into the brain tissue. Between the arachnoid and pia mater is the subarachnoid space, which is filled with cerebrospinal fluid.

Protection of the central nervous system

Meninges

The meninges (Greek for "covering") consist of three connective tissue membranes that overlay the central nervous system. These membranes act to cover and protect the CNS, as well as encase blood vessels and help divide gross areas of the CNS.

The three layers, named from the outermost, include the dura mater, arachnoid mater, and pia mater (Fig. 9.27). The dura mater is a tough, fibrous connec-

tive tissue layer. Surrounding the brain, it consists of two layers, with the outermost layer attached to the periosteum of the cranium. The inner layer serves as a covering over the brain, and extends over the spinal cord where there is only one dural layer. Although the two dural layers over the brain are generally fused, there are several locations where the two layers separate and form dural sinuses. The dural sinuses are blood filled structures that somewhat resemble blood vessels, and which collect venous blood and return it to the internal jugular veins.

There are also areas where the dura mater extends inward from the surface of the brain forming dural folds that help stabilize gross brain structures. The largest of these folds are

- Falx cerebri. This is a sickle-shaped fold of dura that extends down into the longitudinal fissure helping to separate the two cerebral hemispheres. Both the superior sagittal sinus and the inferior sagittal sinus are found within this fold.
- Tentorium cerebelli. This separates the cerebellum from the cerebral hemispheres.
- Falx cerebelli. This divides the two cerebellar hemispheres running along the vermis of the cerebellum.

The arachnoid mater (Greek for "spider") resembles a spider web and lies between the dura mater and pia mater. It forms a loose covering of the brain and never dips into the sulci or fissures. Between the arachnoid mater and pia mater is the subarachnoid space. This space is filled with large blood vessels, as well as cerebrospinal fluid coming from the fourth ventricle. Arachnoid granulations, or villi, project from the arachnoid, through the dura, and into the superior sagittal sinus. Cerebrospinal fluid moves by bulk flow through these granulations and into the general circulation.

Finally, the pia mater closely adheres to the surface of the CNS. It contains many small blood vessels, and the pia mater adheres to these vessels for a short distance as they move into the brain.

Cerebrospinal fluid

A clear and colorless fluid, cerebrospinal fluid has many functions: 1) maintain a constant external environment for cells in the brain, 2) provide a route for removing harmful metabolites from the brain, 3) provide a cushion to protect the brain from trauma, 4) act as the lymphatic system for the brain, and 5) provide a route for peptides that are released at one site and act at a distant site in the brain.

Cerebrospinal fluid is produced mostly from the choroid plexus, a tuft of capillaries found at the top of

Table 9.3.   Comparison of the composition of cerebrospinal fluid and blood.

Chemical	CSF	Blood
Na	145 mmol/L	135–150 mEq/L
K	3 mmol/L	3.9–5.3 mEq/L
Cl	125 mmol/L	97–116 mEq/L
HCO$_3$	22 mmol/L	
P	500 µmole/L	5.5–6.5 mEq/L
Ca	1.2 mmol/L	10.3–11.4 mg/100 ml
Mg	1.0 mmol/L	2.0–3.0 mg/100 ml
Glucose	2.5–4.2 mmol/L	40–120 mg/100 ml
Protein	12–60 mg/dL	7.0–8.3 gm/100 ml
Osmolarity	295 mOsmol/L	
pH	7.31–7.35	7.30–7.54

the third and fourth ventricle, as well as the floor of the lateral ventricles. The remaining CSF is formed from the ependymal cells. Although cerebrospinal fluid originates as an ultrafiltrate of blood, its composition differs from that of plasma in several important ways. It contains less protein, calcium, and potassium, and more sodium, chloride, and hydrogen ions than plasma (Table 9.3).

Blood-brain barrier

Neurons of the brain and spinal cord are very sensitive to alterations in their environment. As such, they are isolated from the systemic circulation by the blood-brain barrier (BBB), which prevents the movement of many molecules into the CNS. The BBB is formed by the endothelial cells lining the blood capillaries. In the periphery, these cells are fenestrated; in the CNS, these cells form tight junctions. The tight junctions are induced by factors produced by astrocytes whose end feet surround the endothelial cells of brain capillaries.

To cross the BBB, a molecule must be either lipid soluble, or must cross via a carrier-mediated transport system. Lipid-soluble compounds readily cross cell membranes, and are thereby readily able to enter the CNS. Such compounds include carbon dioxide, oxygen, steroids, prostaglandins, and alcohol. In contrast, nonlipid-soluble compounds, such as peptides and various antibiotics, do not readily cross the BBB. However, since many essential nutrients for the brain are not lipid soluble, the BBB also possesses many carrier-mediated transport systems that allow such compounds to enter the brain at a rate far greater than that explained by their lipid solubility.

Blood-cerebrospinal fluid barrier

Although the choroid plexus is located within the ventricles, embryologically, it is derived from mesodermal tissue that is outside of the CNS. Therefore, unlike the endothelial cells in most brain capillaries, those in the choroid plexus do not have tight junctions. Instead, the ependymal cells lining the cerebroventricles overlying the choroid plexus have tight junctions, thus forming a barrier between the blood and cerebrospinal fluid.

References

Constantinescu, G.M. 2001. Guide to Regional Ruminant Anatomy Based on the Dissection of the Goat. Iowa State Press, Ames, Iowa.

Constantinescu, G.M. and I.A. Constantinescu, 2004. Clinical Dissection Guide for Large Animals, Horse and Large Ruminants, 2nd edition. Iowa State Press, Ames, Iowa.

Getty, R. 1964. Atlas for Applied Veterinary Anatomy. Iowa State Press, Ames, Iowa.

King, A.S. 1987. Physiological and Clinical Anatomy of Domestic Mammals. Volume 1. Central Nervous System. Oxford University Press, Walton Street, Oxford.

10 Peripheral and autonomic nervous system

Contents

The peripheral nervous system includes that part of the nervous system outside the brain and spinal cord. It is responsible for collecting most of the sensory information that is relayed to the central nervous system. It is also responsible for carrying motor signals to the skeletal and smooth muscles. As discussed in Chapter 8, the peripheral nervous system includes a sensory and motor component (Fig. 8.2). The autonomic nervous system is a branch of this motor component.

Nerves and ganglia

Nerves

Components of a neuron were described in Chapter 8. A nerve, however, is a collection of axons from many neurons, and is found in the peripheral nervous system. Nerves vary in size and are surrounded by a series of connective tissue layers (Fig. 10.1). The epineurium is the outermost layer, consisting of a dense network of collagen fibers. The perineurium is the next innermost layer, and it partitions the nerve into a series of fascicles each containing a bundle of axons. The innermost layer is the endoneurium that surrounds each individual axon.

Arteries and veins enter through the epineurium and branch within the perineurium. Capillaries can penetrate into the endoneurium where they nourish axons and Schwann cells of the nerves as well as the fibroblasts of the connective tissue. Therefore, a nerve consists not only of axons, but its bulk is composed of other tissues, including blood vessels, glial cells and connective tissue.

Classification of nerves

Since the peripheral nervous system has both sensory and motor components, nerves are classified according to their function. Nerves carrying impulses toward

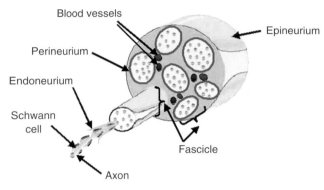

Fig. 10.1. Peripheral nerve. A peripheral nerve consists of many bundles of axons, each called a fascicle. There are three connective tissue layers surrounding various parts of the nerve. The epineurium is the outermost layer wrapping around the entire nerve. The perineurium surrounds each fascicle while the endoneurium surrounds each axon.

the central nervous system (CNS) are called sensory, or afferent, nerves, whereas those carrying impulses away from the CNS are motor, or efferent, nerves. Remember that *e*fferent nerves carry impulses toward an *e*ffector. A nerve that carries impulses in both directions is called a mixed nerve.

Peripheral nerves can function within the autonomic (visceral) nervous system or somatic nervous system. Therefore, they can be further classified as visceral afferent, visceral efferent, somatic afferent, or somatic efferent.

Spinal nerves

Nerves leaving the CNS are called either spinal nerves or cranial nerves. Cranial nerves were discussed in Chapter 8. There is a pair of spinal nerves exiting at each spinal segment. Each spinal nerve has a dorsal and ventral root that enters and exits the spinal cord, respectively (Fig. 10.2). Thus the dorsal roots contain afferent fibers and the ventral roots contain efferent fibers consisting of motor neurons of both the somatic

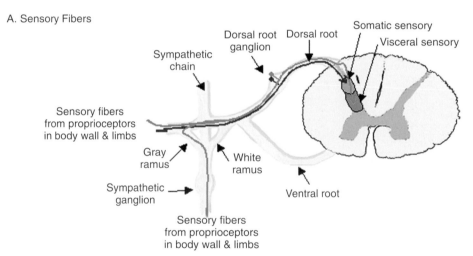

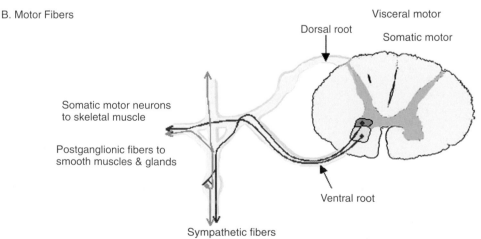

Fig. 10.2. Spinal nerves. A) The sensory neurons from the periphery enter the spinal cord through the dorsal root, and their cell bodies are located in the dorsal root ganglion. These fibers synapse in the dorsal gray horn of the central gray area of the spinal cord. The sensory visceral (autonomic) fibers may or may not pass through the sympathetic chain. B) The motor fibers exit the spinal cord via the ventral root. The visceral motor fibers may enter the sympathetic chain via the white ramus.

and autonomic nervous system. Near the spinal cord, the two roots merge forming a spinal nerve, which is a mixed nerve containing both afferent and efferent fibers. Each dorsal root has a swelling, called the dorsal root ganglion, situated near the spinal cord, which contains the cell bodies of the neurons running through the dorsal root. The dorsal and ventral roots pass through the intervertebral foramen located between adjacent vertebrae; the dorsal root ganglion lies between the pedicles of adjacent vertebrae.

Spinal nerves exit at every vertebra. The first spinal nerve exits superior to the first cervical vertebra while an additional spinal nerve exits inferior to each vertebra. Therefore, cervical spinal nerves are named for the vertebrae immediately following where they exit. Since there are seven cervical vertebrae, there are eight cervical cranial nerves (C1–C8). All other cranial nerves are named for the vertebra immediately preceding where they exit (i.e., T1, T2, etc). After leaving the spinal cord, both the dorsal and ventral roots merge forming a spinal nerve. Shortly thereafter, the spinal nerve branches into the dorsal and ventral ramus. The ventral ramus carries fibers to the skeletal muscles of the body wall and limbs, as well as post-ganglionic fibers to smooth muscles, glands, body walls, and limbs. The dorsal ramus carries similar fibers to the back.

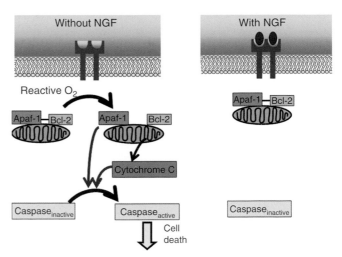

Fig. 10.3. Apoptosis. In a healthy cell, Bcl-2 is found on the outer mitochondria membrane and is bound to Apaf-1. Internal damage to the cell, such as the presence of reactive oxygen species, or lack of neurotrophic factors, such as nerve growth factor (NGF), causes Bcl-2 to release Apaf-1. A related protein called Bax also penetrates the mitochondral membranes, causing the leakage of cytochrome C into the cytoplasm. Released Apaf-1 and cytochrome C bind to inactive caspase. The resulting complex containing cytochrome C, Apaf-1, caspase 9, and ATP is called the apoptosome. Once activated, caspase 9 activates other caspases leading to digestion of structural proteins in the cytoplasm and degradation of chromosomal DNA and phagocytosis of the cell.

Degeneration and regeneration of nerves

Like other cells, neurons die. It is believed that neurotrophic factors are responsible for keeping neurons alive. The presence of these factors suppresses a latent biochemical pathway present in all cells that causes the cells to commit suicide. Cells can die by a process called apoptosis, or programmed cell death, which involves four steps. The cell shrinks, the chromatin condenses, the cell fragments into apoptotic bodies, and the cellular remnants are phagocytized by macrophages or other such cells.

Using sympathetic neurons as a model, a proposed mechanism for apoptosis is as follows (Fig. 10.3). The loss of neurotrophic factors, such as nerve growth factor, decreases activity of the MAP kinase and phosphatidylinositol 3-kindase pathways, resulting in an increase in reactive oxygen species. This leads to an increase in c-jun N-terminal kinases and phosphorylation of c-jun protein. Then there is an increased expression of genes including c-jun, cyclin D1 and c-fos and a decrease in RNA and protein synthesis. There is a decrease in Bcl-2 family proteins. Bcl-2 family proteins are expressed on the outer surface of mitochondria, and are bound to a molecule of Apaf-1. When damage, Bcl-2 family protein release Apaf-1, which activate caspases (Cysteine Aspartate Specific ProteASEs).

Caspases are a family of over a dozen proteins that cleave cellular proteins at aspartate residues.

Cells can also die from trauma or necrotic cell death, a process called necrosis, which is distinguishable from apoptosis. Traumatic death is characterized by an initial swelling of the cell with only modest condensation of the chromatin, and then rapid lysis of cellular membranes without endogenous programmed cell death. Necrotic cells elicit an inflammatory response that recruits macrophages that eliminate the cellular debris. In contrast, during apoptosis individual cells are generally phagocytized prior to releasing their contents.

Ganglia

Ganglia are collections of neuron cell bodies located in the peripheral nervous system. Recall that within the central nervous system, a collection of cell bodies is called a nucleus. The ganglia for afferent (sensory) neurons are located in the dorsal root ganglia discussed above. Somatic motor neurons do not have ganglia since these motor neuron cell bodies are located in the dorsal horn of the spinal cord. However, autonomic motor neurons are associated with ganglia since there are two consecutive nerve fibers associated with each autonomic motor pathway. These autonomic ganglia will be discussed below in the section "Autonomic Nervous System."

Sensory receptors

Sensations are the awareness of a stimulus, whereas perception involves the interpretation of the sensation and occurs in the central nervous system. All senses involve three steps: 1) a physical stimuli, 2) transformation of the stimulus into a nerve impulse, and 3) a response to the sensation in the form of a perception or conscious experience of sensation. Furthermore, all sensory systems give four types of information about the stimuli including modality, location, intensity, and timing, which collectively yield sensation (Table 10.1).

The various modalities of sense include vision, hearing, touch, taste, smell, the vestibular sense of balance, and the somatic senses, including nociception (pain), temperature, itch, and proprioception (posture and movement of body parts). General senses include temperature, pain, touch, pressure, vibration, and proprioception; special senses include olfaction (smell), vision (sight), gustation (taste), equilibrium (balance), and audition (hearing). General sensory receptors are located throughout the body; receptors for special senses are located in specialized structures or organs. General senses are discussed below; special senses are covered in Chapter 11.

Classes of sensory receptors

There are five classes of sensory receptors: mechanical, chemical, nociceptors (*nocere* = to injure), thermal, and electromagnetic. Mechanoreceptors can detect touch, proprioceptive sensation (muscle stretch or contraction), joint position, hearing, and sense of balance. Chemoreceptors function in the sense of itches, taste, and smell. Nociceptors detect pain. Thermoreceptors can sense either hot or cold; photoreceptors sense electromagnetic energy.

These receptors can be further classified by location as exteroceptors, interoceptors, or proprioceptors (from the Latin word *proprius*, meaning "belong to one's own self"):

1. Exteroceptors. These are sensitive to stimuli outside (external) the body. Located near the surface of the body, they can detect touch, pressure, pain, and temperature, as well as special senses such as smell, taste, vision, and auditory.
2. Interoceptors. These receptors monitor the visceral organs and their function. They monitor chemical and temperature changes, as well as stretching within the viscera. Although an animal is not normally consciously aware of their signals, they may produce pain signals alerting the animal of a problem.
3. Proprioceptors. Although these receptors also respond to internal signals, they are restricted to those receptors in muscles and joints that provide information concerning the position of the bones and muscles.

General senses

Mechanoreceptors

Mechanoreceptors detect distortions in their cell membranes such as bending and stretching. There are three classes of mechanoreceptors:

1. Tactile receptors. Responsible for the sensations of touch, pressure, and vibration.

Table 10.1. Sensory receptors and modalities.

Sensory System	Modality	Stimulus	Receptor Class	Receptor Cell Type
Auditory	Hearing	Sound	Mechanoreceptors	Hair cells (cochlea)
Visual	Vision	Light	Photoreceptors	Rods and cones
Vestibular	Balance	Gravity	Mechanoreceptors	Hair cells (vestibular labyrinth)
Somatosensory	Somatic Senses:	Pressure	Mechanoreceptor	III, IV, VI, VII, X, and cervical
	Touch	Displacement	Mechanoreceptor	nerves
	Proprioception	Thermal	Thermoreceptor	
	Temperature	Chemical, thermal or	Chemoreceptor, thermoreceptor,	
	Pain	mechanical	or mechanoreceptor	
Gustatory	Taste	Chemical	Chemoreceptors	Taste buds
Olfactory	Smell	Chemical	Chemoreceptors	Olfactory sensory neurons

2. Baroreceptors (*baro* = pressure). Detect changes in pressure in the walls of blood vessels, as well as the digestive, reproductive, and urinary tracts.
3. Proprioceptors. Detect changes in the position of joints and muscles.

Tactile receptors

Named after the German and Italian histologists who discovered them, the two principle mechanoreceptors located in the superficial skin layers are Merkel discs and Meissner's corpuscles. The Merkel disc receptor is a slowly adapting receptor consisting of a small epithelial cell surrounding a nerve terminal. They are involved in the sense of touch and pressure. Meissner's corpuscles are rapidly adapting and consist of a globular, fluid-filled structure enclosing a stack of flattened epithelial cells around which the sensory nerve is entwined.

The two mechanoreceptors found in the deep subcutaneous layers are the Pacinian corpuscle and the Ruffini ending. Although larger than the receptors found in the superficial layers, these receptors are less numerous. The Pacinian corpuscle, physiologically similar to the Meissner's corpuscle, is a large receptor measuring as long as 2 mm and nearly 1 mm in diameter.

The Pacinian corpuscle, also called a large lamellated corpuscle, is fast-adapting and responds to rapid indentation of the skin but not steady pressure. Since the capsule surrounding this receptor is attached to the skin, this receptor can sense low frequency vibration occurring several centimeters away. These receptors are activated by touching a tuning fork (200–300 Hz) to the skin or bony structure.

Ruffini endings, slightly smaller than Pacinian corpuscles, are slow-adapting. They consist of a capsule surrounding a core of collagen fibers that are continuous with fibers in the surrounding dermis. Dendrites from the sensory neuron are intertwined with the collagen fibers in the capsule. They link the subcutaneous tissue with folds in the skin at the joints and nails. Thus, they sense stretch of the skin bending in these regions.

Vibration is the detection of sinusoidal oscillations of objects in contact with the skin. The various tactile receptors differ in their sensitivity to vibration. Merkel discs are most responsive to low frequency oscillations (5–15 Hz). Meissner's corpuscles are sensitive to mid-range oscillations (20–50 Hz), and Pacinian corpuscles to high frequencies (60–400 Hz). The lowest stimulus intensity to which a receptor produces an action potential is the receptor's tuning threshold. The intensity of the vibration is coded by the number of sensory nerve

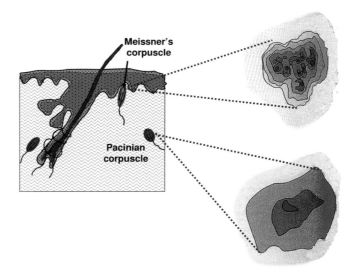

Fig. 10.4. Receptive field. Meissner's corpuscles have a smaller receptive field compared to the move deeply located Pacinian corpuscles.

fibers that are firing rather than the frequency of action potentials within a fiber.

The size of the receptive fields for the various touch receptors differs (Fig. 10.4). Meissner's corpuscles and Merkel discs, located in the superficial skin layers, have small receptive fields. A single dorsal root ganglion cell innervates 10–25 of each of these receptors and produces a receptive field of 2–10 mm in diameter. Therefore, these receptors are responsible for a fine discriminating touch that detects small spatial differences. These receptors are important in a two-point discrimination test. When performed on people, the skin is simultaneously touched by two pointed objects, and the person is asked whether they can detect two objects or a single object. As the two points are moved closer together, the person will eventually be unable to discriminate two objects.

In contrast, each Pacinian corpuscle and Ruffini ending, located in deeper skin layers, is innervated by a single nerve fiber, but its receptive field is large since these receptors can detect changes from mechanical displacement over a large distance. Because of their large receptive fields, these receptors are involved in coarse resolution of touch. The combination of the adaptation rate and size of the receptive field leads to variations in how the tactile receptors respond to stimuli (Fig. 10.5).

In addition to differences in receptive fields of the various tactile receptors, there are also differences in the number of these receptors located throughout the body. The smallest receptive fields, i.e., with the most receptors, are located in the tips of the paws and whiskers.

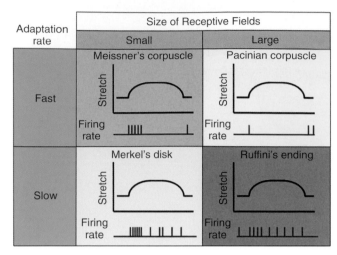

Fig. 10.5. Response of tactile receptors to stretch. The various tactile receptors change their firing rate qualitatively and quantitatively in response to stretch. Whereas Meissner's and Pacinian corpuscles respond quickly but also adapt quickly, Merkel discs and Ruffini's endings adapt more slowly.

Baroreceptors

Consisting of free nerve endings, baroreceptors sense the change in the wall of distensible organs including blood vessels, and a portion of the respiratory, digestive, and urinary tract. When the pressure in the walls of these organs increases, the walls are stretched causing a deformation in the sensory nerves. As the pressure in these organs decreases, the elastic fibers cause the walls to return to their original structure.

Baroreceptors monitor blood pressure in the major vessels, particularly in the carotid artery at the carotid sinus, and the aorta at the aortic arch. Increases in blood pressure at these sites initiates the baroreceptor reflex, in which increased firing rates from these baroreceptors is relayed to the central nervous system, and appropriate adjustments in heart rate and blood pressure are initiated. Baroreceptors in the lungs send information regarding lung inflation to the respiratory rhythmicity centers in the brain stem to regulate breathing. Similarly, baroreceptors in the colon and urinary bladder function in defecation and micturition, respectively. There are also baroreceptors along the gastrointestinal tract that are involved in peristalsis.

Proprioceptors

Proprioceptors monitor the position of joints, and the tension in tendons, ligaments, and muscle. These receptors do not adapt, and they continuously send information to the central nervous system. There are three groups of proprioceptors:

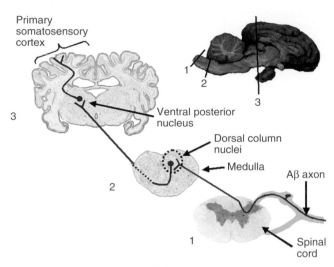

Fig. 10.6. Dorsal column-medial lemniscal pathway. Mechanoreceptor signals enter the spinal cord through the dorsal root where they either synapse on secondary fibers in the gray area or ascend in the dorsal column. Fibers ascending in the dorsal column synapse in the dorsal column nuclei (nucleus gracilus and cuneatus). Fibers from these nuclei immediately decussate, and ascend to the ventral posterior nucleus of the thalamus via the medial lemniscus. From there, fibers ascend to the primary somatosensory cortex.

1. Muscle spindles. Discussed in Chapter 8, these receptors detect the length of skeletal muscles.
2. Golgi tendon organs. Located at the junction between skeletal muscle and its tendon, the Golgi tendon organs detect stretch of the tendons. The dendrites of the receptor neurons branch extensively, wrapping around the collagen fibers of the tendon.
3. Receptors in joint capsules. In order to monitor the position of the body, joint capsules are innervated with free nerve endings that detect pressure, tension, and movement of the joint.

Dorsal column-medial lemniscal pathway (mechanoreceptor pathway)

Axons of skin sensory receptors are designated, in order of decreasing size, as Aα, Aβ, Aδ, and C, which corresponds to axons innervating muscles and tendons called groups I, II, III, and IV, respectively. Aα, Aβ, and Aδ are myelinated; C fibers are unmyelinated. Sensory nerves from the skin do not have Aα fibers. Mechanoreceptors send their messages via Aβ. These fibers enter the dorsal horn of the central gray area of the spinal cord, and branch. One branch synapses on second-order sensory neurons deep in the dorsal horn and are involved in reflexes. The other branch ascends to the brain in the dorsal column-medial lemniscal pathway (Fig. 10.6). This branch enters the ipsilateral dorsal column of the spinal cord. Composed of primary sensory axons, as well as second-order axons from neurons in the central gray area of the spinal cord, these fibers ascend to the dorsal column nuclei at the junction of the spinal cord and medulla where they synapse. The fibers leaving the dorsal column nuclei decussate (cross to the other side) and ascend in the medial lemniscus that courses through the medulla, pons, and midbrain and synapses in the ventral posterior nucleus of the thalamus.

Nociceptors

Pain is mediated by nociceptors. These receptors respond to stimuli that can damage tissue. Some nociceptors respond directly to stimuli, and others respond indirectly since they respond to chemicals released by damaged tissue. The list of chemical intermediates includes histamine, K^+, and proteases released from injured cells, bradykinin, substance P, acidity, ATP, prostaglandins, serotonin, and acetylcholine.

Chemical mediators are released in response to various stimuli. Bradykinin is produced when peptidases released from injured cells cleave the extracellular protein kininogen. Bradykinin acts directly on nociceptors, and it also increases the synthesis and release of prostaglandins from nearby tissue. Tissue acidity can increase when, for example, a galloping horse begins anaerobic metabolism producing lactic acid that leads to an increase in extracellular H^+ ion. Histamine is released when mast cells found in the connective tissue are stimulated, such as during a bee sting. Prostaglandin E_2 is a metabolite of arachidonic acid and is generated by the enzyme cyclooxygenase released from damaged cells. Aspirin and other nonsteroidal antiinflammatory analgesics work by blocking cyclooxygenase and inhibiting the synthesis of prostaglandins.

There are three classes of nociceptor. Mechanical and thermal nociceptors are sensitive to mechanical and thermal stimuli, respectively, whereas polymodal nociceptors respond to traumatized tissue rather than physical properties. Mechanical nociceptors respond to a strong tactile or sharp penetrating stimulus that results in pain. Their firing rate increases with the destructiveness of the mechanical stimuli. Thermal nociceptors respond to extremes in temperature. One group responds to noxious heat above 45°C; the second group responds to noxious cold below 5°C. The polymodal nociceptors respond not only to painful mechanical stimuli such as a strong pinch or puncture, but also to noxious heat and cold, and irritant chemicals. Stimulation of these receptors evokes slow, burning pain. These are the primary receptors in tooth pulp.

Pain signals are carried by lightly myelinated Aδ and unmyelinated C fibers. These fibers have different

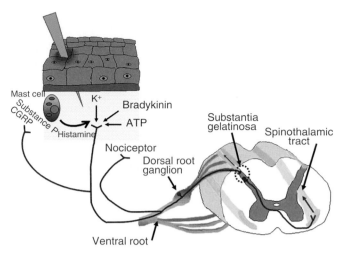

Fig. 10.7. Nociception. Damage to the skin can cause release of certain substances, including ATP, prostaglandins, and bradykinin. These substances can stimulate the nociceptors. Collaterals of the receptors can release substance P and calcitonin generelated peptide (CGRP) that can stimulate mast cells to release histamine. Histamine can stimulate nociceptors as well as cause vasodilation. Hence the redness associated with inflammation. The pain signals are carried by Aδ and C fibers through the dorsal root to the substantia gelatinosa of the central gray area of the spinal cord. Here the fibers release glutamate and/or substance P, which signals secondary fibers. The secondary fibers cross to the contralateral side and synapse on neurons that carry the impulse to the brain via the spinothalamic tract.

conduction velocities; therefore, pain information can produce two different kinds of pain perceptions (Fig. 10.7). The first pain is a fast, sharp pain mediated by Aδ fibers; it is followed by secondary pain that is duller, but longer lasting and mediated by C fibers. Once stimulated, branches of the nociceptor neurons can secrete substance P and calcitonin gene-related peptide, peptide neurotransmitters, from peripheral terminals of collaterals of the primary nociceptive neurons. These two peptides can cause vasodilation as well as release of histamine from mast cells.

Heat, redness, swelling, and pain are the cardinal signs of inflammation. Substance P can cause all of these symptoms. The heat and redness are caused by the vasodilation, swelling is caused by the leakage of proteins and cells from these blood vessels into the interstitial space, and the pain can result by the induced release of histamine that stimulates nociceptors.

Pain pathway

The Aδ and C fibers enter the spinal cord through the dorsal root and synapse in the substantia gelatinosa of the central gray area. The neurotransmitters released at this site are thought to be glutamate and substance P. The glutamate, released from Aδ and C

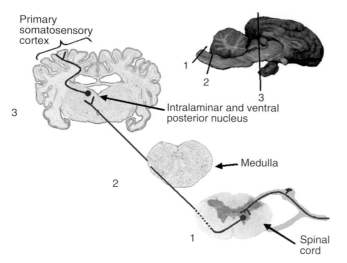

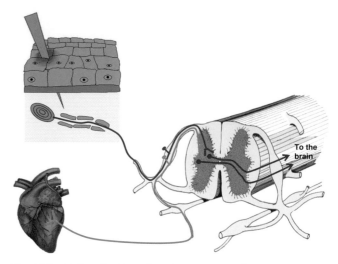

Fig. 10.8. The spinothalamic pathway. Pain and temperature information is carried to the brain via the spinothalamic pathway. Sensory fibers enter the spinal cord by way of the dorsal root and synapse in the central gray area of the spinal cord. They synapse on fibers that decussate and then ascend through the spinothalamic tract to the intralaminar and ventral posterior nuclei of the thalamus where they synapse on fibers that then course to the primary somatosensory cortex.

Fig. 10.9. Referred pain. Referred pain occurs when visceral nociception is perceived as a cutaneous sensation. The classic example of this is angina in which the heart receives insufficient oxygen resulting in pain from this region. However, the body perceives the pain as coming from the upper chest or left arm since cutaneous sensations from this region synapse in the spinal cord near the same region, and the brain is unable to distinguish between the two.

fibers, acts at AMPA-type glutamate receptors and evokes fast synaptic potentials in dorsal horn neurons. Substance P is released from C fibers and evokes slow excitatory postsynaptic potentials. Glutamate and substance P act together to transmit pain signals and, with substance P, enhance and prolong the actions of glutamate. The impulse is then carried by secondary fibers that immediately decussate and then ascend to the brain via the spinothalamic tract (Fig. 10.8).

Many times, shortly after an injury, the site becomes extremely painful and especially sensitive to touch. This is called hyperalgesia and is the body's way of protecting this site from further injury. Primary hyperalgesia is associated with the damaged tissue; however, the surrounding area can also become supersensitive, a process called secondary hyperalgesia. Hyperalgesia is due to the action of various compounds released during injury that make the nociceptors more sensitive.

Nociceptors from the viscera also enter the spinal cord by the same route as those from cutaneous nociceptors. These signals can get mixed within the spinal cord since the afferent fibers from the viscera and somatic area converge on the same projection neurons in the dorsal horn of the spinal cord (Fig. 10.9). This leads to the phenomenon of referred pain in which visceral pain is perceived as a cutaneous sensation. Such is the case with angina in which ischemia in the heart leads to pain in the upper chest and down the left arm.

Thermoreceptors

Thermoreceptors alter their firing rate as a result of changes in temperature. Unlike mechanoreceptors that are silent in the absence of stimuli, thermoreceptors maintain a low, tonic firing rate (2–5 spikes/sec) at normal body temperature. There are separate cold and warm receptors, which can be shown by differential mapping on the skin. These free nerve endings are located in the dermis of the skin, skeletal muscles, liver, and hypothalamus.

Warm receptors begin firing around 30°C, increasing their firing rate up to 45°C, after which their firing rate decreases (Fig. 10.10). Above 50°C, warm receptors stop firing. Instead the animal senses heat pain rather than warmth due to the firing of thermal nociceptors. Cold receptors actively fire at temperatures ranging from 35°C down to 10°C. Below this temperature, cold becomes an anesthetic. For unknown reasons, some cold receptors increase their firing rate above 45°C.

Thermoreceptors are very sensitive to differences in temperature between an object being touched and skin temperature. They respond vigorously to these abrupt changes in temperature and then adapt their firing rate. This can be demonstrated by placing your hand in a beaker of cold water. Notice that with time, the sensations of cold decrease. Then, take your hand and plunge it into a beaker of warm water. Notice that the water will actually feel hot due to the sudden change in temperature.

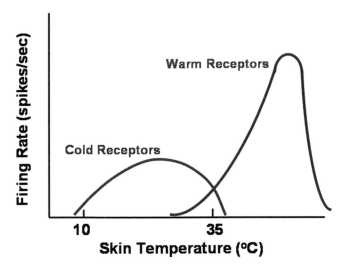

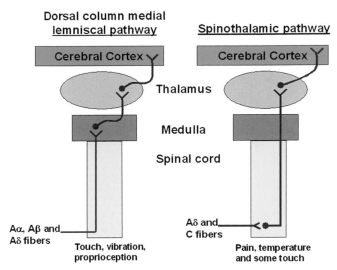

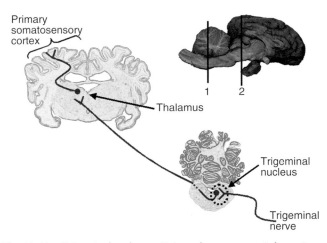

Fig. 10.10.   Thermoreceptors. Thermoreceptors change their firing rate in response to changes in skin or organ temperature. At normal body temperatures (36–38°C), both cold and warm receptors are discharging. As skin temperature decreases below 30°C, warm receptors discontinue firing, whereas cold receptors increase their firing rate, which is maximal at 25°C.

Fig. 10.12.   Pain and temperature pathways. The two major ascending pathways that carry pain and temperature information include the dorsal column-medial lemniscal pathway and the spinothalamic pathway. Note that the dorsal column-medial lemniscal pathway enters the spinal cord through the dorsal root and ascends to the medulla where it synapses on second-order neurons that cross over to the contralateral side and then ascend to the cerebral cortex. In the spinothalamic tract, fibers enter the spinal cord via the dorsal root and synapse on second-order fibers in the central gray area. These second-order neurons cross over to the contralateral side before ascending to the thalamus where they synapse on neurons that then project to the cerebral cortex.

Fig. 10.11.   Trigeminal pathway. Pain and temperature information from the face send information via the trigeminal nerve (cranial nerve V) (A). This information is carried to the trigeminal nucleus and synapses on second-order neurons that decussate and ascend to the thalamus (B) where they synapse on neurons and then ascend to the primary somatosensory cortex.

Thermoreceptor pathway

Cold receptors connect to Aδ and C fibers, whereas warm receptors connect only with C fibers. These fibers synapse in the substantia gelatinosa of the dorsal horn in the spinal cord. The secondary fibers then decussate and ascend in the contralateral spinothalamic tract along with the pain signals.

Pain and temperature information from the face and head reaches the thalamus via the trigeminal pathway (Fig. 10.11). Fibers in the trigeminal nerve synapse on second-order neurons in the spinal trigeminal nucleus

in the brainstem. These fibers decussate and ascend to the thalamus in the trigeminal lemniscus. The pain and temperature pathways are summarized in Figure 10.12.

Chemoreceptors

Chemoreceptors are responsible for detecting changes in concentrations of specific chemicals or compounds. These receptors are also responsible for the special senses of taste (gustation) and smell (olfaction). Taste and olfaction, which are considered special senses whose signals are relayed to the primary sensory cortex, will be discussed separately below. The chemoreceptors whose signals do not travel to the primary sensory cortex will be discussed here. They are responsible for sensing irritating substances on the skin, or nutrients within the gastrointestinal tract or brain, and carbon dioxide or oxygen levels in our blood.

There are chemoreceptors in the respiratory centers of the brain that sense changes in H^+ and CO_2 concentrations. There are also chemoreceptors in the carotid bodies located near the origin of the internal carotid arteries and in the aortic bodies found between the major branches of the aortic arch. These receptors respond to changes in blood pH, CO_2, and oxygen

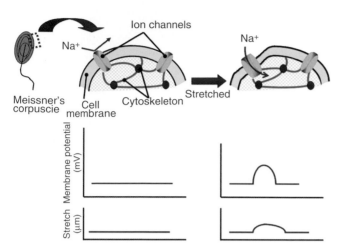

Fig. 10.13. Mechanoreceptor depolarization. Mechanoreceptors respond to physical deformation of the plasma membrane. In this example, a Meissner's corpuscle, located in the skin, is deformed when the skin is pressed. That causes a physical change in the corpuscle membrane, which causes an opening of an ion channel on the plasma membrane. As cations move inward, a receptor potential is generated in the corpuscle.

concentrations. Signals for the carotid and aortic bodies travel to the respiratory centers through the glossopharyngeal (cranial nerve IX) and vagus (cranial nerve X).

Detection of sensory signals

Sensory receptors are morphologically specialized structures that respond to specific stimuli. When stimulated, these receptors transform the stimulus into an electrical signal called a receptor potential, which is a graded potential causing either depolarization or hyperpolarization of the cell. The amplitude and duration of the receptor potential are related to the magnitude and length of time of the stimulus. If the receptor potential is large enough to reach threshold, it is called a generator potential, and causes an action potential to form in the sensory neuron. The process of converting the stimuli into a receptor potential is called stimulus transduction.

The various types of sensory receptors have different mechanisms for transducing the stimulus into a receptor potential. In mechanoreceptors, when there is a conformational change in the tissue in which the receptor resides, it causes a change in the plasma membrane of the mechanoreceptor, thus causing a physical change in the cation channels located in the sensory neuron membrane (Fig. 10.13). This physical change results in the opening of stretch-sensitive channels that increase ion conductance. This leads to depolarization of the neuron and generation of a receptor potential. This mechanism is very similar to the production of an excitatory postsynaptic potential. The

amplitude of the receptor potential is proportional to the intensity of the stimulus. Greater conformational change in the tissue will result in a greater number of channel openings on the mechanoreceptor. When the stimulus is removed, the ion channels close.

Receptors involved in general senses are either free dendritic endings or encapsulated dendritic endings. Free nerve endings are located throughout the body, but are especially abundant in epithelia and connective tissue. They are nonmyelinated, and end in a knoblike swelling, sensitive to touch and pressure. There appears to be no structural differences between those that detect touch and pressure from those that detect temperature and pain. While these are the only sensory receptors on the surface of the eye, there are specialized tactile receptors located throughout the body surface that are probably more important. A summary of the various sensory receptors is shown in Table 10.2.

Surrounding all hairs is a root hair plexus that monitors distortions and movements. Movement of the hair causes a distortion in the sensory dendrites resulting in the production of a receptor potential. These are rapidly adapting receptors. Therefore, they are most important for detecting initial movements, or changes. For example, when a saddle is first placed on a horse these receptors send signals to the brain notifying the presence of the saddle, but rather quickly these receptors adapt and stop sending signals.

Reflexes

Reflexes are automatic, neural responses to specific stimuli. Reflexes work to preserve homeostasis by making rapid adjustments that do not require conscious activity. Therefore, all reflexes involve a sensory receptor and a motor response.

The neural path controlling a reflex is called a reflex arch (Fig. 10.14). The reflex arch begins with a sensory receptor, and ends with the effector. There are four steps to a reflex arch:

1. Stimulus activates receptor. Sensory receptors, such as described above, receive a stimulus that generates a receptor potential, resulting in the production of an action potential in the receptor. If the sensory cell and sensory neuron are separate, the action potential is produced in the sensory neuron.

2. Information processing. The sensory information is transmitted to the central nervous system where it is processed. In a monosynaptic reflex, the sensory neuron synapses directly on a motor neuron releasing an excitatory neurotransmitter and causing the production of an excitatory post-

Table 10.2. Sensory receptors: Structure and function.

Type	Illustration	Function	Adapting	Location
Unencapsulated Free dendritic nerve endings		Nociceptors, thermoreceptors, mechanoreceptors		Most body tissues; dense concentration in connective tissues including ligaments, tendons, dermis, joint capsules, periosteal; epithelia (epidermis, cornea, mucosa, gland)
Merkel discs: modified free dendritic endings	**Merkel cell** **Tactile disc**	Mechanoreceptors, fine touch	Slowly adapting	Basal layer of epidermis of skin
Root hair plexuses		Mechanoreceptors	Rapidly adapting	In and surrounding hair follicles
Encapsulated Meissner's corpuscles		Mechanoreceptors (light pressure, discriminative touch, vibration of low frequency)	Rapidly adapting	Dermal papillae of hairless skin, particularly nipples, external genitalia, fingertips, soles of feet, eyelids

Table 10.2. *Continued*

Type	Illustration	Function	Adapting	Location
Krause's end bulbs				
Pacinian corpuscles (lamellated corpuscles)		Mechanoreceptors (deep pressure and vibration when first applied)	Rapidly adapting	Deep in the dermis and subcutaneous tissue; joint capsules, tendons, ligaments
Ruffini's corpuscles		Mechanoreceptors (respond to deep continuous pressure)	Slowly adapting	Deep in dermis, hypodermis, and joint capsule
Muscle spindles		Proprioceptors	Nonadapting	Skeletal muscle
Golgi tendon organs		Proprioceptors	Nonadapting	Tendons close to skeletal muscle insertion

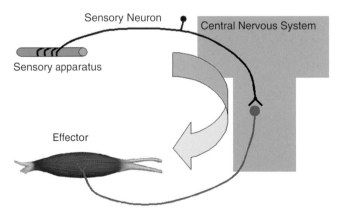

Fig. 10.14. Reflex arch. A reflex arch includes a sensory apparatus, a sensory neuron, a site of information processing or integration, and an effector. The sensory apparatus detects a change that is transmitted via the sensory neuron to the central nervous system. There, the information is processed and a motor response is sent via a motor neuron to the periphery in order to maintain homeostasis.

synaptic potential (EPSP) in the motor neuron. Under normal conditions, EPSPs in motor neurons always result in an action potential in the motor neuron. In a polysynaptic reflex, there are pools of interneurons generally carrying signals to multiple sites (Fig. 10.15). These reflexes generally involve both excitatory and inhibitory neurotransmitters being released from various interneurons (i.e., excitatory interneurons and inhibitory interneurons).

3. Activation of the motor neuron. As a result of the stimulus, a motor neuron is activated to cause contraction in order to establish homeostasis. In the case of polysynaptic reflexes, there are other synergistic muscles that may be stimulated and antagonistic muscles that are inhibited.

4. Response of the peripheral effector. Stimulation of the motor neurons results in release of a neurotransmitter at the synapse between the motor neuron and its effector. This results in contraction

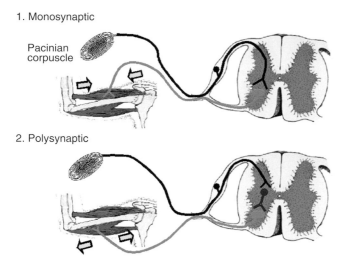

1. Monosynaptic

Pacinian
corpuscle

2. Polysynaptic

Fig. 10.15. Monosynaptic and polysynaptic reflexes. 1. In monosynaptic reflexes, the sensory neuron is activated and carries a signal to the central nervous system where it synapses on an effector neuron. The effector neuron is activated causing an effect to occur in the periphery. 2. In a polysynaptic reflex, the sensory signal synapses on an interneuron in the central nervous system. The interneuron(s) process the information and then synapse on an effector neuron. The interneurons can either be excitatory causing activation of the effector neuron, or they can be inhibitory, thus decreasing the firing rate in the effector neuron.

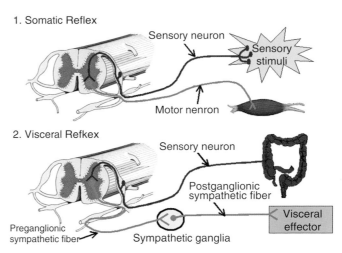

1. Somatic Reflex

Sensory neuron
Sensory stimuli
Motor nenron

2. Visceral Refkex

Sensory neuron
Postganglionic sympathetic fiber
Preganglionic sympathetic fiber
Sympathetic ganglia
Visceral effector

Fig. 10.16. Somatic and visceral reflexes. 1. Somatic reflexes involve a somatic sensory signal that is carried to the central nervous system where it stimulates a somatic motor neuron whose fiber travels to a skeletal muscle and causes contraction. 2. A visceral reflex is polysynaptic. There is either a somatic sensory signal or a visceral sensory signal that is relayed to the central nervous system where it stimulates a presynaptic autonomic fiber, which then exits the central nervous system and synapses on a postsynaptic fiber that then stimulates a visceral effector (i.e., smooth muscle, cardiac muscle, or gland).

of a single muscle in the case of a monosynaptic reflex, or multiple muscles in the case of a polysynaptic synapse.

Classification of reflexes

Reflexes can be classified based on their development, site of information processing, or resulting motor response.

Development of reflex

Animals are born with some reflexes called innate reflexes. Such reflexes involve a development of a genetically programmed response to specific stimuli. Such reflexes generally entail some process vital for life. Examples of such reflexes include suckling, chewing, a withdrawal reflex from painful stimuli, and tracking objects with the eyes. A newborn calf will generally begin suckling almost immediately after birth.

Other reflexes may develop later in life as a result of experience, and are called acquired reflexes. An example of an innate reflex might be salivation in response to the sound of a bell. Like innate reflexes, these responses are quick, automatic, and stereotypic, but they must be learned.

Site of information processing

If the sensory information is processed in the spinal cord, the reflex is called a spinal reflex (e.g., withdrawal reflex). Such reflexes do not require input or processing from the brain; therefore, they are functional in decerebrate animals. The processing of information in the brain results in cranial reflexes.

Resulting motor response

Reflexes that involve the contraction of skeletal muscle are termed somatic reflexes; those that involve smooth muscle, cardiac muscle, or glands are called visceral reflexes (Fig. 10.16). Although the contraction of skeletal muscle is generally under conscious, voluntary control, somatic reflexes involve the involuntary contraction or relaxation of skeletal muscle.

Visceral reflexes are essential for maintaining homeostasis. Some input to the autonomic nervous system is somatosensory. For example, if an animal suddenly cuts itself, this noxious stimulus can activate the sympathetic nervous system, causing local vasoconstriction as well as increased blood pressure and heart rate. Visceral sensory information can also stimulate such reflexes. Sensory information from the thoracic and abdominal region is carried to the brain via the vagus nerve, information from the head and neck via the glossopharyngeal nerves, and visceral chemosensory information (i.e., taste) by the facial nerves.

This sensory information is all carried to the nucleus of the solitary tract.

Spinal reflexes

Monosynaptic reflexes

Skeletal muscle is essential for the control of posture and voluntary movement. The brain sends messages to muscles in order to initiate movement. For example, assume the brain sends a message to the leg of a horse in order to raise the leg and hold it above the ground. After the leg is raised, proprioceptive messages are constantly sent back to the brain from the leg in order to inform the brain as to the location of the leg.

Stretch reflex

The stretch reflex, also called the myotatic reflex from its Greek roots (*myo* = muscle + *tatic* = stretch), is the simplest reflex in the body, and it is an example of a proprioceptive message involved in maintaining posture and muscle tone. It is a monosynaptic reflex providing autonomic control of skeletal muscle. The sensory mechanism involves the muscle spindles, which are small encapsulated sensory receptors located within skeletal muscle that provide information about the changes in length of the muscle.

Anatomy of the muscle spindle

There are two types of muscle fibers within skeletal muscle: extrafusal and intrafusal. Extrafusal muscle fibers are those fibers found outside of the muscle spindle making up the bulk of skeletal muscle, and which are responsible for muscle contraction. In contrast, intrafusal (*intra* = within; *fusal* = spindle) muscle fibers are about one-quarter the size of the extrafusal fibers, are located within the connective tissue capsule that surrounds the muscle spindle, and run parallel to the extrafusal fibers (Fig. 10.17). The middle third of the capsule is swollen, giving it a spindle shape. The central region of each intrafusal fiber lacks myofilaments and is thus noncontractile.

There are two types of intrafusal fibers: nuclear bag fibers and nuclear chain fibers. A typical muscle spindle has 2–3 nuclear bag fibers and a varying number of nuclear chain fibers. Each intrafusal fiber is innervated by both motor and sensory neurons. There are two types of sensory fibers. The primary sensory endings are large type Ia fibers that sense both rate and amount of stretch of the muscle spindle. The secondary sensory endings are small type II fibers that surround the endings of the intrafusal fibers and sense only stretch of the muscle spindle. There are gamma motor neurons

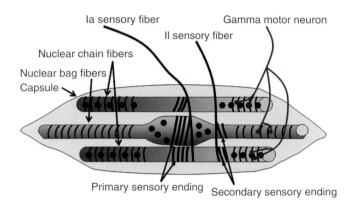

Fig. 10.17. Muscle spindle. A muscle spindle consists of three components: intrafusal fibers, sensory endings, and a motor neuron. There are two types of intrafusal fibers, nuclear chain and nuclear bag fibers. There are two types of sensory endings primary endings and secondary endings. The intrafusal fibers are innervated by a gamma motor neuron.

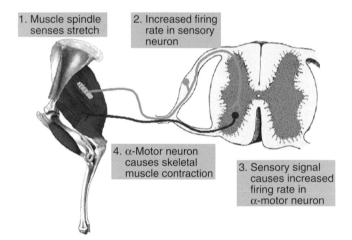

Fig. 10.18. Components of stretch reflex. 1. A muscle spindle senses stretch in the skeletal muscle caused either by contraction of the muscle or tension on the muscle. 2. The sensory endings in the muscle spindle are activated, resulting in an increased firing rate in the sensory fibers from the muscle spindle. 3. The sensory fibers synapse within the spinal cord on the α-motor neurons going to the same muscle. 4. The α-motor neuron is activated, and causes the same muscle to contract. (Leg was adapted from Riegel, R.J. and S.E. Hakola, 1996, Illustrated Atlas of Clinical Disorders of the Horse.)

that innervate each intrafusal fiber, whereas α-motor neurons innervate the extrafusal fibers.

When a muscle is stretched, the intrafusal fibers in the muscle spindle are also stretched. This causes increased activity in the sensory endings. When the muscle shortens, the activity in the sensory endings decreases. Therefore, the components of the stretch reflex include 1) stretch of the muscle spindle, 2) activation of the sensory neurons in the muscle spindle, 3) transmission of the sensory signal to the α-motor neurons located in the dorsal horn in the spinal cord, and 4) stimulation of muscle contraction induced by the α-motor neurons (Fig. 10.18).

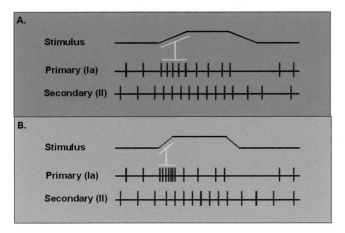

Fig. 10.19. Response of muscle spindles to stretch. A) During stretch of the muscle, both primary and secondary endings in the muscle spindle respond and increase their firing rate. The primary endings give additional information regarding the velocity of stretch as seen here as an increase in firing rate associated with the initiation of stretch. B) Since stretch occurred more rapidly, the primary endings showed increased frequency of firing at the beginning of the muscle stretch compared to that seen in Panel A.

Stimulation of the gamma motor neuron causes the intrafusal fibers to contract, while having no affect on the extrafusal fibers. Contraction of the intrafusal fibers does not contribute to the force of muscle contraction; instead, that is generated by the extrafusal fibers. Stimulation of the gamma motor neurons causes the intrafusal fibers to contract at either end. Since they are attached to the ends of the capsule, this causes the sensory endings to increase their firing rate because they sense stretch.

Muscle spindle and muscle contraction

Since contraction of intrafusal fibers does not contribute to the force of muscle contraction, what is the function of the muscle spindle? When a muscle contracts, there are two phases to contraction. The dynamic phase is the period during which the muscle length is changing; the static phase is when the muscle has stabilized its length. The two sensory endings provide information regarding these phases (Fig. 10.19). When the muscle is first stretched, both the primary and secondary endings increase their firing rate. Since the primary endings are also sensitive to the velocity of stretch, their firing rate also provides information regarding the rate of stretch (or contraction) of the muscle.

Function of the gamma motor neurons

When the α-motor neurons are stimulated, they cause contraction of extrafusal fibers within skeletal muscle.

Since the muscle spindle capsule is anchored within the extrafusal fibers, the muscle spindle becomes flaccid as the two ends of the spindle move closer together (Fig. 10.20). As a result, the muscle spindle becomes insensitive to stretch. To correct this situation, the intrafusal fibers in the muscle spindle are innervated with γ-motor neurons. Stimulation of γ-motor neurons results in contraction of intrafusal fibers, thus causing the muscle spindle to shorten so that it remains responsive to changes in the length of the extrafusal fibers.

Gamma motor neuron loop

Although conscious motor movement is usually initiated by signals carried by the α-motor neuron, there is a second method to initiate contraction of skeletal muscle called the gamma motor neuron loop (Fig. 10.21). Stimulation of a gamma motor neuron causes contraction of intrafusal fibers, which causes the muscle spindle to detect stretch. The sensory endings in the muscle spindle detect the stretch, resulting in an increased firing rate in the sensory neuron. This information is transmitted back to the central nervous system where the sensory neurons synapse directly on the α-motor neurons going to the same muscle. Increased firing rate in the α-motor neuron results in contraction of the muscle in order to reduce the stretch in the muscle spindle.

Polysynaptic reflexes

Tendon reflex

Although the stretch reflex is designed to prevent tearing of skeletal muscle, the tendon reflex, also called the inverse myotatic reflex or reverse myotatic reflex, functions to prevent tearing of tendons (Fig. 10.22). Golgi tendon receptors located within the tendons of the muscle increase their firing rate in response to increased tension in the tendon. When stimulated, afferent signals from the Golgi tendon receptors are transmitted to the spinal cord where these fibers synapse on interneurons. This signal then causes inhibition of contraction of the muscle from which the signal initiated while causing reciprocal activation of antagonist muscles. The result is relaxation of muscle attached to the overstretched tendon, and contraction of antagonist muscles, an affect opposite that of the stretch reflex.

The Golgi tendon reflex is particularly important during quick activities involving rapid changes between flexion and extension. This reflex is designed to prevent the overstretching of the collagen fibers in tendons.

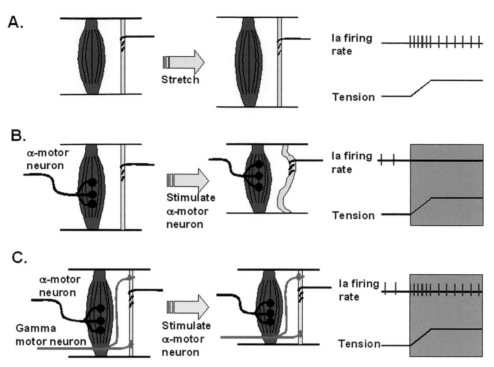

Fig. 10.20. Role of gamma motor neuron in muscle spindle. Although the muscle spindle is actually found deep in the muscle, for clarity the extrafusal and intrafusal fibers have been displayed separately in this figure. A) When the muscle is stretched, there is an increase in firing rate in the sensory neurons. Only the primary endings are displayed in this figure. B) When the α-motor neuron is stimulated, it causes contraction of the extrafusal fibers. Since the muscle spindle is anchored within these fibers, the muscle spindle become flaccid as the extrafusal fibers shorten. C) If the gamma motor neuron is stimulated simultaneously with the α-motor neuron, the intrafusal fibers contract along with the extrafusal fibers thus preventing the muscle spindle from becoming unloaded. Therefore, the muscle spindle is able to maintain its ability to sense stretch within the muscle. (Figure modified from Kandel et al., 2000.)

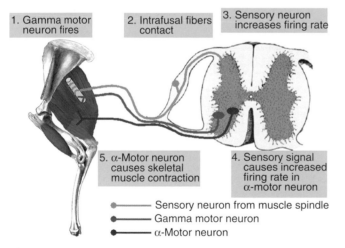

Fig. 10.21. Gamma motor neuron loop. Stimulation of the gamma motor neuron causes shortening of the intrafusal fibers within the muscle spindle. This causes an increased frequency of firing in the sensory neuron that synapses on the α-motor neuron. Stimulation of the α-motor neuron results in contraction of the skeletal muscle. (Leg was adapted from Riegel, R.J. and S.E. Hakola, 1996, Illustrated Atlas of Clinical Disorders of the Horse.)

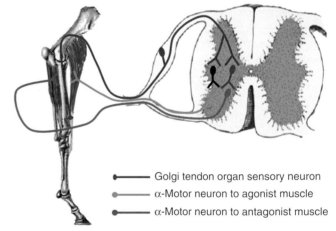

Fig. 10.22. The tendon reflex (inverse myotatic reflex). When the Golgi tendon apparatus within the tendon is stretched, a sensory signal is carried in afferent fibers to the spinal cord where they synapse on interneurons. Inhibitory interneurons synapsing on α-motor neurons going to the muscle where the sensory signal was generated cause relaxation of that muscle. Excitatory interneurons also synapse on α-motor neurons going to antagonist muscles causing them to contract in order to relieve the stretch on the tendons in the agonist muscle. (Leg was adapted from Riegel, R.J. and S.E. Hakola, 1996, Illustrated Atlas of Clinical Disorders of the Horse.)

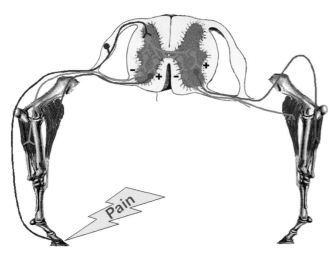

Fig. 10.23. The withdrawal and crossed-extensor reflexes. The withdrawal reflex is initiated as a response to painful stimuli. Stepping on a nail would cause a noxious signal to be transmitted to the central nervous system where it would initiate contraction of the flexor muscles and relaxation of the extensor muscles so that the limb is withdrawn from the painful stimuli. So that the animal does not fall, the crossed-extensor reflex is also initiated, in which the extensors and flexors on the contralateral side are stimulated and relaxed, respectively.

Withdrawal reflex

The withdrawal reflex, also called the flexor reflex, allows for the immediate withdrawal of a body part in response to painful stimuli (Fig. 10.23). A painful stimuli causes a sensory signal to be transmitted to the spinal cord where it causes excitation of α-motor neurons going to flexors in that region while simultaneously inhibiting the extensors in the same region. This allows for the quick withdrawal of the body part.

Crossed-extensor reflex

The crossed-extensor reflex is a polysynaptic reflex in which a signal is sent to the contralateral side of the spinal cord to initiate an extensor reflex at the same time the withdrawal, or flexor, reflex is occurring on the ipsilateral side (Fig. 10.23). As an animal withdraws a limb in response to a noxious stimuli, it would fall if it did not simultaneously support itself on the opposite leg. The crossed-extensor reflex immediately allows the animal to support its weight on the contralateral side as it shifts its weight off the ipsilateral side.

Use of reflexes in diagnosis

Reflexes are routinely examined when assessing the nervous system. They provide a diagnostic tool at the site of a spinal cord, brain, spinal nerve, or cranial nerve injury. Muscle tone is tested by passively manipulating a limb. This can provide an indication of whether the animal has hypotonia (less than normal muscle tone) or hypertonia (excessive muscle tone). Disease of the lower motor neurons, those motor neurons with cell bodies in the brain stem or spinal cord, usually causes hypotonia, whereas hypertonia and spasticity is observed with diseases of the upper motor neurons. When muscles are no longer innervated by the lower motor neurons, they begin to atrophy and lose tone. Upper motor neurons are those neurons with cell bodies in the CNS processing center. These neurons either facilitate or inhibit lower motor neurons, which innervate a single motor unit. When an upper motor neuron, which has a cell body in the CNS processing center, is diseased, this results in facilitation (i.e., lowering the threshold for propagation of the action potential) of the lower motor neurons causing hypertonia.

Table 10.3 gives examples of reflexes used in diagnostics. These reflexes are important in determining the site of injury in an animal.

Autonomic nervous system

Overview

Many activities of an animal are under conscious control. Such activities include voluntary motor movement and generally are not immediately necessary to sustain life. These activities are controlled by the somatic nervous system. In contrast, most physiological and endocrine activities of the body require no conscious activity, but are instead controlled automatically. These activities are generally essential to sustain life and include such activities as blood pressure, heart rate maintenance, and control of blood chemistry. These life-sustaining activities are controlled by the autonomic nervous system that coordinates and integrates the visceral functions of the body. As originally proposed by Claude Bernard and further developed by Walter Cannon, the concept of homeostasis is largely controlled by the autonomic nervous system.

The somatic nervous system, or somatic motor system, is under voluntary control, and regulates the contraction of skeletal muscle. In contrast, the autonomic nervous system, or visceral motor system, is generally not under voluntary control and controls

Table 10.3.　Reflexes used in diagnostics.

Reflex	Stimulus	Afferent Nerves	Spinal Segment	Efferent Nerves	Normal Response
Patellar	Lightly tap patellar tendon	Femoral	L_3, L_4, L_5	Femoral	Extension of knee
Tricep	Tap tricep tendon proximal to olecranon process	Radial	C_6, C_7, T_1, T_2	Radial	Extension of elbow
Bicep	Place finger on distal ends of biceps and brachialis muscles at level of elbow; tap finger with hammer	Musculocutaneous	C_5, C_6, C_7	Musculocutaneous	Flexion of elbow
Flexor- pelvic limb	Painful stimuli (i.e., pinch base of toenail with hemostats)	Tibial, saphenous, femoral	L_4, L_5, S_1	Tibial, saphenous, femoral	Flexion of hip
Crossed-extensor	Initiating flexor reflex	Regional spinal	Regional spinal area	Regional spinal	If animal has upper motor neuron disease, extension of opposite limb
Perineal	Noxious stimuli to anus	Sacral	Sacrum	Sacral	Contraction of sphincter and flexion of tail
Panniculus	Mild stimulation of skin of trunk	Regional spinal	Regional spinal area	Regional spinal	Contraction of cutaneous trunci

visceral effectors, including smooth muscle, cardiac muscle, glandular tissue, and visceral reflexes.

There are some fundamental differences in the arrangement of these two branches of the nervous system (Fig. 10.24). Efferent fibers in the somatic nervous system begin in the primary motor cortex and travel either to cranial nerve nuclei located in the brain or to α-motor neuron cell bodies in the anterior horn of the spinal cord. From there, motor neurons exit the central nervous system and travel to skeletal muscles. Therefore, in the somatic nervous system, the cell bodies of the motor neurons are located within the central nervous system.

Efferent fibers of the autonomic nervous system generally originate in the hypothalamus and travel to either autonomic nerve nuclei in the brain or preganglionic neurons located in the anterior horn of the spinal cord. The preganglionic neurons then leave the spinal cord and synapse on postganglionic neurons located in autonomic ganglia located in the periphery. These neurons are called pre- and postganglionic neurons because they synapse on one another within a ganglion located in the peripheral nervous system. In contrast to the somatic nervous system, the cell bodies of motor neurons of the autonomic nervous system are located outside of the central nervous system within autonomic ganglia.

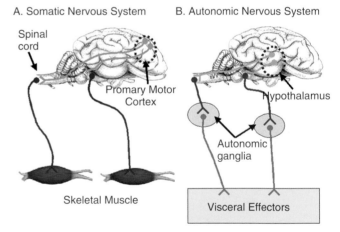

Fig. 10.24.　Organization of the somatic and autonomic nervous systems. A) Motor commands for the somatic nervous system originate in the primary motor cortex. These efferent fibers then synapse either within the brain on nuclei for cranial nerves, or on α-motor neurons within the spinal cord. The α-motor neurons, whose cell bodies are within the central nervous system, exit and travel to the skeletal muscle. B) Motor commands for the autonomic nervous system originate in the hypothalamus. These efferent signals then travel to autonomic nuclei either in the brain or spinal cord where they synapse on preganglionic fibers. These preganglionic fibers leave the central nervous system and travel to autonomic ganglia located in the periphery where they synapse on postganglionic fibers. The postganglionic fibers travel to the visceral effectors such as smooth muscle, cardiac muscle, and glands.

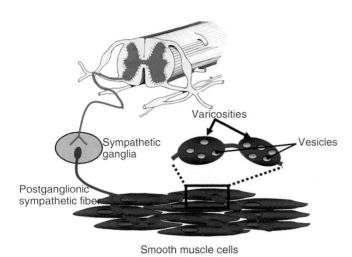

Fig. 10.25. Sympathetic varicosities. Rather than embedding within the smooth muscle cells, postganglionic sympathetic fibers running over smooth muscle cells have swellings along their length called varicosities. Within the varicosities are vesicles containing norepinephrine.

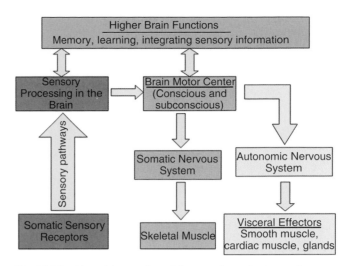

Fig. 10.26. Neural integration of the somatic and autonomic nervous systems. The somatic and autonomic nervous systems can simultaneously elicit various responses as a result of sensory information.

Innervation of target tissue by the autonomic nervous system differs from that of the somatic nervous system. Whereas somatic neurons innervating skeletal muscle have specialized synapses called motor end plates containing specialized presynaptic structures such as an active zone, nerve endings of autonomic neurons have only swellings called varicosities and vesicles containing neurotransmitters (Fig. 10.25). Autonomic neurons can be highly branched with synaptic transmission occurring at multiple sites along an axon terminal.

Overlap of somatic and autonomic functions

Both somatic and visceral sensory information can initiate a visceral reflex (Fig. 10.26). In other words, the two systems work together to maintain homeostasis. For example, if an animal suddenly feels cold, it may activate the somatic nervous system to move to a warmer location but may also activate a visceral reflex that causes vasoconstriction in the skin and piloerection in order to reduce heat loss. If an animal is running hard, not only are neural inputs necessary to tell the skeletal muscles to contract, but visceral reflexes are necessary in order to increase blood flow to the skeletal muscles.

Divisions of the autonomic nervous system

The autonomic nervous system is subdivided into the sympathetic and parasympathetic subdivisions. These subdivisions have opposing effects on most functions.

The sympathetic division, sometimes called the "flight-or-fight" division, generally causes excitation and results in catabolism. This division is activated during periods of stress and exertion. The parasympathetic division is responsible for rest, digestion, and anabolism (i.e., building phase of metabolism). Walter B. Cannon originally suggested that these two divisions work in opposition and function at opposite times; in fact, they are generally both active and work in conjunction to control motor systems.

Included under the autonomic nervous system is the enteric nervous system, sometimes called the "little brain." Located within the walls of the digestive tract, this extensive network of neurons is a largely self-contained system consisting of the myenteric (or Auerbach's) plexus and the submucosal (or Meissner's) plexus that controls digestive functions. While under normal circumstances the other branches of the autonomic nervous system influence the enteric nervous system, if the digestive tract is deinnervated such as occurs during severe spinal injuries, the enteric nervous system is able to maintain digestive functions. The enteric nervous system is discussed in more detail in Chapter 17.

Sympathetic division

The sympathetic division of the autonomic nervous system allows that body to respond to emergency situations resulting from sudden changes in the internal or external environment. It mediates an increase in alertness, heart rate, blood pressure, metabolism, respiration rate, sweating, piloerection, and mobilization of energy within the body. Simultaneously, it decreases activity of the digestive, urinary, and immune systems. It causes an increase in blood flow to the skeletal muscles while decreasing blood flow to the visceral organs.

In other words, the sympathetic nervous system activates those systems and animal needs in order to fight while inhibiting those systems not needed for fighting. If an animal is engaged in a fight, it needs increased blood flow to the skeletal muscles for increased muscular activity. Such blood flow comes at the expense of blood flow to the viscera. If an animal is shunting resources to fight, it does not need to be simultaneously digesting a meal; therefore, blood flow is shifted from the digestive tract to skeletal muscle.

Parasympathetic division

The parasympathetic nervous system stimulates restful activities while inhibiting stress responses. Therefore, it is active during nonstressful conditions. The parasympathetic nervous system promotes activities such as digestion while simultaneously conserving energy and decreasing blood pressure, heart rate, and respiration rate. Metabolic rate is decreased by the parasympathetic nervous system, and the pupils are constricted while the lens is allowed to become more convex in order to accommodate for close vision.

Anatomy of the autonomic nervous system

Sympathetic division

The sympathetic division, also called the thoracolumbar division, exits the central nervous system from the thoracic and lumbar vertebrae. The preganglionic fibers have cell bodies in the intermediolateral horn, sometimes called the lateral horns or visceral motor zones, of the spinal cord (Fig. 10.27). After leaving the spinal cord through the ventral root, the preganglionic sympathetic fibers enter the spinal nerve along with somatic motor fibers. Shortly thereafter, the sympathetic preganglionic fibers separate from the spinal nerve and pass through the white rami to enter the sympathetic chains (paravertebral chain) lying on either side of the spinal cord. Therefore, the preganglionic fibers are short and the postganglionic fibers are long.

Upon entering the sympathetic chain, the myelinated preganglionic fibers can either synapse at that level, or they can travel rostrally or caudally before synapsing. The unmyelinated postganglionic fibers exit the sympathetic chain via the gray rami.

The sympathetic preganglionic fibers innervating the head exit the spinal cord from the first four tho-

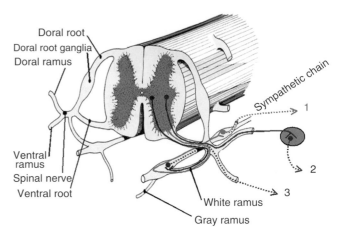

Fig. 10.27. Sympathetic chain and pathways. Preganglionic sympathetic fibers originate in the intermediolateral horn of the thoracic and lumbar vertebrae. These fibers can follow three paths: 1. As shown in green, the fiber can enter the sympathetic chain via the white ramus and continue to a different level within the chain where it then synapses on a postganglionic fiber that leaves the chain via the gray ramus. 2. As shown in blue, the preganglionic fiber can enter the spinal nerve and synapse on a postganglionic fiber in an outlying ganglion (prevertebral ganglion). 3. As shown in red, the preganglionic fiber can enter the sympathetic chain and synapse on a postganglionic fiber at the same level. (Figure modified from Getty, 1964.)

racic segments (T1–T4), enter the sympathetic chain, and ascend to the superior cervical ganglion, the most rostral extension of the sympathetic chain (Fig. 10.28). These fibers stimulate the dilator muscles for the irises of the eye, inhibit nasal and salivary glands, and innervate the muscle that lifts the eyelids. These responses are all typical of those observed during stress. Other fibers from the superior cervical ganglia innervate skin and blood vessels in the head, as well as sending branches to the heart.

Prevertebral ganglia

The preganglionic fibers from T_5 caudally pass through the sympathetic chain before synapsing in prevertebral ganglia. Prior to reaching the prevertebral ganglia, these fibers form nerves called splanchnic nerves (*splanchni* = viscera) that include such nerves as the thoracic greater, lesser and least splanchnic nerves, lumbar splanchnics, and the sacral splanchnics. The prevertebral ganglia include the celiac ganglion and the superior and inferior mesenteric ganglia. These ganglia differ from the paravertebral chain in that they lie anterior to the vertebral column, are unpaired, and occur only in the abdomen and pelvis. The postganglionic fibers from the prevertebral ganglia innervate the gastrointestinal tract and its accessory organs, including the pancreas and liver. These fibers also innervate the kidneys, bladder, and genitalia.

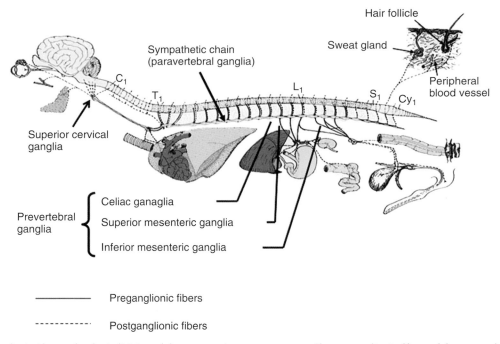

Hair follicle

Sweat gland

Peripheral
blood vessel

Sympathetic chain
(paravertebral ganglia)

C_1

T_1

L_1

S_1

Cy_1

Superior cervical
ganglia

Prevertebral
ganglia

Celiac ganaglia

Superior mesenteric ganglia

Inferior mesenteric ganglia

———————   Preganglionic fibers

- - - - - - - - - -   Postganglionic fibers

Fig. 10.28.   Sympathetic (thoracolumbar) division of the autonomic nervous system. The preganglionic fibers of the sympathetic nervous system originate in the lateral horns of the thoracic and lumbar vertebrae. The fibers exit and travel as shown in Figure 10.2 to outlying ganglia. The postganglionic fibers originate in the outlying ganglia and travel to the target organs. (Figure modified from Getty, 1964.)

Pathways to the adrenal medulla

Embryologically, the adrenal medulla and sympathetic ganglia arise from the same tissue. Therefore, the adrenal medulla is unique in that it consists of postganglionic cells of the sympathetic nervous system. The preganglionic fibers are found in the thoracic splanchnic nerves that pass through the celiac ganglion without synapsing before reaching the adrenal medulla. The postganglionic cells making up the adrenal medulla secrete norepinephrine and epinephrine when stimulated.

Parasympathetic division

The parasympathetic division, or craniosacral division, originates from brain stem nuclei and S2S4 of the sacrum (Fig. 10.29). The preganglionic fibers synapse on postganglionic fibers either on or near the target organ (intramural ganglia). Therefore, the preganglionic fibers are long and the postganglionic fibers short.

The cranial outflow of the parasympathetic nervous system comes from four cranial nerves. These fibers originate in the Edinger-Westphal nucleus, the oculomotor nerve (III), the superior salivary nuclei associated with the facial nerve (VII), the inferior salivary nuclei associated with the glossopharyngeal nerve (IX), and the dorsal vagal nucleus and nucleus ambiguous, both associated with the vagus nerve (X). The oculomotor nerves are responsible for pupil constriction and bulging of the lens as occurs during accommodation when objects are moved closer in the field of vision. The facial nerves stimulate secretory activity from glands in the head such as the lacrimal and nasal glands and mandibular and sublingual salivary glands. The glossopharyngeal nerves activate the parotid salivary glands.

The vagus nerves account for 90% of all preganglionic parasympathetic fibers. They provide input to the neck and all viscera in the thoracic and abdominal cavities. The vagus nerve mostly arises from the dorsal motor nuclei in the medulla, with its fibers synapsing on ganglia located on the target organ walls. These ganglia are not named, but instead collectively are called intramural ganglia, that is, "ganglia within the walls." After passing into the thorax, the vagus sends branches to various nerve plexuses including the cardiac plexuses, the pulmonary plexuses, and the esophageal plexuses supplying the heart, lungs and bronchi, and esophagus, respectively. Upon reaching the esophagus, fibers from the two vagus nerves intermingle and form the anterior and posterior vagal trunks.

The prevertebral fibers from the sacral spinal cord leave via the ventral roots and travel in the pelvic nerve to the pelvic ganglion plexus. These fibers innervate the descending colon, bladder, and external genitalia.

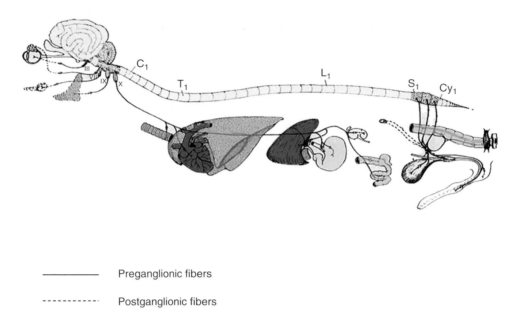

——————   Preganglionic fibers

-----------   Postganglionic fibers

Fig. 10.29.   Parasympathetic (craniosacral) division of the autonomic nervous system. The preganglionic fibers of the parasympathetic nervous system originate in the brain stem and sacral vertebrae. The fibers exit either as cranial nerves from the brain stem or spinal nerves from the sacrum and project to outlying ganglia located on or near the target organ. The postganglionic fibers originate in the outlying (intramural) ganglia and innervate the target organs. (Figure modified from Getty, 1964.)

Physiology of the autonomic nervous system

Neurotransmitters and receptors

The major neurotransmitters in the autonomic nervous system are acetylcholine and norepinephrine. Postganglionic neurons of the parasympathetic nervous system release acetylcholine and are thus called cholinergic neurons; those of the sympathetic nervous system generally release norepinephrine and are called adrenergic fibers. The exception is sympathetic fibers innervating sweat glands, which release acetylcholine.

Both sympathetic and parasympathetic preganglionic fibers generally release acetylcholine that acts at nicotinic receptors to induce fast excitatory postsynaptic potentials in postsynaptic cells.

Cholinergic fibers

Acetylcholine can bind to two types of receptors called nicotinic and muscarinic. These receptors were named for pharmacological compounds that activate these receptors and are thus called agonists. Nicotine, the active ingredient in cigarettes, is the agonist for the nicotinic receptor; muscarine, which is found in poisonous mushrooms, is the agonist at muscarinic receptors.

Nicotinic receptors are found at skeletal muscle end plates, and in autonomic ganglionic neurons in both the parasympathetic and sympathetic nervous systems. Therefore, somatic neurons and all preganglionic neurons release acetylcholine that acts at nicotinic receptors. The binding of acetylcholine to nicotinic receptors always causes excitation of the effector cell. In autonomic ganglion, stimulation of the nicotinic receptors evokes a fast excitatory postsynaptic potential (EPSP), usually triggering an action potential in the postsynaptic neuron.

All cholinergic postganglionic fibers act at muscarinic receptors. These include all parasympathetic fibers as well as those sympathetic fibers innervating sweat glands.

Adrenergic fibers

Postganglionic sympathetic fibers, except those innervating sweat glands, release norepinephrine. The sympathetic postganglionic fibers in the adrenal medulla release both norepinephrine and epinephrine. There are two major classes of adrenergic receptors, alpha (α) and beta (β). Norepinephrine and epinephrine act at both types of receptors. Target organs can have one or both types of receptors. While, in general, activating α-adrenergic receptors causes excitation and activating β-adrenergic receptors causes inhibition, there are notable exceptions to these rules because there are various subclasses of these classes of receptors. A summary of the actions of these receptors is shown in Table 10.4.

Note that norepinephrine can have opposite affects on vasomotor tone, depending on the dose of

Table 10.4. Pharmacology of the autonomic nervous system.

Neurotransmitter	Receptor Types	Major Locations	Effect	Drugs Acting at Receptor	Medical Use
Acetylcholine (ACh)	Nicotinic (ganglion)	Neuromuscular junction; all ganglionic neurons, adrenal medullary cells	Skeletal muscle contraction, excitation of postganglionic cells		
	Mucscarinic				
	M_1	Autonomic nerve terminals	Inhibits ACh and NE release	Pirenzepine (antagonist)	Anti-ulcerogenic
	M_2	Parasympathetic input to heart and smooth muscle	Inhibits heart rate, excitation of smooth muscle	Atropine (antagonist)	Dilation of pupils
	M_3	Glandular tissue	Secretion from glands	Atropine (antagonist)	Reduction of drooling during surgery and Parkinson's disease
Norepinephrine (NE) epinephrine (E)	Alpha				
	α_1	Most all sympathetic target cells except heart	Vasoconstriction, constriction of organ sphincters, dilation of pupils	Prazosin (antagonist)	Hypertension
	α_2	Presynaptic nerve endings (autoreceptors); blood platelets; postsynaptic in CNS	Inhibits norepinephrine release from nerve terminal, promotes blood clotting, relaxes digestive tract smooth muscle	Yohimbine (antagonist)	Delay of ejaculation
	Beta				
	β_1	Heart and coronary blood vessels; kidney; liver; adipose tissue	Increases heart rate and strength of contraction, stimulates rennin release from kidney	Isoproterenol (agonist)	Bronchiole dilator
	β_2	Most sympathetic target cells	Dilation of blood vessels and bronchioles stimulates insulin secretion relaxes smooth muscle of digestive and urinary tracts, relaxes uterus when pregnant, glycogenolysis	Propranolol (antagonist)	Decrease of blood pressure
	β_3	Adipose tissue	Stimulates lipolysis in fat cells	Clenbuturol	Decrease of lipid deposition
Adensosine and ATP	Purinergic P_1	Autonomic effectors	Reduces autonomic response	Theophylline (antagonist)	Bronchodilator
	Purinergic P_2	Smooth muscle	Fast and slow responses to ATP	Pyridoxalphosphate-6-azophenyl-2',4'-disulfonic acid tetrasodium salt (antagonist)	
Nitric oxide (NO)	NO receptor	Smooth muscle, especially blood vessels	Relaxes smooth muscle	Glyceryl trinitriate and nitroprusside (generate NO)	Induction of coronary vasodilation for angina

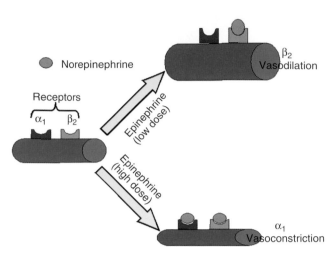

Fig. 10.30. Adrenergic affect on blood vessels. Blood vessels have both α₁ and β₂ receptors on their surface. Epinephrine and norepinephrine have differential effect on blood vessel tone depending on the concentration of the neurotransmitter. When the concentration of these neurotransmitters is low, they stimulate the β₂-adrenergic receptors on the blood vessel walls, causing vasodilation. When the concentration is high, the primary effect is due to stimulation of the α₁-adrenergic receptors, which causes vasoconstriction.

neurotransmitter (Fig. 10.30). When the dose of norepinephrine or epinephrine is relatively low, it causes vasodilation in skeletal muscle. Such a response is seen when an animal is alarmed or experiencing a "fight or flight" response in which there needs to be increased blood flow to skeletal muscle to support its increased metabolic activity. This effect is mediated by the neurotransmitters acting at β₂-adrenergic receptors. In contrast, the same neurotransmitters can cause vasoconstriction when these neurotransmitters are administered at high doses, and the effect is mediated by α₁-adrenergic receptors. This latter response is observed only at doses of neurotransmitters above those present in vivo.

Other neurotransmitters

Acetylcholine (ACh) can also evoke slow EPSPs and inhibitory postsynaptic potentials (IPSP) in postganglionic neurons. These effects are mediated by muscarinic receptors. The slow EPSPs occur when ACh causes the opening of Na⁺ and Ca⁺⁺ channels and the closure of M-type K⁺ channels. Since these K⁺ channels are normally open at resting membrane potentials, their closure results in depolarization. The slow IPSPs result from opening K⁺ channels resulting in hyperpolarization.

Adenosine triphosphate (ATP) is frequently coreleased with norepinephrine at many postganglionic sympathetic neurons. ATP can act at ATP-gated ion

channels (P₂ purinergic receptors) causing excitation. In addition, adenosine, which is produced by the hydrolysis of ATP, can act both pre- and postsynaptically at P₂ receptors. Adenosine reduces the release of norepinephrine and ATP from nerve terminals, particularly after intense sympathetic activity.

Many neuropeptides are also coreleased with norepinephrine and ACh from autonomic neurons. Cholinergic preganglionic fibers may contain enkephalins, neurotensin, somatostatin, or substance P. Cholinergic postganglionic fibers can also contain calcitonin gene-related peptide and vasoactive intestinal peptide (VIP). Corelease of VIP may enhance the effect of ACh since VIP causes vasodilation. For example, when ACh causes salivary gland secretion, VIP enhances blood flow to support the secretory response.

Noradrenergic postganglionic fibers may also release neuropeptide Y. At synapses where the nerve ending is more than 60 nm from the target tissue, neuropeptide Y enhances both the purinergic and adrenergic component of the tissue response. At synapses where the nerve ending is within 20 nm of the target, neuropeptide Y acts presynaptically to inhibit ATP and norepinephrine release. Sympathetic neurons can also contain galanin and dynorphin along with neuropeptide Y.

Interactions of the sympathetic and paraysmpathetic divisions

Both divisions of the autonomic nervous system innervate most organs, with the two divisions having opposite effects. While both divisions are normally active, the effect on the organ is dependent on the relative activity of each division (Table 10.5).

Central nervous system control of the autonomic nervous system

The two divisions of the autonomic nervous system are highly coordinated at the level of the central nervous system. The nucleus of the solitary tract serves an important role in this regard. It receives visceral input from cranial nerves VII, IX, and X, and can then modulate autonomic functions in two ways. First, this nucleus projects to neurons in the brain stem and spinal cord forming circuits to control autonomic function. For example, visceral sensory information transmitted through this nucleus is used to regulate vagal motor control to the stomach and heart. Second, this nucleus integrates autonomic functions with endocrine and behavioral responses largely through its interaction with the hypothalamus.

The hypothalamus was once termed the "head ganglion" of the autonomic nervous system. Early studies

Table 10.5. Parasympathetic and sympathetic effects.

Target Organ	Parasympathetic Effect	Sympathetic Effects
Eye (Iris)	Constricts eye pupils	Dilates eye pupils (α_1)
Eye (ciliary muscle)	Makes lens more convex for accommodation	No effect
Glands (nasal, lacrimal, salivary, gastric, pancreas)	Stimulates secretion	Inhibits secretion, causes vasoconstriction of blood vessels to glands
Sweat glands	No effect	Stimulates secretion via cholinergic fibers
Adrenal medulla	No effect	Stimulates NE and EP secretion
Arrector pili muscles	No effect	Contraction causing erection of hairs and goosebumps
Heart muscle	Decreases heart rate and strength of contraction	Increases heart rate and strength of contractions
Coronary blood vessel	Vasoconstriction	Vasodilation
Bladder/urethra	Contracts bladder wall, relaxes urethra sphincter, voids urine	Relaxes bladder wall, constricts urethra sphincter, inhibits urine release
Lungs	Constricts bronchioles	Dilates bronchioles
Digestive tract	Increases peristalsis and secretion of digestive juices, relaxes sphincters	Decreases digestive motility and secretion
Liver	No effect	Epinephrine stimulates glycogenolysis
Gallbladder	Stimulates contraction	Inhibits contraction
Kidney	No effect	Vasoconstriction, decreases urine output, increases rennin formation
Penis	Erection via vasodilation	Ejaculation
Vagina/clitoris	Erection via vasodilation of clitoris	Reverses peristalsis or contraction of vagina
Blood vessels	Vasodilation via production of nitric oxide	Constricts most vessels, increasing blood pressure; dilates vessels in skeletal muscle, heart, and bronchioles
Blood coagulation	No effect	Increases coagulation
Cellular metabolism	No effect	Increases metabolic rate
Mental activity	No effect	Increases alertness
Adipose tissue	No effect	Stimulates lypolysis

on brain function found that stimulating or lesioning the hypothalamus altered hypothalamic function. Recent studies have revealed that these effects were due to interruption of ascending and descending pathways that course through the hypothalamus traveling between the cerebral cortex and basal forebrain.

The hypothalamus serves a role in regulating five autonomic functions:

1. It regulates blood pressure and electrolyte composition by controlling fluid and salt intake, thus maintaining blood osmolality and volume.
2. It regulates body temperature by controlling the set point for body temperature and activating either heat loss or heat production pathways.
3. It regulates energy metabolism by controlling food intake, digestion, and metabolic rate.
4. It controls an animal's response to stress by regulating adrenal function, blood flow to muscles, and immunological responses.
5. It regulates reproductive functions, including mating, pregnancy, and lactation.

The hypothalamus is well positioned to coordinate these functions since it receives sensory information from most of the body, it is able to compare that information with endogenous set points, and it can then make appropriate adjustments via negative feedback loops to maintain homeostasis. Regarding sensory information, the hypothalamus receives direct input from the visceral sensory system, the olfactory system, and the retina. Information from the retina is used by the suprachiasmatic nucleus to synchronize the internal clock and control circadian rhythms. Pain information is carried to the hypothalamus from the spinal and trigeminal dorsal horns. In addition, the hypothalamus contains sensory neurons that monitor temperature, osmolality, glucose, and sodium levels. Signals from the periphery, such as blood leptin or angiotensin II levels, are also able to reach the hypothalamus because of specialized structures called circumventricular organs, which allow peptides to cross the blood-brain barrier at these sites.

Visceral reflexes

Although the definition of visceral reflexes was discussed above, here we describe specific visceral reflexes. Visceral reflexes control an array of autonomic responses. Some responses are very rapid, such as change in pupil size; others are relatively slow, such as gastric secretions.

Ocular reflexes

The diameter of the pupil and the shape of the lens are controlled by the autonomic nervous system. Sympathetic fibers originating from the superior cervical ganglia innervate the muscles controlling dilation of the pupil; parasympathetic fibers innervate circular muscles constricting the pupil. When excited, the autonomic nervous system inhibits pupillary constriction while it stimulates pupillodilator muscles.

Cardiovascular reflexes

Arterial blood pressure is controlled by both cardiac output and resistance to blood flow. The sympathetic nervous system can increase heart rate, strength of cardiac contraction, and peripheral resistance while the parasympathetic nervous system can decrease heart rate and peripheral resistance, although its affect on peripheral resistance is less than that of the sympathetic nervous system.

Sympathetic vasoconstrictor tone is controlled by adrenergic neurons originating in the ventrolateral medulla that innervate sympathetic vasoconstrictor preganglionic neurons. Stimulation of baroreceptors sends signals to the nucleus of the solitary tract, which excites interneurons in the caudal ventrolateral medulla leading to inhibition of vasomotor neurons and excitation of vagal cardiomotor neurons. This results in a decrease in blood pressure and heart rate.

Norepinephrine is released from sympathetic fibers innervating the heart and acts on the β-adrenergic receptors in the heart to increase heart rate and force of contraction. It acts by increasing the production of cyclic adenosine monophosphate (cAMP) that in turn opens long-lasting (L-type) Ca^{++} channels. Norepinephrine also decreases the threshold for firing of cardiac pacemaker cells (located in the sinoatrial node) leading to increased heart rate.

Acetylcholine is released from parasympathetic fibers innervating the heart and acts on muscarinic receptors in the sinoatrial (SA) and atrioventricular (AV) nodes of cardiac muscle. This causes an increase in K^+ conductance in these cells, which causes hyperpolarization of the SA and AV nodes, thus slowing transmission through these sites. Acetylcholine also increases the threshold for firing the pacemaker cells in the SA node. The strength of contraction of cardiac muscle is also decreased by acetylcholine by decreasing the intracellular cAMP, thus reducing the L-type Ca^{++} current.

Glandular reflexes

The parasympathetic nervous system stimulates gastrointestinal glands such as the nasal, lacrimal, and gastric glands. Glands located in the upper gastrointestinal tract (GIT), particularly in the mouth and stomach, are more strongly stimulated than those in the lower GIT. Glands in the lower part of the GIT are mostly under the control of the enteric nervous system. Salivary glands are under both sympathetic and parasympathetic control. Sympathetic input causes a viscous secretion high in amylase; parasympathetic input causes a watery secretion of higher volume.

In general, the sympathetic nervous system decreases glandular secretions while the parasympathetic nervous system increases glandular secretions. This is because the sympathetic nervous system generally decreases blood flow to glands. The exception is sweat glands, in which the sympathetic nervous system increases sweating. Sympathetic fibers to the sweat glands are cholinergic rather than adrenergic.

Gastrointestinal reflexes

The parasympathetic nervous system stimulates gastric acid secretion, whereas the sympathetic nervous system inhibits such function. The enteric nervous system controls peristalsis. The presence of a bolus of food in the gastrointestinal tract causes stretch in the gut walls generating sensory signals that synapse on interneurons within the gut wall. These interneurons initiate a stimulatory motor signal to the circular muscle layer rostral of the bolus while simultaneously causing inhibition of motor neurons of the circular muscle layer caudad of the bolus. In addition, the interneurons send signals resulting in stimulation of the longitudinal muscle layer caudad of the bolus while inhibiting the longitudinal muscle layer rostral of the bolus.

Urogenital reflexes

Bladder emptying is generally under autonomic control, although there can be some voluntary control. When the bladder is extended, there is a visceral sensory reflex in which parasympathetic postganglionic neurons in the pelvic ganglion plexus promote contraction of the bladder. The sympathetic nervous system promotes bladder smooth muscle relaxation.

References

Getty, R. 1964. Atlas for Applied Veterinary Anatomy. Iowa State Press, Ames, Iowa.

Kandel, E.R., J.H. Schwartz, and T.M. Jessell. 2000. Principles of Neural Science, 4th edition. McGraw-Hill, New York.

Riegel, R.J. and S.E. Hakola. 1996. Illustrated Atlas of Clinical Equine Anatomy and Common Disorders of the Horse, Vol. 1, Musculoskeletal System & Lameness Disorders. Equistar Publication, Limited, Marysville, Ohio.

11

Special senses

Contents

The special senses include smell, taste, vision, hearing, and equilibrium. Unlike the sense of touch that generally involves free nerve endings, special senses are dependent on specific receptor cells localized in the head region of the animal.

Olfaction: The sense of smell

Both smell and taste are chemical senses involving chemoreceptors. Olfaction involves the detection of volatile chemicals in solution.

Anatomy of olfactory receptors

The olfactory epithelium is located in the roof of the nasal cavity along the inferior surface of the cribriform plate of the ethmoid bone and extending along the superior nasal concha and upper part of the middle nasal concha. It consists of olfactory receptors, supporting cells, and basal stem cells.

Olfactory receptors are bipolar neurons (Fig. 11.1). At their apical end, the dendrite forms a knob from which several long cilia project. These cilia lie flat on the nasal epithelium and are covered with a thin mucus layer produced by the supporting cells and olfactory glands. Unlike other cilia, these remain stationary. At their basal end, the axon from the olfactory receptors projects through the cribriform plate and into the olfactory bulb.

The supporting cells are columnar epithelial cells surrounding the olfactory receptors. They provide physical support and cushioning, nourishment, and electrical insulation for the olfactory receptor cells. They also contain a yellow-brown pigment that gives the olfactory epithelium a yellow tint.

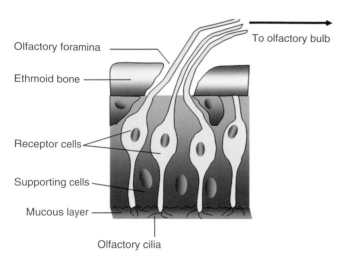

Olfactory foramina

Ethmoid bone

To olfactory bulb

Receptor cells

Supporting cells

Mucous layer

Olfactory cilia

Fig. 11.1. Olfactory receptors. Olfactory receptor cells are interspersed among supporting cells. The olfactory cilia, embedded in the mucous layer of the olfactory epithelia, detect odorants causing the development of a receptor potential in the olfactory cells. Axons project from the olfactory receptors forming the olfactory nerve (cranial nerve I).

Basal stem cells are found between the supporting cells. They continually undergo cell division producing new olfactory receptors. The olfactory receptors live for approximately 1 month before dying and being replaced. This makes these neurons unusual since most neurons are long-lived, and are not replaced.

Olfactory (Bowman's) glands are found in the connective tissue that supports the olfactory epithelium. These glands produce mucus that is carried to the surface of the olfactory epithelium and which dissolves odorants, i.e., chemicals that stimulate the olfactory hairs.

The facial nerve (cranial nerve VII) innervates supporting cells and olfactory glands. When these structures are stimulated by certain chemicals, nerve impulses in the facial nerve can result in stimulation of the lacrimal glands in the eyes and nasal mucous glands. This can cause tearing and a runny nose.

Physiology of olfaction

Odorants dissolve in the mucus membrane of the olfactory epithelium. They bind to protein receptors on the olfactory cilium membrane stimulating G proteins resulting in the activation of adenylate cyclase. Adenylate cyclase then catalyzes the production of cyclic adenosine monophosphate (cAMP), which causes Na^+-channels to open. The influx of Na^+ results in depolarization of the olfactory receptor and the production of a receptor potential.

Olfactory pathway

The unmyelinated axons of the olfactory receptors constitute the first-order neurons, which pass through the numerous olfactory foramina in the cribriform plate of the ethmoid bone. These axons collectively form the right and left olfactory nerves (cranial nerve I). They terminate on secondary neurons located within the olfactory bulbs located just below the frontal lobes of the cerebrum. Neurons from the olfactory bulb extend posteriorly in the olfactory tract, projecting to the lateral olfactory area in the temporal lobe. The olfactory area is part of the limbic system. The olfactory neurons also project to the hypothalamus and other limbic areas, thus explaining how smell can evoke various memories and emotions.

Gustation: the sense of taste

Tongue

The tongue is the muscular organ filling most of the oral cavity. It is composed of interlacing bundles of skeletal muscle fibers, and it is involved in gripping, repositioning food, mixing food with saliva, and forming the compact mass of food called a bolus.

The tongue has intrinsic and extrinsic muscles. The intrinsic muscles confined to the tongue, and not attached to bone, run in several directions allowing the tongue to change shape as necessary for prehension, moving food, and making sounds. The extrinsic muscles attach the tongue to bones of the skull and the soft palate. They allow the tongue to protrude, retract, and move side to side. The lingual frenulum attaches the tongue to the floor of the mouth.

The surface of the tongue is covered with small bumps called papillae (Latin for "bumps"; sing. = papilla). Papillae are named for their shape. Filiform papillae are thorn-shaped giving the tongue roughness and thus aiding in licking and manipulating food. They have a mechanical function. In the ox and cat, they are heavily cornified. Fungiform papillae are mushroom-shaped, scattered among the more numerous filiform papillae, have taste buds, and are thus mechanical and gustatory (Fig. 11.2). Foliate papillae have a series of leaf-shaped ridges, are located on the lateral borders of the tongue, and have a gustatory function. They are absent in the ox. Vallate, or circumvallate, papillae are the largest and least numerous. They are located in a V-shaped row near the back of the tongue. They resemble the fungiform papillae, but are circled by a cleft containing taste buds. Marginal taste buds are found along the edge of the rostral portion of the tongue of newborn dogs, but they disappear when puppies switch to solid food.

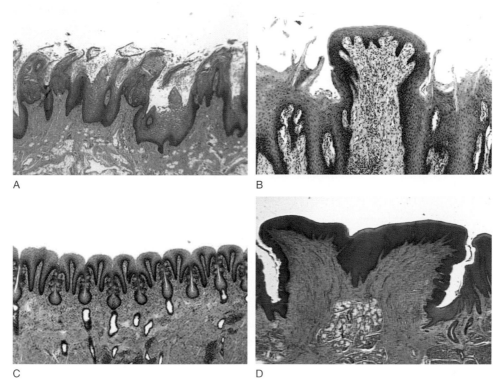

Fig. 11.2. Shape of papillae. A) Filiform papillae, which are thorn-shaped. B) Fungiform papillae, which are mushroom-shaped. C) Filiate papillae, which are leaf-shaped. D) Vallate, or circumvallae papillae, which are similarly shaped to fungiform, but have clefts along the side that contain taste buds.

Taste

Taste is an important sense in animals because it helps identify nutritious feedstuffs from toxic materials. Animals have innate preferences for certain flavors such as those that are sweet, while tending to reject those that are unpleasant such as bitter flavors. Each papilla has one to hundreds of taste buds. Taste buds are also located in the palate, pharynx, epiglottis, and upper third of the esophagus.

Each taste bud is gourd-shaped and consists of three types of taste cells called light, intermediate, and dark cells, as well as basal cells (Fig. 11.3). The different taste cells are believed to be either cells at different stages of differentiation, with the lightest being the most mature, or cells of different cell lineages. The basal cells are thought to be stem cells for the taste cells, which are short-lived. There is a small opening at the surface of the epithelium called the taste pore. Each taste cell has microvilli extending into the taste pore. The microvilli are the only part of the cell exposed to the oral cavity. Each taste cell is innervated by sensory gustatory neurons. The space between the taste cells and sensory neurons appears to act as a synapse. Taste cells are electrically excitable and have voltage-gated Na^+, K^+, and Ca^{++} channels on their surface.

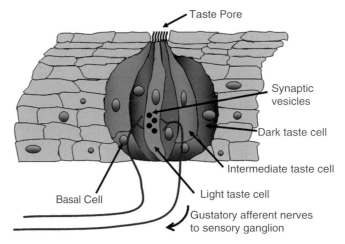

Fig. 11.3. Taste bud. Each taste bud consists of three types of taste cells called dark, intermediate, and light cells. In addition, there are small, round basal cells located at the base of the taste bud. The basal cells are thought to be stem cells that produce taste cells.

Until recently, it was generally believed that animals had four primary tastes, including salty, sour, sweet, and bitter. Recently, a fifth category was added called umami, meaning "delicious" in Japanese. It is stimulated by monosodium glutamate. Foods can provide a different taste by stimulating a varying combination of these five tastes. In addition, volatile components

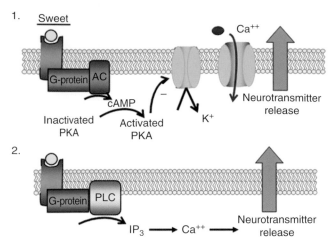

Fig. 11.4. Sweet taste. There are two mechanisms for sweet taste. 1) A sweet tastant binds to a specific receptor inducing the formation of a G protein that activates adenylyl cyclase (AC), thus causing the formation of cAMP. The cAMP activates protein kinase A (PKA) which then closes membrane-bound K^+-channels, thus causing depolarization of the taste cell. This allows voltage-gated Ca^{++} channels to open, and Ca^{++} enters the cell causing the release of the neurotransmitter that excites the gustatory sensory neurons. 2) G proteins activate phospholipase C (PLC), which catalyzes the formation of 1,4,5-triphosphate (IP_3). IP_3 causes the release of calcium from endogenous stores in the endoplasmic reticulum. Ca^{++} then causes the release of the neurotransmitter.

of feedstuffs stimulate the sense of smell that influences the sense of taste.

The binding of taste stimuli, called tastants, to extracellular receptors located on taste cells leads to depolarization of the taste cell either directly or indirectly through the activation of second messengers. The receptor potential induced by depolarization allows the influx of Ca^{++} through voltage-gated Ca^{++} channels. This leads to the release of a neurotransmitter, whose identity is unknown, at the synapse with the sensory gustatory neuron. This neurotransmitter causes excitation in the sensory neuron.

Sweet taste

Sweet taste is initiated by the binding of sweet tastants to receptors. There are two mechanisms for transducing sweet taste stimuli (Fig. 11.4). In the first, the binding of sweet tastants to specific receptors activates a G protein, called gustducin, that activates adenylyl cyclase, causing the formation of cAMP in the cytoplasm. The cAMP then activates protein kinase A, which phosphorylates K^+-selective ion channels located on the basolateral membrane of the taste cells causing them to close. The cAMP-dependent closure of K^+ channels results in depolarization of the taste cells leading to the release of the neurotransmitter that excites the sensory neuron. In the second mechanism, sweet tastants cause production of G proteins leading to activation of phospholipase C, an enzyme that cata-

lyzes the synthesis of inositol 1,4,5-trisphosphate (IP_3). IP_3 causes the release of Ca^{++} from intracellular stores. Calcium then causes the release of the neurotransmitter, which then stimulates the gustatory sensory neurons.

Bitter taste

Bitter taste, often associated with toxic compounds, is elicited by divalent cations, some amino acids, and alkaloids. Some bitter-tasting compounds (such as quinine) are membrane permeable; while others (such as denatorium) are not, suggesting multiple mechanisms for transduction. The mechanisms for bitter taste appear similar to that for sweet tastes (Fig. 11.5). Denatorium causes the increase in intracellular calcium through an IP_3-dependent mechanism. Other bitter compounds activate gustducin that stimulates taste cell phosphodiesterase reducing intracellular cAMP and cGMP levels. Knockout mice, in which the gustducin gene has been deleted, are insensitive to selected bitter tastes. Some bitter compounds are also thought to bind directly to K^+-selective ion channels blocking them. This prevents the movement of K^+ out of the cell, thus causing depolarization and release of the neurotransmitter.

Salty taste

Salty taste is mostly caused by the cation Na^+. Taste cells sensitive to salt have a Na^+-selective ion channel that can be blocked with amiloride (Fig. 11.6). This amiloride-sensitive channel is different than the voltage-gated sodium channels responsible for the upstroke of the action potential. Instead, this channel is not voltage sensitive, and remains open all the time. When an animal consumes feedstuffs high in sodium, this increases the Na^+ concentration outside the salt-sensitive taste cell, and Na^+ then moves down its concentration gradient into the cell causing depolarization.

Taste pathway

Information from taste buds in the anterior two-thirds of the tongue and on the palate travel in the chorda tympani, a branch of the facial nerve (cranial nerve VII). Signals from the taste buds in the posterior third of the tongue are carried via the glossopharyngeal nerve (IX). Taste buds on the epiglottis and esophagus are innervated by the vagus (cranial nerve X). Fibers carrying this information enter the solitary tract in the medulla and enter the gustatory area of the nucleus of the solitary tract. Second-order fibers then ascend to the thalamus synapsing in the parvocellular region of the ventral posterior medial nucleus. This area then projects to the area along the border between the anterior insula and frontal operculum in the ipsilateral

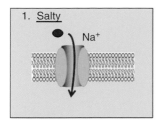

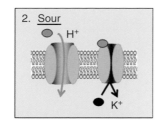

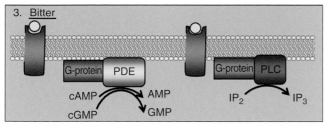

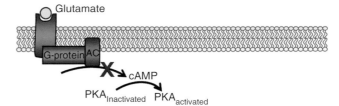

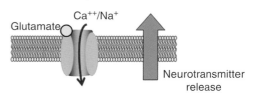

Fig. 11.5. Salty, sour, and bitter taste. 1) Salty taste is elicited by cations, primarily Na$^+$, which enter through a Na$^+$-selective ion channel that can be blocked by amiloride. The entry of Na$^+$ causes depolarization of the taste cell and release of the neurotransmitter, which causes excitation in the gustatory neurons. 2) Sour taste is caused by the entry of H$^+$ ions that permeate amiloride-sensitive Na$^+$ channels; this leads to depolarization of the cell because the cell cannot distinguish between Na$^+$ and H$^+$. Sour taste can also be elicited by H$^+$ binding to and blocking K$^+$-selective channels, preventing the movement of K$^+$ out of the cell. 3) Bitter taste is caused by either increasing intracellular calcium through an IP$_3$-dependent mechanism, or by activating the G protein gustducin that stimulates taste cell phosphodiesterase (PDE), thus reducing intracellular cAMP and cGMP levels.

Fig. 11.6. Umami taste. There are two proposed umami pathways: 1) The first involves a glutamate binding to a receptor which activates a G protein (i.e., a metabotropic receptor). The activated G protein causes a decrease in cAMP levels, resulting in a decrease in the activation of phophokinase A (PKA), and thus a decrease in the metabolic pathway downstream. 2) The second pathway involves an ionotropic receptor in which glutamate interacts with a receptor on the taste bud surface causing the influx of Na$^+$ and Ca^{++}. The resulting depolarization results in neurotransmitter release.

cerebral cortex. Note that this pathway does not cross to the contralateral side.

Sour

The sour taste is caused by the acidity of the feedstuff. The higher the H$^+$ ion concentration, the more sour the flavor. The H$^+$ ions can affect the sour taste receptors in two ways. First, H$^+$ can permeate amiloride-sensitive Na$^+$ channels, which leads to depolarization of the cell since the cell cannot distinguish between Na$^+$ and H$^+$. Second, H$^+$ can bind to and block K$^+$-selective channels preventing the movement of K$^+$ out of the cell.

Umami

Since amino acids are a major part of dietary intake, it should come as no surprise that animals have a taste for amino acids. Studies with glutamate and aspartate show at least two pathways for this taste. Glutamate can activate an ion channel allowing Na$^+$ and Ca^{++} to enter the cell (Fig. 11.6). This inward current causes voltage-gated Ca^{++} channels to open causing depolarization that triggers neurotransmitter release. The second mechanism entails glutamate binding to a G protein coupled receptor, probably resulting in a decrease in intracellular cAMP levels.

Vision

Vision is a major sensation in many animals. This is reflected in the large number of receptors within the eye and the large percentage of the cortex that is devoted to vision. Vision is particularly important in birds. Although the eyes make up only about 1% of the weight of the head in man, they make up approximately 15% in a starling.

Accessory structures of the eye

The accessory structures of the eye include the eyelids, eyelashes, eyebrows, lacrimal (tearing) (Fig. 11.7), and extrinsic muscles of the eye.

Eyelids, eyelashes, and eyebrows

The upper and lower eyelids, or palpebrae, cover the eye during sleep, protect the eye from excessive light and foreign objects, and assist with lubricating the eye (Fig. 11.8). The layers of the eyelid consist of the superficial epidermis, dermis, subcutaneous tissue, fibers of the orbicularis oculi muscle, a tarsal plate, tarsal glands, and conjuctiva. The tarsal plate is a fold of connective tissue giving support to the eyelid. Embedded in the tarsal plate is a row of sebaceous glands called the tarsal, or Meibomian, glands. They secrete fluid that helps prevent the eyelids from adhering from one another. The conjunctiva is a thin, protective mucous membrane consisting of stratified columnar

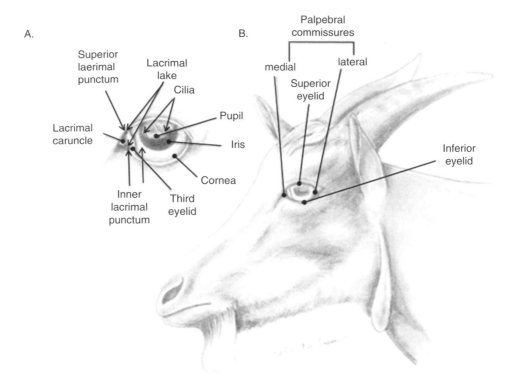

Fig. 11.7. External structures of the eye in the goat. A) Frontal aspect of the eye and lacrimal apparatus. B) Eyelids and eye of the goat. (Reprinted from Constantinescu, 2001. Used by permission of the publisher.)

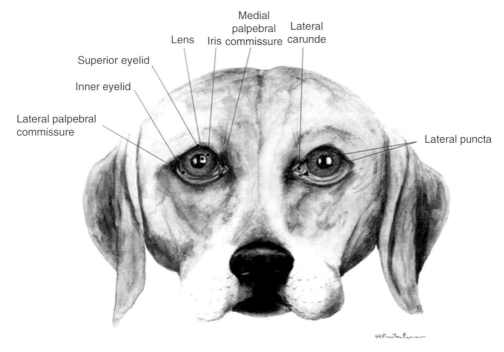

Fig. 11.8. Front view of the eye of the dog. (Reprinted from Constantinescu, 2002. Used by permission of the publisher.)

epithelium with goblet cells and areolar connective tissue. It lines the inside of the palpebrae and the anterior surface of the eyeball, excluding the cornea.

The gap between the two eyelids is the palpebral fissure. At either corner of the eyelid is the lateral and

medial commissure, respectively. A small, reddish elevated area found in the medial commissure is the lacrimal caruncle. It contains both sebaceous (oil) and sudoriferous (sweat) glands.

Domestic species have a nictitating membrane, or third eyelid (Fig. 11.9). This fold of mucous membrane

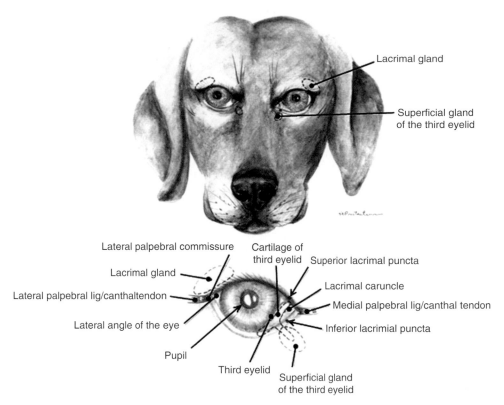

Fig. 11.9. Eye and accessory structures of the dog. (Reprinted from Constantinescu, 2002. Used by permission of the publisher.)

arises from the ventromedial border of the eye. At its base is a serous gland called the gland of the third eyelid.

Located at the margin of the eyelids are the cilia (eyelashes). Located above each eyelid are the eyebrows. Both structures help keep foreign objects, perspiration, and direct sunlight out of the eye. Located at the base of the hair follicles of the eyelashes are sebaceous ciliary glands that release a lubricating fluid. Infection of these glands is a sty.

Lacrimal apparatus

The lacrimal apparatus (Fig. 11.9) consists of a group of structures that produce and drain tears (lacrimal fluid). Lacrimal glands, located in the dorsolateral portion of the orbit, secrete lacrimal fluid through excretory lacrimal ducts that empty onto the surface of the conjunctiva of the upper eyelid. The fluid moves over the anterior surface of the eye and enters two small openings on the upper and lower palpebrae near the medial corner called the lacrimal puncta. From there, the fluid enters the lacrimal canals, two ducts leading into the lacrimal sac. The nasolacrimal duct carries fluid from the lacrimal sac into the nasal cavity just below the inferior nasal concha. Lacrimal fluid contains water, salts, mucus, antibodies, and lysozyme. This fluid protects, lubricates and moistens

the eyeball. The moisture seen on the nose of domestic animals is largely lacrimal fluid.

Extrinsic eye muscles

Movement of the eyeball is controlled by six striated muscles called extraocular muscles, in contrast to intraocular muscles located within the eyeball (Fig. 11.10). The lateral and medial rectus muscles move the eye laterally and medially, respectively. The superior rectus and inferior rectus muscles elevate and depress the eye, respectively. The inferior oblique muscle elevates and turns the eye laterally while the superior oblique depresses and turns the eye laterally.

Anatomy of the eyeball

The receptors for vision reside within the eyeball. The eyeball consists of three layers: 1) fibrous tunic, 2) vascular tunic, and 3) retina (Fig. 11.11).

Fibrous tunic

The fibrous tunic, or external coat of the eyeball, is avascular and consists of the anterior cornea and posterior opaque sclera. The cornea is a transparent layer covering the iris, the colored portion of the front of the

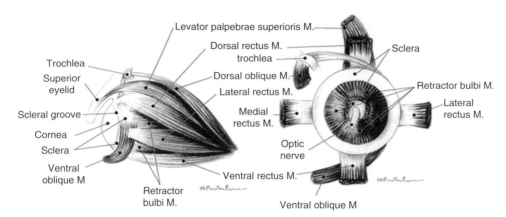

Fig. 11.10. Muscles of the eye of the dog. The left drawing shows the lateral aspect of the eye while the right drawing shows the posterior aspect of the eye. (Reprinted from Constantinescu, 2002. Used by permission of the publisher.)

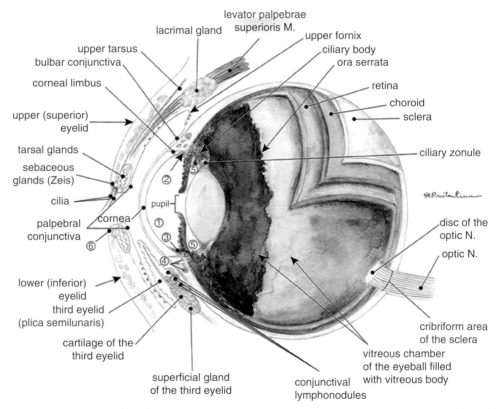

Fig. 11.11. Eye and accessory structures of the dog. (Reprinted from Constantinescu, 2002. Used by permission of the publisher.)

eye. The cornea is curved and therefore helps bend light toward the retina. The cornea consists of three layers. Its outer layer consists of nonkeratinized stratified squamous epithelium, the middle layer consists of collagen fibers and fibroblasts, and the inner layer is simple squamous epithelium. The sclera covers the entire outside surface of the eye with the exception of the cornea. It consists of dense connective tissue and provides rigidity, helping to maintain the shape of the eyeball. The scleral venous sinus (canal of Schlemm)

is located at the junction of the sclera and cornea. Aqueous humor drains into this sinus.

Vascular tunic

The vascular tunic, or uvea, is the middle layer of the eyeball. It consists of three parts: choroid, ciliary body, and iris. The choroid is the highly vascularized, dark brown, posterior portion of the vascular tunic, lining the majority of the inside of the sclera. Its brown pigment is produced by melanocytes, and helps absorb light so that it is not scattered throughout the inside of the eye. The choroid is incomplete where the optic nerve exits the posterior of the eyeball.

Many species of domestic animals, including cats, dogs, horses, and ruminants, have an additional layer in the choroids called the tapetum lucidum. This causes the animal's eyes to appear to glow when shined with a light. The tapetum lucidum reflects light back toward the retina so that the animal can see in low light.

In the anterior, the choroid becomes the ciliary body that extends from the ora serrata, the serrated front margin of the retina, to just posterior of the junction of the sclera and cornea. It consists of the ciliary processes and ciliary muscles. The ciliary processes are folds of tissue containing capillaries that secrete aqueous humor. Extending from the ciliary processes to the lens are zonular fibers (suspensory ligaments). The ciliary muscles are a bundle of smooth muscles that alter the shape of the lens in order to allow for near or far vision.

The iris is the colored portion at the front of the eyeball that is shaped like a disc with a hole, the pupil, in the center. The color of the iris is controlled by its number of pigmented cells. A large number of pigmented cells results in a brown color; a low number results in a blue color. The shape of the pupil can vary. It can be round, elliptical, or slitlike. Cats have an elliptical pupil that opens and closes faster than round pupils.

The iris lies between the cornea in front and the lens in back, and is attached to the ciliary processes. Consisting of circular and radial smooth muscle fibers, the ciliary process regulates the amount of light entering the eye. Parasympathetic signals stimulate the circular muscles to contract during bright light and close vision causing the pupil to constrict. During dim light or distant vision, sympathetic signals stimulate the radial muscles to contract causing the pupil to dilate.

Retina (the sensory tunic)

The innermost layer of the eye is the retina, which lines the posterior portion of the eyeball. The retina consists of two layers: an outer pigmented layer and an inner neural layer. The pigmented layer is a one-cell–thick layer of melanin-containing epithelial cells, similar to the choroid. These cells also act as phagocytes and store vitamin A.

The neural layer of the retina is multilayered, and grows directly out of the brain during embryonic development. It has three major layers: the photoreceptor layer, the bipolar cell layer, and the ganglion cell layer (Fig. 11.12). The outer and inner synaptic layers separate these layers from each other. Before reaching the photoreceptor layer, light must first pass through the ganglion and bipolar cell layers. Light stimulates the photoreceptors found close to the pigmented layer. This generates signals that travel through the outer synaptic layer to the bipolar cells,

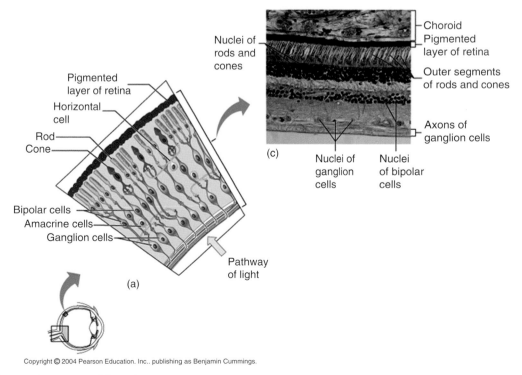

Fig. 11.12. Microscopic anatomy of the retina.

and through the inner synaptic layer to the ganglion cells. Interspersed among these cells are two other types of neurons: horizontal cells and amacrine cells. These latter neurons form lateral connections that modify signals along the photoreceptive pathway.

Axons from the ganglion cells collectively form the optic nerve, which exits the eye at the optic disc. Since the optic disc lacks photoreceptors, it is also called the blind spot. The blind spot normally is not apparent since the brain "fills in" information from this area. However, you can demonstrate its presence to yourself by covering your right eye and gazing at the plus sign below. As you move the position of the book closer or farther from your eye, you will see the large dot disappear:

There are two types of photoreceptors: rods and cones. Rods outnumber cones 20 : 1—except in birds, which have more cones than rods. Rods have a low light threshold, and therefore are effective in dim light allowing for the perception of only shades of gray. Cones have a higher threshold for light and provide for color and high acuity vision.

The macula lutea is an oval region found in the exact center of the posterior of the retina. It contains mostly cones. At its center is a small pit, the central fovea, which contains only cones and where the bipolar and ganglion cells are displaced to the sides. Therefore, light passes unimpeded to the cones. The density of cones in the retina decreases moving from the macula toward the periphery. Since the central fovea has a high concentration of cones, this is the region of the eye with the greatest visual acuity (sharpness of vision). So an animal will focus an object on the fovea to generate greater detail.

The avian retina is avascular, and contains a unique structure called the pecten. This is a black pigmented structure extending from the ventral retina up to just above the area where the optic nerve exits. It is made of blood vessels and pigmented stromal cells, and is thought to serve a nutritive function.

Lens

The lens is a biconvex, transparent, avascular structure that can change its shape in order to focus light on the retina. Located behind the iris, the lens is held in place by the suspensory ligament attaching it to the choroid process.

The lens, enclosed in a thin, elastic capsule, consists of two regions: lens epithelium and lens fibers. The lens epithelium consists of cuboidal cells located on the anterior surface of the lens. These cells differentiate into the lens fibers that form the bulk of the lens.

Arranged like layers of an onion, lens fibers are anuclear, and contain few organelles. Lens fibers are made of folded proteins called crystallins.

Chambers of the eye

The lens divides the eye into the anterior and posterior segments. The iris subdivides the anterior segment into the anterior chamber, located between the cornea and iris, and the posterior chamber, located between the iris and lens. The anterior segment is filled with aqueous humor. It is a clear, watery fluid similar in composition to plasma, which nourishes the lens and cornea. Aqueous humor is continually derived as a filtrate from the capillaries of the ciliary processes entering the posterior chamber. It flows forward through the pupil of the iris into the anterior chamber. From there, it drains into the venous blood via the schleral venous sinus (canal of Schlemm).

Normally produced and removed at the same rate, aqueous humor, along with the vitreous humor discussed below, maintains the intraocular pressure. However, if the drainage of aqueous humor is blocked, intraocular pressure increases causing compression of the retina and optic nerve. This can lead to glaucoma and blindness.

The posterior segment of the eye is the larger of the two segments. It contains vitreous humor, a clear gellike substance. The vitreous humor pushes the retina against the pigmented layer of the choroid allowing the retina to receive a clear image. Unlike aqueous humor, the vitreous humor forms during embryonic development and lasts a lifetime. Running through the center of the vitreous humor from the lens to the optic disc is the hyaloid canal, a narrow channel that is occupied by the hyaloid artery during fetal development. Occasionally, debris called vitreous floaters are visible within the vitreous humor. Such debris may cast a shadow on the retina.

Physiology of vision

The eye can be likened to a camera. The image of an object is focused on the retina by the lens, and the amount of light entering the eye is controlled by the pupil. The retina, lens and pupil are analogous to the film, lens, and aperture of the camera, respectively. Three processes are important in the formation of a clear image: refraction, accommodation, and pupil diameter.

Refraction

When light rays pass from one medium to another of a different density, the speed of light changes. As a

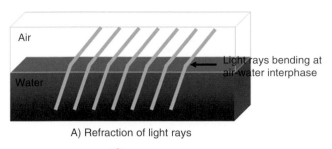

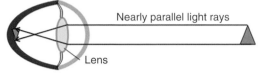

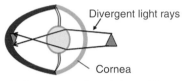

Fig. 11.13. Refraction of light rays. A) Refraction of light rays at the interphase between air and water. B) The refraction of light in order to focus a far object on the retina. C) Note the more spherical shape of the lens necessary to focus a near object on the retina.

result, the light rays are bent, or refracted (Fig. 11.13). For example, when light rays move from air into water, light rays are bent at the interface of the two mediums. With respect to the eye, light rays are refracted, or bent, at the anterior and posterior surfaces of both the cornea and lens. Approximately 75% of the refraction occurs at the interphase with the cornea. Note that images are inverted, both upside down and backward, as they are focused on the retina. The brain reinterprets this image so that objects are not perceived as inverted.

Accommodation

In the eye, the angle at which the light rays are bent depends on the shape of the lens. The more convex the lens, the greater the light rays are bent. As an object is moved closer to the lens, the light rays must be bent at a greater angle in order to focus the image on the retina. The process of increasing the refractive power of the lens is called accommodation. Therefore, as an object moves closer to the eye, the lens must become more rounded, i.e., made more convex, in order to focus the image on the retina.

Accommodation is accomplished by the actions of the ciliary muscle. When the ciliary muscle is relaxed, the zonular fibers surrounding the lens pull on the lens, thus making it fatter, or less convex. When the ciliary muscle contracts, it pulls the ciliary body and

choroid forward, thus decreasing the tension of the zonular fibers on the lens. As a result, because of elastic fibers in the lens, it becomes more convex, i.e., more rounded, which increases its focusing power, causing greater bending of the light rays.

In addition to the accommodating mechanisms described above, some species of birds possess a static mechanism allowing them to keep objects in focus regardless of their distance. This is accomplished from asymmetries in the eye, allowing it to be emmetropic (i.e., light rays focus directly on the retina) in its upper portions while becoming increasingly myopic (i.e., nearsighted) toward its lower portions. This allows a bird to keep objects in the horizon in focus in the upper portion of the eye while simultaneously keeping nearer objects in focus in the lower portion of the eye.

Horses appear to have a limited accommodating ability due to weak ciliary muscles. To compensate, horses have a ramp retina in which the distance between the lens and the retina varies from dorsal to ventral positions. This allows horses to use a form of static accommodation in which they move their head to focus an object at different locations on the retina, depending on the distance of the object from the eye.

The far point of vision is that distance beyond which no accommodation (no change in lens shape) is necessary for focusing. The near point of vision is the closest point at which the animal can focus clearly. It is the point of maximum accommodation of the lens. This point gradually gets farther away as an animal ages.

Refraction problems

A normal eye is said to be emmetropic. As animals age, the lens loses its elasticity, and therefore its ability to accommodate, a condition called presbyopia. When an animal can see close objects but distant objects are blurred, it is called myopia, or nearsightedness. It occurs because the eyeball is too long relative to its focusing power, and therefore distant objects are focused in front of the retina (Fig. 11.14). In hypermyopia, also called hyperopia or farsightedness, the animal can see distant objects but is unable to focus near objects because the eyeball is too short. Therefore, there is not enough accommodating power to focus the light rays of a near object, and the animal instead focuses at a point behind the retina. An irregular curvature in either the lens or cornea results in astigmatism.

Pupil diameter

The amount of light that can enter the eye is controlled by the diameter of the pupil. Circular muscle fibers control the pupil diameter. During the accommoda-

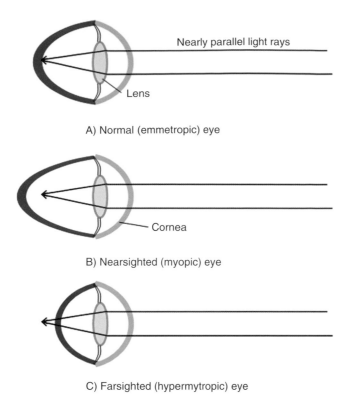

A) Normal (emmetropic) eye

B) Nearsighted (myopic) eye

C) Farsighted (hypermytropic) eye

Fig. 11.14. Refraction problems. A) A normal (emmotropic) eye that can focus light rays on the retina. B) A nearsighted (myopic) eye is too long; thus the light rays from distant objects are focused in front of the retina. C) In a farsighted (hypermyopic) eye, the eyeball is too short so that near objects are focused behind the retina, and the lens does not have enough accommodating power to focus the light rays on the retina.

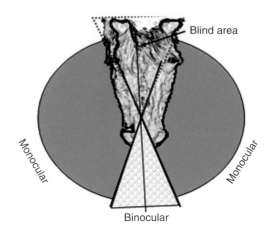

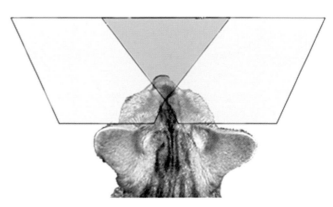

Fig. 11.15. Field of vision. A) There is a blind area immediately between the eyes of a horse and behind the horse's body. B) The cat has a larger binocular area than the horse, but also has a greater blind area behind its body.

tion papillary reflex, parasympathetic signals from the oculomotor nerves cause the pupil to constrict, thus preventing the most divergent light rays from entering the eye. These light rays would fall on the periphery of the retina where they would not be focused properly.

Field of vision

The field of vision is the spatial area that can be seen by a single eye, providing monocular vision. The location of the eyes within the head has an impact on the field of vision. The field of vision of the two eyes generally overlaps, providing an area of binocular vision. The eye location varies between species and within breeds of species. The wider set the eyes, the greater the panoramic field of vision. Herbivores tend to have their eyes set wide, thus providing them with a panoramic field of vision (Fig. 11.15), although they can not see directly in front of the nose or behind their hindquarters.

Photoreception

Photoreception involves the conversion of light energy focused on the retina being converted to an electrical signal carried by the optic nerve. As mentioned before, photoreceptors consist of rods and cones, named for the shape of the outer segment (Fig. 11.16). The outer segment of rods is cylindrical whereas that of the cones is tapered, or cone-shaped. The tips of the rods and cones lie next to the pigmented layer. In birds, oil droplets are also found in cones, which may help filter out UV radiation.

Rods and cones consist of an outer segment involved in photoreception and an inner segment containing the cell nucleus, Golgi complex, and mitochondria. The proximal end of each photoreceptor consists of bulb-shaped synaptic endings containing synaptic vesicles.

Within the outer segments are stacks of membranous discs in which the visual pigments, or photopigments, are embedded. In rods, the discs are discontinuous

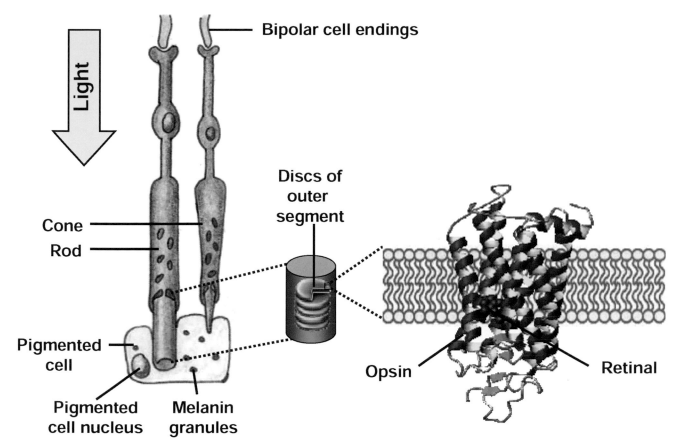

Fig. 11.16. Structure of rods and cones. Rods have a cylindrical outer segment; cones have a conical-shaped outer segment. Note the direction of light and that the tips of the photoreceptors lie near the pigmented layer.

and stacked like pancakes one on top of the other. In cones, the disc membranes are continuous with the plasma membrane, and the interior of the discs is continuous with the extracellular space. In rods, 1–3 new discs are added to the base of the outer segment every hour, thus pushing old discs toward the distal end where they are sloughed off and phagocytized by the pigmented epithelial cells. Cones also renew their discs, but it appears to occur in a circadian rhythm, and is not as well understood.

There is one type of rod and three (four in birds) types of cones, distinguished by different visual pigments. Although rods are more sensitive to light and are stimulated by all visible wavelengths, they perceive only gray tones whereas cones allow for differentiation of color.

Chemistry of visual pigments

The light-absorbing photopigment in rods is rhodopsin. It consists of a glycoprotein called opsin and a vitamin A derivative called retinal. Vitamin A is found in carotenoid-rich vegetables, including carrots, spinach, broccoli, and yellow squash, as well as vitamin A–containing tissues such as liver. Although retinal is the light-absorbing part of all photopigments, the opsins found in each of the three types of cones differ, permitting them to absorb primarily either blue, green, or yellow-orange wavelengths of light.

The photopigments respond to light in the following sequence (Fig. 11.17):

1. In the dark, retinal is found in a bent configuration called 11-cis-retinal, which binds strongly with opsin. In rods, this forms rhodopsin.
2. When exposed to light, cis-retinal is isomerized to all trans-retinal, which is no longer able to bind to retinal. Therefore, trans-retinal and opsin dissociate, thereby forming a colorless photopigment. This process is called bleaching.
3. The enzyme retinal isomerase converts trans-retinal back to cis-retinal.

Light transduction by photoreceptors

In the dark, cyclic GMP (cGMP) binds to sodium channels located on the plasma membrane of the outer segment of the photoreceptor, and keeps them open (Fig. 11.18). The influx of sodium, called the "dark

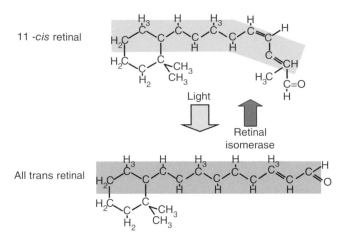

11-*cis* retinal

Light

Retinal isomerase

All trans retinal

Fig. 11.17. Retinal isomers involved in photoreception. In the dark, 11-cis-retinal remains bound to opsin to form rhodopsin. When light strikes the retina, 11-cis-retinal is converted to all trans-retinal in a process called bleaching. All trans-retinal dissociates from opsin and can be isomerized back to 11-cis-retinal in the pigmented epithelium by the enzyme retinal isomerase, which requires ATP.

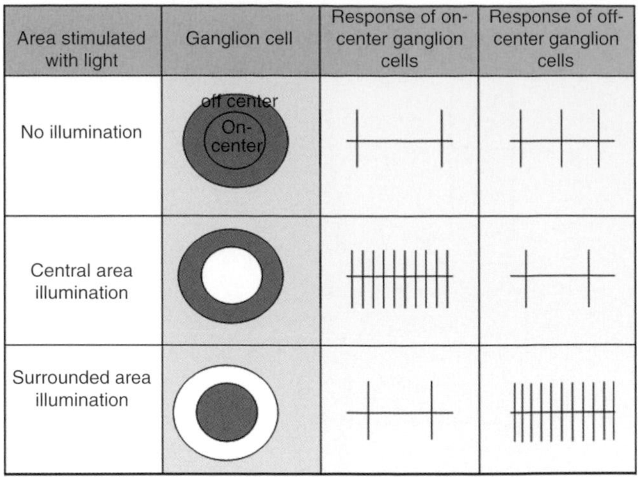

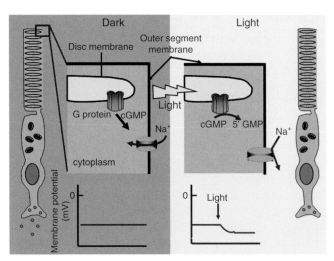

Fig. 11.18. Chemical transduction of light signal. In the dark, cGMP migrates to the plasma membrane and keeps cGMP-gated sodium channels open. When light interacts with rhodopsin found on the disc membrane, it causes 11-cis-retinal to be isomerized to all trans-retinal. Opsin then dissociates from rhodopsin and activates a G-protein. The transducin subunit of the G protein activates phosphodiesterate, which breaks down cGMP to GMP. In the light, since cGMP levels are reduced, the sodium channels close and the cell becomes hyperpolarized causing a decrease in release of the neurotransmitter glutamate. Since glutamate inhibits bipolar cells, decreased release of glutamate disinhibits the bipolar cells, so they develop an action potential.

current," into the photoreceptors depolarizes the membrane. This keeps the Ca^{2+} channels on the synaptic endings open, thus allowing the continuous release of the neurotransmitter, thought to be glutamate, which then interacts with the bipolar cells.

Area stimulated with light	Ganglion cell	Response of on-center ganglion cells	Response of off-center ganglion cells
No illumination	off center On-center		
Central area illumination			
Surrounded area illumination			

Fig. 11.19. Receptive fields of retinal ganglion cells. Ganglion cells have circular receptive fields with the central area being the on-center area and the surrounding area being the off-center area. On-center ganglion cells increase their firing rate when illuminated; off-center cells have an opposite response, and vice versa when the off-center cells are illuminated.

Glutamate induces the production of inhibitory post-synaptic potentials in bipolar cells, thus inhibiting them.

On the disc membrane, the presence of light converts 11-cis-retinal to all trans-retinal, causing opsin to dissociate from the photopigment. Opsin then interacts with a G-protein subunit called transducin. Transducin activates phosphodiesterease, an enzyme that breaks down cGMP to GMP. The breakdown of cGMP causes the sodium channels on the plasma membrane to close. Since sodium entry into the cell decreases while potassium leakage from the cell continues, the cell hyperpolarizes as the membrane potential approaches –70 mV, thus decreasing the release of the neurotransmitter. Since the photoreceptors release an inhibitory neurotransmitter, decreased release of glutamate results in stimulation of bipolar cells. Bipolar cells then stimulate ganglion cells whose axons make up the optic nerve.

Retinal processing of visual information

Only ganglion cells produce action potentials while the amacrine, horizontal, and bipolar cells produce graded potentials. Ganglion cells have circular receptive fields consisting of a circle within a circle (Fig. 11.19). The circular zone at the center is called the on-center area; that on the periphery is called the off-center, or surround, area. The on-center ganglion cells are excited when light illuminates rods or cones in the central area while the off-center area is inhibited. Conversely, light illuminating the off-center area will

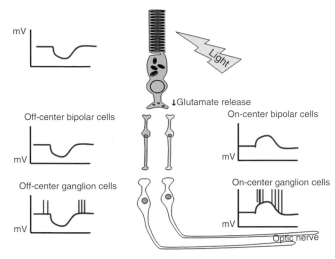

Off-center bipolar cells

On-center bipolar cells

Off-center ganglion cells

On-center ganglion cells

↓Glutamate release

Light

Optic nerve

Fig. 11.20. Off-Center Bipolar Cells.
The on-center and off-center bipolar cells are differentially affected by glutamate. Glutamate opens Na$^+$-channels on off-center bipolar cells allowing the inward movement of Na$^+$, and thus causing depolarization. Acting on on-center cells, glutamate either opens K$^+$-channels or closes cGMP-gated Na$^+$-channels, resulting in hyperpolarization. (Modified from Kandel, Schwartz, and Jessel, 2000.)

inhibit the on-center ganglion cells while exciting the off-center ganglion cells.

Each rod or cone in the on-center area synapses in an on-center and off-center bipolar cell (Fig. 11.20). In the dark, rods and cones are depolarized, and glutamate is released. In light, the rods and cones are hyperpolarized, which closes the voltage-gated Ca^{2+} channels and reduces the release of glutamate. Glutamate affects the on-center and off-center bipolar cells differently. The decreased release of glutamate disinhibits the on-center bipolar cells allowing them to become depolarized. Conversely, decreased glutamate release causes the off-center bipolar cells to become hyperpolarized. These differential effects of glutamate on bipolar cells is due to its effects on different cation channels. On off-center bipolar cells, glutamate opens a Na$^+$-channel allowing Na$^+$ to enter the cell; in on-center bipolar cells, glutamate either opens a K$^+$-channel or closes a cGMP-gated Na$^+$-channel.

Amacrine and horizontal cells function as interneurons providing lateral inputs within the retina. Horizontal cells receive input from the photoreceptors and project to surrounding bipolar cells and photoreceptors, whereas amacrine cells receive input from bipolar cells and project laterally to surrounding ganglion cells, bipolar cells, and other amacrine cells. When the off-center area is illuminated, horizontal cells hyperpolarize the on-center bipolar cells. Similarly, information from surrounding bipolar cells is conveyed to on-center ganglion cells by amacrine cells.

Light or dark adaptation

The eye adapts to a sudden increase in light intensity by decreasing its sensitivity, a process called light adaptation. While light adaptation involves contraction of the pupil to restrict the amount of light reaching the retina, and bleaching of photopigments, the two most important changes occur in the cone photoreceptors. Bright light causes the cGMP-gated channels to close, thus hyperpolarizing the cells to approximately −70 mV. If bright light continues, the cells slowly depolarize to between −70 and −40 mV so that they are again responsive to light. In addition, cones become desensitized so that the smallest change in light intensity that can be detected by the cell increases with prolonged exposure to light.

Dark adaptation is essentially the reverse of light adaptation. When an animal moves to a relatively dark area, photosensitivity is slowly restored as the rod photopigments regenerate. Cones essentially stop functioning in low-intensity light, so animals can perceive only black, white, and shades of gray. Cats have more rods than cones, making their night vision and motion detection superior to that of humans.

Visual pathway

There are many more rods and cones than bipolar cells, so these photoreceptors converge on bipolar cells, which send signals to the ganglion cells. The axons of the ganglion cells project to the back of the eyeball converging to form the optic nerve. At the optic chiasma, fibers from the medial portion of the eye cross to the opposite side and continue via the optic tracts (Fig. 11.21). Therefore, each optic tract contains fibers from the temporal (lateral) aspect of the eye on the ipsilateral side and fibers from the nasal (medial) aspect of the contralateral eye. Each eye is carrying information from the same half of the visual field from each eye. Since the lens reverses all images, the medial half of each retina receives light rays from the lateral portion of the visual field while the lateral half of each retina receives light rays from the medial portion of the visual field. Therefore, the right optic tract carries signals representing the left half of the visual field and the left optic tract carries signals from the right visual field.

The axons of ganglion cells make up the optic nerve, which crosses at the optic chiasma. Most of these axons then travel to the lateral geniculate body of the thalamus, where they synapse on second-order neurons that travel through the internal capsule forming the optic radiation. These fibers project to the primary visual cortex in the occipital lobes.

Some fibers in the optic tract project to the superior colliculi, which is involved in visual reflexes control-

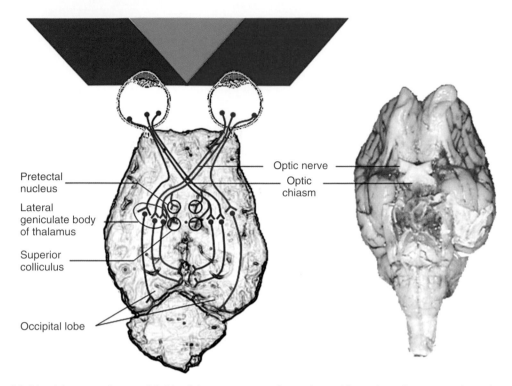

Fig. 11.21. Visual fields of the eyes. The visual fields of the two eyes overlap in the middle, indicated in green. The pathway of signals generated in the retina of the right and left eye are indicated by red and blue lines, respectively.

ling the extrinsic muscle of the eye. Other fibers project to the pretectal nucleus, which is involved in pupil light reflexes, and to the suprachiasmatic nucleus of the hypothalamus, which is involved in circadian rhythms.

Hearing and balance

Anatomy of the ear

The ear consists of three regions: the outer, middle, and inner ear. The outer ear, also called the external ear, collects sound waves and directs them to the middle ear. The middle ear carries these sound waves to the inner ear, and the inner ear contains receptors for hearing and equilibrium.

Outer (external) ear

The outer ear consists of the pinna, or auricle, and the external acoustic meatus (Fig. 11.22). The pinna is a fleshy appendage attached to the lateral surfaces of the skull by muscles and ligaments. It is mobile and funnels sound waves toward the external auditory meatus. Hairs and specialized sebaceous (oil) glands called ceruminous glands that secrete earwax are found near the entrance of the external auditory meatus. The hair and earwax function to restrict the entrance of foreign materials such as dust.

Middle ear

Separated from the outer ear by the tympanic membrane, a thin, semitransparent membrane, the middle ear is an air-filled cavity within the temporal bone (Fig. 11.23). It is separated from the inner ear by two openings, the superiorly located oval window and the round window. Extending from the tympanic membrane to the oval window are three auditory ossicles called the malleus, incus, and stapes, or commonly called the hammer, anvil, and stirrup, respectively. These bones are connected by synovial joints. The handle of the malleus is attached to the inner surface of the tympanic membrane and its head is attached to the body of the incus. The incus articulates with the head of the stapes, whose footplate then fits into the oval windows.

Two small muscles also attach to the auditory ossicles. The tensor tympani muscle restricts the movement and increases tension on the tympanic membrane to minimize damage to the inner ear from loud noises. The stapedius muscle, the smallest skeletal muscle, attenuates large vibrations of the stapes in response to loud noises.

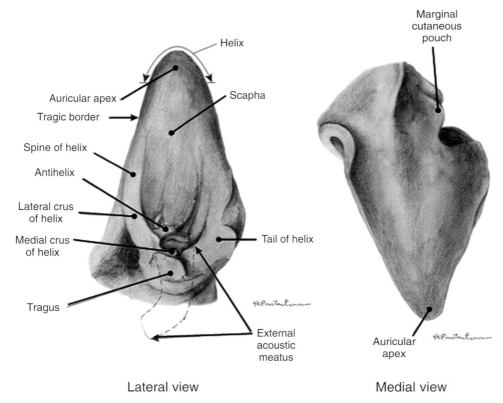

Lateral view   Medial view

Fig. 11.22. Outer ear of the dog. (Reprinted from Constantinescu, 2002. Used by permission of the publisher.)

Inner ear

The inner ear is sometimes called the labyrinth because of its extensive series of canals (Fig. 11.23). It consists of two main sections, an outer bony labyrinth enclosing an inner membranous labyrinth. The bony labyrinth lies in the temporal bone and consists of three areas: 1) the semicircular canals, 2) the vestibule, and 3) the cochlea. The first two contain receptors for equilibrium, and the cochlea contains receptors for hearing. The bony labyrinth is lined with periosteum and is filled with perilymph. Perilymph is similar to cerebrospinal fluid. The membranous labyrinth is lined with epithelium and contains endolymph, which contains a relatively high level of K^+ ions.

The vestibule is the central region of the bony labyrinth. The parts of the membranous labyrinth within the vestibule are the utricle (little bag) and saccule (little sac), which are connected by a short duct. Projecting from the vestibule are three semicircular canals, called the anterior, posterior, and lateral semicircular canals. They lie at a right angle to the other. There is a swollen enlargement at one end of each semicircular canal called the ampulla (saclike duct). The membranous labyrinth within each semicircular canal is called the semicircular ducts, which are continuous with the utricle and saccule.

The cochlea (snail-shaped), a bony spiral canal resembling a snail shell, lies anterior to the vestibule. The cochlea makes nearly three spirals around a bony core called the modiolus. If uncoiled and cut in cross section, the cochlea consists of three channels. Beginning at the oval window, the upper channel is the scala vestibuli. The lower channel is the scala tympani, which ends at the round window. These two channels contain perilymph and are continuous with one another, connecting at the apex of the cochlea, the helicotrema. The third channel, lying between the other two, is the cochlear duct, or scala media. The cochlear duct is separated from the scala vestibuli by the vestibular membrane and from the scala tympani by the basilar membrane.

The spiral organ, or organ of Corti, sits on the basilar membrane. It consists of epithelial cells, supporting cells, and hair cells, the receptors for hearing (Fig. 11.24). There are two groups of hair cells. There is a single row of inner hair cells and three rows of outer hair cells. On the apical (top) surface of each hair cell is a hair bundle consisting of many stereocilia and one long kinocilium, which are in contact with a flexible,

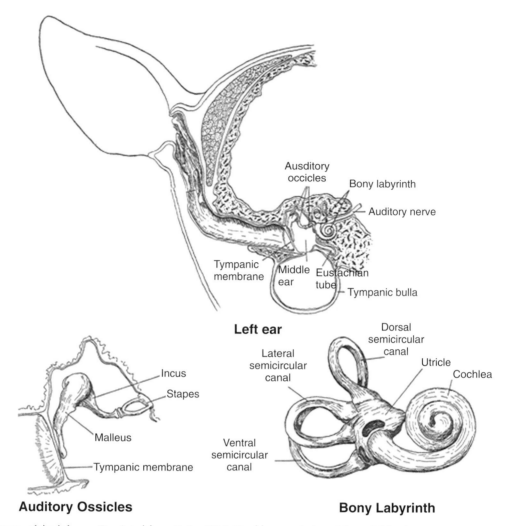

Fig. 11.23. Anatomy of the left ear. (Reprinted from Getty, 1964. Used by permission of the publisher.)

gelatinous membrane called the tectorial membrane. At their basal (bottom) end, each hair cell synapses with first-order sensory neurons and with motor neurons from the cochlear branch of the vestibulocochlear nerve (cranial nerve VIII). The cell bodies of these sensory neurons reside in the spiral ganglion. The inner hair cells synapse with approximately 90% of the first-order sensory neurons; 90% of the motor neurons synapse with outer hair cells.

Sound

Sound waves appear as sine waves traveling through a medium such as air or water. Originating from a vibrating object, the pitch is related to the frequency of the sound wave while the intensity is related to the amplitude of the sound wave. The higher the fre-

quency, the higher the pitch. Similarly, the higher the amplitude, the louder the sound.

Physiology of hearing

The act of hearing can be described as follows:

1. The auricle collects the sound waves into the external meatus.
2. These sound waves strike the tympanic membrane causing it to vibrate.
3. The central region of the tympanic membrane makes contact with the malleus, causing it to vibrate. This causes the incus and stapes to vibrate in succession.
4. The stapes makes contact with the oval window causing it to vibrate. The sound wave is thus

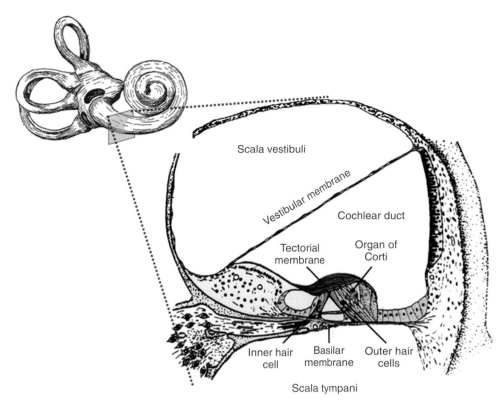

Fig. 11.24. Section through the cochlea. A transverse section through the cochlea reveals its three channels, including the scala vestibule, which is continuous with the scala tympani, and the cochlear duct, which lies in between. The spiral organ (organ of Corti) rests on the basilar membrane. It consists of a single row of inner hair cells and three rows of outer hair cells, which project into the tectorial membrane.

transferred to the perilymph in the scala vestibuli located in the cochlea.

5. This sound wave moves through the scala vestibuli, around the helicotrema, and into the scala tympani, which finally causes the round window to vibrate. This sound wave causes the basilar membrane to move up and down.

6. Since the cilia and kinocilia of the hair cells are embedded in the stationary tectorial membrane, as the basilar membrane oscillates, it causes the cilia and kinocilia on the hair cells to shear.

7. If the hair cells shear toward the kinocilia, the hair cell is depolarized, whereas shearing away from the kinocilia causes hyperpolarization.

Depending on the frequency, or pitch, of the sound wave, it causes different regions of the basilar membrane to oscillate. Higher-frequency sounds cause the basilar membrane closest to the round window to vibrate; lower-frequency waves cause the region near the helicotrema to oscillate. The stimulation of hair cells near the round window is associated with high-pitch sounds; those near the helicotrema are associated with low-pitch sounds.

Physiology of equilibrium

In addition to hearing, the ear is involved in the sense of balance. Receptors in the semicircular canals and vestibule collectively make up the vestibular apparatus, the part of the ear associated with equilibrium. There are two types of equilibrium: static and dynamic. Static equilibrium refers to the maintenance of the position of the body while not moving, whereas dynamic equilibrium is the maintenance of body position in response to sudden movements such as acceleration, deceleration, and rotation.

Otolithic organs within the utricle and saccule

On the walls of both the utricle and saccule is a thickened area called the macula. These are perpendicular to one another and are mostly involved in static equilibrium, but they also have a role in dynamic equilibrium since they respond to linear acceleration, but not to rotation. They provide sensory information about the position of the head in space and thereby function in posture and equilibrium.

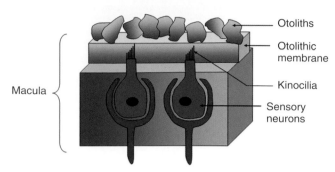

Macula

Otoliths
Otolithic membrane
Kinocilia
Sensory neurons

Fig. 11.25. The macula. The macula is a sensory apparatus found in the utricle and saccule. The sensory neurons have hair cells called stereocilia that project into the gelatinous otolithic membrane. The longest stereocilia is called the kinocilia. Embedded in the otolithic membrane are grains of calcium carbonate called otoliths.

Each macula consists of a bed of supporting cells surrounding scattered hair cells. The hair cells have many sterocilia and a single kinocilium projecting from their apex. The hair cells are embedded in an overlying otolithic membrane (Fig. 11.25). The otolithic membrane is a jellylike mass on which crystals of calcium carbonate called otoliths (ear stones) are present. The otoliths provide inertia to the otolithic membrane, which resists any change in motion.

As the head starts or stops moving in a linear direction, the otoliths cause the otolithic membrane to shear in the opposite direction, much like the head falls backward when one suddenly accelerates forward in a car. This shearing of the otolithic membrane causes the hair cells projecting into the membrane to bend in the opposite direction of movement. When the hair cells bend toward the single kinocilium, they depolarize; bending in the opposite direction causes hyperpolarization. While the hair cells continuously release neurotransmitters, a change in membrane potential alters the release of the neurotransmitter released by these receptors. This changes the rate of impulse in the vestibular nerve, a subdivision of cranial nerve VIII.

Remember, the macula responds only to changes in linear acceleration of the head. The hair cells adapt quickly, so they do not respond while the head is stationary.

The crista ampularis and dynamic equilibrium

The crista ampularis, located in the ampulla of each semicircular canal, is the receptor for dynamic equilibrium. Like the macula, the crista ampularis consists of supporting cells and hair cells. The hair cells have sterocilia and one kinocilium that project into a gelatinous mass called the capula.

The crista ampularis responds to changes in velocity of rotation of the head. The inertia exerted by the endolymph in the semicircular canals causes the hair cells to bend in the opposite direction of movement. As in the macula, this causes either depolarization or hyperpolarization of the hair cells, thus changing the release of the neurotransmitter.

Signals from the semicircular canals are important in vestibular nystagmus, a reflex movement of the eyes. As the head rotates, the eyes drift in the opposite direction as if fixed on an object. After a time, the eyes rapidly jump toward the direction of rotation and establish a new fixation point. This type of eye movement continues until the endolymph comes to rest.

References

Budras, K-D., W.O. Sack, and S. Rock. 2003. Anatomy of the Horse. An Illustrated Text. Schlütersche GmbH & Co., Hannover, Germany.

Constantinescu, G.M. 2001. Guide to Regional Ruminant Anatomy Based on the Dissection of the Goat. Iowa State Press, Ames, Iowa.

Constantinescu, G.M. 2002. Clinical Anatomy for Small Animal Practitioners. Iowa State Press, Ames, Iowa.

Constantinescu, G.M. and I.A. Constantinescu. 2004. Clinical Dissection Guide for Large Animals, Horse and Large Ruminants, 2nd edition. Iowa State Press, Ames, Iowa.

Getty, R. 1964. Atlas for Applied Veterinary Anatomy. Iowa State Press, Ames, Iowa.

Kandel, E.R., J.H. Schwartz, and T.M. Jessel. 2000. Principles of Neural Science. McGraw Hill, New York.

Martini, F.H. 2004. Fundamentals of Anatomy and Physiology, 6th edition. Benjamin Cummings, San Francisco.

Pasquini, C., T. Spurgeon, and S. Pasquini. 1995. Anatomy of Domestic Animals, 8th edition. SUDZ Publishing, Pilot Point, Texas.

Swenson, J.J. and W.O. Reece. 1993. Duke's Physiology of Domestic Animals, 11th edition. Cornell University Press, Ithaca, New York.

12 Endocrine system

Contents

Introduction and overview

As we consider regulation of homeostasis, two closely linked interacting physiological systems, the nervous and endocrine system, are probably most involved. As a general theme, actions mediated by the nervous system are characteristically acute and relatively short-lived, whereas endocrine effects are often slow to develop but can generate responses that continue for hours or even weeks. Some simple examples illustrate these points. Consider what happens with overheating. As the core body temperature rises, the warmer blood flowing to the hypothalamus and other brain areas initiates nerve impulses relayed by efferent spinal nerve tracts to the smooth muscle sphincters of the arterioles controlling blood flow to the dermis. This produces relaxation and therefore increased blood flow so that heat can be lost. Nerve fibers also stimulate the secretion of dermal sweat glands. These events increase flow of warm blood near the body surface, and the release and evaporation of sweat act to lower temperature and thereby return body temperature to its usual limits. These reactions occur very quickly.

Let's now consider how changes in the two hormones calcitonin (CT) and parathyroid hormone (PTH) act to regulate circulating concentrations of calcium. Decreases in calcium stimulate the release of PTH. PTH in turn directly impacts bone and the kidney and indirectly the GI tract. In the bone, PTH stimulates the secretion calcium into extracellular fluids and ultimately blood by promoting the resorption of inorganic bone matrix by osteocytes and osteoblasts. In the kidney, PTH acts on the cells of the distal convoluted tubules of the nephrons to increase the recovery of calcium from the filtrate at the expense of phosphate secretion. PTH also promotes the absorption of calcium from the lumen of the gut because it promotes activation of vitamin D, needed for maximal activity of calcium transport proteins in the gut enterocytes. CT is secreted in situations when circulating calcium concentrations are too high. Its targets are primarily in osseous tissue where it promotes the deposition of calcium. However, it seems clear that the capacity to maintain calcium concentrations within a relatively narrow range is increased by having regulators that act specifically when concentrations are either too low or too high. As you might well predict, responses that require synthesis of enzymes (i.e., bone resorption) or stimulation of transporter proteins (GI tract), are likely to occur over prolonged periods compared with neural effects.

However, it is not accurate to carry this generalization too far. For example, when dairy animals are prepared for milking, auditory cues (clanging of the milking equipment) and/or tactile stimulation to clean the udder and teats for milking machine attachment stimulate the secretion of oxytocin from the posterior pituitary. Upon arrival in the mammary tissue, oxytocin binds to receptors on the myoepithelial cells that surround the mammary alveoli. This causes the contraction of the myoepithelial cells. Since they are arranged in a network around the alveoli, this reduces volume, increases internal pressure, and forces milk into larger ducts and to the teat or nipple end for harvesting. In reality this is a neuroendocrine reflex. That is, neural input to the hypothalamus ultimately causes secretion of oxytocin that promotes milk ejection. It is clear that an intimate relationship between the nervous system and endocrine system is necessary for this event to occur. Moreover, this endocrine-mediated effect is very rapid. The moral is simple; homeostasis is possible only because of the functional coordination between the nervous and endocrine systems.

Cell signaling

The complex interface between the nervous and endocrine systems continues at the cellular level. You have already learned that many neurotransmitters act by binding to receptors on the surface of postsynaptic cells. These binding reactions ultimately induce a biochemical process in the target cells that, if sufficient, causes the generation of an action potential in that cell.

A substance that binds to a receptor is called a ligand, for example, when insulin binds to its specific receptor on the surface of a liver cell. However, this can become complicated. If we stick with the insulin family, there are other hormones called insulinlike growth factors, i.e., insulinlike growth factor one (IGF-I) and insulinlike growth factor two (IGF-II). Based on the names, you would likely suspect that these growth factors must have some attributes that are similar to insulin. You would be correct. These molecules have similar but *not identical* structures. This means that insulin can also bind to specific IGF-I receptors on target cells. However, this usually is not physiologically important because the affinity (a measure of how easily the binding occurs) of the binding is much less than for IGF-I. You can envision the relevance of affinity this way: A ligand with high affinity for a receptor occupies a greater proportion of the receptors at a much lower concentration than if the ligand for the receptor has a low affinity for the receptor. Does this have practical significance? The answer is absolutely yes.

For example, at normal circulating concentrations insulin molecules would rarely interact with an IGF-I receptor. However, with diabetes or other situations when insulin concentrations are chronically increased, the greater abundance of insulin molecules can "overcome" the fact that insulin has low affinity for the IGF-I receptor. As another example, many synthetic steroids have been engineered so that they have greater affinity for receptors than the native molecule, i.e., testosterone versus synthetic anabolic steroids.

The classic definition of a hormone is as follows. A hormone is a signaling molecule that is secreted by a ductless (endocrine) gland into the bloodstream where it travels to a site some distance away and acts on a target cell. Except for the transport period in the bloodstream, this pattern is not different from regulators that are secreted in the extracellular fluid to act on target cells only a few millimeters or μm away from the site of production? At the mechanistic level there are many parallels between the effects of neurotransmitters, classic hormones, and growth factors. Indeed, as understanding has evolved it is now recognized that many growth factor, hormone or neurotransmitter-like molecules can impact target cells at multiple levels.

For example, a paracrine action refers to a molecule released from a signaling cell that acts to impact neighboring cells. An example of this is the production of

Table 12.1. Major structural classes of surface-acting hormone receptors.

Seven-Transmembrane Domain Receptors
β-adrenergic
Parathyroid hormone (PTH)
Luteinizing hormone (LH)
Thyroid-stimulating hormone (TSH)
Glucagon
Growth hormone–releasing hormone (GHRH)
Thyrotropin-releasing hormone (TRH)
Adrenocortotropic hormone (ACTH)
Melanocyte-stimulating hormone (MSH)

Single-Transmembrane Receptors
Insulin
Insulinlike growth factor one (IGF-I)
Epidermal growth factor (EGF)
Platelet-derived growth factor (PDGF)

Cytokine Receptor Super Family
Growth hormone (GH)
Prolactin (Prl)
Leptin
Erythropoietin
Interleukins

Guanyl Cyclase-Linked Receptors
Natriuretic peptides

IGF-I by stromal cells of the mammary gland. This growth factor subsequently stimulates the epithelial cells of the adjacent mammary ducts or alveoli. Autocrine stimulation indicates that the signaling molecule impacts the same cells that produced the molecule. Juxtacrine refers to the stimulation of immediately adjacent cells.

Both neurotransmitter and peptide hormones interact primarily with receptors located in the plasma membrane of the target cells. For these regulators this means that this binding event triggers biochemical changes inside the target cells that are responsible for the hormone effects that are observed. Since the hormone or ligand does not enter the target cell, this pattern of action is known as a second messenger mechanism. In other words the hormone binding to the receptor is the "first" message and the biochemical mediator released inside the target cell is the "second" messenger. Our goal is not to overwhelm you with details, but we think it is important to have some appreciation of the various biochemical pathways that are involved in explaining how surface-acting hormones function. We begin by illustrating some of the types of surface receptors.

As shown in Table 12.1, based primarily on structure these receptors (remember, they are all proteins) can be grouped into the four classes. Seven-transmem-brane domain receptors are one of the largest groups. These receptors all contain an amino terminal piece or domain followed by seven hydrophobic segments that form loops that span the plasma membrane. The last of the seven loops ends in a hydrophilic domain that protrudes into the cytoplasmic portion of the cell. So you can imagine a bit of the receptor protein at the outer surface of the cells and a bit protruding into the cytoplasm of the cell. Most of these receptors rely on the activation of G proteins to elicit their effects. Examples of these are receptors including those for PTH, luteinizing hormone (LH), and melanocyte stimulating hormone (MSH).

A second class of receptors is single-transmembrane domain receptors. These receptors span the plasma membrane and have intrinsic tyrosine kinase activity—in other words, the binding of the ligand to receptor activates enzyme action. Recall that kinases are involved in phosphorylation reactions. This group includes insulin, IGF-I, epidermal growth factor (EGF) and others.

A third group is structurally similar to the second, but the receptors have no intrinsic tyrosine kinase activity. Instead, functional activity depends on ligand binding causing the activation of soluble transducer molecules located in the cytoplasm. In this case, ligand binding causes molecules in the cytoplasm to interact with the receptor, which then produces a cascade of reactions. Receptors for prolactin (Prl) and growth hormone (GH) are this type of receptor.

A fourth group acts via guanylyl cyclase or adenylyl cyclase and synthesis of cGMP or cAMP, respectively. Epinephrine, for example, binds to its surface receptor and in conjunction with a stimulatory G protein activates adenylyl cyclase, which causes the conversion of ATP to cAMP. This pathway was the first example demonstrating the second messenger mechanism of hormone action. Figure 12.1 provides a schematic view of the structural variations between these types of surface receptors.

Mechanisms of cell surface hormone signaling

In addition to classification based on structure, receptor proteins for hormones, growth factors, and neurotransmitters are also defined by the signal transduction method that is employed. Ion-channel–linked receptors common in the nervous system are involved in rapid signaling, usually between electrically excitable cells. G protein–linked receptors function by modifying the activity of a separate plasma membrane anchored protein, which may be an enzyme or may act as an ion channel (Fig. 12.2). Briefly, interac-

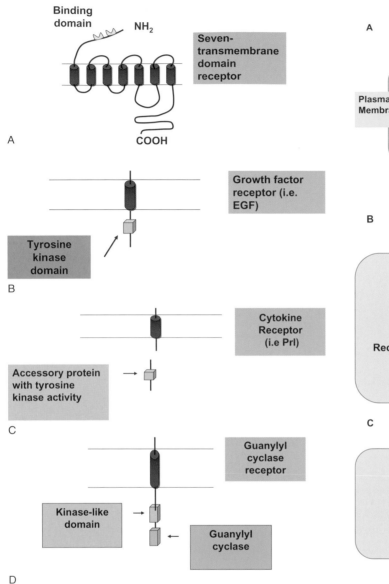

Fig. 12.1. A schematic view of the structural variations between types of cell surface receptors. From top to bottom are illustrations of (A) a seven-transmembrane domain receptor, (B) a single-transmembrane domain receptor with kinase activity typical of many growth factors, (C) receptors with no intrinsic tyrosine kinase activity but activation by soluble transducer molecules, and (D) receptors dependent on guanylyl cyclase or adenylyl cyclase and synthesis of cGMP or cAMP.

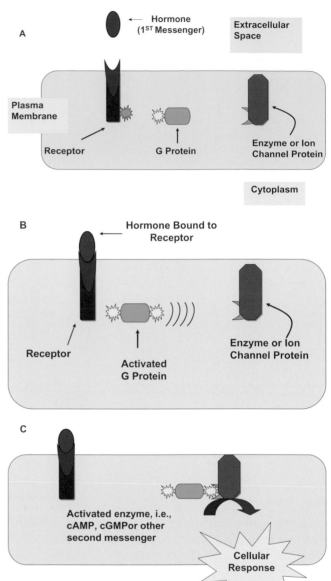

Fig. 12.2. Example of a G protein–linked hormone mechanism of action. Activation of the receptor is induced by the binding of the hormone (1st messenger) (Panel A). This leads to a conformational change in the cytoplasmic tail of the receptor to allow binding of a complementary G protein and activation (Panel B). This activated complex links to a second membrane-bound protein (enzyme or ion channel) to increase the intracellular concentration of an intracellular mediator (second messenger), which is responsible for the effect associated with hormone action (Panel C).

tion between the receptor and the anchored membrane protein is mediated by the action of a third protein, a trimeric GTP-binding protein (G protein). If this target protein is the enzyme type, activation alters the concentration of an intracellular mediator (e.g., cyclic GMP, cyclic AMP, diacylglycerol, or inositol triphosphate). It should be understood that G protein hormone-mediated effects can be inhibitory or stimulatory. The illustration in Figure 12.3 depicts a response

if a stimulatory G protein variant (G_s) is activated in response to hormone binding. The result is an increase in the intracellular concentration of a second messenger molecule.

Let's suppose, however, that the illustrated target cell also has receptors for another hormone whose effect is mediated by an inhibitory G protein variant

(G$_i$) and that the second messenger molecule is the same. In this case hormone binding to the receptor would activate G$_i$ with the effect of inhibiting the production of the second messenger. This suggests that the overall response of the cell to these two hormones would depend on the relative concentration of the two receptors on the cell surface and ratio of circulating concentrations of the two hormones in the blood available to interact. This possibility is illustrated in Figure 12.3.

As Figure 12.3 suggests, complex interactions control the concentrations of even a single second messenger molecule in target cells. Just imagine the possible control points. Using this illustration as an example, what regulates the rate of synthesis of G proteins or the rate at which cAMP molecules are degraded? What about the rate of synthesis of the adenylyl cyclase enzyme or expression of the receptor subtypes? On the other side of the coin how many molecules of the hormones are available in the blood to bind to the receptors on the cell surface? Overlap in signaling pathways, changes in secretion of hormones, and alterations in expression of cell receptors provide many opportunities for regulation of cell response to hormones or growth factors.

Common membrane enzymes regulated by G proteins include adenylyl cyclase and phospholipase C. Changes in the activity state of adenylyl cyclase depend on G$_s$ or G$_i$ proteins to influence capacity of the enzyme to convert ATP to cyclic AMP (cAMP). Cyclic AMP binds to a cytosolic protein, cyclic AMP dependent protein kinase (A-Kinase). This allows regulatory protein (subunits) to detach from inactive A-Kinase. These active enzymes cause phosphorylation of proteins unique to particular target cells. These phosphorylated proteins have potent biochemical effects, including activation of other enzymes or gene activation.

Other G proteins function by activating (or inhibiting) the inositol phospholipid-signaling pathway. Effects are initiated by hormone receptor binding which allows binding to an inactive G protein. Binding of GTP displaces GDP and the G protein is activated. Activated G protein translocates within the plasma membrane and activates phospholipase C (PLC). PLC cleaves the phospholipid phosphoinositol 4,5-bisphosphate (PIP2) to yield diacylglycerol (DAG) and inositol 1,4,5-triphosphate (IP3). DAG activates specific protein kinases and IP3 triggers the release of Ca2+ ions. Increased Ca2+ stimulates activity of specific enzymes, thus acting as a second messenger or it binds the regulatory protein calmodulin.

Other binding reactions lead to the activation of guanylate cyclase. This enzyme catalyzes the conversion of GTP into cyclic GMP (cGMP), which can act as

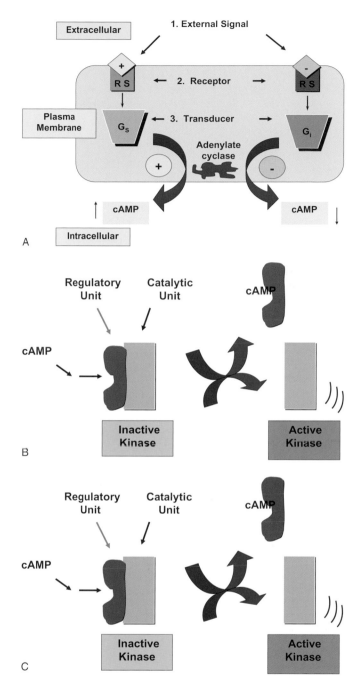

Fig. 12.3. Stimulatory versus inhibitory G proteins. In this example the target cell expresses receptors for two hormones, both of which impact the synthesis of the second messenger cyclic AMP. However, one induces the activation of a stimulatory G protein (G$_s$) and the other an inhibitory G protein (G$_i$). This suggests that the balance between the actions of these two antagonistic pathways controls pathways affected by cAMP abundance. What would you predict if the expression of receptors for one of the hormones suddenly tripled? The lower portion of the figure illustrates a possible model for activation of a kinase enzyme with increased free cAMP concentrations. The cAMP binds to a regulatory subunit allowing the catalytic subunit to phosphorylate its substrate protein. Changes in phosphorylation state can either stimulate or inhibit the actions of the target protein (depending on the particular protein).

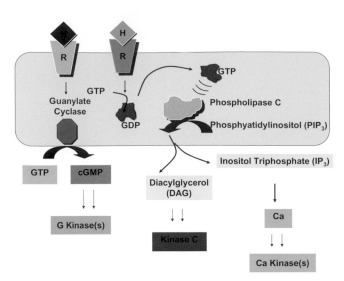

Fig. 12.4. Phospholipase C signaling pathways. A variety of second messengers, DAG, IP3, and Ca, can be produced by factors that stimulate phospholipase C in the plasma membrane.

a second messenger like cAMP. Some of these other second messengers are illustrated in Figure 12.4. To finish our discussion of G proteins, if the target protein acts as an ion channel, activation acts to change permeability of the membrane for that ion. The G protein-linked receptors make a very large family of surface receptors, including the oxytocin receptor we discussed earlier related to the milk ejection reflex.

A third class of surface-acting signaling molecules is composed of the enzyme-linked receptors. Essentially, the binding of the hormone to the receptor activates the receptor (or directly linked protein) so that it is capable of phosphorylating cellular proteins. Phosphorylation alters activity of the affected protein. Some agriculturally relevant signaling molecules include the mammary active regulators IGF-I, insulin, EGF, and vascular endothelial growth factor (VEGF); these are all examples of tyrosine-specific protein kinases (Butler et al., 1998: Adams et al., 2000).

To illustrate some of the cellular and molecular detail of these receptor types we focus on the interaction of IGF-I and its receptor. IGF-I is an excellent example of a receptor kinase. Second, IGF-I is important in animal agriculture and medicine. IGFs are intimately tied to normal development (muscle growth, mammary growth, and reproduction), diabetes, and some cancers. In animal agriculture, growth is critical and use of GH as a tool to increase milk production and development is also linked to IGFs (Akers, 2006). Figure 12.5 illustrates an example of one of these receptor types, specifically the insulin and insulinlike growth factor receptors.

IGF-I and IGF-II regulate cell growth, cell differentiation, maintenance of cell function, and prevention of apoptosis. Research with IGF-I and IGF-II was initially centered on the somatomedin hypothesis, which proposed that these growth factors mediated somatotropin (GH) effects on postnatal growth. Since those early experiments, the view has evolved that the IGFs are also important local actors. These peptides can interact with several related cell surface receptors. The primary signaling receptor for IGF-I (IGF-IR) is a tyrosine kinase receptor structurally similar to the insulin receptor. Members of this family of proteins share a heterotetrameric structure. IGF-IR binds with IGF-I with high affinity (Kd ~1 nM), but affinity for insulin binding is about 500 times lower.

IGF-II binds with high affinity to a receptor that is identical with a receptor for mannose-6-phosphate, but the receptor has no known intracellular signaling function. The affinity of this receptor for IGF-I is about a hundredfold lower than for IGF-II and it does not recognize insulin.

For IGF-I binding to its receptor to be effective, two cellular processes must come together. First, the binding reaction must transmit a signal through the plasma membrane to regulatory molecules located on the cytoplasmic face of the membrane. Second, a signal is needed to cause localization and interaction of the internal receptor domain with downstream effector molecules of the signal transduction cascade. Activation of IGF-IR produces intracellular molecules that mediate at least four distinct, but overlapping, signaling pathways. This likely explains multiple effects linked to IGF-I activation reported in various cell types or in the same cell type under differing physiological conditions.

In addition to receptors and the intracellular signaling cascade, there are also six IGF-I binding proteins (IGFBPs) and nine related proteins (IGFBP-rP) that affect the actions of IGF-I (Clemmons, 1998).

Mechanisms of action for prolactin (Prl) and growth hormone (GH), two protein hormones with long-recognized importance in growth and development and mammary function have only recently been elucidated. Prolactin receptor (PrlR) and growth hormone receptor (GHR) are simple proteins with a single transmembrane domain. The hormone has two sites capable of binding to its receptor protein. Initially the hormone binds (site 1) to create an inactive complex. This hormone-receptor complex then diffuses within the membrane to bind with a second receptor (site 2). This causes receptor homodimerization and formation of an active complex. (Fig. 12.6). Although it had been known that stimulation with Prl or GH caused tyrosine phosphorylation of a number of cellular proteins, the cytoplasmic domains of the receptors have no inherent enzymatic activity. This means that hormone binding and dimer formation must activate other kinases. A breakthrough came with the discovery

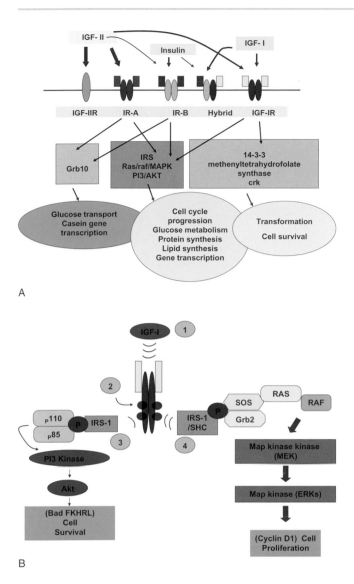

Fig. 12.5. Diagram of components of the insulin and IGF family of proteins and receptors. Panel A illustrates binding of IGF-I, IGF-II, and insulin to related receptors. The thickness of the arrows varies with affinity of binding. Phosphorylation signaling cascades linked to binding of ligands to different receptors. Cellular events most closely related to receptor binding are shown, but the overlap in binding, signaling, and response is also apparent. The example is on activities in mammary tissue, but similar responses also occur in other tissues. Panel B illustrates some of the details of the signal transduction pathways for IGF-I. Of course, the process is initiated by binding of IGF-I to its receptor (1); this leads to autophosphorylation tyrosine residues of the β subunits of the receptor (2, blacked circles). This phosphorylation cascade allows for binding of IRS proteins (3) and their phosphorylation. This change makes available binding sites for recruitment of other intracellular signaling molecules (i.e., the p85 and p110 subunits of PI3 Kinase), resulting in enzymatic activity that converts membrane-bound lipids like 3,4-inositol phosphate into active second-messenger molecules (inositol triphosphate). These molecules combine with phosphoinositide-dependent kinase-1 to activate AKT. AKT signaling is linked with IGF-I stimulation of protein synthesis. PI3K-linked signaling is associated with inhibition of apoptosis (as described in the text) as well as IGF-I stimulation of glucose transport. In addition to this pathway, IRS-1 with SHC binds to the receptor and is phosphorylated as well (4). Activation of MAPK (Mitogen-activated Protein Kinase) signaling proceeds through recruitment of a complex composed of Grb2 and son of sevenless (SOS), which is recruited from the cytoplasm to the cell membrane. This allows SOS to come in close position to RAS (a GTP-binding protein named for the RAS gene first identified in viruses that cause sarcoma in rats). This catalyzes a RAS GTP/GDP exchange. This then activates RAF kinase, which in turn activates MAPK or MEK1. Targets of this cascade include members of the ETS and forkhead transcription factor families. Regulation ultimately of these transcription factors explains how IGF-I binding to its receptor can produce alterations in gene expressions that modify proliferation, differentiation, and apoptosis in target cells. Figures adapted from Hadsell and Bonnette (2000), Hadsell, et al. (2002), Clemmons and Maile (2003), or LeRoith and Roberts (2003).

that Janus tyrosine kinase 2 (JAK2) is activated after receptor dimerization. This kinase belongs to a family with four members—JAK1, JAK2, JAK3, and Tyk2—each of which act in signaling of various cytokine receptors. For PrlR and GHR, JAK2 is especially important. With PrlR, JAK2 is constitutively associated with the receptor, but with GHR the enzyme associates with the receptor only after hormone binding and dimer formation (Goffin and Kelly, 1997; Hynes et al., 1997).

The signaling pathway depends on JAK2-induced phosphorylation of a transcription factor(s) called signal transducers and activators of transcription (STATs); one of these, STAT5, is specifically for Prl stimulation of the casein gene expression in mammary tissue. When GH, Prl, or IGF-I are added to cultures containing pieces of rat and bovine mammary tissue, STAT5 DNA binding is increased.

It is sometimes easy to dismiss these detailed bio-chemical studies as esoteric. However, basic information derived from studies with our domestic species will yield techniques to improve the control of growth and performance of our animals in unexpected ways. This is a very complex and important area of research. Our goal is not to overwhelm you with details of cell signaling but to give you an appreciation of the intricate, even elegant myriad of controls that are possible in regulation of hormone and growth factor action after they bind to their respective receptors.

Mechanisms of internal hormone cell signaling

Steroid hormones, thyroid hormones, retinoids, and vitamin D are structurally diverse small hydrophobic molecules that pass across the plasma membrane of target cells to act internally.

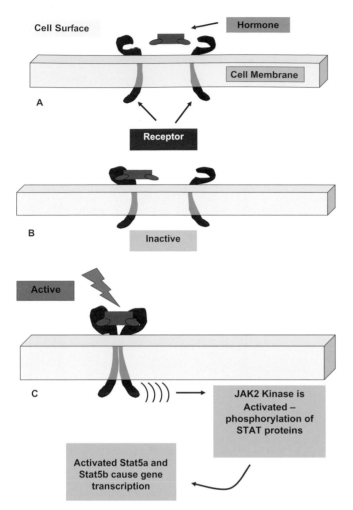

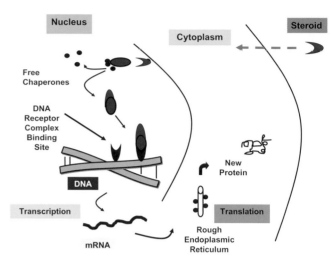

Fig. 12.6. Ligand-induced receptor homodimerization. The hormone first binds with the receptor to create an inactive complex (A). Binding with a second receptor produces a dimer (B). This produces an activated complex (C). The active complex stimulates JAK2 kinase, which phosphorylates Stat proteins. As a dairy example, Stat5a and Stat5b are closely involved in Prl stimulation of specific milk protein gene transcription. Receptor activation can also stimulate other signaling pathways, including mitogen-activated protein (MAP) kinase and protein C kinase (PKC).

Fig. 12.7. Steroid hormone mechanism of action. The hormone diffuses into the nucleus and binds to a receptor-chaperonin complex. Binding allows the chaperone proteins to dissociate and the activated hormone receptor combination binds to specific sites on the DNA. This triggers the transcription of certain genes and production of new mRNA. The new mRNA is translated and new proteins made. The new proteins are responsible for the biological effects of the hormone.

These receptors are believed to have evolved from a gene superfamily and they all act at the cell nucleus. The receptor proteins for these hormones have a hydrophobic region near the C-terminal end of the protein that binds directly to the hormone. A more hydrophilic domain of the receptor binds to DNA when the hormone-receptor complexes translocate to the nucleus. These segments of the receptor are homologous between the various steroid family receptors. Specifically, there are nine highly conserved Cys residues that occur in Cys-X-X-Cys. These repeated sequences create what are called the zinc-finger arrangement so that loops of the protein structure are highly stable. Hormone receptor complexes bind to either DNA directly (promoter regions of genes) or to transcription factors that then interact with genes. Binding releases associated proteins called chaperones so that the newly formed hormone-receptor complex can attach to a specific region of the DNA. This association allows transcription of the gene(s) adjacent to this binding site. Thereafter, transcription of the specific gene(s) occurs and the new mRNA is processed and transported to the ribosome for translation. These newly minted pro-teins are responsible for the hormone effects observed (Fig. 12.7). A reasonable view is that steroid hormone family receptors are essentially ligand-activated transcription factors. A general rule is that responses to these hormones are slower than for the surface-acting peptides.

Evidence for extracellular or surface actions for steroid hormones includes reports of specific binding of radiolabeled steroid hormones to cell membranes and very rapid response that can occur following addition of steroid hormones to target cells. For example, testosterone rapidly stimulates transport of glucose, calcium, and amino acids into kidney cells. There is also evidence for binding of steroid hormones to Gamma Amino Butyric Acid (GABA) receptors in nerve cells and associated rapid changes in ion flow into the cells. Thus some effects linked with steroid hormone action may well depend on surface actions. The point here is to remind you that endocrine research is ongoing, so it is foolish to make dogmatic conclusions about hormone mechanisms of action. New findings and discoveries have to be incorporated into our understanding.

Estrogen, progesterone, cortisol, triiodiothyronine, retinoids, and others are potent stimulators of target cells in domestic animals. Effects of a variety of steroid family hormones will be discussed in subsequent sections as well as in other chapters. The essential feature of this section is to emphasize the primary differences in the mechanism of action for surface-acting versus other hormones.

Receptors and regulation

As you have surmised from your reading to this point, controlling the actions of hormones and growth factors is critical in homeostasis. Alterations in internal cell signaling are important, but it is also important to appreciate general factors that affect the ability of hormones to function. Hormones elicit their biological effects by binding with high-affinity receptors. Ligand binding to its receptor is governed by the law of mass action:

$$[H]+[R] \underset{k-1}{\overset{k+1}{\rightleftarrows}} [HR]$$

In this expression, *[H]* is the hormone concentration, *[R]* is the receptor concentration, and *[HR]* is the concentration of the hormone receptor complex; *k + 1* and *k − 1* are rate constants for creation and dissolution of the [HR] complex, respectively. At equilibrium conditions these terms can be written as follows:

$$\frac{[H][R]}{[HR]} = \frac{k-1}{k+1} = KD$$

KD is the equilibrium dissociation constant, which describes the affinity of the ligand-receptor interaction. The lower the value, the higher the affinity. In practical terms high affinity means that low concentrations on the ligand (hormone or growth factor) are sufficient to bind to the receptor. On average when the concentration of the hormone is equal to the value for the affinity of the receptor, 50% of the receptor will be bound. Typical affinity estimates for common receptors are in the range of 10^{-9} to 10^{-10} M/L. For example, the affinity of prolactin receptor for membranes of mammary cells is about 2×10^{-9} M/L. At the level of the bloodstream this means a concentration of ~50 ng/ml would equal this value. This is relevant because normal blood (basal) concentrations range from a low of about 5 ng/ml to a high of about 75 ng/ml. So the affinity of the receptor ensures that normal

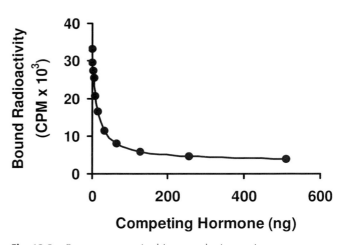

Fig. 12.8. Receptor assay. In this example, increasing concentration of nonradiolabeled prolactin (competing hormone) displaces binding of radiolabeled prolactin to receptors on cell membranes prepared from mammary glands of lactating sheep.

circulating concentrations of prolactin can effectively impact target cells.

You might ask how it is possible to measure the affinity of various receptors for their hormone ligands or to measure very low circulating concentrations of hormones. As is often the case technology advances were critical. Soon after techniques were developed for the radiolabeling of hormones it became clear to a number of researchers that measuring the amount of isotope bound to a target tissue, cells, or cell fractions could be used to estimate the number of receptors. Radiolabeling refers to the incorporation of a radioactive isotope into the hormone. For proteins, iodine is the most common isotope used for this purpose. Analogous to thyroid hormones, which have dietary iodine incorporated into the ring structure of its tyrosine amino acids, test-tube reactions are used to chemically incorporate radiolabeled iodine. If this is done using either I^{125} or I^{131} isotopes of iodine, the protein is effectively labeled or tagged. Assuming the protein is still biologically active, that is that the site where the iodine molecule(s) incorporated does not impair the binding reaction; the newly labeled protein can be used to measure the quantity of receptor in a tissue or cell preparation. This is typically done by allowing the iodinated hormone ("hot" or "tracer" hormone) to bind and then in parallel tubes adding an excess of non-radiolabeled ("cold") hormone. The difference in binding of isotope between samples with and without the competing cold hormone is a relative indicator of receptor number. Figure 12.8 is an example illustrating prolactin receptor binding in the membranes from the ovine mammary gland.

In this example, a series of tubes, all containing equal amounts of cell membrane suspended in buffer, was incubated with the same quantity of radiolabeled hormone (64,500 counts per minute, cpm, per tube equal to 1 ng). Notice in the absence of competition that the membranes bound about half of the total added ~38,000 cpm. Sets of tubes then received increasing quantities of cold hormone ranging from 0 (total binding tubes) to 512 ng per tube. The data presented are the average of three samples at each concentration. After a period of time to reach equilibrium, the tubes were centrifuged. The membrane formed a pellet in the bottom of the tube and the liquid was removed. The amount of radioactivity remaining in the pellets was then measured by placing the samples in a gamma counter. This machine measures the amount of radioactivity in cpm. As you can see, addition of increasing amounts of cold hormone displaced about 90% of the bound radioactivity once the hormone concentration reached about a hundredfold excess (~100 ng) compared with the quantity of radioactively labeled material added. Notice that adding greater quantities of cold hormone have very little further effect. The radioactivity that cannot be competed away even in the presence of excess cold is called nonspecific binding. The radioactivity that is displaced (specific binding) reflects the number of receptor molecules in the sample. In addition, if displacement is studied using either a graded concentration of cold displacement or a saturation of binding using known graded increasing concentrations of tracer, it is possible to calculate the affinity of the binding reaction as well as to estimate the number of receptors.

Specifically, if it is assumed that total receptor concentration R0 = [HR] + [R], the equation given above can be rearranged to give the following expression

$$\frac{[HR]}{[H]} = \left(\frac{[HR]}{KD}\right) + \frac{[RO]}{KD}$$

This is the Scatchard equation, which provides that when the ratio of bound over free ligand ([HR]/[H]) is plotted against bound ligand concentration ([HR]), the slope of the line is defined by $-1/KD$, the y-intercept by R0/KD and the x-intercept by R0. These computational methods, based on knowledge of bound and free concentrations of hormone determined experimentally, give information about the apparent affinity of the receptor and the total concentration of receptors in the preparation. Examples of a saturation curve and Scatchard plot are illustrated in Figure 12.9.

In practice the affinity of a given receptor for its ligand is generally stable; however, the number of receptors can vary dramatically in response to treatments or physiological status. Thus a major mechanism for regulating the effects of a hormone or growth factor is to alter the number of target cell receptors that are synthesized. This is really fundamental when you

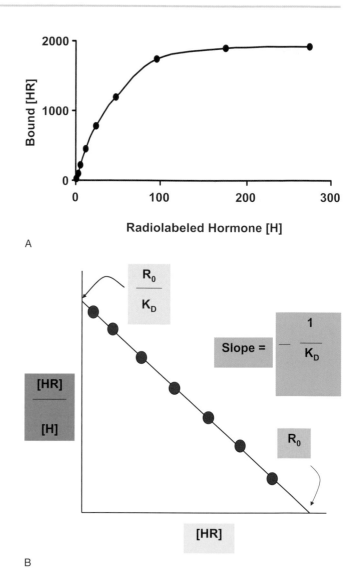

Fig. 12.9. Saturation binding and Scatchard plot. A hypothetical ligand saturation curve (upper) and Scatchard analysis of receptor binding (lower) is shown. The K_D represents the dissociation constant, R0 the total receptor concentration and [HR] and [H] concentrations of the bound and free ligand, respectively.

consider the initial equation describing the law of mass action given above. If the number of available receptors is reduced, and the hormone concentration stays the same, the number of hormone receptor complexes that can be formed is correspondingly reduced. This also suggests that changes in the other element of the equation, hormone concentration or [H], are also important in determining responsiveness. Indeed, circulating concentrations of many hormones are dramatically altered with time or in response to physiological stimuli. For example, in monogastric species, consumption of a meal high in carbohydrates stimulates the secretion of the hormone insulin. This means that the capacity of insulin to drive glucose into storage is improved because of the increased blood concentration. Even if the concentration of insulin receptors is not changed, the effect of insulin is enhanced; this is the essence of the law of mass action. With more insulin, the odds of generating the [HR] complexes are improved. As time passes, the peak in insulin concentrations decreases, so its affect is diminished because of reduced receptor binding.

To summarize, not only are there complex changes in signal transduction pathways that modify hormone responses, changes in hormone receptor number or hormone concentration also modify effectiveness. A change in the number of receptors can result from the synthesis of more hormone receptors, i.e., more mRNA, transcription, and translation, or in some cases by simply making available receptors that were previously unavailable. Such receptors might be bound to other proteins that mask the hormone-binding site. If this inhibitor is removed, the number of available hormone receptors is increased and, everything else being equal, response to the hormone enhanced. As we discuss specific endocrine organs we will provide some examples of changes in receptor number that correspond with alterations in function.

One common response to prolonged increases in circulating concentrations of a particular hormone is receptor down-regulation. This is essentially a homeostatic response to prevent overstimulation. These mechanisms are vital but not foolproof. For example, hypersecretion of growth hormone prior to puberty can lead to gigantism, but after puberty acromegaly can occur. In some breeds of beef cattle, large size and muscle development is at least partially attributed to alteration in the growth hormone–insulinlike growth factor axis. This suggests there has essentially been genetic selection for what was initially a mutation in growth control.

In other cases, increased secretion of a hormone stimulates the synthesis of other hormone receptors. For example, late in gestation as parturition approaches, circulating concentrations of estrogen increase. This leads to an increase in production of oxytocin receptors in the uterus. This increase in estrogen-induced expression of oxytocin receptors means that uterine receptors are available at the appropriate time to promote the birth process, but are not expressed earlier in gestation.

Molecules that bind to receptors with high affinity are classified as either agonists or antagonists. Agonists are ligands that trigger the usual response associated with hormone action. However, if you used the pharmaceutical industry as an example, many drugs act to either mimic or block naturally occurring ligand-binding reactions. The same general idea applies to hormone receptor interactions. Some synthetic versions of steroid hormones are much more potent than the corresponding naturally occurring versions. This

may reflect an increased affinity of the receptor for the analog compound so that more [HR] complexes are maintained therefore enhancing response. Other possibilities are that the analog is longer lived, i.e., not subject to normal degradation pathways or some other mechanism. Antagonists bind to the receptor but fail to activate usual effector mechanisms. Since they occupy the receptor, normal agonists are prevented from action so hormone response declines.

In a few cases, receptors are available in several fold surplus relative to those required for a maximum physiological response. Having these spare receptors seems a waste but it is suggested that this allows a seeming mismatch between low circulating concentrations of the hormone and relatively low affinity receptors to still be effective. Going back to the law of mass action, by increasing the number of available receptors, this guarantees that an adequate number of receptors will be bound for appropriate action despite the presence of less than saturating concentrations of hormone in circulation.

Measuring circulating hormone concentrations

The development of radioimmunoassay (RIA) techniques in the late 1960s and early 1970s ushered in a golden age for the study of endocrine regulation of lactation, reproduction, and growth in domestic animals. Although bioassays had served to establish general themes (changes in pituitary Prl, GH, FSH, or LH in correspondence with major reproductive events, e.g., puberty, pregnancy, lactation), widespread availability of RIA methods for Prl, GH, oxytocin, progesterone, estrogen, and other hormones allowed study of hormone secretion on a scale previously unimagined. These techniques replaced the bioassays and allowed the accurate measurement of circulating blood or tissue concentrations of many hormones. Hormones and growth factors are typically present in only picogram (pg) or nanogram (ng) quantities per milliliter of plasma. For the first time, it became possible to determine correspondence between the secretion rate and pattern of secretion. As an offshoot of methods for radiolabeling purified hormones for use in biochemistry and receptor-binding studies, RIA methods were subsequently developed.

A brief history explains the idea behind the RIA. Dr. Rosalyn Yalow, who was working at the Veterans Administration Hospital, Bronx, New York, was considering the possibility that some of her diabetic patients were producing antibodies against insulin. To test this idea she reasoned that if this were true it could be tested by incubating blood serum from suspect patients with radioactively tagged or labeled insulin.

This was about the time when techniques for radiolabeling proteins for receptor studies were also developed. The idea was that if antibodies against insulin were present, they would bind to the insulin and thereby prevent insulin from having its normal physiological effects. After an incubation period with added radiolabeled insulin, the samples were passed over a gel filtration column. The key point is that antibodies are very large proteins compared to insulin. Radiolabeled insulin that is not bound to an antibody would pass through the column more slowly than insulin in the bound state. Specifically, small molecules are retarded in the column (they can migrate into all small spaces that make up the gel matrix), but large complexes of antibody + insulin would quickly be eluted from the column. Second, Dr. Yalow could estimate rates of passage by measuring the amount of radioactivity in fractions that eluted from the column. If the sample contained antibodies, the rate of passage would be much faster with a control sample. She did find that some diabetic patients made antibodies against insulin.

However, our focus is on what happened later. She and her collaborators started to work on the question of whether antibodies might not be used to somehow measure hormone concentrations. This is similar to the example shown in Figure 12.8, which illustrates the competition of radiolabeled Prl on receptor protein binding sites by adding increasing amounts of nonradiolabeled Prl. Essentially, could antibodies be used to first bind radiolabeled hormone and the rate of competition be used to estimate the amount of hormone in an unknown sample? The answer turned out to be yes. This was a major accomplishment. In fact, Dr. Yalow shared the Nobel Prize for medicine in 1977 for her pioneering efforts to develop RIA for protein hormones. The other winners that year were Drs. Andrew Schally and Roger Guillemin for their competing efforts to discover hypothalamic hormones that control secretion of anterior pituitary hormones.

Several things are required to develop an RIA for measuring hormone concentration. First a source of purified hormone is needed. This was fortuitous in Dr. Yalow's research since insulin has been purified from porcine or bovine pancreatic tissue since the 1930s for use in diabetic patients. (Because of recombinant DNA technology, much of the insulin currently in clinical use utilizes the human insulin gene spliced into *E. coli*). By the way, this biotechnology revolution has altered much more than possibly an esoteric study of endocrinology; an increasing number of agricultural products are produced in this manner—bovine GH or bST to increase milk production or the rennet used in cheese making readily come to mind.

The purified hormone is needed to make the radiolabeled tracer and is used to generate a standard curve in the assay procedure. A source of purified hormone is also necessary to produce antibodies that recognize the hormone under study. The antibody (often simply a dilution of serum from an immunized host animal) that specifically binds to the hormone is called the primary or first antibody. A common RIA technique is called the double antibody RIA. This procedure requires the use of another antibody solution. For example, if guinea pigs were immunized against bovine insulin, the animals would have antibodies that recognize or bind bovine insulin in their bloodstream. Blood or serum samples from these animals could be used to provide the first antibody source needed in an RIA. As part of the procedure, there is also a need for more general antibodies that recognize any guinea pig antibody—in other words, anti–guinea pig gamma globulin antiserum (gamma globulin is the class of proteins to which antibodies belong). Most often a large animal (sheep or goat) is used for this purpose. Briefly, the sheep or goat is immunized with a mixture of purified guinea pig gamma globulins. It is important to realize that these antibodies recognize antibodies from the guinea pig. They do not recognize the hormone (bovine insulin in our example). The purpose of these second antibodies is to create a complex that can be precipitated by simple centrifugation. They are added in excess so that all of the available primary antibody molecules are captured. Since the tracer is competed from binding sites on the first antibody, much of the tracer can be lost when the tubes are decanted following centrifugation. Table 12.2 summarizes these required reagents. Let's now consider the procedure of how the double antibody RIA assay is performed.

A normal procedure requires the creation of a standard curve and dilution of unknown samples followed by addition of the reagents in a prescribed sequence. Here is a typical pattern:

Table 12.2.   Materials needed for RIA procedures.

Reagent	Purpose
Purified hormone	Preparation of a standard curve Making of radiolabeled hormone (tracer) Use in immunization procedure
Tracer	The radiolabeled hormone
1st or primary antibody	Often diluted blood serum from an immunized animal; rabbits or guinea pigs are frequently used
2nd antibody	Usually diluted blood serum from an immunized sheep or goat—for example, sheep anti-rabbit gamma globulin
Assay buffer	Usually a phosphate buffer solution to maintain pH and conditions appropriate for the binding reactions to take place

Day 1.   Label tubes and add dilutions of standards and unknowns in assay buffer to appropriate tubes (usually 500 µl total volume).

Day 2.   Add tracer (a dilution of radiolabeled hormone ~30,000 cpm per tube; usually 100 µl).

Day 2.   Add diluted first antibody to all tubes except total count and background tubes (usually 100 µl).

Day 3.   Add diluted second antibody to all tubes except the total count tubes (usually 100 µl).

Days 3–6.   Incubate the assay tubes at 4°C.

Day 7.   Add cold assay buffer (usually 1 ml) and immediate centrifuge all tubes except the total count tubes. Decant the liquid and measure the radioactivity remaining in each tube.

There are now variations on this basic procedure, for example many commercial RIA kits use tubes that have the first antibody bound to the surface of the tube. This eliminates the need for the second antibody and centrifugation but basic principles remain the same. The fundamental idea is that competition of tracer bound to the primary antibody by hormone in unknowns to be evaluated is compared with the competition that occurs when known amounts of purified non-radiolabeled hormone is added to assay tubes. In other words, the amount of radioactivity remaining in tubes containing unknown samples is compared against a standard curve. Although most procedures now rely on computer programs to crunch the numbers and calculate concentrations rather than interpolation of results from a graphical plot of the standard curve, the ideas can be readily illustrated this way. Let's consider a set of results (Table 12.3) from an RIA standard curve for bovine insulin and some radioactivity values for some unknown samples.

The values listed are averages for replicates of 3–4 tubes or duplicates for the total count tubes. Total

count tubes are simply the average of two tubes that contain 100 µl of the tracer solution but nothing else. These tubes are set aside and counted along with the other assay tubes to provide a measure of how much of the tracer was added to each of the assay tubes. Remember, all the tubes had 100 µl of the same diluted solution of tracer at the start of the assay or ~33,000 cpm each in this example. Radioactivity is more accurately described in terms of disintegrations per minute (dpm) because this takes into account the efficiency of the counting device. However, use of cpm is acceptable to describe relative differences in radioactivity, especially if there are no issues with variation in counting between samples. This is not typically an issue with higher energy isotopes like I^{125}. Tubes 3–4 received all of the same solutions as the other assay tubes except buffer instead of 100 µl of first antibody solution. Because the tracer is an iodinated protein, it can stick nonspecifically to surfaces. The radioactivity or cpm remaining in these tubes provides a measurement of background or nonspecific binding. The values for percent binding have the background cpm subtracted prior to calculation. Tubes 6–9 are called total binding tubes because they contain tracer and all the necessary antibodies but no competing hormone—that is, neither added standard nor unknown. Notice that in the absence of any competition, about 39% of the total tracer added is bound to the antibody TB/TC × 100 (12,950/32,650 × 100 = 39.7%). For the purpose of creating the standard curve, this total binding or zero competing value provides a reference point for comparison to create the standard curve and is called the 100% binding value.

Now consider the radioactivity values for tubes 10–12 to 31–33. For those that had 0.1 ng of non-radiolabeled insulin added, the radioactivity is slightly less than for the total binding tubes (12,950 versus 11,551), which expressed as a percent of the total binding sample is 88.7%. As you scan down the listing with increasing amounts of non-radiolabeled (cold) insulin added, the remaining radioactivity becomes progressively less. For example, with the addition of 6.4 ng of cold insulin, bound radioactivity equals 2,507 cpm or 15.7% of total binding. Clearly, there is a negative relationship between the concentration of competing cold insulin and the amount of tracer bound to the antibody. Data for tubes 34–36 are the average for replicated samples (100 µl of serum) taken from a cow prior to the infusion of glucose. Bound radioactivity averages 10,369 cpm or 79.2% of total binding. Data for tubes 37–39 is the average for replicate samples (100 µl of serum) from the same cow 10 minutes following an IV infusion of glucose. Bound radioactivity averages 7,256 cpm or 54.1% of total binding. Could you now extrapolate from the standard curve to estimate the ng of insulin in each of these samples?

Table 12.3.   Example bovine insulin RIA data.

Tube No.	Description	Radioactivity Remaining (cpm)	% Bound
1, 2	Total Count	32,650	
3–5	Background	555	
6–9	Total Binding	12,950	100.0
10–12	Std 0.1 ng/tube	11,551	88.7
13–15	Std 0.2 ng/tube	9,981	76.0
16–18	Std 0.4 ng/tube	8,800	66.5
19–21	Std 0.8 ng/tube	7,311	54.5
22–24	Std 1.6 ng/tube	5,564	40.4
25–27	Std 3.2 ng/tube	4,026	28.0
28–30	Std 6.4 ng/tube	2,507	15.7
31–33	Std 12.8 ng/tube	1,856	10.5
34–36	Unknown 1	10,369	79.2
37–39	Unknown 2	7,256	54.1

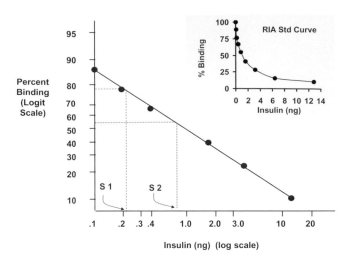

Fig. 12.10. RIA standard curve standard plot. The insert shows the relationship between percent binding and amount of added insulin on a simple arithmetic plot. Conversion to Logit-Log transformation of the same data produces a straight-line relationship that simplifies extrapolation for calculating unknown values (S 1 and S 2).

Figure 12.10 shows a plot (insert) of percent of radioactivity bound versus ng of cold insulin added. Although this simple plot clearly shows this negative relationship, it is mathematically more complex to extrapolate from this curve. However, a simple transformation serves to linearize the shape of the curve so that extrapolation is simpler. Specifically, concentrations of cold hormone are expressed on a log scale (x-axis), and the percent binding (y-axis) as a logit transformation. In practice these calculations are usually done via computer program, but comparing the two plots (Fig. 12.10) illustrates the utility of the transformation. For example, consider the data for unknown 1 (tubes 34–36; 10,369 cpm; 79.2% binding) and the corresponding dashed line (S1) in Figure 12.10. The intersection with the x-axis suggests that this corresponds to ~.22 ng of insulin in 100 μl of serum or 2.2 ng/ml, i.e., each ml (0.22 ng × 10 = 2.2 ng/ml). The second unknown (S2) suggests an intersection at about .85 ng, so this corresponds with .85 ng/100 μl or 8.5 ng/ml. This indicates a nearly fourfold increase in serum insulin within 10 minutes after administration of glucose.

The RIA methodology has been a powerful technology to measure not only hormones but other proteins and molecules. For isotope labeling some steroids are labeled with tritium (^{3}H) or carbon (^{14}C). In addition, to producing antiserum to detect steroids and other small poor antigens, the molecules are often linked with larger proteins or peptides. Although traditionally hormones were tagged with radioactivity, a number of other immunoassay techniques have evolved to avoid the use of isotopes and costs associ-

ated with possible safety issues or waste disposal. In these assays, the antigen is linked to an enzyme, fluorescent tag, or chemiluminescent label to produce the tracer solution. For example, many enzyme-linked immunoabsorbent assays (ELISAs) that depend on antibody-coated microtiter plates and enzyme-labeled reporter antibody can be as sensitive as traditional RIA procedures.

Despite the advancements allowed by use of the RIA it is nonetheless important to remember that the method depends on antibody-antigen binding, so it is possible with highly specific antibodies (e.g., monoclonal antibodies) that fragments of hormones might be detected in addition to intact molecules. Since the method does not distinguish biologically active hormones, some caution in interpretation of results is also warranted.

Endocrine and growth factor signaling

By this point you might be wondering, how can I build a framework to put some of this seemingly bewildering array of first and second messengers, receptor types, and signaling cascades to really understand relationships with physiology? Traditionally, hormones were classified based on their effects. One such classification scheme is illustrated in Table 12.4. For example, glucocorticoids (cortisol and relatives) were named for their capacity to affect carbohydrate metabolism, hence the metabolic classification. The pituitary hormones were named because of their trophic effects—that is, their capacity to induce secretions of hormones in other endocrine glands. However, GH, for example, has impacts on metabolism, growth, cardiac function, and secretion of IGF-I from the liver. Prl is associated with more than 100 specific physiological activities. Other hormones were named based on their gland of origin, i.e., thyroid hormones. Although such classifications have logic, there can be confusion and problems. For example, the actions of the glucocorticoids can be much more diverse than just those that impact carbohydrate metabolism. These affects are only a subset. Second, it is possible that structurally similar hormones can signal target cells by a common receptor. For example, as illustrated in Figure 12.5, insulin and IGF-I have distinct receptors. The affinity of insulin for the IGF-I receptor is lower than for IGF-I, but, for example, what would happen in a diabetic state with elevated concentrations circulating insulin? Despite the lower affinity it is likely that under these conditions insulin could more likely signal via its native receptor as well as IGF-I.

These complications and the burgeoning data coming from molecular biology and cell biology studies suggests that hormones and growth factors

Table 12.4. Functional classification of hormones.

Class	Examples	Actions
Kinetic	Oxytocin, epinephrine	Uterine contractions, milk ejection Pigment secretion
Metabolic	Cortisol Insulin Triiodothyronine	Carbohydrate mobilization Glucose uptake Metabolic rate
Morphogenic	Estrogen GH Testosterone	Gamete production, tissue development, sex characteristics General body growth Gamete production, secondary sex characteristics
Behavior	Estrogen Testosterone Prl	Estrus Aggression Nest building and other maternal actions

would be more logically classified based on the receptor through which these molecules signal target cells. This has certainly revolutionized our understanding of cell signaling; we now understand that there are broad families of hormones and growth factors that share similar mechanisms of action. For example, until the structural details of the receptors became available, who would have combined leptin, Prl, and erythropoietin into the same class of molecules? This does not mean that we plan to abandon a traditional discussion of the major endocrine glands and their products. It is, however, important to appreciate that understanding of the endocrine system and its physiology is an area of rapidly evolving research and study.

The hypophyseal-pituitary axis

For many years, the pituitary gland was called the master endocrine gland. This was because of the large number of hormones that it produces and their widespread physiological effects throughout the body. However, since negative feedback loops and secretion of hypothalamic hormones ultimately regulate secretion of the pituitary hormones, the question of master and servant is a real one. Regardless, the pituitary hormones are essential and critically important in control of animal function directly related to animal agriculture productivity, i.e., rate of growth, muscle development, reproduction, and lactation. This is where we will begin our survey of major endocrine glands, their products, and their actions.

Secretion of the hormones of the anterior pituitary is tightly linked to secretion of other hormones that are produced by cells located in nuclei of the hypothalamus. Although these releasing hormones (or releasing inhibiting hormones in some cases) are produced only in very small amounts, they are able to

impact the activity of cells of the pars distalis because of a unique arrangement of blood vessels between the hypothalamus and the anterior pituitary. This is called the hypothalamic-hypophyseal portal blood system. Simply stated, venous blood that drains from the hypothalamus mixes with arterial blood and passes to the anterior pituitary before it goes into the general venous circulation. The importance of this special anatomical relationship was confirmed by elegant experiments in the 1960s and 1970s that showed that placing a foil barrier between the hypothalamus and pituitary markedly inhibited the secretion of all of the anterior pituitary hormones except Prl. Although the secretion of the hypothalamic releasing hormones was not prevented by this procedure, diversion of these secretions into the general circulation diluted the concentrations so much that the capacity of regulating secretion of anterior pituitary hormones was lost. Of course the pituitary gland must also receive oxygenated arterial blood. Arterial branches of the circle of Willis supply most of this blood.

The pituitary overview

The pituitary gland, or hypophysis, is located at the very base of the brain in a depression of the sphenoid bone of the lower skull called the sella turcia. This obviously provides a great deal of protection for this important endocrine gland. It is divided into three divisions or lobes. The largest is the adenohypophysis, or anterior pituitary. Much of the anterior lobe contains cords of closely compacted epithelial cells, which secrete many of the more familiar pituitary hormones, i.e., GH, Prl, FSH, etc. This hormone-synthesizing region, called the pars distalis, accounts for most of the tissue mass. However, a smaller tongue of tissue extends up and around the pituitary stalk to form a

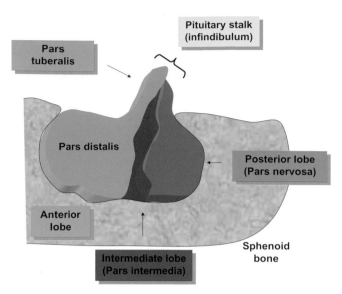

Fig. 12.11. Pituitary gland anatomy.

part of the anterior lobe called the pars tuberalis. A smaller region of tissue, the pars intermedia or intermediate lob, is sandwiched between the anterior pituitary and the second largest division called the posterior pituitary, or pars nervosa. As you might have guessed from its name, this region of the pituitary gland has a very different cellular structure than the anterior lobe. The cells of the region are, in fact, neurosecretory cell nerve endings and associated supporting cells. The hormones of the posterior pituitary are actually synthesized by cell bodies of the hypothalamus but released from the neural cells that populate the posterior pituitary. Figure 12.11 illustrates the basics of the pituitary gland.

Many of the pituitary hormones are called trophic hormones. This refers to the fact that these hormones generally stimulate the secretion of hormones by other endocrine glands in addition to other biological effects. For example, consider follicle-stimulating hormone (FSH). In females, FSH stimulates the ovarian follicles, which synthesize and secrete estrogen and/or progesterone (following ovulation). In males, FSH and LH are involved in spermatogenesis but they also promote testosterone production. There are often many overlapping biological actions between hormones. The secretion of one hormone can enhance the action of another. This is called a synergistic effect. In other situations, secretion of one hormone is necessary for another to be effective; this can be described as a permissive effect. In fewer situations, two hormones can have opposing or antagonistic effects. It is important that the secretion of the anterior pituitary hormones be adequately controlled. We'll discuss the importance of the hypothalamus shortly, but secretion of these

hormones is controlled by negative feedback loops. This type of regulation can involve the anterior pituitary hormones directly, i.e., continued secretion of high amounts of the hormone negatively impacts the pituitary to reduce further synthesis and/or secretion of the hormone. In other cases the negative feedback involves the target stimulated by the particular trophic hormone. Negative feedback can also occur by altering the rate of secretion of the hypothalamic hormones that stimulate the secretion of the anterior pituitary hormones. We'll provide examples of these feedback loops as we discuss individual hormones.

The epithelial cells of the anterior pituitary, specifically the pars distalis, were first described based on their morphology and staining characteristics. For example, some populations of the cells stained with basic dyes were identified as basophils. Other populations stained with acidic dyes were dubbed acidophils. Cells that stained poorly with either class of dyes were identified as chromophobes. Various physiological experiments or pathological events that tracked changes in reproduction or growth or other factors slowly led to an appreciation of cell types that were connected with the secretion of specific hormones. For example, lactating animals were shown to have pituitaries with an increased number of acidophils. This was coupled with increased Prl secretion, thus linking Prl secretion with acidophils. Generally, acidophils include both somatotrophs that secrete GH or somatotropin and lactotrophs that secrete Prl. Under usual circumstances the acidophils account for 50 to 70% of the cells. The basophils include the FSH and LH secreting gonadotrophs, corticotrophs that secrete adrenocorticotropic hormone (ACTH), and thyrotrophs that secrete thyroid-stimulating hormone (TSH). More recent studies have utilized specific immunocytochemical techniques to localize specific hormones to particular pituitary cells. Results of these studies suggest that some cells may secrete more than one hormone. For example, Prl and GH staining has been noted in the same cells. Such cells are called mammosomatotrophs. In humans, they are most frequently noted within pituitary tumors. Regardless, this suggests that the cells of the pars distalis may display much more plasticity with respect to secretion of hormones than was once thought. Table 12.5 provides a listing of the anterior pituitary hormones and their major trophic targets.

Secretion of these pituitary hormones is closely coupled with the hypothalamus. Figure 12.12 illustrates relationships between the hypothalamus and the pituitary gland. The key idea is that particular groups of nerve cells (nuclei) in the hypothalamus secrete hormones that act on the adjacent anterior pituitary. For example, growth hormone releasing hormone (GHRH) is a 44 amino acids peptide produced in the arcuate nucleus from a larger precursor molecule of 107 or 108 amino acids. Most of the activity of the GHRH resides in the first 29 amino acids of the molecule; experiments have shown that infusions of the truncated version are as effective as the full-length version of the molecule. Many of the hypothalamic peptides appear in other places in the body. For example, D cells of the pancreatic islet cells also secrete the tetradecapeptide somatostatin (GHIH). These hormones and their corresponding pituitary target hormones are listed in Table 12.6.

The hypothalamic hormones were first described because of their effects on the anterior pituitary hormones. It is now known that many of these substances also function as neurotransmitters. The reverse is also true. A number of molecules first described as neurotransmitters also function as classic hormones. That is the same substance that might act as neurotransmitter, neural hormone, or classic hormone. As a student, this adds confusion but also indicates how difficult it is to make hard and fast rules to categorize whether a messenger is a hormone or a neurotransmitter.

Table 12.7 provides some further detail about the structure of hypothalamic hormones and posterior pituitary hormones. Many of these peptides are very small molecules compared with many other proteins hormones. A comparison of the nonapeptides oxytocin and vasopressin shows the similarity of structure of these molecules, i.e., only two amino acids differ and they have essentially identical cyclic structures, yet their biological responses are distinct. GHRH and CRH are larger but relatively simple peptide chains. PIH is now known to be dopamine, which is similar in structure to epinephrine and norepinephrine. Somatostatin, like several of the hypothalamic hormones and neurotransmitters is found not only in the hypothalamus but also in the D cells of pancreatic islets, enterocytes of the GI tract, and C cells (parafollicular cells) of the thyroid gland. There are also several structural variants of somatostatin. Somatostatin 14 is predominant in the hypothalamus, but somatostatin 28 is found in the cells of the intestinal tract. In addition to its role in regulating GH secretion, somatostatin inhibits the secretion of insulin, glucagon, gastrin, and secretin. Somatostatin also regulates the secretion of

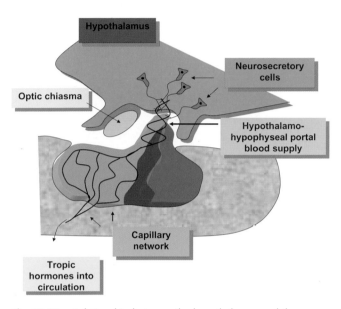

Fig. 12.12. Relationship between the hypothalamus and the anterior pituitary.

Table 12.5. Hormones of the anterior pituitary gland.

Hormone	Abbreviation	Tropic Target
Growth hormone	GH or STH	Liver
Prolactin	Prl	None
Adrenocorticotropin	ACTH	Adrenal Cortex
Thyroid-stimulating hormone	TSH	Thyroid
Follicle-stimulating hormone	FSH	Ovary—Testes
Luteinizing hormone	LH	Ovary—Testes

Table 12.6. Hormones of the hypothalamus.

Hormone	Abbreviation	Pituitary Target
Thyrotropin-releasing hormone	TRH	TSH secreting cells (Prl—lactotrophs?)
Gonadotropin-releasing hormone	GnRH	Gonadotrophs (FSH-LH)
GH-inhibiting hormone (somatostatin)	GHIH	Somatotrophs (GH)
GH-releasing hormone	GHRH	Somatotrophs (GH)
Corticotropin-releasing hormone	CRH	Corticotrophs (ACTH)
Prolactin-inhibiting hormone (dopamine)	PIH	Lactotrophs (Prl)
Prolactin-releasing hormone	PIH	? (TRH)

Table 12.7. Hypothalamic and neurohypophysis hormone structures.

Hormone	Structure
TRH (tripeptide)	(pyro)Glu-His-Pro-NH$_2$
GNRH (decapeptide)	(pyro)Glu-His-Trp-Ser-Try-Gly-Leu-Arg-Pro-Gyl-NH$_2$
GHIH (tetradecapeptide)	Ala-Gyl-Cys-Lys-Asn-Phe-Phe-Trp-Lys-Thr-Phe-Thr-Ser-Cys (disulfide bonds: S—S)
GHRH	44 amino acids—derived from 107 AA precursor
CRH	41 amino acids—derived from 196 AA precursor
PIH	HO, HO—〈ring〉—CH$_2$CH$_2$NH$_2$ (dopamine)
Oxytocin (nonapeptide)	Cys-Try-Ile-Gln-Asn-Cys-Pro-Leu-Gly-NH$_2$ (disulfide bonds: S—S)
Vasopressin (nonapeptide)	Cys-Try-Phe-Gln-Asn-Cys-Pro-Arg-Gly-NH$_2$ (disulfide bonds: S—S)

Table 12.8. Neuroendocrine messengers as hormones and neurotransmitters.

	Hormone Secreted by Endocrine Gland	Hormone Secreted by Neurons	Neurotransmitter
Dopamine	Yes	Yes	Yes
Norepinephrine	Yes	Yes	Yes
Epinephrine	Yes		Yes
Somatostatin	Yes	Yes	
GNRH	Yes	Yes	Yes
TRH		Yes	Yes
Oxytocin	Yes	Yes	Yes
Vasopressin	Yes	Yes	Yes
Glucagon	Yes		Yes
Cholecystokinin	Yes		Yes

TSH because of its capacity to enhance the negative feedback of thyroid hormone on the thyrotrophs of the anterior pituitary. Similarly, TRH acts to increase secretion of Prl. Table 12.8 provides a listing of neuroendocrine messengers with overlapping and diverse activities.

Negative feedback loops

Secretion of most of the anterior pituitary hormones is controlled at multiple levels. As Table 12.6 shows, control begins in the hypothalamus with the synthesis and secretion of the hypothalamic hormones into the hypophyseal portal blood supply. Because these agents reach their target cells in the pars distalis with minimal dilution, they are very effective. One means of regulation is to alter the rate at which these hypothalamic hormones are made. Changes in higher brain function that impact the hypothalamus also alter production of many of these agents and thereby activity of the pituitary.

An interesting example of this is the Bruce Effect. As first described in rodents, this is an example of a pheromone (a hormonelike agent that acts between individuals) that blocks implantation of a newly fertilized ovum in the uterus. If a newly mature male is introduced into a rodent population soon after mating by the previous dominant male, newly fertilized females fail to maintain their pregnancies. How does this occur? First, a little background is needed to understand how failure occurs. Development of follicles, and then a dominant follicle, and finally ovulation depends on secretion of pituitary FSH and LH. Estrogen and then progesterone from the ovary are essential to prepare the uterus to accept the newly fertilized ovum for implantation. Secretion of FSH and LH are controlled by GHRH from the hypothalamus. When the new male is introduced to the newly mated female, she responds to a pheromone secreted in his urine. This agent acts on her brain to block production of hypothalamic GHRH. This lowers FSH and LH secretion, which minimizes steroid hormone production and thereby prevents implantation. It is known that the agent acts through the olfactory system because females that have their olfactory nerves blocked do not display this response. Second, the new male does not have to be physically present. Simply exposing the animals to urine from the male can elicit the effect.

Let's now consider some less exotic examples of regulation anterior pituitary hormones. Since there are multiple interacting steps for these trophic anterior pituitary hormones—hypothalamus → pituitary → endocrine organ target → target hormone secretion—there are many opportunities for negative feedback. In the simplest case, the secretion of a hormone by an endocrine gland builds up in the bloodstream. As the concentration increases, the hormone affects the secreting cells to reduce the amount that is being made and/or secreted. This can be called simple or primary level negative feedback. Since the effects of hormones are generally proportional to their concentrations in blood, it follows that physiological systems would have evolved to ensure normal functioning that could be maintained by carefully monitoring and regulating circulating concentrations of hormones. Since the primary factor that affects the circulating concentration is the rate of secretion, negative feedback loops have evolved to monitor concentrations of hormones at their point of origin. This is complicated by these interactions between the hypothalamus, pituitary, and target endocrine gland. Figure 12.13 illustrates feedback loops that act to regulate the secretion of pituitary hormones.

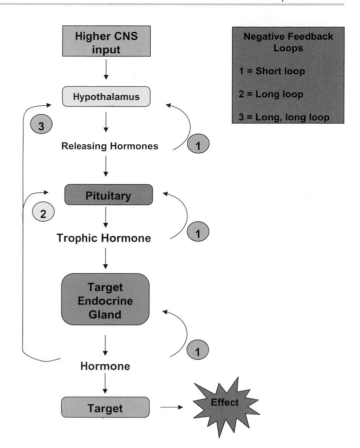

Fig. 12.13. Negative feedback loops and pituitary hormones.

Hormones and cells of the posterior pituitary

The neurohypophysis, or posterior pituitary, is chiefly composed of neurosecretory cells and supporting cells. The axons have their origins primarily with the paraventricular and supraoptic nuclei of the hypothalamus. Fundamentally, the posterior pituitary is an extension of the hypothalamus with the nerve endings within the posterior lobe. However, these neurons differ from other neurons in several ways. Like other neurons they are innervated by other nerve cells located in higher brain regions. Unlike other neurons these cells release their neurotransmitter-like molecules into the bloodstream. This means that the targets for these agents can literally be positioned anywhere in the body. In this way secretions from these cells are acting as classic hormones.

One of the first experiments to indicate the importance of these hormones was work from the late 1800s that showed that the injection of an extract from the pituitary gland increased blood pressure. This effect was traced to the posterior lobe of the gland and is one of the primary effects of the hormone now known

as vasopressin. Evidence for the presence of a second hormone of the posterior lobe, oxytocin, was deduced from experiments by Gaines in 1915. He showed that injection of posterior pituitary extracts caused milk ejection in lactating animals (Fig. 12.14). Structures of oxytocin and vasopressin were reported in 1954 when du Vigneaud's Nobel Prize–winning work elucidated the amino acid sequences of these peptides. In fact, this was the first example of research providing the amino acid sequence and structure of any peptide.

In cows and other mammals sensory receptors are abundant in the skin of the mammary gland and especially in the teat, or nipple. In response to preparation of the udder for milking or nuzzling of the offspring, nerve impulses travel via afferent nerves (branches of the inguinal nerve) to the dorsal root ganglia of the spinal cord and ultimately ascend the spinal cord along the dorsal funiculus to the midbrain. Branches project the paraventricular and supraoptic nuclei of the hypothalamus. Ultimately, associated nerve cells, which synapse with the neurosecretory cells of the paraventricular or supraoptic nuclei, act to either inhibit or facilitate this pathway. A predominance of cholinergic activity excites or facilitates but stimulation of local adrenergic neurons impair oxytocin secretion. It has long been recognized that stress at the time

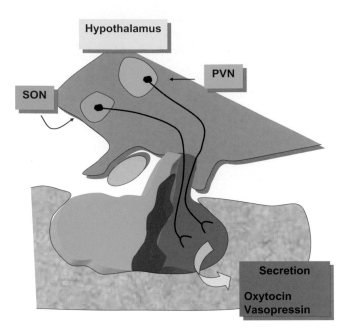

Fig. 12.14. Posterior pituitary pathways. Neurosecretory cells from the Paraventricular nucleus (PVN) and Supraoptic nucleus (SON) of the hypothalamus send axons to the neurohypophysis for secretion of vasopressin and oxytocin, respectively.

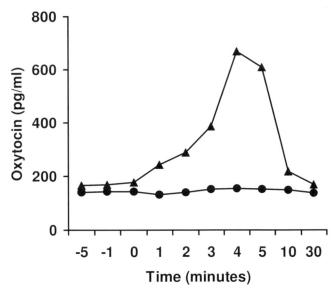

Fig. 12.15. Serum oxytocin at milking. Serum oxytocin measured in two cows in the period just before and after milking. For one cow (●) there is no measurable change in oxytocin concentration but for the other cow (▲) oxytocin is increased fourfold within 4 minutes. Milk yields were normal for each animal. Adapted from Lefcourt and Akers (1983).

of milking interferes with the milk ejection reflex. Failure of oxytocin to be secreted as an explanation for impaired milk letdown is called central inhibition. Since it is likely that stress causes stimulation of the sympathetic division of the autonomic nervous system, it is also possible that increased sympathetic nervous system mediated vasoconstriction (via β-adrenergic receptors) on the sphincters of the metarterioles in the mammary capillary beds act to shunt oxytocin-laden blood away from the alveoli. Since the oxytocin acutely secreted at milking has a short half-life ~5 minutes failure of delivery to the myoepithelial cells (peripheral inhibition) may also explain failures of milk ejection. The often-repeated advice for careful, gentle handling of animals at milking or suckling is based on sound physiology.

Regardless, measurement of oxytocin with RIA confirms bioassay data showing large variations in oxytocin response to milking or suckling in dairy animals. In goats and cows as many as 40% of the animals show no change in oxytocin with milking stimulation. Moreover, milk yields of the mammary glands of goats transplanted under the neck were normal despite the lack of innervation or apparent milk ejection response. Perhaps for animals, such as sheep and goats with large gland cisterns relative to mammary size, milk ejection is not essential for adequate milk removal. On the other hand, it is very clear that adequate oxytocin release is critical to obtain milk from rodents and pigs, for example. Figure 12.15 illustrates changes in blood

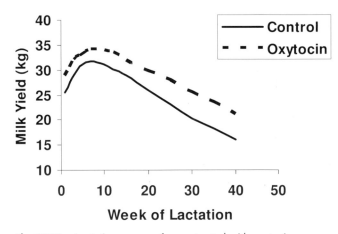

Fig. 12.16. Lactation curves of cows treated with oxytocin. Placebo or oxytocin was administered at the time of milking. Data adapted from Nostrand et al. (1991).

oxytocin in response to 4 min of milking in two cows. One animal shows an abrupt increase in blood oxytocin and the other cow shows essentially no response at all, and yet milk yields were normal. Regardless, oxytocin is widely used in veterinary medicine as an aid to induced uterine contractions or milk ejection. There is also evidence (Fig. 12.16) that oxytocin treatments can increase long-term milk production in dairy cows.

Although vasopressin was named based on observed impacts on blood pressure, its major physiological effect is as an antidiuretic agent. It acts on the kidney to enhance water retention. When concentrations are elevated, more concentrated urine is produced and more water is retained. This increases interstitial fluid and then blood volume, and consequently blood pressure rises. Thus vasopressin is frequently called antidiuretic hormone (ADH). This more accurately reflects a major physiological action. However, ADH also has some direct pressor effects due to its capacity to stimulate contraction of vascular smooth muscle cells. Most species express arginine vasopressin, but closely related arginine vasotocin is synthesized in many birds.

Secretion of ADH is controlled by osmoreceptors located primarily in the hypothalamus, but receptors are present in the stomach and esophagus. If the osmolarity of blood or interstitial fluids is increased this promotes impulses by hypothalamic neurons to increase ADH secretion. The end result is retention of water and consequently reduced osmolarity. A drop in blood volume also activates volume receptors within the atria or the carotid sinus. This reduces activities of neurons that normally send inhibitory signals to the hypothalamus. Problems with ADH are most often the result of hyposecretion. When this becomes chronic, large quantities of very dilute urine are produced. This is called diabetes insipidus. In diabetes mellitus, urine production is also elevated but this is because of excess glucose that acts to draw water into urine. Frequent drinking is a symptom of both diseases. Diabetes insipidus can be caused by a failure to secrete ADH (hypothalamic problem) or by failure of the kidney to respond to ADH (nephrogenic defect).

Both oxytocin and ADH are synthesized from precursor molecules called preprohormones-prepro-pressinphysin for vasopressin and prepro-oxyphysin for oxytocin in large cell bodies (magnocellular nuclei) in the hypothalamus. As the molecules are transported down the axons to the posterior pituitary, cleavage takes place to yield oxytocin or ADH. The proteins, neurophysin I or neurophysin II, are also secreted along with oxytocin or ADH. The neurophysins were initially thought to act as carrier proteins for the peptides, but there are currently no known specific function attributed to these proteins.

Hormones of the anterior pituitary

Our earlier discussion briefly outlined the names and hypothalamic partners for the anterior pituitary hormones. We'll now consider major physiological actions and some of the structural details of each of these hormones. Given the importance of these hormones in regulation of growth, development, lactation, and reproduction, it is apparent that these agents are critical to understanding and improving animal agricul-ture. To illustrate this idea consider the importance of these hormones in mammary development and function and therefore the dairy industry specifically and management of mammals more generally.

The endocrine system perhaps more than any other physiological system, is central in all aspects of mammary development (mammogenesis), onset of lactation (lactogenesis), and maintenance of milk secretion (galactopoiesis). Experiments beginning in the 1920s (Stricker and Grueter, 1928) showed that milk secretion could be induced in virgin rabbits by injecting an anterior pituitary extract. In 1933, Riddle, Bates, and Dykshorn purified the protein responsible for the milk secretion response observed by Stricker and Grueter, they named it prolactin (Prl). Even now, the widely touted and utilized galactopoietic effect of somatotropin or GH to increase milk production in lactating dairy cows had its foundation in studies by Asimov and Krouze in the 1930s. They showed that injections of pituitary extracts consistently increased milk production in lactating cows. Scientists describing and quantifying the potent effects of the pregnancy on mammary growth and changes in the mammary gland at puberty spurred others to isolate and identify the steroid hormones estrogen and progesterone. Advances in purification techniques and understanding of steroid hormone chemistry allowed further studies leading to the production of these steroids for widespread animal testing.

Although the existence of mammogenic and lactogenic substances from the pituitary had long been known, the efforts of Lyons and colleagues in the 1940s to purify larger quantities of Prl and GH were essential. Soon thereafter, specific roles for these hormones in the regulation of mammogenesis in rodents were delineated in classic ablation replacement experiments (Lyons, 1958; Nandi, 1958). In an extensive series of studies, triply operated (adrenalectomized, ovariectomized, and hypophysectomized) rats and mice were treated with various combinations of purified hormones to see whether normal mammary development could be restored. Injections of estrogen and GH together caused proliferation of mammary ducts. However, treatment with estrogen, progesterone, Prl, and GH were needed for lobulo-alveolar development. The maximum ductular and lobulo-alveolar development, although still less than in pregnancy, was obtained in animals also given glucocorticoids. For some strains of mice GH and Prl were both capable of stimulating lobulo-alveolar development. Interestingly, it was not until the 1960s that it was conclusively shown that human Prl and human GH were distinct proteins.

British researchers, focused on efforts to improve and maintain milk supplies during World War II, initiated many endocrine studies on mammary development and function in dairy animals (Cowie et al., 1980). For example, the effects of estrogen and progesterone on mammogenesis were extensively evaluated in attempts to induce lactation in nonpregnant animals. Although difficulties with needed surgeries and expense continue to limit use of ablation replacement experiments to study mammary development and function in cattle, Cowie et al. (1966) studied hypophysectomized-ovariectomized goats and showed that mammary development comparable to midgestation could be obtained in animals treated with a combination of estrogen, progesterone, Prl, GH, and ACTH. Such experiments served to confirm that at least general effects attributed to these hormones on mammary development in rodents also applied to mammary development in dairy animals.

Somatotropin (GH)

By the 1920s, it was discovered that crude extracts prepared from homogenates of bovine pituitary glands could stimulate the growth of rats. The active agent was named *somatotropin* after the Greek word for "growth." Soon thereafter, the ability of such extracts to promote milk secretion in pseudopregnant rabbits and milk production in lactating goats were reported. Some of the more extensive early experiments with cows by the Russians Asimov and Krouze in the 1930s involved the treatment of more than 2,000 cows with crude anterior pituitary extracts. Soon after, as part of efforts to increase food production during World War II, the British scientist Folley (1956) also studied effects of GH on milk production in cows and goats. They identified GH as the primary active galactopoietic component in bovine pituitary extracts. Other studies established dose-response curves, confirmed that relative responses were greater in declining lactation and that gross milk composition was unaffected, and confirmed the generally potent effect of GH on milk yield in dairy ruminants. They concluded that use of pituitary GH would be highly profitable to individual farmers but that an inadequate supply limited the impact that GH could have in stimulating the national milk supply. For example, approximately 25 pituitaries are needed to produce enough GH for a typical daily treatment. These studies were a prelude to subsequent studies and ultimately large-scale use of recombinant bovine GH (bGH) in dairy cows (Etherton and Bauman, 1998; Bauman, 1999).

GH, like Prl, is a single-chain protein and the proteins share about 50% structural homology. GH is also structurally similar between species, e.g., bovine GH is 192 amino acids (23,000 MW), but biologically activity within species is characteristically distinct. As the name suggests, GH is closely associated with body growth. For example, soon after its characterization, it was hoped that bovine GH (bGH) might supply material to treat humans with impaired growth caused by hyposecretion of human GH (hGH). However, it was soon discovered that bGH had no effect in primates. Some human patients were ultimately treated with hGH derived from cadavers, but supplies were limited and unfortunately some samples contained agents (viruses and possibly prions) that made them harmful. More wide-scale therapeutic use of GH in humans had to wait until recombinant hGH became available.

Somatotropin, or GH, depending on the tissue, can act directly or indirectly to coordinate biochemical adaptations that chronically alter the metabolism of carbohydrates, lipids and proteins. Although generalizations can be misleading, under most circumstances elevations in GH act to increase available nutrients by promoting mobilization of tissue stores. For example, GH tends to increase protein synthesis by promoting the uptake of amino acids while at the same time decreasing protein catabolism and promoting lipid mobilization. This acts to make fatty acids preferential fuel sources. Somatotropin directly or indirectly coordinates metabolic adaptations that promote increased milk production in the lactating dairy cow. These adaptations involve chronic alterations in carbohydrate, lipid, and protein metabolism in a number of tissues and serve to preferentially direct nutrients toward the mammary gland. This coordinated regulation to support the priorities of a physiological state is called homeorhetic regulation.

In farm animals, this has been studied rather extensively in dairy cows because of the capacity of GH treatments to enhance milk production. In some of the early short-term studies, GH markedly increased serum triglycerides. A common belief related to nutrient regulation at the time of these studies was that nutrient use largely involved a competition between organs for needed substrates. This means that an increase in milk production in response to, for example, treatment with GH would require either an increase in the metabolism of the mammary gland to better "fight" for nutrients or reduction in nutrient use by other tissues to support increased nutrient demands of the mammary cells for milk synthesis and secretion. Mechanisms for GH's actions were generally thought to depend on acute effects to "push" metabolism of peripheral tissue to reduce competition and thus favor the lactating mammary gland. On the surface many acute effects of GH seem to support this model. These GH-stimulated responses include glycotropic (reduced response to insulin in glucose tolerance testing), diabetogenic (hyperglycemia and glycouremia), and lipolytic (increases in blood nonesterified fatty acids) activity. Given these effects, a number of researchers were concerned that GH induction of these responses would promote metabolic problems in lactating cows. There was concern that acute mobilization of adipose tissue, particularly in postpartum animals already in a negative energy balance, might suffer increased metabolic disorders—ketosis, fatty livers. However, these "extra" nutrients were preferentially directed toward the mammary gland for use in increased milk production.

About this time the concept of homeorhesis came to be applied to the high milk production of genetically superior dairy cows. The overriding idea was that homeorhesis does not act to defeat homeostasis but rather that chronic changes in physiological controls allow coordination of physiological processes to support major physiological events (the definition of homeorhesis). Examples include physiological support for fetal development and reproductive performance, or in this case a sustained high level of milk production while at the same time preserving homeostasis. The preponderance of evidence suggests that GH enhances milk production largely by partitioning nutrients to support milk production, by both direct and indirect actions, but GH does not alter digestibility of nutrients. In dairy cows given exogenous GH, metabolism is altered in an organ-specific fashion to establish nutrient flux toward the mammary gland. Increased appetite and dietary intake interact to moderate some of the demand for nutrients some days after the start of treatments.

The somatomedin hypothesis

The primary function of GH is promotion of linear growth, but many of its growth promoting effects are indirect because of its ability to stimulate the liver to produce insulinlike growth factor–one (IGF-I). This is called the somatomedin hypothesis. Initially, IGF-I and IGF-II were called somatomedins, to account for their relationship with GH action. However, once structures of the molecules were delineated it became clear that the molecules were similar to insulin; hence the new names. Regardless, it is now certain that many actions originally attributed to GH are mediated by IGF-I. But it should not be forgotten that many tissue also express GH receptors. The liver is the primary source for IGF-I in circulation, but IGF-I is also produced locally in many tissues. It may be that locally produced IGF-I is as important as circulating IGF-I. The importance of non-liver sources became clear from knockout mouse studies. In these experiments, genetic engineering techniques were used to block or knock out normal liver IGF-I synthesis. Despite this these animals exhibited essentially normal growth and development. This suggests that for many situations local production of IGF-I can replace and/or supplement circulating IGF-I supplied by the liver.

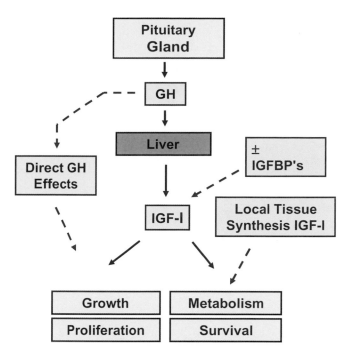

Fig. 12.17. The somatomedin hypothesis. Relationships between secretion of pituitary GH and liver IGF-I are illustrated by the solid black arrows. Dashed red arrows indicate direct effects of GH, significance of local tissue production of IGF-I, and the role of IGF-I–binding proteins to control biological actions of IGF-I.

Other complications include the discovery of a family of IGF-I binding proteins (IGFBPs). These molecules also appear in circulation and are produced locally in many tissues. Depending on conditions, these proteins can either inhibit or enhance biological effects associated with IGF-I. Some of these relationships are illustrated in Figure 12.17. The black arrows illustrate the pathways associated with the "classic" somatomedin hypothesis, and the red dashed arrows, illustrate more recent findings related to local production of IGF-I and IGFBPs.

Figure 12.18 demonstrates synthesis of IGF-I by stroma cells in the bovine mammary gland. In this instance stromal tissue and isolated mammary epithelial cells were tested for the presence of mRNA for IGF-I. These results suggest that IGF-I mRNA detected in samples of mammary parenchymal tissue is actually synthesized by stromal tissue cells that surround the developing mammary ducts.

The physiological relevance of GH becomes apparent in situations with either hyper- or hyposecretion. Hypersecretion of GH prior to puberty produces gigantism because of rapid, prolonged proliferation of growth plate chondrocytes. If excess secretion is initiated after closure of the epiphyseal plates of the long bones the result is acromegaly. This is characterized by enlargement of extremities and facial bones. Failure to produce sufficient GH in young animals leads to

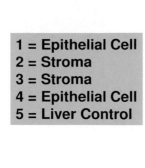

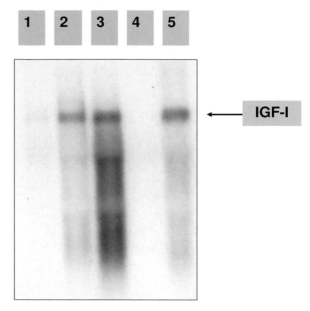

1 = Epithelial Cell
2 = Stroma
3 = Stroma
4 = Epithelial Cell
5 = Liver Control

Fig. 12.18. Expression of IGF-I. Shown is a northern analysis of IGF-I mRNA expression of mammary epithelial cells or stromal tissue prepared from a heifer mammary. Notice there is a signal for IGF-I in samples of mammary stroma and liver RNA but not in mammary epithelial cell RNA. Data adapted from Berry et al. (2003).

production of stunted development and a type of dwarfism. Given its importance to growth, it should be no surprise that there is a great deal of interest in understanding effects of GH related to growth and development in farm animals. For example, do strains or lines of naturally rapid growing animals produce more GH? Could administration of exogenous GH or perhaps immunization against somatostatin be used to promote GH secretion and more rapid growth? Aside from indirect effects of GH on chondrocytes and protein accretion, changes in GH secretion are certainly important in both short-term and more chronic changes in metabolism.

GH secretion

Figure 12.19 illustrates average concentrations of GH and insulin in the blood of cows during the lactation cycle. In early lactation the rapid increase in milk production causes the animals to exhibit a negative energy balance. In other words, feed intake does not keep up with demands. After about 90 days of lactation, peak milk yields are past, feed intake continues to rise, and the animals begin to go into a positive energy balance. In the later stages of lactation body condition increases and the animals begin to deposit excess energy in the form of subcutaneous fat. Changes in average concentrations of blood insulin and GH mirror these physiological changes. Insulin of course is typically elevated

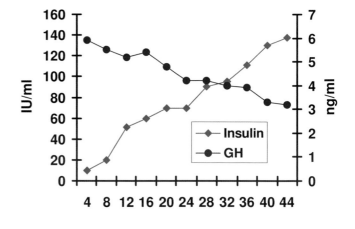

Week of Lactation

Fig. 12.19. Insulin and GH during lactation. Basal insulin and GH in serum of cows during lactation. Adapted from Koprowski and Tucker (1973).

to drive glucose into storage, but GH is elevated to mobilize nutrients. In early lactation insulin concentrations are suppressed while GH is elevated. Toward the end of lactation this situation is reversed.

Secretion of GH is not constant. Instead it is secreted in bursts or pulses so that with frequent blood sampling blood concentrations periodically spike. In younger animals and in males, the frequency of these

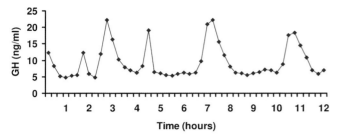

Fig. 12.20. Pattern of GH secretion. In this Holstein heifer calf, note there are several apparent secretory episodes during this 12 hr period of time. Samples were collected at 15 min intervals for assay. Average GH concentration was 9.4 ng/ml.

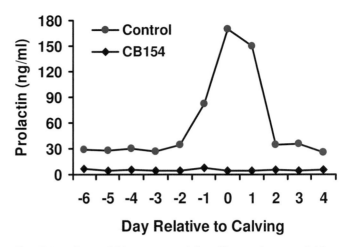

Fig. 12.21. Serum Prl in cows at calving. Changes in serum Prl in cows given ergrocryptine (CB 154) around the time of calving are shown. Note the usual surge in Prl secretion at calving is blocked and that average Prl concentrations before and after calving is reduced but secretion of Prl is not completely inhibited. Adapted from Akers et al. (1981).

events is more common and the amplitude of these secretory spikes greater. This results in higher average or basal GH concentrations as well. Like many hormones there are also intrinsic overall patterns of secretion that follow circadian and ultradian rhythms (Lefcourt et al. 1995). Figure 12.20 illustrates changes in serum GH over the course of 12 hr in a Holstein heifer calf.

Prolactin

As its name suggests, Prl has undoubtedly been the most intensely studied hormone related to lactation and mammary growth. However, it is very clear that Prl exhibits a very wide variety of physiological actions. For example, increased secretion of Prl is associated with onset of nest building and brooding in birds. Prl is also important in kidney and immune system function. In the past 20 years it has been established that native Prl is really part of a family of structurally related protein isoforms or variants. The Prl gene is transcribed not only in the lactotropes of the anterior pituitary gland but also by cells in the placenta, hypothalamus, mammary gland, and in lymphocytes. Moreover, either as it is secreted or after interaction with target cells, some Prl is enzymatically modified to become cleaved, phosphorylated, or glycosylated. Thus, the pleiotropic actions of Prl may ultimately be attributed to the presence of these different isoforms of the hormone. As suggested, (Das and Vonderhaar, 1997), the signaling pathway for Prl stimulation of cell differentiation compared with that for Prl signaling of cell proliferation needs to be deciphered to truly appreciate the role of Prl in one of its specific target tissues the mammary gland.

At least three distinct forms of the Prl receptor are also known to exist. The three forms of the receptor exhibit differences in their cytoplasmic domains. The long form is 90 kDa and differs from the short form (40 kDa) because of differential splicing of mRNA transcribed from the Prl receptor gene. An intermediate version of the receptor is a deletion mutant of the long form that lacks 198 amino acids in the cytoplasmic domain. The intermediate form of the receptor is more sensitive to Prl and a major form of the receptor found in the Prl also belongs to a superfamily of structurally related proteins that include GH and placental lactogen. This realization has facilitated the study of intracellular signaling pathways because the structural similarities suggest parallel similarities in mechanisms of action.

As a specific example, expression of the Prl receptor in the bovine or ovine mammary gland increases dramatically near the time of parturition in concert with lactogenesis, and this level of expression is generally maintained during lactation. But there is no evidence for expression of different forms of the receptor to suggest that possible mammogenic versus lactogenic effects on mammary growth or function in ruminants is associated with a particular Prl receptor subclass (Smith et al., 1993).

Some of the best evidence for the importance of increased periparturient secretion of Prl in stage II lactogenesis in cows has come from experiments in which the administration of a dopamine agonist has been used to inhibit Prl secretion and correspondingly impair lactation. In ruminants where postpartum milking continues, administration of the dopamine agonist α-bromoergocryptine (CB154) reduced basal prolactin concentration about 80% and prevented the usual periparturient rise as well as milking-induced Prl rise during the first week postpartum. Differences in Prl secretion in control and CB154-treated cows are shown in Figure 12.21. Milk production was reduced

Table 12.9. Mammary biochemistry after prolactin suppression.

	Treatment			
	Prepartum	Postpartum	CB154	CB154 + Prl
Lactose synthesis (μg/h/100 mg)	39 ± 63	552 ± 70	327 ± 63	628 ± 81
α-Lactalbumin (μg/mg/protein)	1.7 ± .04	5.4 ± 0.4	2.8 ± 0.4	6.8 ± 0.5
RNA (g)	23.6 ± 2.1	87.2 ± 16.8	56.0 ± 7.9	91.5 ± 12.8
DNA (g)	27.9 ± 2.9	46.0 ± 3.8	40.1 ± 3.8	42.2 ± 3.8

Adapted from Akers et al. (1981). Control animals were killed 10 days before or after parturition. CB154 was administered for 12 days prior to expected parturition through parturition. Animals given Prl were infused continuously for 6 days immediately before parturition.

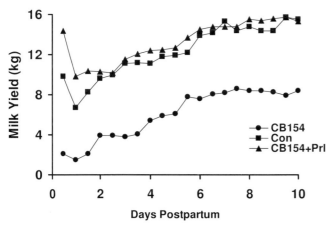

Fig. 12.22. Milk production after suppression of Prl. Milk production per milking in control, CB154-treated, and CB154+Prl-treated cows is shown. Note the marked decrease in milk yield of cows given CB154 and that milk yield is restored to normal for cows also given Prl. Data adapted from Akers et al. (1981).

45% during the first 10 days postpartum. Lost milk production was associated with reduced synthesis of α-lactalbumin, lactose, and fatty acids, as well as impaired structural differentiation of the mammary secretory cells. Selected effects are summarized in Table 12.9. Cows treated with exogenous Prl in addition to the agonist (to replace the periparturient surge in prolactin) showed no loss of milk production or effects on milk component biosynthesis or alveolar cell differentiation. An effect of Prl suppression and replacement during the periparturient period on milk production in multiparous cows is shown in Figure 12.22. Clearly, Prl is important in mammary cell differentiation and lactogenesis (Akers et al., 1981).

Prolactin secretion

Prl secretion, like GH, is episodic but it also is acutely increased by a variety of stimuli. Average concentrations are higher with warm temperatures and longer photoperiods. Manipulation of the photoperiod has also been used to increase livestock productivity for many years. Examples include manipulation of the photoperiod to increase egg production in chickens or to manipulate breeding activity in seasonal breeders such as horses and sheep. Early studies noting the positive effect of the photoperiod on Prl secretion prompted a landmark investigation by Peters et al. (1978), on the effects of an increased photoperiod on milk production in cows. They showed that exposure of lactating cows to a long-day photoperiod between September and April in Michigan significantly increased milk yields (2.0 kg/d) compared with cows exposed to the ambient photoperiod. This effect has been confirmed by numerous other research groups in North America and Europe, in latitudes ranging from 39 to 62° N. In cattle, increasing the duration of the daily photoperiod from 8 hr light:16 dark to 16 hr light:8 dark increases Prl concentrations in the blood several fold. It is, however, important that animals experience at least a minimal dark cycle, since animals on a continuous lighting regimen appear to revert to a short-day photoperiodic response pattern. However, recent work suggests that increases in milk production are likely mediated by changes in the IGF-I axis rather than Prl (Dahl et al., 2000).

In various species (cow, goat, sheep, human, and rat) stimuli associated with milking or sucking promote the secretion of Prl. However, secretion of Prl or other hormones in response to milking or suckling does not directly depend on the removal of secretions because teat stimulation alone can also induce Prl secretion in nonlactating animals. Little is known about the development of this neuroendocrine reflex, but it is affected by stage of development. For example, in an experiment with 3-, 6-, and 10-month-old heifers, three of six 3-month-old heifers showed a moderate increase in blood Prl with mimic hand milking, but only two of six showed an increase for the 6-month-old heifers and none of six for the heifers at 10 months of age. In contrast, with heifers tested during gestation all of the heifers responded and Prl secretion increased monotonically as gestation advanced (Fig. 12.23). The response continues into lactation with Prl routinely

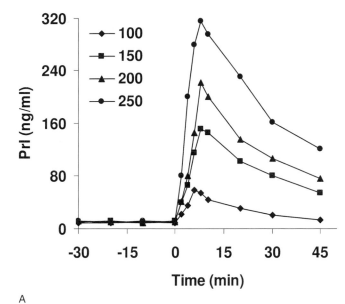

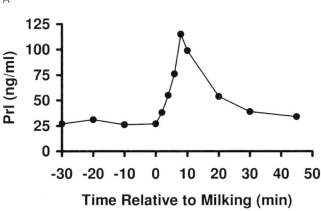

A

B

Fig. 12.23. Prl secretion after teat stimulation. Panel A shows changes in serum Prl concentrations before, during, and after teat stimulation of pregnant Holstein heifers sampled at 100, 150, 200, or 250 days of gestation. Note the monotonic increase in response with advancing gestation. The lower panel shows Prl secretion in heifers in response to machine milking 30 days postpartum. Data adapted from Akers and Lefcourt (1982).

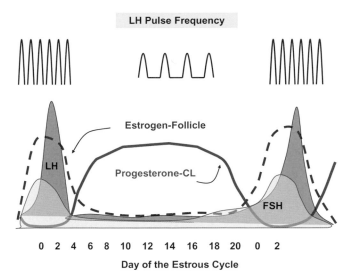

Fig. 12.24. Hormones during estrus cycle. Relative changes in concentrations of estrogen, progesterone, FSH, LH, and LH pulse frequency during the estrus cycle in the cow is illustrated.

secreted with each milking, but in cows the magnitude of the response declines with advancing lactation (Akers and Lefcourt, 1982).

Follicle-stimulating hormone and luteinizing hormone

It is fitting that follicle-stimulating hormone (FSH) and luteinizing hormone (LH) be discussed together. In both males and females together, these gonadotropins regulate reproductive physiology. Both hormones have an α and β chain. In fact, thyroid-stimulating hormone (TSH) shares this structural similarity. For

each of these hormones, the biological action of the hormones depends on the β chain. FSH has a major effect on the growth and development of ovarian follicles. This is closely linked with the capacity of the hormone to induce secretion of estrogen by the theca cells surrounding developing oocytes. As the waves of follicles develop during the estrus cycle of the cow, for example, only one of a cohort of follicles becomes dominant. This follicle proceeds to enlarge and develop so that it becomes the follicle destined for ovulation. Closely tied with FSH control of estrogen secretion and changing sensitivity of the hypothalamus, there is an acute increase in secretion of LH, which promotes ovulation of the dominant follicle. This is the ovulatory surge in LH. This not only causes rupture and release of the egg, it also promotes remaining follicular cells to differentiate into luteal cells and create a corpus luteum (yellow body). This luteinization process explains how the hormone gets its name. More importantly, as these cells are luteinized they begin to secrete progesterone, which prepares the uterus to accept a fertilized oocyte. In the absence of fertilization, the corpus luteum of CL degenerates. Figure 12.24 illustrates relative changes in secretion of estrogen and progesterone during the estrus cycle and relationship to changing secretion of LH.

A preovulatory surge in the LH begins about 24 hr prior to ovulation in most domestic species (cow, goat, sheep, and pig); this triggers critical changes in the follicle that impact its endocrine activity and culminate in ovulation. Poorly characterized factors in the granulosa cells prevent the premature conversion of the cells into luteal tissue until after ovulation. Increased LH allows for the resumption of meiosis by the oocyte and removes the block on luteinization of the granulosa cells. This effectively converts the cells from predominate estrogen production to progesterone secretion as illustrated in Figure 12.24. The process actually begins in the period before ovulation, but the LH surge hastens the decline in estrogen secretion and concomitant rise in progesterone secretion. Indeed, the progressive increase in secretion of estrogen by the rapidly developing follicles just before ovulation acts to signal the hypothalamus, and ultimately the anterior pituitary, that conditions are appropriate for ovulation.

Secretion of FSH and LH is controlled by release of GnRH from the hypothalamus. Secretion of GnRH occurs in bursts or spikes so that the corresponding secretion of FSH and LH also occurs episodically. However, at least two clusters of nerve cells or nuclei in the hypothalamus (ventromedial and arcuate nucleus) produce GnRH in a tonic release center. This secretion pattern produces short-lived pulses of GnRH sometimes compared with the drip, drip of a leaking faucet and corresponding brief bursts of FSH and LH secretion.

As illustrated by the pulse frequency for LH illustrated at the top of Figure 12.24, gonadotropin secretion is increased during the follicular phase of the estrus cycle but decreased during the luteal phase. Acute control to allow for increased pulse frequency but decreased pulse amplitude allows for final growth and development of the dominant follicle. The rapid increase in estrogen creates a positive feedback at the level of the hypothalamus. Increased estrogen from the rapidly developing follicle induces increased GnRH pulses. This produces more FSH secretion, thus more estrogen, and further GnRH secretion. This cycle is broken by the maturation of the follicle and the LH surge. As estrogen concentrations decline, the positive feedback is lost, and inhibitory progesterone concentrations increase. This likely explains the rapid rise and equally rapid decline in LH. However, since, generally, GnRH stimulates the secretion of both LH and FSH, what explains the abrupt LH surge without a corresponding peak in FSH secretion?

This is explained by the presence of a second cluster of hypothalamic nuclei (preoptic nucleus, anterior hypothalamic area, and suprachiasmatic nucleus) called the surge or preovulatory center. The cells in this area appear to respond to a threshold level of estrogen. As the estrogen concentration increases rapidly just before estrus, this induces a flood of GnRH secretion (like turning on a faucet compared with the drip, drip of the tonic center) and a corresponding marked increase in LH called the ovulatory peak. Although GnRH usually stimulates secretion of both FSH and LH, it is thought that secretion of inhibin by the follicle at this time suppresses FSH secretion.

In males, LH plays a major role in regulation of testosterone secretion by the Leydig cells located in the interstitial tissue surrounding the seminiferous tubules of the testes. Within the tubules, FSH stimulates development and function of the Sertoli cells that nourish and regulate developing spermatozoa.

Thyroid-stimulating hormone

Like FSH and LH, TSH is a glycoprotein that shares a similar structure having an α and a β chain. The α subunits are identical and the β chains confer biological specificity. During synthesis the chains are produced separately and then are joined as glycosylation occurs in the Golgi. Mature TSH ultimately binds to receptors in the thyroid to promote thyroid uptake of iodine, iodination to produce triiodothyronine (T_3), and thyroxine (T_4) by the follicular cells of the thyroid gland. These events are triggered as a consequence of activating adenylyl cyclase and subsequently synthesis of cyclic AMP. With more prolonged stimulation, the thyroid gland is enlarged and follicular spaces are filled with stored thyroglobulin. Further details will be described in our discussion of the thyroid hormones.

Secretion of TSH is regulated by both stimulatory and inhibitory influences. The most direct control is from hypothalamic TRH that promotes secretion. However, somatostatin also acts as a potent inhibitor of secretion. Under usual circumstances, negative feedback from T_4 at the level of the pituitary and T_3 at the level of the hypothalamus provides acute control. However, since TSH and the thyroid hormones are so critical in metabolism it should not be surprising that other metabolically active hormones have an impact. For example, estrogen enhances the effect of TRH on secretion of TSH but GH and glucocorticoids dampen the effectiveness of TRH. At higher areas of the brain the activities of bioaminergic and peptidergic neurons also impact secretion of TRH and therefore TSH. For example, dopaminergic agonists (bromocriptine) inhibit TSH secretion but antagonists increase TSH release. Well-known effects of cold and stress to increase metabolic rate begin with alterations in neural activity that ultimately impacts hypothalamic secretion of TRH. This cascade of events then leads to secretion of TSH and then T_3, which is ultimately responsible for increased metabolism.

Adrenocortropic hormone (ACTH)

ACTH is a 39-amino-acid peptide processed from a larger precursor molecule called pro-opiomelanocortin (POMC), illustrated in Figure 12.25. In the corticotrophs of the anterior pituitary, the mRNA from the POMC gene directs the synthesis and processing of the transcript to yield at least eight biologically active fragments. ACTH primarily stimulates the secretion of glucocorticoids from the cortex of the adrenal gland. Two of the fragments are derived from ACTH. The first 13 amino acids of ACTH are β-MSH and the ACTH 18–39 corticotropin-like intermediate lobe peptide (CLIP). The larger precursor POMC appears in the intermediate lobe of the pituitary in many species and is associated with secretion of melanocyte-stimulating hormone (MSH). Biological effect of adrenal steroids will be considered in a subsequent section.

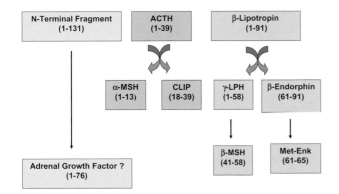

Fig. 12.25. Processing of pro-opiomelanocortin. Abbreviations include corticotropin-like intermediate lobe peptide (CLIP), melanocytes-stimulating hormone (MSH), lipotropin (LPH), and methynine-enkaplin (Met-Enk).

Although ACTH is the focus, a family of diverse peptides is derived from POMC. Secretion of ACTH is greatly impacted by neural factors and hormones. These agents ultimately modify the secretion of CRH, which, like GnRH, is secreted in an episodic pattern. In many species there is also a diurnal rhythm in the ACTH secretion pattern and therefore a diurnal secretion of adrenal steroids. Negative feedback loops, involving cortisol, are important in control of ACTH. One mechanism is sensitive to the rate of change in circulating glucocorticoids (fast feedback) and another responds to the absolute concentration of cortisol in a thresholdlike response (slow feedback). These effects are mediated at both the pituitary and hypothalamus. Furthermore, a host of stresses (pain, hypoxia, cold exposure, etc.) can override the usual rhythmic secretion of ACTH. This is classically thought of as the part of the fight-or-flight reactions and the need for nutrient mobilization, and it is associated with more prolonged secretion of glucocorticoids.

The thyroid gland

Located just below the larynx, the thyroid has left and right lobes medial to the midline of the ventral surface of the trachea. A sliver of tissue called the isthmus connects the lobes. The thyroid gland is composed of clusters of follicles whose internal surfaces are lined by a layer of simple cuboidal epithelial cells. Triiodothyronine (T_3) and thyroxine (T_4) is synthesized by the follicular cells and stored as part of a larger protein (thyroglobulin) within the lumenal spaces of the follicles. This stored material is called colloid. Figure 12.26 shows the histological structure of thyroid glands of a sheep and a cat. The follicular cells predominate but

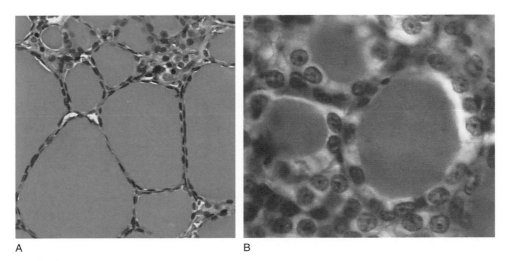

A   B

Fig. 12.26. Thyroid histology. Panel A is a low-power (20×) view of a sheep thyroid. The follicles are filled with colloid and the epithelial cells are compressed. Panel B (40×) is the thyroid from a cat. Here, the cells are more cuboidal and are actively reabsorbing colloid to make T_3 and T_4 available. Images courtesy of Dr. Lutz Slomianka.

in the spaces between follicles, parafollicular or C cells occur. C cells synthesize calcitonin, which is involved in calcium metabolism.

Biosynthesis of triiodothyronine and thyroxine

The critical elements required for thyroid hormone synthesis are the amino acid tyrosine and iodine. As iodine is absorbed into the follicular cells, it becomes attached to the ring structure of tyrosine amino acids that are part of the thyroglobulin sequence of amino acids. Each tyrosine is capable of becoming iodinated with two iodide atoms. When this occurs the result is diiodotyrosine, but attachment of a single atom produces monoiodotyrosine. The subsequent coupling of two diiodotyrosines produces thyroxine or T_4. The coupling of one diiodotyrosine and one monoiodotyrosine yields triiodothyronine or T_3. When the intestinal cells absorb iodine, it is converted to iodide for use in the thyroid. Thyroglobulin is a very large glycoprotein (5,496 amino acids) that has about 40 tyrosine residues. The follicular cells have an active transport system that very efficiently sequesters iodide so that intracellular concentrations can be 200-fold greater than that in circulation. Structures of thyroid hormones are shown in Figure 12.27.

Pathways for the synthesis, storage, and release of thyroid hormones are illustrated in Figure 12.28. The process can be divided into six steps: 1) uptake of I, 2) oxidation of iodide and iodination of tyrosine residues in the thyroglobulin, 3) linking of the DIT and MIT to create T_3 and T_4, 4) proteolysis of thyroglobulin to produce free T_3 and T_4, 5) deiodination of iodotyrosines in the follicular cells for reuse, and 6) 5'-deiodination of T_4 to generate T_3.

Biological effects of thyroid hormones

Thyroid hormones are the major regulators of basal metabolism. Thyroid hormones increase oxygen consumption and therefore heat production because they stimulate oxidative phosphorylation. This is called a calorigenic effect, a response especially useful when animals are exposed to cold stressful situations. Of course, increasing energy demands require nutrient fuel. Small amounts of thyroid hormones promote glycogen storage, but glycogenolysis is stimulated as concentrations rise. Other effects include increased absorption of glucose and promotion of glucose uptake by cells. Thyroid hormones also impact lipid metabolism but especially lipolysis. Fitting their ability to increase metabolism, the thyroid hormones also

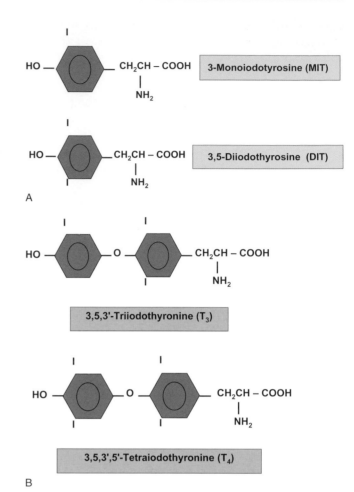

Fig. 12.27.   Structures of thyroid hormones.

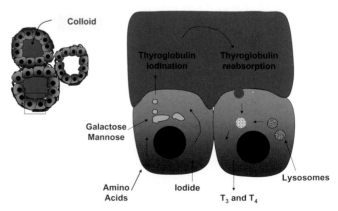

Fig. 12.28.   Iodination of thyroid hormone. A cluster of follicles is shown on the left and on the right an enlargement of two cells. In the cell on the left, amino acids allow synthesis of the thyroglobulin followed by posttranslational modification and packaging in the Golgi. Once thyroglobulin is secreted, iodination is completed. Secretion of TSH promotes the resorption of the iodinated thyroglobulin, the fusion with lysosomes, and ultimately the releases of T_3 and T_4.

enhance the effects of sympathetic nervous system stimulation. This is believed to be occurring by thyroid hormone stimulation of synthesis of β-adrenergic receptors in tissues that are targets for epinephrine and norepinephrine. This mechanism also likely explains the enhanced force of cardiac contractions when thyroid hormones are elevated.

Other effects of thyroid hormones are evident during growth and development. For example, classic experiments showed that thyroxine causes differentiation of tadpoles into frogs. Thyroidectomy or treatment with antithyroid drugs caused the animals to grow into very big tadpoles but metamorphosis was blocked. The situation is less drastic in mammals, but thyroid hormones are nonetheless essentially for normal development of the nervous system.

Given the myriad of effects attributed to thyroid hormones, it should not be a surprise that deviations from a normal or euthyroid state impacts physiology generally and homeostasis in particular. Hypothyroidism or a deficiency slows metabolic processes. In young animals development and growth is impaired, and in primates serious permanent failure of neural development produces mental retardation leading to cretinism. Hypothyroidism in mature animals produces lethargy. For example in humans, deposition of glycosaminoglycans in the skin causes puffiness and clinical symptoms called myxedema. Causes of hypothyroidism vary but can be classified as 1) primary (thyroid failure), 2) secondary (pituitary TSH problem), 3) tertiary (hypothalamic defect), or 4) quaternary (peripheral resistance to action of the hormones). This later case is frequently related to autoimmune disease in which a generation of antibodies against thyroid cells, thyroid hormone receptors, or thyroglobulin impairs function. Among domestic species, lactating dairy cows are typically hypothyroid so that peripheral deiodination of T_4 to produce the more potent T_3 is especially important to maintain function of many target tissues. Hypothyroidism is also common in dogs. The cause is not well understood but detection of antibodies against thyroglobulin in many of these animals suggests that autoimmune disease plays a role. Hyperthyroidism is relatively common in older cats and is usually associated with appearance of benign thyroid tumors.

Fortunately, because of the common structure of thyroid hormones across species, radioimmunoassays originally developed for human testing are appropriate for animal testing. A common functional test is to measure concentrations of plasma T_3 for T_4 in response to injections of TSH or TRH. In correspondence with variations in metabolic rate with season, the data in Figure 12.29 illustrate secretion of T_3 and T_4 following TRH injections in cows during winter compared with

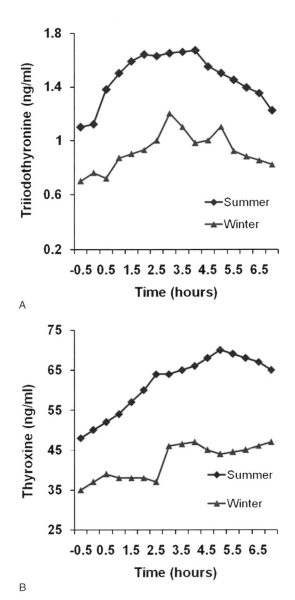

Fig. 12.29. Thyroid hormone responses to TRH. Lactating cows were injected with TRH (25 μg/100 kg body wt.) and blood collected to monitor changes in T_3 and T_4. Secretion of both hormones was reduced in winter. Data adapted from Perera et al. (1985).

summer. After a delay, TRH produced modest increases in circulating T_3 and T_4 in lactating cows. This reflects the time delay required for TRH to first stimulate the secretion of TSH by the anterior pituitary gland and for TSH to induce the process of colloid reabsorption by the thyroid follicular cells. There is also an evident seasonal variation in the response to TRH in these cows. Mean concentrations of T_3 and T_4 before administration of TRH were lower in cows sampled during winter and response to TRH was reduced. These reductions likely reflect greater utilization of thyroid hormones to enhance thermogenesis during the winter. Concentrations of T_4 were about fiftyfold greater than T_3. This is similar to other domestic animals and suggests that substantial T_3 formation occurs outside of the thyroid gland by the deiodination of T_4. Tissues with high levels of deiodination enzymes include the liver and kidneys. The mammary gland also expresses a deiodinase that increases with the onset of lactation and in response to other hormones known to stimulate milk production. This provides an enhanced local tissue concentration of mammary T_3 available to stimulate metabolic activity to support high levels of milk production despite the fact that lactating cows are typically in a hypothyroid state.

Thyroid hormones do not circulate freely in the serum but are bound to plasma proteins. The most predominant is thyroxine-binding globulin, but its concentration is relatively low, so despite its high binding affinity, substantial amounts of T_3 and T_4 also circulate bound to albumin. A third protein, thyroxine-binding pre-albumin is especially good at sequestering T_4. Although only free thyroid hormones are able to pass into target cells to bind with nuclear T_3 receptors, the hormones have the potential for long-lasting effects, in part because of their very long half-life. Whereas most hormones are rapidly degraded or taken from circulation (half-lives of minutes), T_3 and T_4 have long half-lives: ~1 and 7 days, respectively. Since T_3 is the essential biologically active thyroid hormone, deiodinase reactions to convert T_4 are physiologically important. It is reasonable to view the relatively larger quantities of circulating T_4 as a local tissue source for T_3 in target cells. Two primary deiodination pathways act to convert T_4 to either biologically potent T_3 (5'-deiodinase enzyme) or to reverse T_3 (5-deiodinase enzyme), which is biologically inert. Thus the increased 5-deiodinase can be viewed as a degradation pathway or increased 5'-deiodinase as an activation pathway. These conversions are illustrated in Figure 12.30.

Given the importance of thyroid hormones in regulation of metabolism, it was only natural for animal scientists to consider whether administration of thyroid hormones might be used to improve metabolic rate to support enhanced growth or development. For example, involvement of the thyroid gland in maintenance of lactation has been known since reports in the early 1900s showing that milk yield was reduced in thyroidectomized goats. By the 1930s it was shown that thyroidectomy of dairy cows reduced milk yield; and conversely that treatment with T_4 increased milk yield by approximately 20%. Because T_4 is also efficacious when fed, these reports stimulated much interest in the practical utilization of the hormone to increase milk production in cattle. This became economically feasible by the relatively low

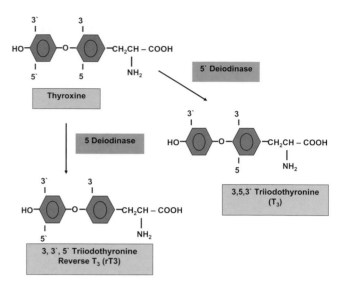

Fig. 12.30.   Structure and nomenclature for conversion of thyroxine.

cost manufacture of thyroxine and other thyroactive iodinated proteins. However, results of multiple studies showed that while feeding thyroxine (or iodinated proteins) increased milk production by 10–40%, the galactopoietic effect was of variable duration and milk production returned to normal or below-normal levels despite continued treatment.

The galactopoietic effect of thyroxine supplementation depends on a general increase in body metabolism. Thus it is not effective when cows are in early lactation and (negative energy balance) and already mobilizing body reserves to meet the energy demands of lactation. A general increase in body metabolism at this time would be counterproductive to meeting the nutrient demands of lactation. It was concluded that thyroxine treatment should not be initiated before midlactation and that the energy density of the diet should be increased during treatment because feed intake does not increase in proportion to increased energy utilization. Furthermore, upon withdrawal of treatment, a hypothyroid condition ensues that exacerbates the usual decline in milk yield in late lactation. Despite the initial interest in thyroid hormone supplementation to increase milk yield, the temporary nature of the milk yield response and frequent undershoot below normal production afterward led to the conclusion that its adaptation would be of minimal value.

Although T_4 is the predominant thyroid hormone in the circulation, it essentially serves as a prohormone because it has little if any biological activity. The most metabolically active thyroid hormone, T_3, is produced by enzymatic 5'-deiodination of T_4 within the thyroid and peripheral tissues. Changes in the extrathyroidal activity of thyroxine-5′-deiodinase (5′-D) alter localized T_3 availability. Activity of the enzyme also varies with physiological state. For example, with onset of lactation in rodents and ruminants, there is an increase in 5′-D in mammary gland and a decrease in liver. These changes are believed to maintain a euthyroid state in the lactating mammary gland despite the fact that the body is hypothyroid as a whole. The transfer of iodine, iodinated nonhormonal compounds and thyroid hormones through the mammary gland into the milk further exacerbates a systemic hypothyroid condition. Maintenance of a euthyroid state in the lactating mammary gland in the midst of a functional hypothyroid condition is consistent with increasing the metabolic priority of the mammary gland and providing T_3 to heighten the effect of other galactopoietic hormones. For example, this occurs in response to treatment of cows with exogenous bST (Capuco et al., 1989).

The relationship between GH and thyroid hormones is not limited to GH-induced alterations in 5′-D during lactation and galactopoiesis. There is a close relationship between thyroid hormones, thyroid hormone metabolism, and GH and IGF-I synthesis. Mechanistically, T_3 can alter hepatic GH receptor binding and thus enhance GH stimulation of IGF-I synthesis. Alternatively T_3 can also increase IGF-I synthesis in the absence of GH. It is worth noting that in those situations when GH does not stimulate IGF synthesis (e.g., during food restriction, fetal development, sex-linked dwarfism, and hypothyroidism) there is evidence for T_3 deficiency. In addition, T_3 serves as a regulator of GH synthesis by the pituitary. Conversely, GH can alter synthesis of 5′-D and therefore peripheral production of T_3 (Capuco et al., 1989).

Calcitonin

It would be difficult to overstate the physiological relevance of the thyroid hormones, but before we leave the thyroid gland behind, two other hormones are also synthesized in the thyroid or the parathyroid glands. Calcitonin is a 32–amino acids peptide whose major function is to inhibit the enzymatic action of osteoclasts in compact bone to reduce resorption of the inorganic matrix surrounding the cells. Parafollicular or C cells of the thyroid synthesize and secrete calcitonin in response to changes in serum Ca concentration. As concentrations rise—hypercalcemia—the cells increase calcitonin secretion, but with hypocalcemia hormone secretion is inhibited so that degradation of bone matrix is enhanced and Ca concentrations can return to normal. Although therapeutic use of calcitonin is limited in animals, in humans it is used in patients with Paget's disease (associated with abnormal bone resorption) and in some cases of osteoporosis.

Parathyroid hormone

Parathyroid hormone or PTH works with calcitonin to provide even greater control over calcium metabolism and ultimately improved homeostasis. The parathyroid glands usually occur in four pairs located near the poles of the two lobes of the thyroid gland. They are typically small clusters of tissue ~50 mg each. Cells that are actively synthesizing and secreting PTH are called chief cells. PTH is initially produced as a precursor (preproPTH) of 115 amino acids that has 25 amino acids cleaved in transit from the RER to the Golgi. Once in the Golgi, removal of 6 additional amino acids results in creation of biologically active PTH that is secreted in secretory vesicles by exocytosis.

The primary effect of PTH is to increase calcium and decrease phosphate concentrations in extracellular fluids. These effects are mediated by actions in multiple tissues. Since compact bone is the most abundant mineral reserve in the body, it is a major target tissue. An early effect of PTH is to stimulate the passage of calcium out of osteocytes and osteoblasts. Soon after, PTH activates osteoclast activity, which leads to increased enzymatic resorption of hydroxyapatite. Since the hydroxyapatite is essentially calcium, phosphate, and water, this action increases serum calcium and phosphate. Second, PTH acts on the distal convoluted tubules of the kidney nephrons to increase calcium absorption from the filtrate and simultaneously on the proximal convoluted tubules to decrease phosphate reabsorption. This improves calcium status without a corresponding increase in serum phosphate. In addition, PTH enhances the kidney tissue production of α1-hydroxylase, an enzyme that is needed for conversion of 25 hydroxy vitamin D3 into its more biologically active 1,25 dihydroxy analog. This is important because 1,25-(OH)2-vitamin D acts hormonelike to stimulate the synthesis of calcium binding—transport proteins in the intestinal epithelial cells. Over the course of several hours or days this increases absorption of calcium from the gut and therefore increases serum calcium. Given its myriad of actions, it is reasonable to assume that PTH plays a more prominent role in calcium homeostasis than calcitonin.

In domestic animals the most common disturbance in calcium metabolism typically occurs at the time of parturition and is most frequent in dairy cows (milk fever) and dogs. Affected animals exhibit severe hypocalcemia and often severe neuromuscular dysfunction. The animals frequently become recumbent (cows

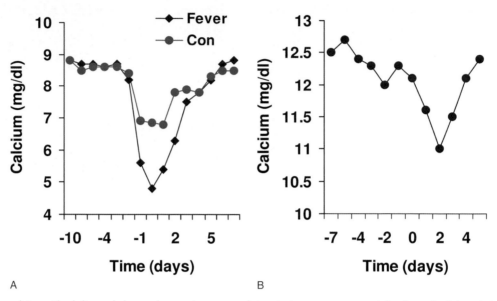

Fig. 12.31. Serum calcium. The left panel shows changes in serum calcium in Jersey cows around the time of calving. Animals that exhibited milk fever (diamonds) showed lower minimum values compared with herdmates (con) that did not exhibit milk fever. Data adapted from Goff et al. (1995). The right panel illustrates periparturient serum calcium for mares. The decrease in calcium of small magnitude and minimum values occurs 2 days after foaling. Data adapted from Martin et al. (1996).

typically are immobilized) and in dogs, for example, there are often involuntary muscle spasms referred to as tetany or eclampsia. The problem arises from the sudden demand for calcium needed for milk production so that serum concentrations are no longer maintained within usual homeostatic limits. Treatment typically involves infusion of glucose and calcium. After treatment, animals generally recover mechanisms to maintain calcium concentrations.

The etiology of milk fever is complex but it does not seem to involve a failure of PTH secretion. However, it may be that responsiveness of PTH target tissues (receptor expression) or vitamin D activation is impaired. In dairy cows, a common management recommendation is to feed diets that are low in calcium in the period before calving. The idea is to induce mobilization mechanisms prior to the dramatic increase that occurs with the onset of lactation so that the increased demand can be met. Figure 12.31 illustrates changes in serum calcium around the time of parturition in horses and cows. Both exhibit a decrease but it is relatively more dramatic in cows and especially in those that exhibited milk fever symptoms. Also, the lowest serum calcium level in the mares does not occur until 2 days postpartum.

The adrenal gland

Despite their small size the adrenal glands, located at the superior pole of each kidney, are critical regulators of metabolism. The outer portion of each gland, the cortex, is responsible for the production of two broad classes of steroid hormones, the mineralocorticoids of which aldosterone is a prime example and glucocorticoids represented by cortisol. The center of the gland, the medulla, is derived from neural tissue. It is essentially postganglionic tissue that is part of the sympathetic division of the autonomic nervous system. When stimulated it secretes epinephrine, a structural cousin of the neurotransmitter norepinephrine. Both of these regions are important in adaptation necessary to respond to stress and to maintain homeostasis. When animals are under prolonged stress it is not uncommon that the adrenal glands become enlarged. However, under extreme situations the capacity to respond can be lost, resulting in exhaustion. In the 1930s Sir Hans Selye was among the first to focus on the role of the adrenal to combat stress. He studied the response of adrenalectomized animals to injury or stress and pioneered what came to be called the general adaptation syndrome. His hypothesis consisted of three phases: 1) alarm reaction, 2) stage of resistance, and 3) stage of exhaustion. This can be envisioned by considering the pathways responsible for glucocorticoid secretion and biological responses to glucocorticoid release. First, stress induces neural stimulation leading to hypothalamic secretion of CRH. This results in secretion of ACTH, which produces glucocorticoid secretion. An early effect of glucocorticoid release is mobilization of glycogen reserves to increase circulating glucose. Other tissues are progressively catabolized to provide fatty acids or amino acids for energy production. If these actions provide the necessary nutrients to respond to the stress alarm, repairs are made and conditions return to normal. When stress continues but is manageable, a new "set point," or stage of resistance is achieved. However, with more extreme or prolonged stress, a new balance cannot be achieved so that signals for more glucocorticoid release cannot be answered by the adrenal cortex. This is the stage of exhaustion.

The adrenal cortex is organized into three zones (Figs. 12.32, 12.33). Just below the protective capsule that surrounds the gland, is the zona glomerulosa, it typically accounts for about 20% of the cortical cells. Here, the cells are organized into more or less spherical clusters; the name comes from *glomerulus*, Latin for "little ball." The zona fasciculate is the largest region and the cells are typically arranged into columns. Between the columns there are long fenestrated capil-

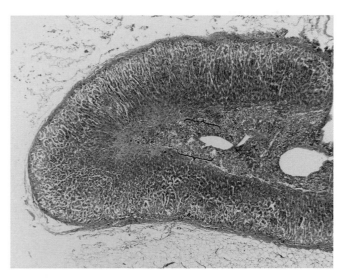

Fig. 12.32. Adrenal gland. Note the central area (medulla, brackets) and the outer cortex, H&E staining, 2× magnification.

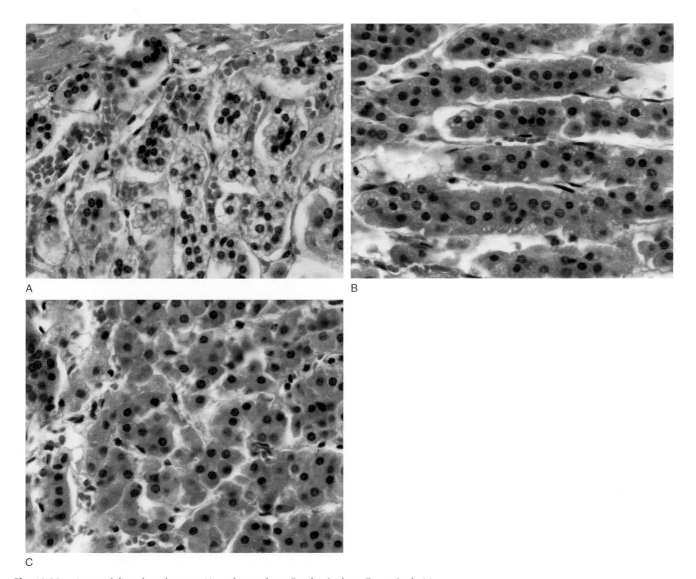

A

B

C

Fig. 12.33. Areas of the adrenal cortex (A = glomerulosa; B = fasciculata; C = reticularis).

laries. The innermost region of the cortex, the zona reticularis, is about the size of the zona glomerulosa and the cells are arranged in an irregular network.

The major hormones made in the adrenal cortex are cortisol or corticosterone (typical glucocorticoids), androgens (testosterone or testosterone-like), and aldosterone (mineralocorticoids). The zona glomerulosa is primarily responsible for the synthesis of aldosterone. Although we discussed some of the basics of steroid hormone structure earlier, some review is in order. Steroid synthesis begins with cholesterol. Much of the needed cholesterol comes from uptake from plasma lipoproteins, but synthesis directly from acetate also occurs. A critical, rate-limiting step involves the conversion of cholesterol to pregnenolone. In the two inner zones of the cortex this is stimulated by ACTH. This conversion occurs within the mitochondria and involves two hydroxylation steps along with cleavage of the side chain of the cholesterol. The pregnenolone passes out of the mitochondria for further processing. Differences in steroid synthesis between zones of the adrenal cortex reflect differences in the enzymes present. The greatest differences are between the zona glomerulosa and the inner zones. This explains why aldosterone is the predominant product of the glomerulosa. Specifically, the zona glomerulosa lacks 17α-hydroxylase activity, so it cannot produce either 17α-hydroxypregnenolone or 17α-hydroxyprogesterone. This is relevant because these molecules are the immediate precursors for cortisol and adrenal androgens. Furthermore, only the zona glomerulosa can convert corticosterone to 18-hydroxycortisosterone and aldosterone. Synthesis of aldosterone is largely controlled by the renin-angiotensin system of the kidney. This will be discussed in greater detail in our study of the urinary system. However, the essential point is that decreases in renal blood pressure leads to the production of angiotensin II which among other actions stimulates the secretion of aldosterone. Aldosterone then acts to increase resorption of sodium by the distal convoluted epithelial cells of the kidney nephrons. Increased recovery of sodium from the urinary filtrate, allows the companion recovery of more water (via osmosis) so that interstitial fluid volume and subsequently blood volume is increased. This returns blood pressure to normal, thus shutting off the trigger for increased aldosterone secretion in the first place. Secretions and regulation of the zona glomerulosa and two inner zones of the adrenal cortex are quite distinct. Some of the pathways for synthesis of various steroids in the adrenal gland are illustrated in Figure 12.34.

ACTH rapidly stimulates secretion of glucocorticoids from the inner zones of the adrenal cortex along with increases in DNA, RNA, and protein synthesis.

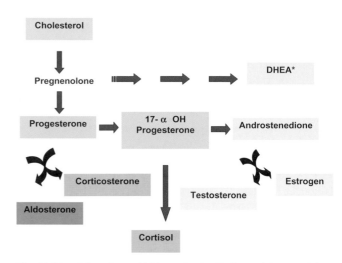

Fig. 12.34. Adrenal steroid biosynthesis. Cholesterol is essential, but conversion to pregnenolone allows subsequent production of sex steroids (yellow), glucocorticoids (tan), and mineralocorticoids (pink). *DHEA is dehydroepiandrosterone sulfate.

With chronic stimulation there is hyperplasia and hypertrophy of the cortical cells. Binding of ACTH to cortical cell receptors activates adenylyl cyclase leading to increased concentrations of cAMP. This activates intracellular phosphoprotein kinases. This ultimately stimulates the rate-limiting conversion of cholesterol to pregnenolone to allow for steroidogenesis. ACTH secretion is controlled by secretion of CRH from the hypothalamus so that changes in ACTH are closely paralleled by changes in cortisol or corticosterone secretion (depending on the species). However, neuroendocrine control of adrenal cortical activity is complex. Three levels of regulation include 1) circadian rhythm, 2) stress response, and 3) feedback inhibition. A circadian rhythm is superimposed on the typical episodic secretion of glucocorticoids that occurs throughout the day. This reflects CNS activity that controls both the number and magnitude of CRH and ACTH secretory episodes during the day. In primates, glucocorticoid secretion is usually low in the late evening and with the onset of sleep, but as dawn or wakefulness begins CNS activity and correspondingly CRH and ACTH secretory events increase in number and magnitude so that glucocorticoid concentrations increase. This pattern of low activity during sleep and increased activity during early day is relatively fixed, but substantial relative variability occurs. This inherent rhythm is impacted by physical and mental stresses and various disease conditions. Stress responses are usually tied with corresponding increases in release of epinephrine and thyroid hormones. This family of reactions allows for metabolic effects to maintain homeostasis. For example, increased glycogenolysis and gluconeogenesis provide fuel to synthesize ATP in stressful fight or flight situations. In conjunction with secretion of epinephrine from the adrenal medulla, a major effect in adipose tissue is increased lipolysis and release of glycerol and fatty acids for energy production.

Glucocorticoids impact multiple tissues. In excess they inhibit collagen synthesis by fibroblasts. This can produce thinning of the skin, easy bruising, and slow healing of wounds. Impaired bone formation can occur from reduced cell proliferation and extracellular matrix protein synthesis required for deposition of inorganic components of bone. This can clearly impact mineral metabolism as well as growth and development. One of the effects of glucocorticoids, inhibition of neutrophils, is used therapeutically to lessen inflammation. These potent effects demonstrate the dramatic problems that accompany situations where either too much or too little of the adrenal steroids are produced.

Routine control over glucocorticoid secretion depends on negative feedback at multiple levels (see Fig. 12.13). In particular, increased concentrations of glucocorticoids inhibit secretion of CRH from the hypothalamus as well as ACTH from the pituitary. In fact, two distinct negative feedback responses have been described. A fast-feedback glucocorticoid-induced inhibition of ACTH secretion occurs that is directly related to the rate of increase in glucocorticoid secretion. This phase occurs within minutes and acts to reduce both basal and ACTH-stimulated increases in adrenal glucocorticoids. A delayed-feedback inhibition subsequently suppresses both CRH and ACTH secretion. At the extreme, prolonged administration of glucocorticoids suppresses CRH and ACTH secretion and the adrenal cortex atrophies. Addison's disease or adrenocortical insufficiency occurs when there is a failure of the adrenal cortex to produce sufficient amounts of mineralocorticoids or glucocorticoids. The consequences of this are clearly dramatic. Symptoms can include muscle weakness, fatigue, anorexia, hypotension, hyponatremia, and hypoglycemia. With companion failure of aldosterone production, additional symptoms include dehydration hyperkalemia and acidosis. Causes include destruction or dysfunction of the adrenal cortex. For example, tuberculosis can destroy the adrenal cortex, as can autoimmune disorders. Other causes reflect failures at the level of the hypothalamus (impaired secretion of CRH) or pituitary (impaired secretion of ACTH). Before adrenal steroids became available for therapy, primary adrenocortical insufficiency was fatal.

The opposite problem, chronic secretion of excess glucocorticoids, leads to an array of problems called Cushing's syndrome in humans. The most common cause is excess glucocorticoid therapy. This again emphasizes the importance of careful use of these potent steroids. Classic Cushing's syndrome is often caused by pituitary or adrenal abnormalities that lead to excess concentrations of ACTH, i.e., tumor products. Cushing's disease has multiple effects on tissue metabolism and organ function. This is expected given the widespread distribution of glucocorticoid receptors. Obesity can occur with alterations in distribution of adipose tissue, i.e., moon face and appearance of a "buffalo-hump" are symptoms that can develop over time. Hypertension, glucose intolerance, and gonad dysfunction are also manifestations of the disease.

As concerns with animal health and welfare and perceived problems attributed to stress have emerged in recent years, tools to quantitatively measure stress have been sought. Certainly there are behavior attributes and production-related measures (absence of chronic disease, rate of gain, milk production, etc.) that can be linked with disruption of homeostasis tied to stress, but many of these are poorly defined. It is also true that some level of stress is necessary, even desirable, for normal physiological responses and health. As indicated earlier, during short-term stress secretion of glucocorticoids and epinephrine allow mobilization of nutrients necessary for homeostasis. The problems arise with severe chronic stress and consequences of prolonged secretion of glucocorticoids, i.e., immunosuppression and atrophy of tissues. However, measuring changes in circulating concentrations of glucocorticoids, responses to an ACTH challenge, and/or secretion of epinephrine provide a generally accepted quantifiable stress index for animals. Paradoxically, it is possible that the process (handling, needle sticks, and restraint) of taking frequent blood samples (often necessary because of the episodic nature of glucocorticoid secretion) can be stressful in itself. This has led to development of remote blood sampling devices or sampling of other body fluids (saliva or urine), but these samples may also require confinement or handling that can confound results. Möstl and Palme (2002) described the assay of metabolites of cortisol in feces as a tool to noninvasively monitor secretion of glucocorticoids as a possible stress index. The concentrations of these cortisol metabolites in feces reflect a kind of "average" glucocorticoid production over a period of hours that is likely species-specific. For example, in sheep and cattle changes in fecal concentrations of 11,17-dioxoandrostane are correlated with changes in blood levels of cortisol following treatment with a bolus challenge of ACTH but with a 10–12 hour delay (Palme et al., 1999).

The endocrine pancreas

The two primary endocrine products of the pancreas are insulin and glucagon. Both hormones are simple proteins synthesized in small clusters or islands of cells nested within the exocrine tissue of the pancreas. The German pathologist Paul Langerhans discovered these clusters of cells, now called the islets of Langerhans, in 1869. They represent only a small fraction of the mass of the pancreas (1–2%). Each individual islet (~0.4 mm in diameter) contains only a few thousand cells but they are nonetheless critical for homeostasis. Four cell types can be distinguished within the islets. Glucagon-producing α cells are about 20% of the total. Insulin-secreting β cells are the most abundant constituting 60 to 80% of the total. Somatostatin-producing δ cells are infrequently observed (3–10% of the total), but pancreatic polypeptide–secreting PP or F cells are rare (~1% abundance).

Insulin is a small protein, with a molecular weight of about 6,000 daltons. It is composed of two chains held together by disulfide bonds, but it is synthesized as a precursor molecule in which a fragment called the C-peptide is removed to produce the biologically active molecule. The amino acid sequence of insulin is highly conserved. For example, it is still common for diabetic patients to be treated with porcine insulin. In fact, the first case of treatment of a human diabetic with insulin was in 1922.

Insulin synthesis begins with translation of its mRNA as a single-chain precursor called preproinsulin. As it passes into the cisternal space of the RER, removal of its signal peptide produces proinsulin. Proinsulin has three domains: an amino-terminal B chain, the A chain carboxy terminal region, and a connecting peptide in the middle called the C peptide. Once it passes into the cisternal space of the RER endopeptidases excise the C peptide, to produce mature insulin. Insulin and free C peptide are packaged in the Golgi into secretory granules, which accumulate in the cytoplasm. When the β cell is stimulated, insulin and C peptide are secreted from the cell by exocytosis. However, C peptide has no known biological activity.

Secretion of both insulin and glucagon is closely tied to circulating concentrations of glucose. For optimal health and maintenance of homeostasis, blood glucose concentrations must be maintained within fairly narrow boundaries. In the case of the β cells, extracellular glucose is transported into the cells by facilitated diffusion involving specific glucose transporter proteins. Because its uptake depends on diffusion, the greater the extracellular glucose concentration, the greater the corresponding intracellular concentration. As concentrations reach a threshold value this produces a change in membrane depolarization and

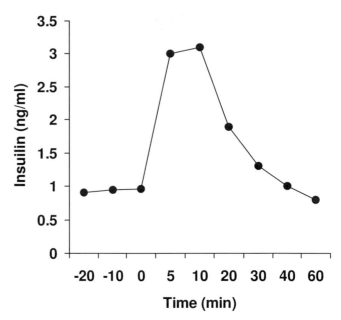

Fig. 12.35.   Insulin after glucose. Cows were infused with glucose (0.1 g/kg body wt.) at time zero. Data adapted from Denbow et al. (1986).

subsequently an influx of extracellular calcium. The precise mechanism(s) responsible for depolarization are not well defined but may depend on metabolism of glucose that is taken up into the cell and alterations in the ATP : ADP ratio within the cytoplasm. Regardless, the increase in free calcium is believed to be a primary stimulator of exocytosis of insulin containing vesicles.

It is clear that increased glucose concentrations markedly increase secretion of insulin in normal animals. This is particularly evident in monogastric animals after feeding of a high-carbohydrate meal. Figure 12.35 illustrates the increase in insulin in cows that were given a bolus injection of glucose into the jugular vein. In this case the experiment was done to compare pancreatic responsiveness among cows in various seasons. There is plainly an abrupt increase in serum insulin following a glucose challenge even in ruminants.

Although secretion of insulin acts to lower blood glucose by promoting the uptake of glucose into most cells and particularly increased glycogenesis in liver tissue, control of blood glucose concentration does not simply depend on changing secretion of insulin. When blood glucose concentration drops, the islets secrete glucagon. Glucagon stimulates the breakdown of glycogen and promotes gluconeogenesis. As a generalization, increases in blood insulin concentrations act to drive energy substrates into storage in tissues and glucagon the mobilization of fuel substrates. This association is illustrated in Figure 12.36.

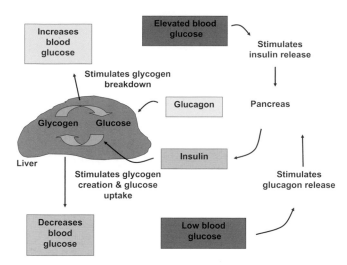

Fig. 12.36. Regulation of blood glucose. When glucose is elevated, the pancreas releases insulin. This promotes the uptake of glucose and glycogen formation in the liver, thus reducing blood glucose and promoting hypoglycemia. Glucagon is released when blood glucose is low. This stimulates glycogen breakdown, thereby returning glucose concentration to normal, a hyperglycemic response.

Problems with regulation of blood glucose concentrations are relatively common in humans and animals. Naturally occurring diabetes is probably the most common endocrine disorder diagnosed in dogs, with estimates for the frequency of diabetes ranging from a high of 1 in 100 to 1 in 500. Diabetes mellitus is a complex disease that is manifested by inappropriate hyperglycemia. Symptoms and problems result from a failure of insulin secretion, failure of biological action of insulin, or both. It is useful but somewhat arbitrary to classify diabetes as either insulin-dependent (type I) or non–insulin-dependent (type II). In type I diabetes, insulin is very low or absent, plasma glucagon is typically elevated, and the β cells fail to respond to stimuli known to stimulate insulin secretion in healthy animals. Typical symptoms include polyuria and polydipsia as well as weakness and fatigue and often polyphagia with weight loss. The increased urination is a consequence of osmotic diuresis related to hyperglycemia. Thirst and polydipsia occur as a consequence of hyperosmotic state of body fluids. Since glucose is poorly utilized in the absence of insulin, ketosis and subsequently ketoacidosis occur as fatty acids are catabolized to supply energy demands. Wasting of muscle mass can also happen as muscle proteins are degraded to supply amino acids for glucose and ketone bodies. Ironically, it is as if the body is starving, despite the presence of large quantities of blood glucose. Without insulin, the capacity of cells to capture blood glucose is impaired yet energy demands remain. To add insult to injury, so to speak,

the β cells of the islets also require insulin to sense that glucose concentrations are adequate. This means that the α cells are stimulated to secrete glucagon; this further worsens the problems by promoting glycogenolysis and gluconeogenesis. With acute insulin deficiency the increased energy demands and failure to utilize glucose, ketones (acetoacetate, β-hydroxybutyrate, and acetone) rapidly increase. Along with reduced renal blood flow (reduced extracellular fluid volume) and associated reduced renal excretion, hydrogen ions also can accumulate. This can lead to dramatic ketoacidosis. Continuing increases in blood osmolarity (>330 mosm/L) and progressive acidosis produce coma and ultimately cardiovascular collapse and death.

Clearly, the primary treatment option is to monitor blood glucose to minimize drastic swings with careful attention to diet and replacement of missing insulin with exogenous treatments. Fortunately, recent advancements in molecular biology and biotechnology have made multiple options available. Many patients still are treated with porcine or bovine insulin, but recombinant human insulin is also available. There are also multiple forms of insulin available for therapy, i.e., short acting (so-called regular insulin), as well as intermediate and long-acting formulations. This has increased the opportunity to better control blood glucose, particularly with respect to meals.

With less acute episodes but chronic hyperglycemia of diabetes, a variety of pathological changes can occur during the course of the disease. Vascular diseases include both microvascular and macrovascular problems. In capillaries and smaller precapillary arterioles there is frequently a thickening of the basement membrane. These can be especially problematic in the retina, leading to retinopathy and progressively failed vision; in the kidney, progressive disease produces pathological problems in the peritubular capillary beds surrounding the nephrons. In larger vessels, diabetes is believed to accelerate atherosclerosis and all of the associated problems, i.e., increased incidence of myocardial infarction, stroke, and peripheral gangrene, which seems to be largely unique to diabetic patients.

Diabetes is also associated with increased incidence of cataracts. Increased blood glucose is believed to contribute to formation of cataracts by promoting glycosylation of lens proteins and by increasing concentrations of sorbitol within the lens tissue. Sorbitol is a by-product of glucose metabolism. As it accumulates this promotes osmotic changes that ultimately promote swelling and fibrosis. Changes in the cornea and lens are frequently rapid and are a consistent ocular manifestation of diabetes. A decrease in corneal sensitivity is often observed as the disease progresses. Corneal nerves are important in producing protective responses (tear production and eyelid closure) so that diabetic-related impairment of these responses can have important consequences. Table 12.10 shows the results of Cochet-Bonnet aesthesiometer measurement to compare the sensitivity of the corneal touch threshold (CTT) in diabetic, compared with normal, dogs. This test utilizes an instrument that has 6.0 cm length of monofilament nylon that is pushed against the cornea until there is a slight deflection. Reducing the length of the filament in 0.5 cm segments until a blink reflex is recorded continues the process. This length is recorded and converted to a force value (g/mm2)—in other words, the force required to elicit the blink response (from 0.4 to 15.9 g/mm2) depending on the length from 6.0 to 0.5 cm. Testing is done to compare various regions of the cornea, i.e., central (C), nasal (N), dorsal (D), temporal (T) and ventral (V) and averaged for both eyes. These data show a consistent pattern of reduced sensitivity (i.e., greater force required to elicit the blink response) in diabetic, compared with clinically normal, dogs.

In type II diabetes, the problem is failure of insulin to be biologically active. However, this is typically a milder form of the disease in that it is heterogeneous with respect to symptoms and the degree of biological failure. This also influences treatment options. Simplistically, type I diabetes treatment requires replacement of missing insulin. This situation is more complex with type II because treatment options depend on the relative contribution of still-functional β cells and the degree of insulin insensitivity. For example, type II is more common in obese animals. This in part reflects the fact that adipose tissue has abundant insulin receptors and is a key tissue in control of energy balance and homeostatic alterations in carbohydrate metabolism. Therefore, a common treatment scheme is to promote weight loss and to control episodes of hypo- or hyperglycemia with diet.

Other hormones and growth factors

As you have concluded by now, a host of hormones and growth factors are involved in physiological processes. In this chapter, we have chosen to focus on some of the major endocrine organs and selected growth factors. Indeed, entire courses of study are devoted to endocrinology or even narrow families of related messengers. As we discuss specific systems, we will briefly describe the properties and actions of some of the other hormones and growth factors. Some examples include 1) leptin, a hormone produced by adipose tissue that affects appetite; 2) erythropoietin, a kidney-derived hormone that responds to a reduction in blood oxygen and stimulates synthesis of red blood cells; and 3) atrial naturetic peptide, a hormone from the heart that impacts blood pressure by affecting sodium resorption. Table 12.11 gives a listing of some of these other hormones and growth factors and some relevant physiological features.

Table 12.10. Corneal touch threshold in diabetic and normal dogs.

Region of Cornea	Diabetic	Normal
Central	2.9	1.8
Nasal	4.0	2.2
Dorsal	5.1	2.8
Temporal	5.1	2.8
Ventral	6.5	5.1

Data adapted from Good et al. (2003).

Table 12.11. Selected growth factors.

Growth Factor	Abbreviation	Properties
Epidermal growth factor	EGF	Proliferation of epithelium derived from epidermis, mammary development, cancer, and development. At least 10 family members (EGF, TGF-α, heregulins) bind to type I receptor kinases (ErbB-1,2).
Transforming growth factor	TGF-β	Family of at least five proteins, i.e., TGF-β1,2,3, etc., involved in modification of the extracellular matrix (ECM) to influence tissue development. Secreted bound to glycoproteins that are cleaved for activation.
Fibroblast growth factor	FGF	Related family of 20 peptides, strong affinity for heparinlike glycosaminoglycans of the ECM. Many members are likely stromal tissue–derived mitogens.
Leptin		Produced primarily in adipocytes, involved in control of feed intake as well as other developmental processes.
Transforming growth factor	TGF	Member of superfamily of proteins that typically inhibit epithelial cell growth, important expression of ECM proteins, and glandular morphogenesis.
Atrial natriuretic peptide	ANP	Produced by heart atrium secreted in response to stretch along with a related factor brain natriuretic factor (BNP). Responses include vasodilation, inhibition of aldosterone secretion, and diuresis to normalize blood pressure.

Some of the growth factors that have particular significance in animal research are briefly discussed in the following sections. To serve as examples we have focused on several that are known to be important in mammary development or function. This is because lactation and mammary development are important in all mammals and especially relevant with respect to the dairy industry. Second, some of the factors we have selected for discussion have been in the news in recent years because of relationships with cancer generally and with breast cancer specifically. This does not mean that these agents do not have more general roles in most animals; rather, our focus on the mammary gland gives us a common theme for this discussion and makes for relevant examples to illustrate some of the biological properties of these agents.

Last, it is difficult to overstate the significance of technical advancements in cell and molecular biology that have allowed a major expansion in our understanding of structural relationships between various messengers. Based on detailed structural analysis at the DNA, RNA, and protein levels, messengers not previously identified as being related have come to be grouped into families of molecules. In some cases, messengers are grouped based on structure of the protein, but other ligands are grouped based on similarity of the receptors to which they bind. For researchers this is a time of astonishingly rapid advancements and accumulation of enormous detailed information. Unfortunately, for students and others it can also be confusing as more details emerge to allow reclassification or new understanding. Again, our goal in this section is not to provide a comprehensive review of the myriad of growth factors but to illustrate the properties of some of these agents that are relevant in animal agriculture or are a part of recent medical news.

IGF family

While we have discussed the somatomedin hypothesis and the role of IGF-I as it relates to the actions of GH, it has become increasingly clear that the IGF family of growth factors, receptors, and binding proteins play critical roles in many specific physiological processes including mammary and ovarian development. IGF-I and IGF-II are widely expressed endocrine-, autocrine-, or paracrine-acting peptides that regulate cell growth, cell differentiation, maintenance of cell function, and prevention of apoptosis in multiple cell types. Research with IGF-I and IGF-II was initially centered on the somatomedin hypothesis (Hadsell et al., 2002). Since these early experiments, with the somatomedins now called the IGFs, the view

has evolved that the IGFs are also important local acting autocrine or paracrine stimulators of cell function. The primary signaling receptor for the IGF-I peptide is a tyrosine kinase receptor (IGF-IR) structurally similar to the insulin receptor (see Figure 12.5). The receptor is widely distributed and is now known to have important roles in normal cell growth and development. Moreover, abnormal stimulation of IGF-IR is implicated in appearance and continuing development of a variety of different types of tumors. In particular, the strongly antiapoptotic activity of the receptor is recognized as being relevant in tumor genesis. However, other related effects, including effects on cell-cell and cell-extracellular matrix interactions, are also likely important in both normal and abnormal tissue development. Our focus is on normal development, but much of the recent basic work to understand functions of IGFs and IGF-IR are derived from cancer-oriented studies.

In the cow, normal circulating concentrations of insulin 1–5 ng/ml would have little ability to signal via IGF-IR. IGF-I can also bind to the insulin receptor but with much less affinity (~thousandfold). The situation is further confounded by the existence of hybrid receptors between IGF-IR and the native insulin receptor (IR), which has a higher affinity for IGFs than for insulin. IGF-II binds with high affinity to a receptor that is identical with a receptor for mannose-6-phosphate, but the receptor has no known intracellular signaling function. The affinity of this receptor for IGF-I is about a hundredfold lower than for IGF-II and it does not recognize insulin. There are as many as five distinct types of insulin/IGF-I hybrid receptors. The IR isoforms (IR-A and IR-B) and IGF-IR have the ability to form both homo- and heterotetramers. This clearly can change the diversity of signaling induced by binding of insulin or IGFs. Signaling pathways and biological effects are best characterized for IGF-IR and IR-B, but experiments in cell culture model systems support the idea that combinations of native and hybrid receptors allow both overlapping and unique physiological effects. In general, stimulation of either IGF-IR or IR-B is associated with cell cycle progression, but stimulation of IR-B is more closely related to metabolic events and stimulation of IGF-IR with mitogenesis. These major properties were illustrated in elegant molecular studies in which the cytoplasmic domains for IR-B and IGF-IR receptors were swapped. In the normal situation, there are overlapping as well as specific signaling events associated with activation of IR-B or IGF-IR (Hadsell and Bonnette, 2000).

Studies with rodents in which various elements of the IGF-I axis were deleted have confirmed that IGF-I and/or IGFI-R are essential for normal mammary development (Kleinburg et al., 2000). Since animals homozygous for absence of the IGF-IR do not survive after parturition, these experiments required the transplantation of the fetal mammary analog from ~day 18 fetuses into the cleared mammary fat pads of syngeneic hosts. Growth of rudimentary mammary structures from IGF-IR–null mice, compared with tissue from wild-type mice, was minimal. In mice without expression of IGF-I, the development of terminal end buds required replacement with IGF-I. Neither estradiol or GH alone (classic mammary-acting hormones) nor the combination had any affect on prepubertal mammary development in these knockout mice. These and related rodent experiments show that in normal peripubertal mammary development, GH acts to bind to GH receptors in the stromal tissue. This is associated with local production of IGF-I, which, in turn, promotes the development of the mammary ducts. Certainly overexpression of recombinant IGF-I in the mammary glands of transgenic mice promotes premature development of alveolar buds in prepubertal animals (Weber et al., 1998).

In addition to IGF-I and IGF-II there are six IGF-binding proteins (IGFBPs) and nine related proteins (IGFBP-rP) that affect the actions of IGF-I and II. The IGFBPs are well characterized and bind IGF-I with ~tenfold higher affinity than the IGFBP-rPs. The IGFBPs have several functions, including prolonging the half-life of IGF-I, transporting IGF-I from the circulation, and localizing IGF-I to potential target cells (Clemmons, 1998; Duan 2002). Locally produced IGFBPs provide a mechanism to target or localize IGFs within particular tissues or cells and thereby alter biological responses to IGFs. It is worth taking a moment to discuss this idea of binding proteins and how they can be studied. A typical procedure is to separate solutions of proteins suspected to contain binding proteins by standard SDS-PAGE electrophoresis. These proteins, which are next separated in columns or lanes based on molecular weight and/or charge, are then transferred to a membrane (essentially like a sheet of paper). This membrane is subsequently washed in an appropriate buffer and then incubated in a solution containing I^{125} radiolabeled IGF-I or IGF-II. The iodinated protein is allowed to bind, and then the membrane is washed and exposed to x-ray film. The position of proteins that bind to the IGF appears as black dense bands on the developed film. These bands can then be photographed and/or scanned and evaluated for the level of density. When specific antibodies to the binding proteins for a particular species are available, these ligand blots can be supplemented using western blotting. Figure 12.37 gives an example of an IGF-I ligand blot binding protein prepared from conditioned medium collected from bovine mammary epithelial cells. In this example, there is abundant expression of IGFBP-2 and IGFBP-3 (as confirmed by western blotting) and a lower molecular weight

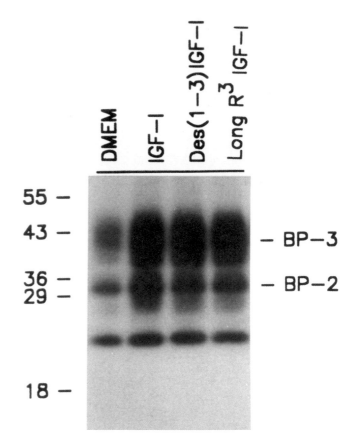

Fig. 12.37. IGF-I binding proteins. Effects of incubation of bovine mammary cells with IGF-I or selected IGF-I analogs are shown. Adapted from Romagnolo et al. (1994).

binding protein that is probably IGFBP-4 based on molecular weight (Romagnolo et al., 1994). The secretion of these binding proteins is increased when the cells are incubated with native IGF-I or two analogs of IGF-I that exhibit reduced capacity to interact with binding proteins.

Along with locally produced IGF-I made by epithelial cells (see Figure 12.18), as illustrated by experiments with bovine mammary tissue (Weber et al., 2000), mammary cells also synthesize several IGFBPs, including IGFBP-1, 2, 3, and 5. IGFBP-3 is usually touted as an inhibitor of responses to IGF-I. For example, Figure 12.38 shows increased proliferation of mammary tissue following treatment with estrogen, GH, or the combination, and the associated mirror image shows a decrease in tissue concentrations of IGFBP-3. This suggests that at least some of the proliferation induced with these classic mammogenic hormones is mediated by a local reduction in mammary tissue IGFBP-3. There is also increased tissue IGF-I, again suggesting the importance of IGF-I axis molecules in regulation of mammary development (Berry et al., 2001).

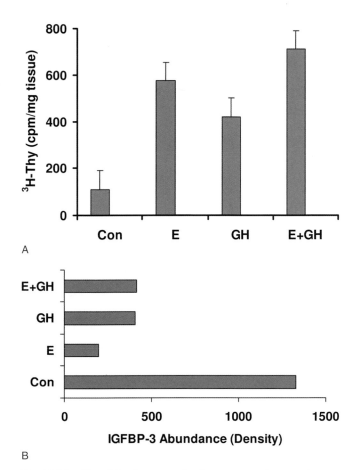

Fig. 12.38. Thymidine incorporation in mammary tissue and IGFBP-3. Panel A shows increased DNA synthesis in mammary tissue of heifers treated with placebo (Con), estradiol (E), growth hormone (GH) or both (E+GH). Panel B illustrates the relative abundance of IGFBP-3 in mammary tissue from these same animals. Note that increased proliferation appears negatively correlated with decreased tissue IGFBP-3. Adapted from Berry et al. (2001).

In addition to its effects related to mammary development and function in farm animals, the IGFs and binding proteins are also critical in ovarian development. In fact, in all mammalian species studied, IGF-I stimulates the granulosa cell growth and steroidogenesis. However, changes in local concentrations of IGFs are not as critical as marked alterations in the tissue concentrations of IGFBPs. These changes are responsible for enhanced availability of free IGF-I during terminal follicular growth and then increase synthesis of IGFBP-2, 4, and 5 to promote atresia. Specifically, as reviewed by Monget et al. (2002), in the ewe, sow, cow, and mare, intrafollicular concentrations of IGFBP-2, -4, are markedly decreased from the 1 to 2 mm follicles to the larger preovulatory follicles. By contrast, intrafollicular concentrations of these same IGFBPs as well as IGFBP-5 in the ruminants greatly increase in atretic follicles. This pattern of change is due to two events:

variation in mRNA expression and selected degradation caused by expression of intrafollicular proteases. These examples simply illustrate two areas of tissue and cell development that are impacted by this important family of growth factors.

EGF family

Epidermal growth factor (EGF) was discovered by accident in 1960 when unexpected biological activity (not attributed to nerve growth factor) occurred following injections of extracts of murine salivary glands into test animals. These effects were associated with precocious eyelid opening and tooth eruption in neonates. Subsequent studies showed that preparations of EGF stimulated the proliferation of isolated epidermal cells and epidermal tissue explants. Study of a human epidermal cancer cell line (A-431) was fundamental in subsequent studies because these mutated cells greatly overexpressed receptors for EGF ($\sim 3 \times 10^6$ receptors per cell). This property allowed for the isolation and structural characterization of the receptor. The availability of relatively large quantities of the receptor also led to the discovery that the addition of EGF to isolated membranes stimulated the phosphorylation of both endogenous membrane proteins as well as many exogenously added proteins. It was subsequently shown that the receptor protein was a 170 kDa transmembrane glycoprotein whose external domain formed the binding site for EGF and whose cytoplasmic domain possessed tyrosine kinase activity. EGF bound to the external portion of the receptor activates the cytoplasmic or catalytic domain of the receptor to produce autophosphorylation and, subsequently, phosphorylation of cytoplasmic substrates essential for EGF action. These observations were important because they were among the first to directly link ligand binding, receptor activation, and phosphorylation as general mechanisms of action for many growth factors.

This family of proteins contains at least 10 members, including EGF, heparin binding EGF, transforming growth factor α (TGF-α), amphiregulin, neuroregulins (four subtypes), and several heregulins. Each of these structurally similar proteins acts by binding to one of several related membrane receptors called type I receptor tyrosine kinases (RTK) or the ErbB family of receptors. The usual EGF receptor is called ErbB-1, but at least four variants are known. Certain receptors in the family, ErbB-2 [also called HER2 or Neu], contribute to the aggressive phenotype of some human breast carcinomas and related poor prognosis. A homologue of EGF, TGF-α was first isolated from the medium of oncogene-transformed cells, and a transforming avian retrovirus subsequently was shown to code for synthesis of an abbreviated form of the EGF receptor. EGF and TGF-α are highly expressed in early embryonic development. Amphiregulin and HB-EGF are secreted heparin-binding growth factors. The ErbB family of receptor kinases is essential for development of the nervous, cardiovascular, gastrointestinal, and other systems.

Dysfunction of these receptors is common in many forms of carcinogenesis, which explains much of the emphasis for work in this area. A direct connection between the ErbB family and cancer was established with the breakthrough that the retroviral oncogene v-ErbB, which is transduced by the avian erythroblastosis virus, is a form of an avian EGF receptor. This then led to subsequent discoveries showing that overexpression of ErbB agonist proteins and/or overexpression or inappropriate expression of ErbB receptors were important in a variety of human cancers. In fact, a humanized monoclonal antibody against ErbB-2 called Herceptin was the first such product approved for human use. It was designed specifically for breast cancer patients with tumors that overexpress ErbB-2 (Stern, 2003; Harris et al., 2003).

EGF is important in normal mammary gland development in mice and likely other species as well. In particular, there is compelling evidence to suggest that estrogen (a potent mammogenic hormone from the ovary) likely induces local production of EGF agonists [EGF itself, TGF-α, or amphiregulin] and that these agents are important in alveolar development. Receptors for EGF are present in regions of rapidly growing mammary ducts, including the surrounding stromal cells. The importance of these proteins in mammogenesis in farm animals is less well established, but specific EGF receptors are found in mammary tissue from sheep and cows (Plaut, 1993) and expression of EGF mRNA has been shown for bovine mammary tissue (Koff and Plaut, 1995). Ligand binding assays using either radiolabeled EGF or TGF-α show a single class of high-affinity binding sites in mammary tissue of sheep and cows during gestation and into lactation. However, the number of receptors is greater during midpregnancy than during late pregnancy or during lactation. Expression of TGF-α occurs in the bovine and amphiregulin occurs in ovine mammary tissue. Addition of either TGF-α or EGF stimulates DNA synthesis in explants from midpregnant heifers, in epithelial cells from heifers or pregnant cows and sheep. Figure 12.39 shows the effect of EGF on DNA synthesis in mammary explants prepared from tissue taken from midpregnant heifers, either before or after xenotransplantation into nude mice. For freshly prepared explants, concentrations of EGF of less than 10 nM only stimulated DNA synthesis after 2 days in culture. For xenotransplanted tissues, priming of mice with estrogen and progesterone for 10 days increased the

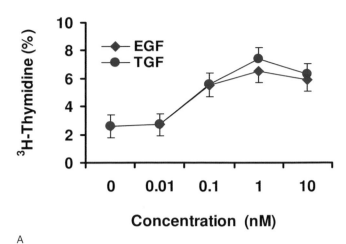

A

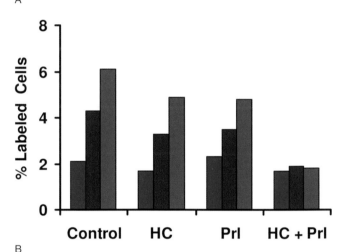

B

Fig. 12.39.   EGF and cell growth. Panel A shows an autoradiographic analysis of EGF or TGF-α stimulated DNA synthesis in bovine mammary tissue explants from midpregnant Holstein heifers. Tissues were incubated for 2 days in the presence of the growth factors. DNA synthesis was measured during the last 6 hours of culture by measurement of tritiated thymidine incorporation. Panel B shows the effect of hydrocortisone (HC) and Prl on EGF-induced DNA synthesis in bovine mammary alveolar epithelial cells for tissue explants maintained in athymic nude mice. Mice were primed for 10 days with estrogen and progesterone and then treated for 2 days with placebo (Control), HC, or Prl. Xenografted tissues were removed and cultured for 2 days with no EGF (dark blue), 0.1 nM EGF (burgundy) or 1 nM EGF (pink). Note the lack of effect of EGF for tissues when mice were treated with HC + Prl. Data adapted from Sheffield (1998).

sensitivity of the tissue to EGF when explants were removed and tested in culture. Interestingly, treatment of the mice with hydrocortisone or Prl for the final 2 days of transplantation slightly reduced the subsequent response to EGF but treatment with hydrocortisone (synthetic glucocorticoids) + Prl blocked any effect of EGF on DNA synthesis. This response suggests that mammogenic effects of EGF may be more important for mammary ductular development than for lobulo-alveolar formation in cattle. Failure of EGF to stimulate DNA synthesis in mice given hydrocortisone and Prl suggests that differentiation of the alveolar cells is incompatible with EGF-induced growth. Intramammary infusion of EGF stimulated DNA synthesis in udders of pregnant heifers but it is not clear whether this represents augmentation of a normal response to naturally occurring EGF in the bovine mammary gland or a pharmacological effect.

For tissues that synthesize EGF or its related ligands, these growth factors are made as transmembrane glycoproteins. The EGF-like sequences are external to the plasma membrane. Requirements for secretion are not completely understood, but they involve the action of a protease that cleaves the membrane-bound protein for release of the EGF (or relative) into the interstitial fluid. Induced overexpression of TGF-α under control of mammary promoters in rodents leads to the appearance of mammary tumors. This fits with measurements showing that some spontaneous human mammary tumors also express large amounts of TGF-α or EGF receptor. It is also important to remember that responses of cells or tissues in culture may not necessarily reflect the response of tissue in the complex environment of the intact animal. Presence of EGF receptors, ligands, and demonstrated response of ruminant mammary cells to EGF support a role for these growth factors in mammogenesis, but much more information is needed to determine exact roles. In short, it is not known whether the EGF family of proteins and receptors are largely permissive or whether they have an essential direct impact in ruminant mammary development.

The EGF family is also important in the growth and development of hair, so there is much interest in impacts of these growth factors on wool and other animal hair products. Specifically, the hair follicle has two closely aligned epithelial cell layers. The inner root sheath cells produce TGF-α but do not express EGF receptor (ErbB-1), but the opposite is true for the outer root sheath (receptors but no TGF-α). For normal growth it is essential that newly formed TGF-α be processed for release and then rapidly bound by receptors in the outer sheath of cells. In the case of EGFR or TGF-α–null mice, which are engineered without the receptor and/or ligand, hair follicle formation is disturbed. When this local TGF-α escapes capture, it acts as an attractor of other cells into the region of the hair follicle so that the hair coat is abnormal and whiskers are wavy (Mann et al., 1993).

FGF family

FGFs constitute a family of 20 small peptide growth factors that share a highly homologous core of 140 amino acids and strong affinity for heparin and heparinlike glycosaminoglycans (HLGAGs) of the extracellular matrix (ECM). FGF signaling and interactions with the ECM has attracted the attention of numerous cancer researchers because of the potential role of the FGFs in promoting the progression of some tumors from a hormone-dependent to a hormone-independent pattern of growth. Others are attracted to FGF studies from observations that development of many cancers positively correlates with local tissue secretion of proteases and changes in pH, which might act to change concentrations of biologically available FGFs in the local tissue environment. Both FGF-1 (also known as acidic FGF or aFGF) and FGF-2 (also known as basic FGF or bFGF) were first identified from extracts of bovine pituitary glands based on the capacity of the proteins to stimulate DNA synthesis in cultured fibroblasts. Members of this family of growth factors are linked by structural similarities and capacity to bind heparin or HLGAGs, and not specificity by their growth-stimulating activity. By convention they continued to be designated as FGFs despite the fact that not all of the proteins actually stimulate proliferation of fibroblasts. Consequently, several members of the FGF family have emerged as stroma-derived mitogens, which may act in a paracrine manner—for example, in the mammary gland—to locally influence epithelial cell proliferation and glandular morphogenesis (Hovey et al., 1999; Powers et al., 2000).

Although the FGFs function after they appear in the extracellular environment via binding to high-affinity cell surface receptors, neither FGF-1 nor FGF-2 are synthesized with a leader peptide sequence. You may recall from our discussion of cell physiology that the leader sequence is a strand of hydrophobic amino acids at the amino terminal of the newly synthesized peptides that serve to control the secretion destination of the protein. That determines whether the protein will be retained within the cell or secreted. The leader peptide is recognized by a signal recognition particle (SRP), which temporarily halts translation and serves to transport the translation complex to the endoplasmic reticulum (ER). At this point protein synthesis resumes and the nascent peptide chain is vectored into the cisternal space of the ER where it subsequently passes to the Golgi for packaging into secretory vesicles for secretion from the cell. This feature has attracted cell biologists to the study of these FGF variants to decipher this secretion mechanism. Because FGFs are also involved in wound healing it has been suggested that mechanical damage provides a mechanism for release of FGF from endothelial cells, but such a mechanism would seemingly lack the regulation necessary for secretion of FGFs in many other situations—for example, whether they play a role in normal glandular development.

FGF-1 likely functions as a paracrine mitogen for epithelial cells. For example, transgenic mouse experiments that target overexpression of a defective FGF receptor to the mammary gland showed that lobulo-alveolar development was distinctly impaired. Of the various rat mammary cell types, fibroblasts express the greatest level of FGF-1 mRNA in vitro. Appearance of mRNA and protein within both the intact mouse mammary gland and epithelial-cleared mammary fat pad strongly supports the idea that FGF is stromal in origin. At least three of the known FGF variants—FGF-1, FGF-2, and FGF-7 (also known as keratinocyte growth factor, KGF)—are proposed to be involved in ruminant mammary development. These FGFs and their receptors are expressed during mammogenesis, lactation, and mammary involution. The highest levels of expression were in glands of virgin heifers and in primiparous heifers during involution.

Although FGF-2 mRNA expression is greatest in the stromal tissue, immunocytochemical studies show that the FGF-2 protein associates with myoepithelial cells. This distribution may simply reflect the high affinity of FGF-2 for specific components of the ECM, further supporting its proposed role as a paracrine/autocrine mitogen for myoepithelial cells. Synthesis of FGF-2 in the mouse mammary fat pad is hormonally regulated based on observations that expression is greatest during late pregnancy in correspondence with the appearance of higher tissue concentrations of the protein at this time. Expression is also increased in the bovine mammary gland in late gestation. Interaction between epithelium and the surrounding stroma likely influence paracrine FGF-2 expression; in rodents and ruminants expression is greater in the stroma adjacent to the developing parenchymal tissue.

Transforming growth factor family

The TGF-β group of proteins is made up of at least five multifunctional proteins that have functions ranging from modification of the ECM, to induction of differentiation of target cells, to stimulation of proliferation in multiple cells types and tissues. Based on continuing genetic and molecular studies, it is now known that TGF-βs are only part of a superfamily of at least 40 members of structurally related proteins that include the TGF-βs, activins/inhibins (important in gamete production, i.e., first identified based on their activity in regulation of FSH secretion), and bone morphogenetic proteins (BMPs). At least 28 genes encode for various elements of this family of proteins and companion receptors. Three of the variants—TGF-β1, TGF-β2, and TGFβ-3—stimulate connective tissue formation and are chemotactic for fibroblasts. They can indirectly promote proliferation of mesenchymal cells but can inhibit growth of epithelial cells in vivo and in vitro. These varied effects of TGF-βs suggests that they are likely important in tissue development and function. TGF-β1 is the best-described of these proteins related to mammary function. Blood platelets provide the most concentrated source of TGF-β1, but it is believed to be produced by nearly every cell type in the body. Biologically active TGF-β1 is a 25 kDa disulphide-linked homodimer. When secreted it is bound to a large 75 kDa glycoprotein called the latency-associated peptide (LAP). Activation of the latent form by proteases, alkalinization, or chaotropic agents is necessary for TGF-β1 to bind to its receptor, so control of this reaction is an important regulator of TGF-β1 action. Unregulated epithelial cell proliferation is obviously an undesirable trait of tumor formation, so it should not be surprising that actively-growing cells must be controlled to prevent hyperplasia. For example, most of the mammary associated effects of TGF-βs are inhibitory (Plaut et al., 2003).

Effects of TGF-β are mediated by binding to specific cell surface receptors (designated type I, II, or III receptors) present on most cell types. The type I and type II receptors are directly involved in signal transduction; the type III receptor is thought to enhance binding of TGF-β to one of the other receptor subtypes. In heifers, for example, the ductal epithelial cells of the mammary gland show extensive presence of type I and type II receptors by immunocytochemical localization of antibody to the receptors.

The specific role of TGF-β1 in ruminant mammary development is unknown, but concentrations of TGF-β1 in serum ranged from 7 to 30 ng/ml, and receptors for TGF-β1 are increased during the peripubertal period corresponding with rapid mammary development. Related studies show that TGF-β1 inhibits the proliferation due to addition of IGF-I, IGF-II, des (1–3)-IGF-I, EGF, or amphiregulin. TGF-β1 also affects the morphology of bovine mammary organoids in culture (Ellis et al., 2000). The possibility that IGFBP-3 (or fragments) might have IGF-I receptor independent actions in mammary cells, via binding to the type V TGF-β receptor, coupled with TGF-β induction of IGFBP-3, makes for an intriguing overlap between the growth-stimulating actions of the IGF-I axis and the inhibitory effects of the TGF-β family of molecules. TGF-β members are important in early embryonic development and maintenance of homeostasis in adult tissue by affecting cell growth, differentiation of epithelial cells, and apoptosis.

The signaling cascade for TGF-β, like the other growth factors, involves binding of the ligand to cell surface receptors. These receptors are transmembrane serine/threonine kinases. A current model is that binding induces the creation of a receptor complex composed of the type I and type II receptors. Receptor II then acts to phosphorylate receptor I. The phosphorylated form of receptor I is activated to generate the intracellular signal responsible for the effect of the growth factor. Specifically, cytoplasmic Smad proteins in target cells are substrates for the activated receptor, and these serve as signaling modulators. Interestingly, Smad proteins were named based on work that arose from comparative molecular studies. Specifically, Drosophila geneticists isolated a gene called *Mad* while others working on *C. elagans* identified a gene they called *Sma*. It was soon realized that these were the same gene products, so a combined naming convention was evolved—*Smad*. Smads are widely expressed throughout development and in virtually all tissues.

Regulation of specific genes can be either positive or negative, depending on the conditions specific to a particular target cell. In TGF-β signaling, I-Smads block signaling by recruiting so-called Smurf ubiquitin ligases to capture various Smad proteins and target them for degradation. Generally, the activity of many cellular proteins is controlled by selective proteolysis through the ubiquitin-proteosome pathway. In summary, Smads can be thought of as transcriptional co-modulators whose activity is controlled by various receptors of the TGF-β superfamily of receptors via induction of nuclear accumulation of Smads (Moustakas et al., 2003).

Leptin

Evidence for an adipose tissue–derived homeostatic regulator of feed intake has accumulated for a number of years (Ahima and Flier, 2000; Ingvartsen and Andersen, 2000. These studies built on the proposals by Kennedy (1953) stating that the amount of energy stored in adipose tissue mass represents a steady state between energy needs and energy derived from feed intake. Since adipose tissue tends to be relatively stable for long periods in many mammals, he suggested that there must be a regulatory mechanism that effectively monitors changes in energy stores to elicit the needed change in feed intake to "restock" adipose reserves when demand is higher but to conversely reduce "deliveries" during periods of lower energy demand.

This concept of a circulating fat-derived regulator of feeding behavior was bolstered by the discovery of genetic mutations in mice, obese (ob) and diabetes (db) phenotypes. Both of these recessive mutations lead to hyperphagia, decreased activity, and early onset of obesity. Parabiosis of wild-type mice with ob/ob mice suppressed the weight gain in the defective mice, but parabiosis of wild-type mice with db/db mice caused marked hyperphagia and weight gain in the normal mice. This led to the idea that the ob gene locus was essential for the production of a circulating satiety factor and that the db locus encoded for a molecule capable of responding to this circulating agent. The product of the ob gene was subsequently named leptin (from the Greek word *leptos* for "thin"), because of the effects of the protein to reduce feed intake and body weight when injected into leptin-deprived or normal animals. Leptin satisfied many of the requirements of the adipose tissue regulator envisioned by Kennedy many years ago. Specifically, leptin is proposed to prevent obesity by reducing feed intake and increasing thermogenesis by affecting the hypothalamus. These initial reports stimulated tremendous interest in leptin as an obesity preventative or weight-control agent in humans. However, like many aspects of homeostatic or homeorhetic regulation, simple answers are not often sufficient. Although leptin can provide a signaling pathway between adipose tissue and the central nervous system for monitoring of adipose tissue stores, the wide distribution of leptin receptors indicated that leptin affects many tissues and physiological systems.

Leptin is a 16 kDa protein primarily produced in adipose cells, and in nonruminants circulates both in a free form and bound to other proteins in circulation. Energy stores influence expression of the leptin gene, as shown by increased adipose tissue leptin mRNA and serum concentrations in obese mammals. There is also a positive correlation between body fat stores and leptin concentrations in blood, and secretion occurs with a circadian rhythm and may show episodic secretion. Although adipose tissue is the major source of leptin, relatively lower levels of expression are found in many other tissues. It may be that local tissue production of leptin is also important in addition to effects mediated by changes in circulating concentrations.

Cloning studies of the leptin receptor (Ob-R) indicate that there are at least six leptin receptor isoforms derived by alternative splice variants of the mRNA coding for the receptor. The receptor belongs to the family of cytokine receptors, which includes receptors for interleukins and Prl. Each of the leptin isoforms has identical extracellular ligand binding domains but they differ at the carboxy terminal end of the molecule or the cytoplasmic portion. Differences among the isoforms mean that there can be a great deal of variation in the signaling cascade stimulated by the binding of leptin to a particular receptor. Since expression of receptor isoforms is not uniform among target tissues, this adds an additional layer of complexity to understanding the physiological effects of leptin stimulation.

Unfortunately, studies in domestic animals and especially dairy animals are limited (Houseknecht, et al., 1998). However, fasting increases the expression of the Ob-RL receptor in the sheep hypothalamus. Interestingly, leptin is also increased in the serum of animals fed high-energy diets, which may be related to decreased mammary development that can occur in these animals. Moreover, leptin appears in milk and is present in cultured bovine mammary epithelial cells. The cells also express mRNA for leptin and were impacted by additions of insulin and IGF-I, both of which are known mediators of mammary function. This suggests that leptin may be an autocrine- or paracrine-signaling molecule in the mammary gland (Smith and Sheffield, 2002).

Leptin may also be involved in regulation of onset of puberty in heifers and ewes. It is well known that age of puberty, within limits, is affected by dietary energy intake, rate of growth, and accumulation of adipose tissue in the body. Given the role of leptin in adipose tissue metabolism it is attractive to suggest that leptin is also important in this process. Short-term fasting of peripubertal heifers decreases leptin gene expression, circulating leptin, and luteinizing hormone (Williams et al., 2002). Leptin can modify activity of the hypothalamic-pituitary axis as well as the endocrine pancreas, depending on nutritional conditions in cattle and sheep.

In conclusion, we have provided an overview of major hormones—their sources, properties, and actions. We have also provided some examples of the details related to how target cells respond to hormones, growth factors, and similar regulators. These are complex and difficult topics, but it is important to slowly develop some appreciation of the intricate interrelationships between these messengers and tissues. It is difficult to overstate the relevance of the endocrine system in physiological regulation.

References

Adams, T.E., V.C. Epa, T.P.J. Garrett, and C.W. Ward. 2000. Structure and function of the type 1 insulin-like growth factor receptor. CMLS. Cell. Mol. Life. Sci. 57: 1050–1093.

Ahima, R.S. and J.S. Flier. 2000. Leptin. Annu. Rev. Physiol. 62: 413–437.

Akers, R.M. 2006. Major advances associated with hormones and growth factor regulation of mammary growth and lactation in dairy cows. J. Dairy Sci. 89: 1222–1234.

Akers, R.M. and A.M. Lefcourt. 1982. Teat stimulation-induced prolactin release in non-pregnant and pregnant Holstein heifers. J. Endocrinol. 96: 433–442.

Akers, R.M., D.E. Bauman, A.V. Capuco, G.T. Goodman, and H.A. Tucker. 1981. Prolactin regulation of milk secretion and biochemical differentiation of mammary epithelial cells in periparturient cows. Endocrinol. 109: 23–30.

Akers, R.M., S.E. Ellis, S.D. Berrya. 2005. Ovarian and IGF-I control of mammary development in prepubertal heifers. Domestic Anim. Endo. 29: 259–267.

Akers, R.M., T.B. McFadden, S. Purup, M. Vestergaard, K. Sejrsen, and A.V. Capuco. 2000. Local IGF-I axis in peripubertal ruminant mammary development. J. Mammary Gland Biol. Neoplasia 5: 43–51.

Asimov, G.J. and N.K. Krouze. 1937. The lactogenic preparations for the anterior pituitary and the increase of milk yield in cows. J. Dairy Sci. 20: 289–306.

Bauman, D.E. 1999. Bovine somatotropin and lactation: From basic science to commercial application. Domestic Anim. Endo. 17: 101–116.

Baumrucker, C.R., C.A. Gibson, and F.L. Schanbacher. 2003. Bovine lactoferrin binds to insulin like growth factor binding protein-3. Domestic Anim. Endo. 24: 287–303.

Berry, S.D., R.D. Howard, P.M. Jobst, and R.M. Akers. 2003. Interactions between the ovary and the local IGF-I axis modulate mammary development in prepubertal heifers. J. Endocrinol. 177: 295–304.

Berry, S.D., T.B. McFadden, R.E. Pearson, and R.M. Akers. 2001. A local increase in the mammary IGF-I : IGFBP-3 ratio mediates the mammogenic effects of estrogen and growth hormone. Domestic Anim. Endo. 21: 39–53.

Butler, A.A., S. Yakar, I.H. Gewolb, M. Karas, Y. Okubo, and D. LeRoith. 1998. Insulin-like growth factor-I receptor signal transduction: At the interface between physiology and cell biology. Comp. Biochem. Physiol. Part B 121: 19–26.

Capuco, A.V., J.E. Keys, and J.J. Smith. 1989. Somatotropin increases thyroxine-5'-monodeidonase activity in lactating mammary tissue of the cow. J. Endocrinol. 121: 205–211.

Clemmons, D.R. 1998. Role of insulin-like growth factor binding proteins in controlling IGF actions. Mol. Cell. Endocrinol. 140: 19–24.

Clemmons, D.R. and L.A. Maile. 2003. Minireview: Integral membrane proteins that function coordinately with insulin-like growth factor I receptor to regulate intracellular signaling. Endocrinol. 144: 1664–1670.

Cowie, A.T., I.A. Forsyth, and I.C. Hart. 1980. Hormonal Control of Lactation. Heidelberg: Springer-Verlag Berlin.

Cowie, A.T., J.S. Tindal, and A. Yokoyama. 1966. The induction of mammary growth in the hypophysectomized goat. J. Endocrinol. 34: 185–195.

Dahl, G.E., B.A. Buchanan, and H.A. Tucker. 2000. Photoperiodic effects on dairy cattle: a review. J. Dairy Sci. 83: 885–893.

Das, R. and B.K. Vonderhaar. 1997. Prolactin as a mitogen in mammary cells. J. Mammary Gland Biol. Neoplasia 2: 29–39.

Denbow, C.J., K.S. Perera, F.C. Gwazdauskas, R.M. Akers, R.E. Pearson, and M.L. McGilliard. 1986. Effect of season and stage of lactation on plasma insulin and glucose following glucose injection in Holstein cattle. J Dairy Sci 69: 211–216.

Duan, C. 2002. Beyond Carrier Proteins—Specifying the cellular responses to IGF-I signals: Roles of IGF-binding proteins. J. Endo. 175: 41–54.

Ellis, S.E., S. Purup, K. Sejrsen, and R.M. Akers. 2000. Growth and morphogenesis of epithelial organoids from peripheral and medial mammary parenchyma of prepubertal heifers. J. Dairy Sci. 83: 952–961.

Etherton, T.D. and D.E. Bauman. 1998. The biology of somatotropin in growth and lactation of domestic animals. Physiol. Rev. 78: 745–761.

Folley, S.J. 1956. The Physiology and Biochemistry of Lactation. Oliver and Boyd, Edinburgh, Scotland.

Goff, J.P., T.A. Reinhardt, and R.L. Horst. 1995. Milk fever and dietary cation-anion balance effects on concentrations of vitamin D receptor in tissues of periparturient dairy cows. J. Dairy Sci. 78: 2388–2394.

Goffin, V. and P. Kelly. 1997. The prolactin/growth hormone receptor family: Structure/function relationships. J. Mammary Gland Biol. Neoplasia. 2: 7–18.

Good, K.L., D.J. Maggs, S.R. Hollingsworth, R.H. Scagliotti, and R.W. Nelson. 2003. Corneal sensitivity in dogs with diabetes mellitus. Am. J. Vet. Res. 64: 7–11.

Hadsell, D.L. and S.G. Bonnette. 2000. IGF and insulin action in the mammary gland: Lessons from transgenic and knockout models. J. Mammary Gland Biol. Neoplasia 5: 19–30.

Hadsell, D.L., S.G. Bonnette, and A.V. Lee. 2002. Genetic manipulation of the IGF-I axis to regulate mammary gland development and function. J. Dairy Sci. 85: 365–377.

Hansen, R.K. and M.J. Bissell. 2000. Tissue architecture and breast cancer: The role of extracellular matrix and steroid hormones. Endocrine-Related Cancer 7: 95–113.

Harris, R.C., E. Chung, and R.J. Coffey. 2003. EGF receptor ligands. Exp. Cell Res. 284: 2–13.

Houseknecht, K.L., C.A. Baile, R.L. Matteri, and M.E. Spurlock. 1998. The biology of leptin: A review. J. Anim. Sci. 76: 1405–1420.

Hovey, R.C., T.B. McFadden, and R.M. Akers. 1999. Regulation of mammary gland growth and morphogenesis by the mammary fat pad: A species comparison. J. Mammary Gland Biol. Neoplasia 4: 53–68.

Hynes, N.E., N. Cella, and M. Wartmann. 1997. Prolactin mediated intracellular signaling in mammary epithelial cells. J. Mammary Gland Biol. Neoplasia 2: 19–27.

Ingvartsen, K.L. and J.B. Andersen. 2000. Integration of metabolism and intake regulation: A review focusing on periparturient animals. J. Dairy Sci. 83: 1573–1597.

Kennedy, G.C. 1953. The role of depot fat in the hypothalamic control of feed intake in the rat. Proc. R. Soc. Ser. B139: 578–592.

Kleinburg, D.L., M. Feldman, and W. Ruan. 2000. IGF-I is an essential factor in terminal end bud formation and ductal morphogenesis. J. Mammary Gland Biol. Neoplasia 5: 7–19.

Koff, M.D. and K. Plaut. 1995. Detection of transforming growth factor-alpha like messenger RNA in the bovine mammary gland. J. Dairy Sci. 78: 1903–1908.

Koprowski, J.A. and H.A. Tucker. 1973. Bovine serum growth hormone, corticoids and insulin during lactation. Endocrinol. 93: 645–651.

Laud, K., I. Gourdou, L. Belair, D. H. Keisler, and J. Djiane. 1999. Detection and regulation of leptin recptor mRNA in ovine mammary epithelial cells during pregnancy and lactation. FEBS Lett. 463: 194–198.

Lefcourt, A.M. and R.M. Akers. 1983. Is oxytocin really necessary for efficient milk removal in dairy cows? J. Dairy Science 66: 2251–2259.

Lefcourt, A.M., J. Bitman, D.L. Wood, and R.M. Akers. 1995. Circadian and ultradian rhythms of peripheral growth hormone concentrations in lactating dairy cows. Domestic Anim. Endo. 12: 247–256.

LeRoith, D. and C.T. Roberts, Jr. 2003. The insulin-like growth factor system in cancer. Cancer Letters 195: 127–137.

LeRoith, D., C. Bondy, S. Yakar, J. Lui, and A. Butler. 2001. The somatomedin hypothesis, 2001. Endo. Rev. 22: 53–74.

Lyons, W.R. 1958. Hormonal synergism in mammary gland growth. Proc. Royal Soc. B149: 303–325.

Lyons, W.R., C.H. Li, and R.E. Johnson. 1958. The hormonal control of mammary growth. Recent Prog. Horm. Res. 14: 219–254.

Mann, G.B., K.J. Fowler, A. Gabriel, E.C. Nice, R.L. Williams, and A.R. Dunn. 1993. Mice with a null mutation of the TGF alpha gene have abnormal skin architecture, wavy hair, and curly whiskers and often develop corneal inflammation. Cell 73: 249–261.

Martin, K.L., R.M. Hoffman, D.S. Kronfeld, W.B. Ley, and L.D. Warnick. 1996. Calcium decreases and parathyroid hormone increases in serum of periparturient mares. J. Anim. Sci. 74: 834–839.

Monget, P., S. Fabre, P. Mulsant, F. Lecerf, J. Elsen, S. Mazerbourg, C. Pisselet, and D. Monniaux. 2002. Regulation of ovarian folliculogenesis by IGF and BMP system in domestic animals. Domestic Anim. Endo. 23: 139–154.

Möstl, E. and R. Palme. 2002. Hormones as indicators of stress. Domestic Anim. Endo. 23: 67–74.

Moustakas, A., S. Souchelnytksyi, and C. Heldin. 2003. Smad regulation in TGF-β signal transduction. J. Cell Sci. 114: 4359–4369.

Nandi, S. 1958. Endocrine control of mammary gland development and function in the C3H/He Crgl mouse. J. Natl. Cancer Inst. 21: 1039–1360.

Nostrand, S.D., D.M. Galton, H.N. Erb, and D.E. Bauman. 1991. Effects of daily exogenous oxytocin on lactation milk yield and composition. J. Dairy Sci. 74: 2119–2127.

Palme, R., C. Robia, C.S. Memann, S.J. Hofer, and E. Möstl. 1999. Measurement of faecal cortisol metabolites in ruminants: A non-invasive parameter of adrenocortical function. Wien Tierarztl Mschr 86: 237–241.

Perera, K.S., F.C. Gwazdauskas, R.M. Akers, and R.E. Pearson. 1985. Season and lactational effects on response to thyrotropin releasing hormone injecting in Holstein cows. Domestic Anim. Endocrinol. 2: 43–52.

Peters, R.R., L.T. Chapin, K.B. Leining, and H.A. Tucker. 1978. Supplemental lighting stimulates growth and lactation in cattle. Science 199: 911–912.

Plaut, K. 1993. The role of epidermal growth factor and transforming growth factors in mammary development and lactation. J. Dairy Sci. 76: 1526–1538.

Plaut, K., A.J. Dean, T.A. Patnode, and T.M. Casey. 2003. Effect of transforming growth factor-beta (TGF-β) on mammary development. J. Dairy Sci. 86: E16–E27.

Powers, C.J., S.W. McLeskey, and A. Wellstein. 2000. Fibroblast growth factors, their receptors and signaling. Endocrine-Related Cancer 7: 165–197.

Riddle, O., R.W. Bates, and S.W. Dykshorn. 1933. The preparation, identification and assay of prolactin—A hormone of the anterior pituitary. Am. J. Physiol. 105: 191–216.

Romagnolo, D., R.M. Akers, J.C. Byatt, E.A. Wong, and J.D. Turner. 1994. IGF-I-induced IGFBP-3 potentiates the mitogenic actions of IGF-I in mammary epithelial MD-IGF-I cells. Molec. Cell. Endo. 102: 131–139.

Rosen, J.M., S.L. Wyszomierski, and D. Hadsell. 1999. Regulation of milk protein gene expression. Annu. Rev. Nutr. 19: 407–436.

Sheffield, L.G. 1998. Hormonal regulation of epidermal growth factor receptor content and signaling in bovine mammary tissue. Endocrinol. 139: 4568–4575.

Silva, L.F.P., M.J. VandeHaar, M.S. Weber Nielsen, and G.W. Smith. 2002. Evidence for a local effect of leptin in bovine mammary gland. J. Dairy Sci. 85: 3277–3286.

Sjogren, K, J.O. Jansson, O.G. Isaksson, and C. Ohlsson. 2002. A transgenic model to determine the physiological role of liver-derived insulin-like growth factor I. Minerva Endocrinol. 4: 299–311.

Smith, J.J., A.V. Capuco, I.H. Mather, and B.K. Vonderhaar. 1993. Ruminants express a prolactin receptor of $M^{\circledR}$ 33,000–36,000 in the mammary gland throughout pregnancy and lactation. J. Endocrinol. 139: 370–479.

Smith, J.L. and L.G. Sheffield. 2002. Production and regulation of leptin in bovine mammary epithelial cells. Domestic Anim. Endo. 22: 145–154.

Stern, D.F. 2003. ErbBs in mammary development. Exp. Cell Res. 284: 89–98.

Stricker, P. and R. Grueter. 1928. Action du lobe anterieur de l'hypophyse sur la montée laiteuse. CR Soc. Biol. (Paris) 99: 1978–1980.

Weber, M.S., P.L. Boyle, B.A. Corl, E.A. Wong, F.C. Gwazdauskas, and R.M. Akers. 1998. Expression of ovine insulin-like growth factor-I (IGF-I) stimulates peripubertal development of alveolar buds in mammary glands of transgenic mice. Endo. 8: 251–259.

Weber, M.S., S. Purup, M. Vestergaard, R.M. Akers, and K. Sejrsen. 2000. Regulation of local synthesis of insulin-like growth factor-I and binding proteins in mammary tissue. J. Dairy Sci. 83: 30–37.

Williams, G.L., M. Amstalden, M.R. Garcia, R.L. Stanko, S.E. Nizelski, C.D. Morrison, and D.H. Keisler. 2002. Leptin and its role in the central regulation of reproduction in cattle. Domestic Anim. Endo. 23: 339–349.

13 Cardiovascular system

Contents

The cardiovascular system (*cardio* = heart; *vascular* = blood vessels) consists of three components: blood, the heart, and blood vessels. Blood is essential for transporting nutrients and wastes, thermoregulation, immunity, and acid-base balance. The heart and blood vessels help deliver the blood throughout the body.

Functions and composition of blood

Functions of blood

The study of blood, blood-forming tissues, and blood disorders is called hematology. Since animals consist of multiple layers of cells, they cannot rely on simple

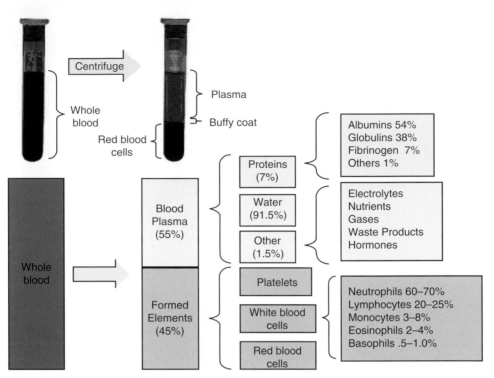

Fig. 13.1. Blood components. Centrifugation of whole blood containing an anticoagulant results in the separation of red blood cells, a buffy coat containing white blood cells and platelets, and plasma.

diffusion to deliver nutrients and remove wastes. Instead, the blood is necessary for these functions. Blood is a connective tissue consisting of materials suspended in a nonliving liquid matrix called plasma. Blood has three main functions: transportation, regulation, and protection.

Transportation

Blood transports O_2 and CO_2 between the lungs and the tissues. In addition, blood transports absorbed nutrients from the gastrointestinal tract to the liver and other cells; hormones from endocrine glands to target cells; waste products from cells to excretory sites including the liver, kidneys, and skin; and heat throughout the body.

Regulation

Blood serves a major role in maintaining homeostasis. Blood helps regulate pH via buffers, body temperature by either carrying excess heat to the skin for dissipation or by vasoconstricting to conserve heat, and osmotic pressure by maintaining blood protein and electrolyte levels.

Protection

Blood plays many roles in immunity. Some blood cells are phagocytic; others produce antibodies. Blood proteins such as complement and interferons are important in immunity. In addition, blood helps maintain homeostasis by clotting to prevent blood loss.

Physical characteristics of blood

Blood is denser and thicker than water. It contains both cellular and liquid components. The cells (formed elements) and cell fragments are suspended in plasma. Although fibers typically seen in connective tissue are not present, during the clotting process, dissolved proteins combine to form fibrous strands.

When centrifuged, the components of the blood will separate into three distinct compartments (Fig. 13.1). The formed elements move toward the bottom of the tube; the plasma appears near the top. Packed at the bottom of a centrifuged tube will be the erythrocytes, or red blood cells. Sitting on top of this layer will be a thin, whitish layer called the buffy coat. This layer contains leukocytes, or white blood cells, and platelets, which are cell fragments. The top layer is the plasma.

The percentage of a blood sample that is erythrocytes is called the hematocrit. An abnormally high hematocrit is called polycythemia, which is an indication that there are too many erythrocytes per milliliter of blood. Such blood can carry elevated amounts of oxygen, but it has a greater viscosity, making it harder for the heart to pump such blood. Polycythemia can also be an indication of dehydration since decreased fluid volume will also result in an increased number of erythrocytes per ml of blood. Conversely, a low hematocrit reading indicates anemia, meaning that there are not enough erythrocytes, and thus a low level of hemoglobin, in the blood. This can result in an increased cardiac output as the animal attempts to deliver adequate oxygen to the tissues.

In dogs and horses, the spleen stores erythrocytes. In fact, horses can store up to 50% of the erythrocytes in the spleen. Therefore, when the animals exercise, the spleen can inject erythrocytes into the circulation, increasing the hematocrit by nearly 25% percent.

Box 13.1 Blood doping

In sports, the term *doping* was first used to describe the illegal drugging of racehorses at the beginning of the 20th century. Today, the term *blood doping* includes the transfer of autologous or homologous erythrocytes and the use of synthetic erythropoeitin (EPO) to increase the number of red blood cells. Synthetic EPO was developed as a treatment for anemia resulting from cancer therapy. Injecting EPO under the skin can increase the hematocrit, thus increasing the oxygen-carrying capacity of the blood. Recently, it was discovered that horses have been doped using drugs designed for Alzheimer's and Parkinson's disease, which increase blood flow to the brain, thus restoring function.

In race horses, using a "milkshake" was a popular practice for enhancing performance. The practice is thought to have begun in Australia in Standardbreds. A milkshake consisted of several ounces of sodium bicarbonate dissolved in a gallon of water. Sometimes confectionery sugar, electrolytes, or nutritional substances including creatine were added. The thought was that giving a milkshake 4–8 hours prior to a race would enhance performance.

Plasma

Consisting of over 90% water, plasma also contains nutrients, gases, hormones, waste products, electrolytes, and proteins. The nutrients include various components absorbed from the gastrointestinal tract or produced in the liver, including glucose, amino acids,

and lipids. Oxygen and CO_2 are transported in the blood as are hormones produced in endocrine glands. Plasma proteins are the most abundant plasma solute. They can function as carriers for other nutrients such as transferrin that carries iron, act in immunity (immunoglobulins), and help in blood clotting (fibrinogen). The liver synthesizes most plasma proteins.

Formed elements in mammals

Formed elements of blood include erythrocytes (red blood cells, RBCs), leukocytes (white blood cells, WBCs) and platelets. RBCs and WBCs are whole cells, whereas platelets are cell fragments. There is only one type of RBC, but there are five types of WBC, including neutrophils, lymphocytes, monocytes, eosinophils, and basophils (Table 13.1). WBCs are grouped into either granulocytes or agranulocytes, depending on whether they contain obvious membrane-bound cytoplasmic granules. Granulocytes include neutrophils, eosinophils, and basophils. Agranulocytes include lymphocytes and monocytes. The number of various blood cells within the blood is shown in Table 13.2.

Types of blood cells in mammals

Erythrocytes

Erythrocytes, or red blood cells, are approximately 7–8 µm in diameter. They are shaped like biconcave discs, thus increasing their surface area to volume ratio. They are flexible, and able to deform in order to move through capillaries. Erythrocytes in mammalian species lack a nucleus and organelles. Avian red blood cells, however, are nucleated. Certain glycolipids found on the plasma membrane of RBCs account for the various blood groups. Since RBCs lack organelles, they are unable to reproduce. They must produce ATP anaerobically because they lack mitochondria.

Erythrocytes are filled with hemoglobin (Fig. 13.2). Hemoglobin is a specialized protein that functions in oxygen transport. Each hemoglobin molecule consists of four polypeptide chains (two alpha and two beta), each of which contains a nonprotein heme portion. An iron ion (Fe^{2+}) is bound in the center of each heme molecule, and can reversibly bind with one oxygen molecule.

Although most carbon dioxide is transported in the plasma as bicarbonate, about 13% is transported bound to hemoglobin as carbaminohemoglobin. In addition, hemoglobin binds nitric oxide (NO), a gas formed by endothelial cells, which functions as a neurotransmitter that causes vasodilation. As hemoglobin delivers oxygen, it can simultaneously release NO,

Table 13.1. Summary of formed elements in blood.

Cell Type		Picture	Description	Cells/mm³	Life Span	Function
Erythrocytes			Biconcave, anucleated discs; 3–7 µm in diameter, depending on species	4–6 million	100–120 days	Transport oxygen and carbon dioxide
Leukocytes						
Granulocytes						
	Neutrophils		Multilobed nucleus; small granules; 10–12 µm in diameter	3,000–7,000	6 hr–few days	Phagocytize bacteria and some fungi
	Eosinophils		Bilobed nucleus; red granules; 10–14 µm in diameter	100–400	8–12 days	Kill parasitic worms; destroy IgE-antigen complexes, inactivate histamine from allergic reactions
	Basophils		U- or S-shaped nucleus; 8–10 µm in diameter	20–50	Few hours to few days	Release histamine and other inflammatory mediators; contain heparin
Agranulocytes						
	Lymphocytes		5–17 µm in diameter	1,500–3,000	Hours to years	Involved in cell-mediated and humoral immunity
	Monocytes		14–24 µm in diameter	100–700	Months	Phagocytosis; develop into macrophages after leaving capillaries
Platelets			Granule-containing cytoplasmic fragments; 2–4 µm in diameter	150,000–400,000	5–10 days	Seal torn blood vessels

Table 13.2. Blood cell numbers (cells/μl).*

Species	Erythrocytes	Total WBC	Neutrophils	Lymphocytes	Monocytes	Eosinophils	Basophils
Dog	6–8 million	6,000–17,000	3,000–11,500	1,000–5,000	0–1,200	100–1,200	0–100
Cat	6–8 million	5,500–19,500	2,500–12,500	2,700–6,700	0–800	0–1,500	0–100
Horse	7–12 million	5,500–12,500	2,700–6,700	1,500–5,500	0–800	0–900	0–200
Cow	6–8 million	4,000–12,000	600–4,000	2,500–7,000	0–800	0–2,400	0–200
Sheep	10–13 million	4,000–12,000	700–6,000	2,000–9,000	0–800	0–1,000	0–300
Pig	6–8 million	11,000–22,000	3,200–10,000	4,500–13,000	200–2,000	100–2,000	0–400

* Values from Swenson and Reece (1993) and Thrall et al. (2004).

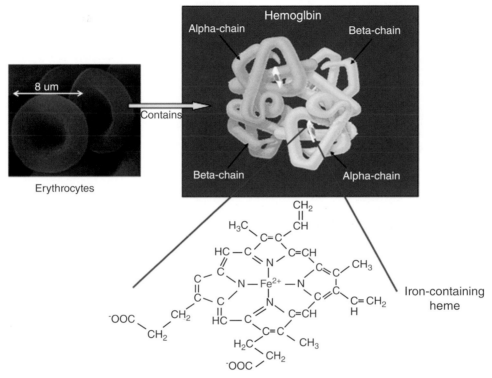

Fig. 13.2. Erythrocytes and hemoglobin structure. Erythrocytes (red blood cells) contain hemoglobin. Hemoglobin consists of four polypeptide chains, 2 alpha and 2 beta, each having a iron-containing heme molecule attached.

which dilates the capillaries allowing more blood, and therefore more oxygen, to be delivered.

Erythrocyte life cycle

Erythrocytes live about 120 days (Fig. 13.3). They get damaged as they squeeze through capillaries, and since they lack a nucleus and other organelles, they are unable to replace damaged structures. Damaged erythrocytes are removed from circulation by fixed phagocytic macrophages in the spleen, bone marrow, and liver. Once destroyed, the following steps occur:

1. The globin and heme portions are separated.
2. Globin is hydrolyzed into its component amino acids, which are then used for synthesis of other proteins.

3. The iron (Fe^{2+}) removed from the heme binds to the plasma protein transferrin and is transported through the bloodstream to muscle fibers, liver cells, and macrophages in the spleen where it is stored attached to ferritin. Since Fe^{2+} and Fe^{3+} can damage molecules in the body, they are transported and stored bound to transferrin and ferritin.
4. When mobilized, the Fe^{3+}-transferrin complex transports iron to bone marrow where erythrocyte precursor cells internalize it via receptor-mediated endocytosis and use it to synthesize hemoglobin. Vitamin B_{12} is needed for hemoglobin synthesis.
5. The non-iron portion of heme is converted to biliverdin, a green pigment, and then to bilirubin, a yellow-orange pigment.

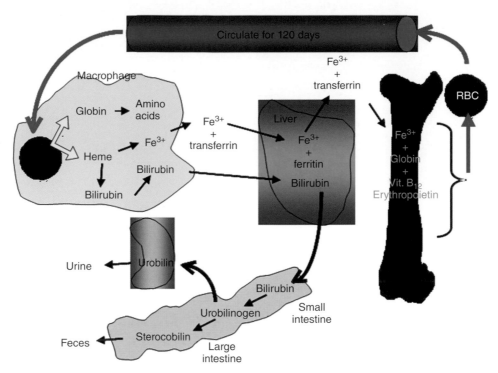

Fig. 13.3. Erythrocyte life cycle. Erythropoietin stimulates the production of new erythrocytes in red bone marrow. The erythrocytes circulate in the blood and have a life span of about 120 days. When worn out, they are phagocytized by macrophages in the spleen, liver, or red bone marrow. The iron in the heme molecule is recycled while the remainder of the heme molecule is metabolized and excreted.

6. Bilirubin is transported to the liver where it is secreted by liver cells into the bile.
7. Bile is released into the small intestine. In the large intestine, bilirubin is converted by bacteria into urobilinogen, which is converted to stercobilin, a brown pigment giving feces their characteristic color.
8. A small fraction of the urobilinogen is reabsorbed in the large intestine and converted to urobilin, a yellow pigment, which is excreted in the urine.

Leukocytes

Leukocytes, also called white blood cells, are the only blood cells that are truly complete cells containing nuclei and organelles. They do not contain hemoglobin. They generally account for only 1% of the blood volume, but they are an important component of the immune system.

They possess properties that allow them to carry out immune functions. WBCs leave the circulatory system by a process called emigration. Emigration involves several steps:

1. Near the site of inflammation, the endothelial cells lining the capillaries display cell adhesion molecules called selectins on their surface. Neutrophils have other cell adhesion molecules called integrins on their surface that recognize selectins. This causes the WBCs to line up along the inner surface of the capillaries near the inflamed site, a process called margination.
2. WBCs can move out of the capillaries through a process called diapedesis.
3. After leaving the bloodstream, they migrate via amoeboid action following a chemical signal produced by damaged tissue, a process called positive chemotaxis.
4. Neutrophils and macrophages become phagocytized and then ingest bacteria and dispose of dead matter.

Granulocytes

Neutrophils

Neutrophils account for 50–70% of WBCs. Twice as large as erythrocytes, their cytoplasm stains a pale lilac with very small granules. The granules stain with both basic and acid dyes. Some granules are considered lysosomes containing hydrolytic enzymes, and others contain antibiotic-like proteins called defensins. Since the nuclei consists of 3–6 lobes, these cells are often called polymorphonuclear leukocytes.

Attracted to sites of inflammation via chemotaxis, neutrophils are the first cells to be attracted by chemotaxis to leave the bloodstream. After leaving the capillaries, they are attracted to bacteria and some fungi. Neutrophils phagocytize these foreign cells and then undergo a process called a respiratory burst. Oxygen is converted to free radicals such as bleach (hypochlorite, OCl^-), superoxide anion (O_2^-), or hydrogen peroxide. The defensin-containing granules merge with the phagosomes, and the defensins act like peptide "spears" producing holes in the walls of the phagocytized cells. The neutrophils then die.

Eosinophils

Eosinophils account for 2–4% of all leukocytes. They contain large, uniform-sized granules that stain red-orange with acidic dyes. The granules do not obscure the nucleus, which often appears to have two or three lobes connected by strands. The granules contain digestive enzymes, but they lack enzymes that specifically digest bacteria.

Eosinophils function against parasitic worms that are too large to phagocytize. Such worms are often ingested or invade through the skin and move to the intestinal or respiratory mucosa. Eosinophils surround such worms and release digestive enzymes onto the parasitic surface.

Basophils

Accounting for only 0.5–1.0% of leukocytes, these are the rarest WBCs. Slightly smaller than neutrophils, they contain histamine-filled granules that stain purplish-black in the presence of basic dyes. The nucleus stains dark purple, and is U- or S-shaped. When bound to immunoglobulin E, these cells release histamine. Histamine is an antiinflammatory chemical that causes vasodilation and attracts other WBCs to the site.

Agranulocytes

Lymphocytes

Accounting for 25% of the WBCs, these cells contain a large, dark-purple–staining nucleus. The nucleus is typically spherical, slightly indented, and is surrounded by pale-blue cytoplasm. Lymphocytes are classified as either large (10–14 μm) or small (6–9 μm). The functional significance of the difference in size is unclear.

Monocytes

Monocytes are 12–20 μm in diameter and account for 3–8% of leukocytes. They contain a kidney- or horseshoe-shaped nucleus. They contain very small blue-gray–staining granules that are lysosomes.

After leaving the bloodstream, monocytes become macrophages. Some become fixed macrophages, such as alveolar macrophages located in the lungs and Kupffer cells located in the liver. Others become wandering macrophages that move throughout the body and collect at sites of infection and inflammation.

Platelets

Platelets, which are fragments of cells, consist of plasma membranes containing numerous vesicles but not nucleus. When there is a tear in a blood vessel, platelets coalesce at the site and form a platelet plug. Chemicals released from their granules aid in blood clotting.

Box 13.2 Complete blood count (CBC)

If an animal is ill, often a blood sample will be taken in order to conduct a complete blood count (CBC), or hemogram. A CBC includes a hematocrit; descriptions of any abnormalities in blood cell shapes, size, color, or appearance; an assessment of blood hemoglobin; and a count of white blood cells. An increase in white blood cell count indicates an infection whereas a decreased count may indicate weakness from a long illness. A decrease in lymphocyte numbers is observed at the beginning of an infection or following the use of steroid medications. An increase in the number of lymphocytes can indicate prolonged illness or leukemia. When total neutrophil numbers are increased, it is usually a sign of a bacterial infection or some form of extreme stress. The quantities increase in the blood when the animal is suffering from an infection with parasites or has allergies. If a dog or cat experiences extreme or prolonged stress, eosinophil numbers decrease. If the platelet numbers are decreased, it may indicate that the animal has either used up a large quantity of the available cells in clot formation or that their number may be low and the animal is at great risk if bleeding.

Formation of blood cells

The formation of new blood cells is called hemopoiesis, or hematopoiesis. Prior to birth, hemopoiesis begins in the yolk sac and later occurs in the liver, spleen, thymus, and lymph nodes of the fetus. After birth, it occurs in red bone marrow, which is found between the trabeculae of spongy bone. This is found predominately in the axial skeleton, pectoral and pelvic girdles, and proximal epiphyses of the humerus and femur.

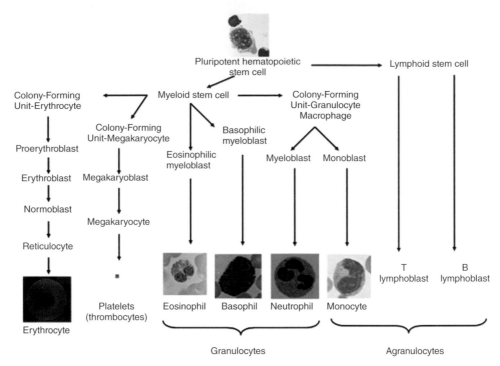

Fig. 13.4. Formation of blood-formed elements. Blood cells are produced from pluripotent hematopoietic stem cells. (Modified from Tortora and Grabowski, 2003.)

Within the red bone marrow are pluripotent stem cells. These can proliferate, or differentiate, into different blood cells, macrophages, reticular cells, mast cells, and adipoctyes. Macrophages are part of the innate immune system. Reticular cells form reticular fibers that serve as part of the matrix supporting red bone marrow cells (Fig. 13.4).

Pluripotent stem cells produce two other stem cells: myeloid stem cells and lymphoid stem cells. Myeloid stem cells differentiate within the red bone marrow to produce erythrocytes, platelets, monocytes, neutrophils, eosinophils, and basophils. In contrast, lymphoid stem cells begin in the red bone marrow but finish differentiating in lymphatic tissue forming lymphocytes. In addition, lymphocytes produce numerous cytokines, small glycoproteins that act as signals to modify other cells.

Myeloid cells produce progenitor cells. These cells are restricted, meaning that they are committed to becoming selected blood cells and cannot reverse to become stem cells. As shown in Figure 13.2, some of these progenitor cells become colony-forming units. Colony-forming units give rise to precursor cells, indicated by names ending in -*blast*.

Erythrocyte formation

Erythropoiesis is the production of erythrocytes in the red bone marrow. Hematopoietic stem cells divide to produce myeloid stem cells, which transform into pro-erythroblasts (Fig. 13.4). Proerythroblasts give rise to erythroblasts, which synthesize hemoglobin, and then are transformed to normoblasts. When the normoblast contains about 34% hemoglobin, it ejects most of its organelles, becoming a reticulocyte, the precursor of an erythrocyte. The process of hematopoietic stem cell to reticulocyte takes about 3–5 days. Reticulocytes are released into the bloodstream where, within 2 days, they release their ribosomes and become erythrocytes.

Erythropoietin (EPO), a glycoprotein produced mostly in the kidney, stimulates erythropoiesis. Although there is generally a small amount of EPO circulating in the bloodstream, hypoxia causes the kidney to produce EPO. Hypoxia can be caused by a reduced number of erythrocytes, reduced availability of oxygen such as might occur at increased altitudes, or increased tissue demand for oxygen. In contrast, excess erythrocytes or oxygen in the bloodstream reduces EPO synthesis.

Leukocyte formation

Hematopoietic stem cells produce lymphoid stem cells, which produce T and B lymphocytes. Leukopoiesis is the production of white blood cells. It is stimulated by various cytokines, generally produced by macrophages and T lymphocytes. Cytokines are glycoproteins, and they include interleukins and colony-stimulating factors. An abnormally low level of white blood cells is termed leukopenia, which can be caused by radiation, shock, or chemotherapeutic agents.

Platelet formation

Platelet formation is stimulated by the hormone thrombopoietin (TPO). Thrombopoietin causes myeloid stem cells to develop into megakaryocyte–colony forming cells, which then become megakaryoblasts. Megakaryoblasts are large cells that later splinter into 2,000 to 3,000 fragments. Each fragment has a cell membrane and is called a platelet, or thrombocyte.

Formed elements and blood cells in birds

Although most of the formed elements in birds are similar to those in mammals, there are some notable differences. Formed elements of blood in birds include erythrocytes, leukocytes, and thrombocytes, the avian equivalent of platelets. Like mammals, the avian leukocytes are divided into granulocytes and agranulocytes. Avian granulocytes include eosinophils, basophils, and heterophils (equivalent to mammalian neutrophils). Avian agranulocytes include lymphocytes and monocytes. The number of various blood cells within the blood is shown in Table 13.2.

Thrombocytes

Thrombocytes are found in birds, reptiles, amphibians, and fish. Unlike platelets, they are nucleated. Thrombocytes are smaller than erythrocytes, and in good preparations, a small eosinophilic vacuole appears as an orange dot located at one end of the nucleus. Whereas mammalian platelets are derived from megakaryocytes, such precursors are lacking in birds. There remains some debate as to whether avian thrombocytes arise from antecedent mononucleated cells or multinucleated cells. Avian thrombocytes have a similar function to mammalian platelets.

Heterophils

Heterophils function similarly to mammalian neutrophils. In some avian species they are the most common peripheral leukocyte. They are typically round, with colorless cytoplasm and many eosinophilic, rod-shaped to spherical granules. The granules may partially obscure the nucleus, which usually has two or three lobes and coarsely aggregated, purple chromatin. Often in blood smears the heterophil sometimes has a distinct ruby-colored central granule since the rod-shaped granules are dissolved, leaving the central one only.

Box 13.3 Heterophil/lymphocyte ratio in birds

While in many animals increased plasma corticosteroids are used as an indication of stress, it was shown that the blood ratio of heterophils (H) to lymphocytes (L) is also a good measure of stress. It was noted that when corticosterone is added to the feed of chickens, the number of blood lymphocytes increased while the number of heterophils decreased. The ratio of H/L is now commonly used as an indicator of prolonged stress in birds. Increased plasma corticosterone levels are an indication of acute stress in birds whereas H/L rations are a better indicator of long-term stress. One will not observe a change in H/L ration until approximately 12 hours after exposure to stress.

Hemostasis

Hemostasis is a series of responses that stop bleeding. As blood vessels are damaged or torn, hemostasis quickly controls the bleeding. The hemostasis response is rapid, localized, and well controlled so as not to spread throughout the body. Hemostasis entails three mechanisms: 1) vascular spasms, 2) platelet plug formation, and 3) blood clotting (coagulation). If bleeding is not stopped for any reason, an animal will hemorrhage and lose blood.

Box 13.4 Aspirin and gastric bleeding

In some conditions, such as arthritis, aspirin may be prescribed to treat dogs and cats. Aspirin belongs to a class of drugs called nonsteroidal antiinflammatory drugs (NSAIDs). Dogs are particularly sensitive to the gastrointestinal effects of NSAIDs, which include pain, bleeding (i.e., gastric hemorrhaging), and ulceration. Coated aspirin may help with the gastrointestinal effects. Aspirin can be given with food, 1–2 times a day.

Since cats cannot break down this drug as quickly as dogs, they are more sensitive to aspirin than dogs. Thus, time between doses is generally increased with cats. Cats are typically dosed at intervals of 48–72 hours.

Acetaminophen and ibuprofen are generally not recommended for dogs. These drugs can be fatal to cats.

Vascular spasm

When blood vessels become injured, the vessels constrict. This vascular spasm is triggered by injury to the vascular smooth muscle, chemicals released from endothelial cells and platelets, and reflexes involving local pain receptors.

Platelet plug formation

Platelets contain a large number of chemicals, including clotting factors, ADP, ATP, Ca^{2+}, serotonin, enzymes that produce thromboxane A2, fibrin-stabilizing factor, and platelet-derived growth factor (PDGF). They also contain lysosomes and mitochondria. Fibrin-stabilizing factor helps strengthen blood clots. PDGF is involved in proliferation of vascular endothelial cells, vascular smooth muscle fibers, and fibroblasts, all of which help repair damaged vessels.

A platelet plug forms as follows:

1. Platelet adhesion. Platelets adhere to the collagen fibers of the connective tissue exposed in a damaged vessel wall.
2. Platelet release reaction. Adhesion to the vessel wall causes the platelets to become activated. They extend processes that allow them to contact and interact with adjacent platelets. They also liberate their vesicular contents in a process called the platelet release reaction. ADP and thromboxane A help activate neighboring platelets. Serotonin and thromboxane A cause vasoconstriction by causing the vascular smooth muscle to contract, thus decreasing blood flow.
3. Platelet aggregation. Released ADP makes adjacent platelets sticky, causing more and more platelets to adhere at the injured site.
4. Platelet plug. As more platelets adhere, a platelet plug forms.

Blood clotting

When blood clots, it forms a straw-colored liquid called serum and a gellike mass called a clot. The clot consists of insoluble protein fibers called fibrin that trap other formed elements of the blood.

Clotting, or coagulation, involves a series of chemical reactions resulting in fibrin thread formation. Clotting factors include calcium ions, inactive enzymes produced in the liver and released into the circulatory system, and chemicals released from platelets and damaged tissue. Clotting factors are generally named by Roman numerals indicating the order of their discovery, not their order in the clotting process.

The formation of a clot in an unbroken blood vessel is called a thrombosis, with the clot being called a thrombus. The movement through the blood of a clot, air bubble, fat from a broken bone, or debris is called

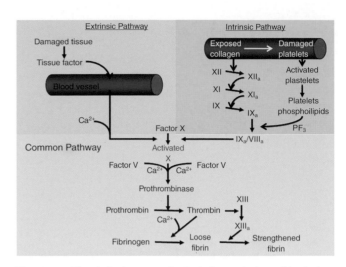

Fig. 13.5.   Blood-clotting cascade. Both the extrinsic and intrinsic pathways result in formation of Activated Factor X that then combines with Factor V to form the active enzyme prothrombinase.

an embolus. These often lodge in the lungs producing a pulmonary embolism.

Clotting consists of three stages (Fig. 13.5): 1) two pathways, called the intrinsic and extrinsic pathways, leading to the production of prothrombinase, 2) conversion of prothrombin to thrombin, catalyzed by prothrombinase, and 3) thrombin catalyzing the conversion of fibrinogen into insoluble fibrin.

Extrinsic pathway

The extrinsic pathway is quicker and has fewer steps than the intrinsic pathway. Damaged tissue releases a tissue protein called tissue factor (TF), or thromboplastin, that initiates the formation of prothrombinase. Since TF comes from outside the blood, this pathway is called the extrinsic pathway. In the presence of Ca^{2+}, TF initiates a series of reactions resulting in the formation of factor X. Factor X then combines with factor V to form the active enzyme prothrombinase.

Intrinsic pathway

In the intrinsic pathway, all the factors necessary for blood clotting are present in (i.e., an intrinsic part of) the blood. The intrinsic pathway relies on the production of PF_3, a phospholipid associated with the external surface of aggregated platelets. Like the extrinsic pathway, the intrinsic pathway results in the production of factor X.

Common pathway

Both the intrinsic and extrinsic pathways use a common pathway after the activation of factor X. Prothrombin is converted to thrombin by prothrombinase. Thrombin then catalyzes the conversion of fibrinogen to fibrin. Activated factor XIII catalyzes the polymerization of cross-linked fibrin.

Role of vitamin K

Although vitamin K is not directly involved in clot formation, it is needed for the synthesis of four clotting factors by hepatocytes. These include factors II (prothrombin), VII, IX, and X. Vitamin K is normally synthesized by bacteria found in the large intestine and is absorbed through the intestinal wall along with other lipids.

Clot retraction and repair

Beginning about 30–60 minutes after clot formation, the clot becomes more stable through a process called clot retraction. Platelets contain actin and myosin, and these contractile proteins begin to contract, similar to muscle contraction. This platelet contraction pulls on surrounding fibrin strands, thus squeezing serum from the clot and pulling the ruptured edges of the vessel closer together. The platelets release factor XIII that helps strengthen the fibrin clot. Simultaneously, PDGF released by degranulating platelets stimulates smooth muscle and fibroblasts to divide and repair the damaged site. The fibroblasts form a connective tissue sheath over the injured area. Vascular endothelial growth factor then causes the endothelial cells to multiply and restore the blood vessel lining.

Fibrinolysis

A clot is not permanent. Following healing, the clot is removed by a process of fibrinolysis. The major clot-busting enzyme is plasmin, which is produced when the blood protein plasminogen is activated by tissue plasminogen activator secreted by endothelial cells. Plasminogen can also be activated by activated factor XII and thrombin released during the clotting process. Plasmin digests the fibrin threads and inactivates fibrinogen, prothrombin, and factors V, VIII, and XII.

Factors limiting clot growth and formation

Since blood clotting involves a positive feedback system, there must be systems in place to localize clot formation. Clots are prevented from spreading by 1) rapid removal of clotting factors, and 2) inhibition of activated clotting factors. Fibrin absorbs thrombin into the clot, thus limiting its site of action. Thrombin that escapes into circulation is inactivated by antithrombin III, an anticoagulant produced in the liver. Endothelial cells and WBCs produce prostacyclin, a prostaglandin that opposes the action of thromboxane A2. Prostacyclin inhibits platelet adhesion.

Heparin, produced by mast cells and basophils, is an anticoagulant that combines with antithrombin increasing its effectiveness. Protein C, also produced in the liver, inactivates factors V and VIII and enhances the activity of plasminogen activators.

Thrombolytic agents

Thrombolytic agents are chemicals injected to dissolve blood clots. Streptokinase, produced by streptococcal bacteria was one of the first commercial thrombolytic agents. More recently, a genetically engineered version of tissue plasminogen activator has been used.

Aspirin can inhibit vasoconstriction and platelet aggregation. It does so by blocking the synthesis of thromboxane A2.

Blood groups and crossmatching

Blood groups

On the surface of erythrocytes are various glycoproteins and glycolipids that act as antigens. Because of these isoantigens or agglutinogens, blood is categorized into various blood groups, each of which can have various blood types. In humans, the most common blood groups are the ABO blood group and the Rh blood groups, whereas animals have a variety of different blood groups.

Cattle have 11 major blood groups systems including A, B, C, F, J, L, M, R, S, T, and Z. The B group has over 60 different antigens. The J antigen is not a true antigen, but instead is a lipid found in body fluids that adheres to erythrocytes.

The antigen groups or blood types in dogs are known as the DEA system. They include DEAs 1.1, 1.2, and 3–8. DEAs 1.1 and 1.2 account for 60% of the canine population. Dogs having DEA 1.1 or 1.2 are considered A-positive; other dogs are considered A-negative. A-negative dogs do not have antibodies against A-positive blood.

Cats have three AB blood groups. Type A is most common, accounting for 95% of short- and longhair domestic cats. Type B is less frequent, and Type AB is rare. Cats with type-A blood have antibodies against A isoantigens whereas type-B cats have alloantibodies (i.e., antibodies found against antigens in some members of the same species) against B isoantigens.

There are seven blood groups in sheep including A, B, C, D, M, R, and X. The B group is highly polymorphic, and the R system is similar to the J system in cattle.

Five blood groups have been identified in goats: A, B, C, M, and J, with J being similar to that of cattle.

Crossmatching

Crossmatching is a procedure to determine whether donor blood is compatible with the recipient's blood. There are two types of crossmatches. In major crossmatching, the donor erythrocytes are compared to the recipient serum to determine whether either acquired or naturally occurring antibodies are present in the recipient serum against the donor erythrocytes. Minor crossmatching compares donor serum to recipient erythrocytes, checking for preformed antibodies in donor serum that could hemolyze recipient red cells. Minor crossmatching is less important since the donor serum is markedly diluted after transfusion, decreasing the risk of a significant reaction.

The heart

Anatomy of the heart

Location and exterior landmarks

The heart is an inverted cone-shaped structure located in the mediastinum, a mass of tissue occupying the medial region of the thoracic cavity extending from the sternum to the vertebral column, and between the lungs. The apex, or "pointed" end of the heart is directed caudoventrally; the base, or top of the heart, is directed dorsocranially.

The cranial and caudal sides of the heart can be located by other structures. The auricles point left, with the pulmonary trunk located between the two auricles. The aortic arch projects caudally.

The coronary groove partially encircles the heart except at the conus and indicates the separation of the atria and ventricles. The conus is the expanded outflow of the right ventricle into the pulmonary trunk. The interventricular grooves indicate the divisions between the two ventricles. The two auricles are visible on the left side of the heart, with the pulmonary trunk between them.

Pericardium

The membrane surrounding the heart is the pericardium. It consists of the fibrous pericardium and serous pericardium. The fibrous pericardium is a tough, inelastic, dense irregular connective tissue sac with one end attaching to the diaphragm and the other open end fusing with the connective tissue surrounding the blood vessels entering and leaving the heart.

The fibrous pericardium anchors the heart within the mediastinum and prevents overfilling of the heart. Inside the fibrous pericardium is the serous pericardium, consisting of a parietal and visceral layer. The parietal layer lines the internal surface of the fibrous pericardium; the visceral layer, also called the epicardium, is an integral part of the heart wall.

Inflammation of the pericardium is called pericarditis. This results in decreased production of serous fluid, and a roughened serous membrane. As a result, the beating heart can be heard with a stethoscope rubbing against the serous layer (pericardial friction rub). In severe cases, inflammation leads to excess fluid production, which compresses the heart and decreases its pumping ability.

Layers of the heart

The heart wall consists of three layers: epicardium, myocardium, and endocardium. The epicardium is the outermost layer, and it is the visceral layer of the pericardium. It consists of a thin, transparent layer of mesothelium and connective tissue. The middle layer, or myocardium, is cardiac muscle and makes up the bulk of the heart. The innermost endocardium is a thin layer of connective tissue providing a smooth lining for the chambers of the heart and valves. The endocardium is continuous with the endothelial lining of the large blood vessels attached to the heart.

Cardiac muscle is also called involuntary, striated muscle. Like skeletal muscle, it contains actin and myosin that is organized into sarcomeres.

Fibrous skeleton of the heart

The heart also contains dense connective tissue surrounding the valves, forming a fibrous skeleton (Fig. 13.6). In addition to forming a point of attachment for the valves, the fibrous skeleton serves to eclectically insulate the atria from the ventricles.

Box 13.5   Dilated cardiomyopathy

Dilated cardiomyopathy (DCM) is a disease characterized by dilation or enlargement of the heart chambers resulting in an abnormally large heart. This disease eventually results in heart failure, since the damaged heart muscle is too weak to efficiently pump blood to the rest of the body. DCM is very common in dogs, representing the most common reason for congestive heart failure (CHF). The left ventricle is most always involved. Since the myocardium cannot work effectively to pump blood out of the heart, subsequent backup of blood into the left atrium and ultimately into the lungs occurs commonly. This backup of blood into the lungs results in pulmonary edema and is a sign of congestive heart failure.

The treatment of dogs with dilated cardiomyopathy varies with the severity of heart failure and specific organ damage. Treatment may include oxygen administration, fluid therapy, and administration of drugs that improve breathing (bronchodilators) and drugs that modify heart function, such as control of the arrhythmias. If low doses of anti-arrhythmic drugs are effective, the heart can often be stabilized. Serious ventricular arrhythmias that can only be controlled by high doses of anti-arrhythmic drugs have a poorer prognosis.

Heart chambers and vessels

The heart has four chambers. Two atria located superiorly, receive blood and pump it to the ventricles. Two ventricles located posteriorly pump the blood away from the heart (Fig. 13.6). The atria are separated by the interatrial septum; the ventricles are separated by the interventricular septum. There is an oval depression on the interatrial septum called the fossa ovalis (Fig. 13.7), a remnant of the foramen ovale, which is an opening between the atria in the fetus that closes shortly before birth.

Atria

The atria are the receiving chambers of the heart. Protruding from the atria are the auricles, which increase the atrial volume. The auricles are lined with pectinate muscles making them appear as if they were raked with a comb. The atria are relatively small and thin-walled, since they need to pump blood only to the ventricles.

Blood enters the right atrium from three veins: 1) the superior vena cava returns blood from the body regions in front of the diaphragm, 2) the inferior vena

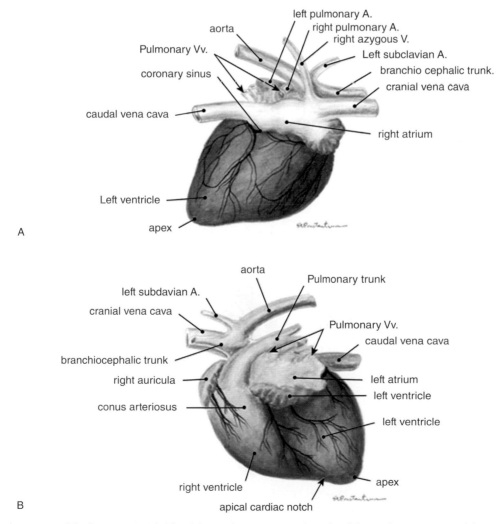

Fig. 13.6.   External structure of the heart. A) Atrial side of the cat heart. B) Auricular side of the cat heart. (Reprinted from Constantinescu, 2002. Used by permission of the publisher.)

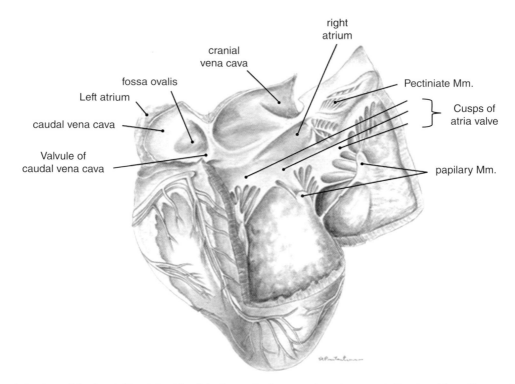

right
atrium

cranial
vena cava

fossa ovalis

Left atrium

caudal vena cava

Valvule of
caudal vena cava

Pectiniate Mm.

Cusps of
atria valve

papilary Mm.

Fig. 13.7. Internal structure of the heart. The right side of the heart of a large ruminant is opened. (Reprinted from Constantinescu and Constantinescu, 2004. Used by permission of the publisher.)

cava returns blood from areas posterior of the diaphragm, and 3) the coronary sinus collects blood draining the myocardium (Fig. 13.6). Blood passes from the right atrium into the right ventricle through the tricuspid valve, so named because it consists of three leaflets or cusps.

Blood enters the left atrium via four pulmonary veins. Blood passes from the left atrium to the left ventricle via the bicuspid, or mitral, valve, named because it has two cusps.

Ventricles

The ventricles form the bulk of the heart. The right ventricle wall is thinner than the left since it has to pump blood only through the lungs via the pulmonary trunk. The left ventricle pumps blood to the body via the aorta, the largest artery in the body.

Blood leaves the right ventricle via the pulmonary valve. The left ventricle forms the apex of the heart. Blood leaves the left ventricle via the aortic valve. During fetal development when there is no pulmonary respiration, there is a temporary blood vessel called the ductus arteriosus that shunts blood from the pulmonary trunk into the aorta. This vessel closes shortly after birth, leaving a remnant called the ligamentum arteriosum.

Inside the ventricles are muscle bundles called the papillary muscles, which serve as attachments for the chordae tendineae, tendinous cords attaching to the atrioventricular valves. The papillary muscles and chordae tendineae assist in valve function.

Box 13.6   Feline dilated cardiomyopathy

Hypertrophic cardiomyopathy (HCM) is a heart (cardio-) muscle disease (myopathy) in which the muscular walls of the left ventricle thickens (hypertrophy). The left ventricular walls may hypertrophy secondarily to other diseases such as systemic hypertension, or the hypertrophy can be a primary disease in itself.

HCM is diagnosed when thickening of the left ventricular walls is not caused by another disease. As HCM progresses, it can alter the heart structure and impair its functioning in several ways, including the following: 1) Ventricular chamber size may be reduced, thus limiting its ability to fill with blood; 2) Ventricular wall stiffness usually increases, which impairs the ability of the ventricle to relax, preventing it from filling efficiently; 3) There may be an increase in ventricular pressure during relaxation (diastole), causing blood to back up into the vessels of the lungs and subsequent congestive heart failure, which includes pulmonary edema and/or pleural effusion (seepage of vascular fluid into the lungs and/or pleural spaces).

Because the left ventricle is unable to fill adequately, less blood is pumped out to the body with each heartbeat. If the blood supply to other vital organs is inadequate, heart rate may increase as the body attempts to compensate. A decrease in blood flow to the kidneys can result in an increased release of rennin, which increases blood volume, increasing the pressures on the left side of the heart and contributing to congestive heart failure.

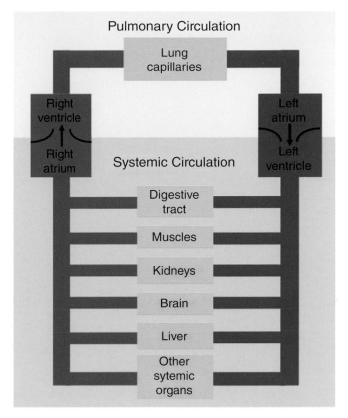

Fig. 13.8. Systemic and pulmonary circulation. The right side of the heart pumps deoxygenated blood to the pulmonary circuit while the left side of the heart pumps oxygenated blood throughout the body.

Pathways of blood through the heart

The heart acts as two pumps, side by side. The pulmonary circuit carries blood to and from the lungs and the systemic circuit transports blood throughout the remainder of the body (Fig. 13.8).

The right side of the heart receives deoxygenated blood from the body. This blood passes into the right atrium, through the tricuspid valve, and into the right ventricle. It is then pumped to the lungs via the pulmonary trunk. In contrast to other major arteries and veins in the body, the pulmonary artery carries oxygen-poor blood while the pulmonary vein carries oxygen-rich blood.

The left side of the heart receives freshly oxygenated blood arriving from the lungs via the pulmonary vein. The blood passes from the left atrium to the left ventricle via the bicuspid valve. Blood is then pumped from the left ventricle into the aorta, passing through the aortic valve.

Heart valve operation

Atrioventricular valves

The atrioventricular (AV) valves lie between the atrium and ventricles. When open, the cusps of the valves push into the ventricles, allowing blood to flow from the atrium to the ventricles. While the AV valves are open, the papillary muscles and chordae tendineae are relaxed. When the ventricles contract, pressure in the ventricles increases and pushes blood back toward the atria. This blood pushes the cusps of the valves back toward the atria, closing the valves. Simultaneously, the papillary muscles contract, pulling on the chordae tendineae. The chordae tendineae prevent the cusps of the AV valves from everting into the atria. Damage to the AV valves or chordae

tendineae allows regurgitation of blood through the AV valves.

Semilunar valves

The semilunar valves include the aortic and pulmonary valves, which allow blood to pass from the ventricles into the aorta and pulmonary vein, respectively. These valves are made of three crescent-shaped cusps. As the pressure in the ventricles exceed that in the arteries, blood passes from the heart into the arteries. As the ventricles relax, the backflow of blood catches the cusps and causes these valves to close, thus preventing the movement of blood back into the ventricles.

There are no valves located at the entrance of the venae cavae into the right atrium or pulmonary veins into the left atrium. So as the atria contract, a small amount of blood can backflow into these veins. However, contraction of the atria compresses the area where the veins attach, thus minimizing the backflow of blood.

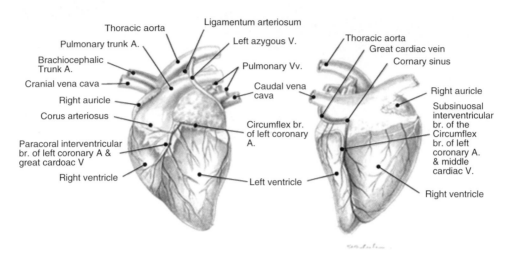

Fig. 13.9. Coronary circulation of goat heart. (Reprinted from Constantinescu, 2001. Used by permission of the publisher.)

Pulmonary, systemic, and coronary circulation

Pulmonary circulation

The pulmonary circulation transports deoxygenated blood from the right ventricle to the lungs where it picks up O_2 while delivering CO_2. The right side of the heart is responsible for the pulmonary circuit. Deoxygenated blood returning from the body enters the right atrium and passes into the right ventricle. The right ventricle pumps the blood into the pulmonary artery and into the pulmonary capillaries. Oxygenated blood is returned to the left atrium via the pulmonary vein.

Systemic circulation

The systemic circulation distributes oxygenated blood throughout the body. Blood is pumped from the left ventricle into the aorta, and then into smaller systemic arteries. These arteries give rise to arterioles that lead to systemic capillaries. Exchange of nutrients occurs across the capillary walls. Blood enters the systemic venules and then into systemic veins that return the blood to the right atrium.

Coronary circulation

The myocardium, or heart muscle, receives nutrients via the coronary circulation (Fig. 13.9). Blood leaves the aorta and passes into the left and right coronary arteries arising at the base of the aorta and encircling the heart in the atrioventricular groove. The left coronary artery has two branches. The anterior interventricular artery travels in the anterior interventricular sulcus and supplies the interventricular septum and

ventral walls of both ventricles. The circumflex artery supplies the left atrium and dorsal walls of the left ventricle.

The right coronary artery also divides into two branches. The marginal artery supplies the lateral right side of the heart, and the posterior interventricular artery travels to the heart apex and supplies the posterior ventricular walls.

After passing through the capillaries, venous blood in the heart collects in the cardiac veins. These veins carry blood to the coronary sinus, which empties into the right atrium.

Cardiac muscle and the cardiac conduction system

Cardiac muscle

Cardiac muscle is also called involuntary, striated muscle. Cardiac muscle fibers are shorter and less circular than skeletal muscle fibers. They generally contain a single nucleus, although occasionally two are present. Cardiac muscle fibers connect with neighboring fibers via thickening of the sarcolemma called intercalated discs (Fig. 13.10). These discs contain desmosomes that hold the fibers together and gap junctions that allow action potentials to move among cardiac muscle fibers. The gap junctions allow the cardiac muscle fibers to act as a functional syncytium, so that the atria and ventricles can contract as a unit.

Cardiac muscle fibers contain larger, more numerous mitochondria than skeletal muscle. The mitochondria account for 25% of the cell volume in cardiac muscle while only occupying 2% in skeletal muscle. Like skeletal muscle fibers, cardiac muscle contains

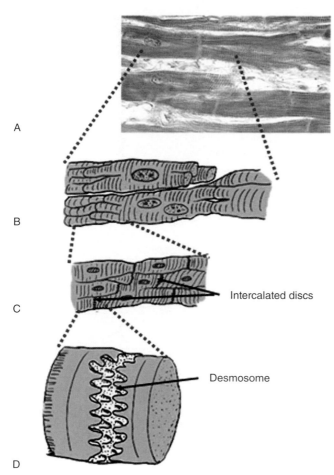

A

B

C

Intercalated discs

Desmosome

D

Fig. 13.10. Cardiac muscle A) Histological section of cardiac muscle. B) Drawing of a longitudinal section of cardiac muscle showing the branched cardiac muscle fibers. C) A close-up of the intersection of adjacent cardiac muscle fibers and their intervening intercalated discs. D) A close-up of the intercalated disc showing a desmosome.

sarcomeres. However, the T tubules in cardiac muscle fibers are wider and less abundant than in skeletal muscle. In addition, there is only one T tubule per sarcomere in cardiac fibers, entering at the Z disc, whereas there are two per sarcomere in skeletal muscle fibers entering at the junction of the A and I bands. The sarcoplasmic reticulum is also less extensive in cardiac muscle fibers.

The conduction system

The heart contains specialized cardiac muscle fibers that can self-generate an action potential, and are therefore called autorhythmic fibers. These cells do not require extrinsic neural input, and they can continue to generate an action potential even when the heart is removed from the body. These autorhythmic cells act as a pacemaker, establishing the basic electrical activity in the heart.

In addition, there are specialized cardiac muscle fibers that form a conduction system that provides a path for electrical excitation to travel throughout the heart (Fig. 13.11). This conduction system helps the heart pump in a coordinated manner so that blood can be pumped throughout the body.

Cardiac electrical activity is propagated through the heart conduction system in the following manner:

1. Located in the wall of the right atria near the entrance of the inferior vena cava is the sinoatrial (SA) node. The cells in the SA node do not maintain a stable resting membrane potential, but instead spontaneously depolarize 75 times/min. Since this is faster than in other areas of the heart, the SA node becomes the pacemaker, establishing the sinus rhythm.

2. Depolarization of the SA node results in an action potential that is propagated throughout the atria via the gap junctions between neighboring cardiac muscle fibers.

3. The action potential reaches the atrioventricular (AV) node, located in the inferior portion of the interatrial septum, above the tricuspid valve. The AV node delays the action potential about 0.1 sec before it travels to the ventricles. The delay occurs because the AV fibers are smaller, and have fewer gap junctions. This delay allows the atria time to complete their contraction before the ventricles contract.

4. From the AV node, the action potential moves to the AV bundle, also called the bundle of His, located in the superior portion of the interventricular septum. There are no gap junctions between the atria and the ventricles, which are instead insulated from each other by the fibrous skeleton of the heart. This necessitates that the action potential travel through the AV node to reach the ventricles.

5. The action potential continues in the right and left branches. These continue through the inferior portion of the interventricular septum toward the apex of the heart.

6. The right and left branches carry the action potential to the Purkinje fibers, which complete the pathway to the heart apex and then turn superiorly, running up the outer walls of the ventricles toward the atria. Purkinje fibers supply the papillary muscles as well as the ventricular muscles.

The rate at which the SA node depolarizes can be influenced by hormones and the autonomic nervous system. If acetylcholine is released by the parasympathetic nervous system, the SA node slows while release of epinephrine by the sympathetic nervous system accelerates the SA node.

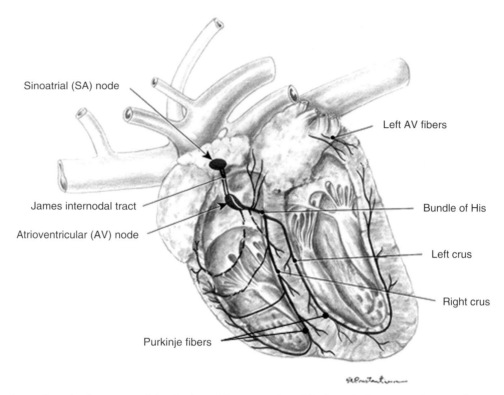

Sinoatrial (SA) node

Left AV fibers

James internodal tract

Bundle of His

Atrioventricular (AV) node

Left crus

Right crus

Purkinje fibers

Fig. 13.11. Excitation and conducting system of the dog heart. The pacemaker of the heart is the sinoatrial (SA) node. A wave of depolarization spreads from the SA node throughout the atria. This wave of depolarization then passes through the atrioventricular (AV) node where it is delayed from proceeding to the ventricles. From the AV node, the wave of depolarization travels down the bundle of His located in the intraventricular septum, and then into the Purkinje fibers. (Modified from Constantinescu, 2002.)

Mechanisms of heart contraction

Action potentials generated in the heart by the SA node travel throughout the heart via the conduction system as described above. The mechanism of contraction of cardiac muscle fibers is described below (Fig.13.12):

1. Depolarization. As a cardiac muscle fiber is stimulated by a neighboring action potential, voltage-gated fast Na^+ channels open. This allows a rapid influx of Na+ from the extracellular fluid, which results in depolarization of the cardiac muscle fiber from $-90\,mV$ to $+30\,mV$. These channels quickly become inactivated and close.
2. Plateau. As the voltage-gated fast Na^+ channels close, voltage-gated slow Ca^{2+} channels open in the sarcolemma and sarcoplasmic reticulum (SR). The influx of Ca^{2+} from the extracellular space (20%) causes a large release (80%) of Ca^{2+} from the SR. Simultaneously, the membrane permeability to K^+ decreases. As a result, the membrane remains depolarized at around $0\,mV$ for about $0.25\,sec$, compared to about $0.001\,sec$ in skeletal muscle.
3. Repolarization. After the relatively long plateau phase, voltage-gated K^+ channels open, allowing potassium ions to flow out of the cell and the membrane to repolarize. The cell returns to its resting membrane potential of about $-90\,mV$.
4. Refractory period. The refractory period, or time during which the next contraction cannot be triggered, is relatively long in cardiac muscle compared to skeletal muscle. The refractory period prevents cardiac muscle from developing tetanus, and thereby it allows the heart to act as an effective pump rather than developing a sustained contraction.

The mechanism of contraction of cardiac muscle fibers is similar to that in skeletal muscle fibers. As intracellular Ca^{2+} concentrations increase, Ca^{2+} binds to troponin, causing the tropomyosin to move and thus uncovering the myosin binding sites on the actin filaments. Myosin then binds to actin, and the actin is pulled across the myosin filament. Drugs that alter the movement of calcium into the cardiac muscle fibers can affect the strength of heart contraction.

ATP production

Cardiac muscle has little capacity for anaerobic cellular respiration; thus, cardiac muscle relies almost

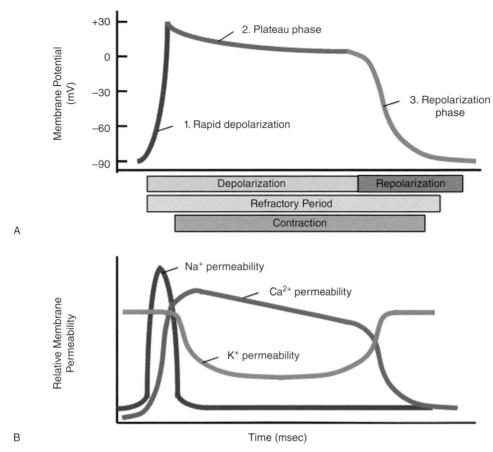

Fig. 13.12. Action potential in cardiac muscle fibers. A) The action potential in cardiac muscle fibers has a plateau phase not seen in skeletal muscle fibers. B) The influx of Na^+ causes the rapid depolarization phase while increased Ca^{2+} permeability leads to the plateau phase. Efflux of K^+ results in repolarization.

entirely on aerobic respiration. Therefore, cardiac muscle needs a continuous supply of O_2, which arrives via the coronary circulation or is released from myoglobin inside the cardiac muscle fibers. Cardiac muscle can produce ATP from the oxidation of fatty acids, glucose, lactic acid, amino acids, and ketone bodies.

Cardiac muscle also contains creatine phosphate, which can be used to produce ATP. The enzyme creatine kinase can catalyze the transfer of a phosphate group from creatine phosphate to ADP to produce a new molecule of ATP. If the heart is damaged, it releases creatine kinase into the bloodstream, which is often measured as an indicator of heart damage.

Electrocardiogram

The propagation of the action potentials through the heart produces electrical currents that can be detected on the surface of the body. A recording of these electrical activities is called an electrocardiogram (ECG or EKG). An ECG represents all of the electrical activity

in the heart rather than a single action potential (Fig. 13.13).

Two electrodes are generally placed on each forelimb, and one on the left hindlimb. The potential difference between electrodes is measured using different combinations of electrodes. By comparing these various recordings, it is possible to determine whether there are abnormalities in the conduction system or whether the heart is damaged.

Each segment of the ECG is generated from a specific area of the heart in sequential manner (Fig. 13.14). A typical ECG has three characteristic waves with each heart beat. The first, or P wave, is a small upward deflection reflecting atrial depolarization (Fig. 13.13). It is generated as the SA node depolarizes, and the action potential spreads throughout the atria. The second wave, or QRS complex, begins with a downward deflection, and then rises sharply and ends with a downward deflection. The QRS complex represents ventricular depolarization. Its shape is complex because the movement of the wave of depolarization through the ventricle changes direction throughout

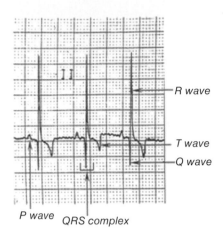

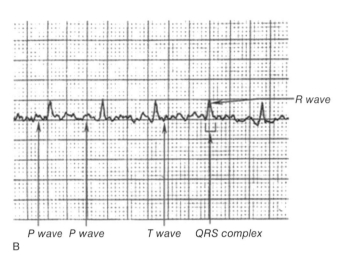

Fig. 13.13. Normal electrocardiogram. A) Dog. B) Cat. (Reprinted from Constantinescu, 2002. Used by permission of the publisher.)

the wave. The third wave is the T wave, and it represents ventricular repolarization. Since repolarization is slower than depolarization, the T wave is longer than the QRS complex.

Within the ECG, it is also possible to examine various intervals or segments. The P–Q interval is the time between the beginning of atrial excitation and the beginning of ventricular excitation. Therefore, it represents the time for the action potential to travel through the atria, the AV node, and the remainder of the conduction system. This interval can lengthen if there is coronary heart disease or scar tissue in the heart. The S–T segment begins with the S wave and ends with the beginning of the T wave. It represents the time when the ventricle is depolarized during the plateau phase. The T wave can be elevated in acute myocardial infarction. The Q–T interval is the period from the beginning of ventricular depolarization through ventricular repolarization. It can be lengthened by myocardial damage or myocardial ischemia.

Heart sounds

Auscultation involves listening to body sounds, usually with a stethoscope. Four sounds are created during each heart beat, and two of these sounds are clearly audible. These sounds are typically described as "lub-dup." The first sound, *lub,* is the AV valves closing. This occurs at the beginning of systole as the ventricular pressure increases above the atria pressure, causing the AV valves to close as blood begins returning to the atria. This sound is louder and longer than the second sound. The *dup* sound is caused by the semilunar valves closing at the beginning of ventricular diastole. The two other sounds, which are less audible, are due to the blood turbulence during ventricular filling and atrial systole.

Heart murmurs include clicking, rushing, or gurgling sounds. Although not always due to a problem, heart murmurs generally indicate a valve disorder. If the valve is stenotic, meaning it has a narrowed opening, a click may be audible when the valve should be fully opened. In contrast, if a swishing sound is heard when the valve should be closed, it may indicate that blood is able to backflow through the valve.

The cardiac cycle

The total of events associated with the movement of blood during one heartbeat is called the cardiac cycle (Fig. 13.15). The contraction and relaxation periods are called systole and diastole, respectively. The following steps describe the cardiac cycle:

1. Mid-to-late diastole. While the heart is relaxed, blood passively returns to the atria and into the ventricles through the opened AV valves. Approximately 70% of ventricular filling occurs during this time.

2. Atrial systole. During atrial systole, the atria contract while the ventricles remain relaxed. Atrial systole begins with depolarization of the SA node, causing an action potential to spread throughout the atria, appearing as the P wave on an ECG. As the atria contract, the remaining 30% of blood is forced through the opened AV valves and into the ventricles. The volume of blood in the ventricles is referred to as the end diastolic volume (EDV).

3. Ventricular systole. While the atria are relaxed (atrial diastole), the ventricles contract, appearing as the QRS complex on an ECG. As the volume in the ventricles decreases, ventricular pressure increases, causing the AV valves to close. For a fraction of a second, all the heart valves are closed, resulting in the isovolumetric contraction phase. When ventricular pressure exceeds the pressure in

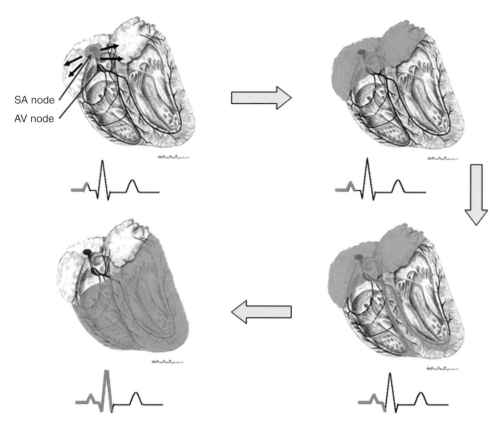

SA node
AV node

Fig. 13.14. Heart excitation and the ECG tracing. The green shading indicates the relationship between the area of the heart depolarizing coincident with the portion of the ECG produced by that depolarization. (Figure modified from Constantinescu, 2002.)

the large arteries, the semilunar valves are forced open, leading to the ventricular ejection phase.

4. Early diastole. Immediately following the T wave (i.e., ventricle repolarization), the ventricles relax, and the amount of blood remaining in the ventricles is referred to as the end systolic volume (ESV). As the pressure in the ventricles decreases, blood in the aorta and pulmonary arteries begins to return to the heart, causing closure of the semilunar valves. As these valves close, it causes a transient increase in aortic blood pressure called the dicrotic notch.

If the heart rate is 75 beats/min, the cardiac cycle is about 0.8 sec. Atrial systole lasts about 0.1 sec, ventricular systole lasts about 0.3 sec, and the remainder of the cycle is the quiescent period.

Cardiac output

The amount of blood pumped by the heart can be altered in response to metabolic changes caused by such factors as exercise, environmental temperature changes, or blood loss. The amount of blood pumped by either the right or left ventricle per minute is called the cardiac output (CO). CO is equal to stroke volume (SV), the amount of blood pumped by the ventricle per heart beat multiplied by the heart rate:

$$\begin{array}{ccccc} CO & = & SV & \times & HR \\ (mL/min) & & (mL/beat) & & (beats/min) \end{array}$$

SV is equal to end diastolic volume (EDV) minus end systolic volume (ESV). The heart pumps approximately 60% of the blood in its chambers with each beat.

Factors that can alter stroke volume will alter CO. Cardiac reserve is the difference between an animal's maximum CO and its resting CO.

Box 13.7 Canine heartworms

Canine heartworms, *Dirofilaria immitus*, are common in the hearts and major heart blood vesicles of dogs throughout the world. The male worms are a few inches in length; the female worms are about double the size and cause most of the damage. The worms are transferred from dog to dog through the bite of an infected mosquito. Mosquitoes transfer microscopic larva that migrate through the body and arrive at the heart several months later where they mature into adult worms. Damage to the dog's heart is due to adult worms.

The first sign of heartworm disease is often premature aging in which dogs gray prematurely around the muzzle and forelegs. Then their activity level decreases and their coats lack luster. Further progression results in a chronic dry cough most noticeable at night when the dog is resting or in a sitting position. At the same time, the dog's heart and pulmonary arteries enlarge due to mechanical obstruction of the worms, inflammation, and valvular damage to the heart.

Until recently, the only medicine available to cure infected dogs of heartworms contained arsenic. More recent medications have an added ingredient, pyrantel pamoate, which prevents infestation with hookworms and roundworms as well.

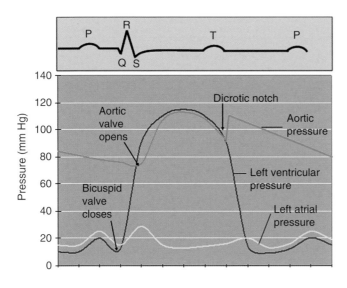

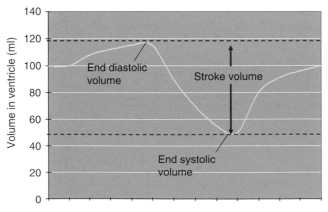

Fig. 13.15. Cardiac cycle. The top of the figure shows a typical ECG. The middle graph displays simultaneous changes in left atrial and ventricle pressure, and aortic pressure. The bottom graph shows changes in ventricular volume during the cardiac cycle.

Regulation of stroke volume

The heart will pump all the blood returning during systole. Three factors regulate stroke volume: preload, contractility, and afterload.

Preload

Preload is the amount of stretch on the heart prior to contraction. Within limits, greater stretch of the heart results in more forceful contraction. This is known as the Frank-Starling law of the heart. Cardiac muscle fibers are normally shorter than their optimal length for generating force. As a result, stretch of these fibers results in increased contractile force.

The preload is directly proportional to the volume of blood in the ventricles, or EDV. Two factors affect EDV: 1) duration of ventricular diastole, and 2) venous return, the amount of blood returning to the heart. As heart rate increases, duration of diastole shortens, resulting in a smaller EDV and a smaller SV. Although the decreased stroke volume can be offset by the increased heart rate, if heart rate becomes too rapid, there is insufficient preload and cardiac output declines. In contrast, during exercise, venous return increases because of increased squeezing of skeletal muscle on the veins. Consequently, SV increases.

Contractility

Contractility is the strength of contraction at a given preload, and it is independent of muscle stretch and EDV. Although preload is the major intrinsic factor regulating SV, contractility is influenced by extrinsic factors. Substances that increase contractility are called positive inotropic agents while those that decrease contractility are called negative inotropic agents.

Positive inotropic agents generally stimulate Ca^{2+} influx into the cytosol of cardiac muscle fibers, strengthening the force of contraction. Such agents include digitalis, glucagon, thyroxine, norepinephrine, and epinephrine (Fig. 13.16). Negative inotropic agents, which impair Ca^{2+} inflow, include anoxia, acidosis, increased extracellular K^+ levels, and calcium channel blockers.

Afterload

The pressure that must be exceeded by the ventricles before blood can be ejected through the semilunar valves is called afterload. Any factor that increases afterload will increase ESV and decrease stroke volume. Such factors include hypertension or narrowing of the arteries, as in arteriosclerosis.

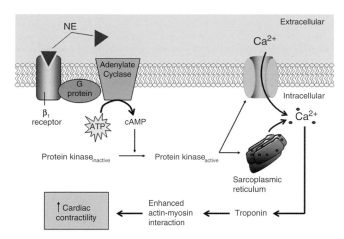

Fig. 13.16. Mechanism of norepinephrine-induced increase in heart contractility. Norepinephrine (NE), or epinephrine, binds to β1-adrenoreceptor on the cardiac muscle fibers. That activates a G protein, which activates adenylate cyclase, thus producing cAMP. cAMP then activates protein kinase, which causes increased cytosolic Ca^{2+}, coming both from the extracellular space and the sarcoplasmic reticulum. Ca^{2+} increases contractility.

Regulation of heart rate

Cardiac output depends on heart rate and stroke volume. Changes in heart rate (HR) are important in short-term regulation of cardiac output. Factors that increase HR are positive chronotropic factors; those that decrease heart rate are negative chronotropic factors. The most important factor controlling heart rate is the autonomic nervous system.

Autonomic nervous system regulation

The cardiovascular center in the medulla oblongata influences heart rate. This center receives input from sensory receptors, the limbic system, and the cerebral cortex. It directs the output from both the parasympathetic and sympathetic divisions of the autonomic nervous system.

The cardiovascular center receives sensory input from several areas. Proprioceptors monitor the positions of the limbs and joints. Increased movement of joints such as during exercise sends signals resulting in a rapid rise in heart rate. Chemoreceptors monitor blood chemical changes that can lead to changes in heart rate. Baroreceptors are located in the aortic arch and carotid arteries. Sudden changes in pressure in these regions cause changes in heart rate.

Activation of the sympathetic nervous system by either emotional or physical factors causes increased heart rate. This activation occurs via the cardiovascular center, which can stimulate heart rate via fibers from the spinal cord that stimulate the cardiac accelerator nerves extending from the spinal cord to the SA

node, to the AV node, and throughout the myocardium. The sympathetic nerve fibers release norepinephrine (NE), which binds to β_1 adrenergic receptors in the heart. NE accelerates the rate of depolarization of the SA node and increases Ca^{2+} influx into cardiac myofibers, increasing contractility. Both of these effects result in enhanced pumping of blood during systole.

Although large increases in heart rate decrease end diastolic volume and stroke volume, moderate increases in heart rate are associated with increased contractility, which maintains stroke volume, and therefore CO increases.

Activation of the parasympathetic nervous system sends signals to the heart via the vagus nerve (cranial nerve X). The vagus nerve terminates in the SA node, AV node, and atrial myocardium. Parasympathetic fibers release acetylcholine, which decreases the spontaneous rate of depolarization of the SA node. Parasympathetic input has little affect on contractility.

Chemical regulation of heart rate

Chemicals can have a profound affect on the heart. The major chemicals affecting the heart are hormones and cations.

Hormones

Epinephrine and norepinephrine are both released from the adrenal medulla, and, acting as neurohormones, increase heart rate and contractility. Thyroid hormones also increase heart rate and contractility.

Cations

Extracellular and intracellular cation concentrations are important in maintaining resting membrane potentials. Therefore, it should come as no surprise that alterations in cation concentrations will affect heart function. Elevated blood Na^+ concentrations decrease heart rate and contractility by interfering with Ca^{2+} influx into the cardiac muscle fiber. Increased blood K^+ also decreases heart rate and contractility, but it does so by inhibiting the formation of the action potential. Increasing blood Ca^{2+} levels increases heart rate and contractility by leading to increased intracellular Ca^{2+}.

Blood vessels and hemodynamics

Structure and function of blood vessels

There are five main types of blood vessels: arteries, arterioles, capillaries, venules, and veins. Arteries carry blood away from the heart as they branch or

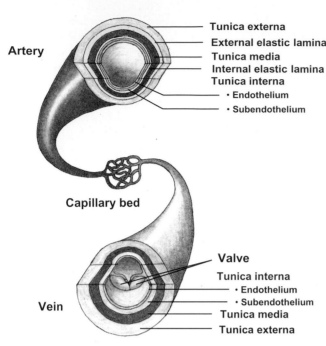

Fig. 13.17. Blood vessel walls.

Arteries

The arteries near the heart are called elastic arteries because they contain a large proportion of elastic fibers in the tunica media. They are large in diameter, therefore providing little resistance to blood flow. They expand to accommodate blood ejected from the ventricles. As the blood pressure decreases, these vessels recoil, thus helping to maintain pressure. They are sometimes called conducting arteries because they carry blood to more muscular, medium-sized vessels. Elastic arteries include the aorta, and the brachiocephalic, common carotid, subclavian, vertebral, pulmonary, and common iliac arteries.

The medium-sized arteries are called muscular arteries because they contain more muscle and less elastic fibers in the tunica media. Being more muscular, they have greater capacity to vasoconstrict. They are sometimes called distributing arteries because they deliver blood to various parts of the body.

Arterioles

The smallest of the arteries, arterioles deliver blood to the capillaries. Large arterioles contain all three tunics, with the tunica media having considerable smooth muscle and few elastic fibers. The smallest arterioles consist of simply a layer of endothelial cells surrounded by scattered smooth muscle cells. A metarteriole connects an arteriole with 10–100 capillaries making a capillary bed.

diverge into smaller arterioles that then carry blood to the capillaries. Blood leaving the capillaries enters venules, which merge into the larger veins that ultimately enter the heart.

Blood vessel walls

Except in the smallest vessels, there are three layers, or tunics, surrounding the blood vessel lumen (Fig. 13.17). The tunica interna, or tunica intima, is the innermost layer. In intimate contact with the blood, this layer contains the endothelium consisting of simple squamous epithelium lining the lumen. These epithelial cells sit on a loose connective tissue basement membrane called the subendothelial layer. The endothelium is continuous with the endocardium lining the inside of the heart.

The middle layer, or tunica media, consists of a circular layer of smooth muscle, and elastin. Stimulation of the vasomotor nerve fibers by the sympathetic nervous system causes vasoconstriction in which the lumen diameter decreases. Relaxation of the smooth muscle results in vasodilation, or an increase in lumen diameter.

The outer layer is the tunica externa, or tunica adventitia, is composed of loosely woven collagen fibers. This layer reinforces and protects the vessels, and it is the site where nerve fibers and lymphatic vessels enter to provide nourishment.

Capillaries

Capillaries, also called exchange vessels, are the smallest vessels. Their walls consist of only a tunica interna. Although capillaries are found in most places in the body, they are lacking in epithelium, the cornea and lens of the eye, and cartilage.

True capillaries originate from arterioles or metarterioles. At their origin is a ring of smooth muscle called the precapillary sphincter (Fig. 13.18). When contracted, the sphincter restricts the flow of blood into the capillary bed. Normally, blood flow within a capillary bed is intermittent due to changing vasomotor tone in the precapillary sphincter.

There are three types of capillaries: continuous, fenestrated, and sinusoidal (Fig. 13.19). Found in skin and muscles, the most common type is continuous, in which the endothelial cells form an uninterrupted layer with tight junctions between cells. However, there are intercellular clefts, or gaps, between neighboring cells allowing for exchange of nutrients. Within the brain, continuous capillaries lack intercellular clefts, and therefore form a structural barrier between the blood and brain, called the blood-brain barrier.

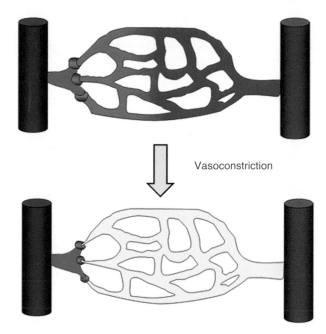

Vasoconstriction

Fig. 13.18. Precapillary sphincters. Constriction of precapillary sphincters restricts the blood flow within a capillary bed.

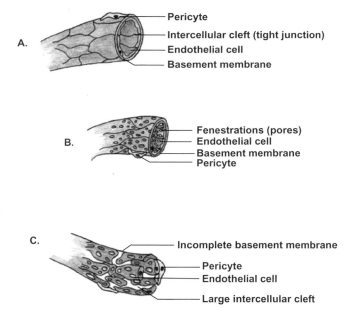

A.
— Pericyte
— Intercellular cleft (tight junction)
— Endothelial cell
— Basement membrane

B.
— Fenestrations (pores)
— Endothelial cell
— Basement membrane
— Pericyte

C.
— Incomplete basement membrane
— Pericyte
— Endothelial cell
— Large intercellular cleft

Fig. 13.19. Types of capillaries.

Fenestrated capillaries are similar to continuous capillaries, but they also have pores, or fenestrations, in the endothelial cells that allow substances to move out of the vessels. Such capillaries are found in the kidneys, villi of the small intestine, choroids plexus, ciliary processes of the eyes, and endocrine glands.

Sinusoidal capillaries have large, irregularly shaped lumens, and their endothelial cells have large fenestrations. They also lack a complete basement membrane, and thus they are very leaky. Such capillaries are found in the liver, bone marrow, lymphoid tissue such as the spleen, anterior pituitary, and parathyroid glands.

Venules

The smallest venules found close to capillaries consist of a tunica interna and a tunica media with a few smooth muscle cells. As the venules enlarge, they may contain a tunica externa.

Veins

Veins have the same three layers as arteries, but their thicknesses vary. The tunica interna and tunica media are thinner. The tunica externa is the thickest layer, containing collagen and elastic fibers. In the largest veins, the tunica externa also contains a longitudinal smooth muscle layer.

Unlike other vessels, veins also contain venous valves (Fig. 13.20). Formed from the tunica interna,

these one-way valves point toward the heart. The contraction of skeletal muscle during movement and increased thoracic pressure associated with respiration squeezes the veins, forcing blood towards the heart. As the skeletal muscle relaxes, the backflow of blood is prevented by the venous valves.

Because veins have a large lumen and thin walls, they can contain a large blood volume. Because veins can contain up to 65% of blood volume, they are called capacitance vessels.

Anastomoses

Most tissues receive blood from multiple arteries. The merging of these multiple sources results in an anastomosis. Such mergers provide alternate routes by which tissue can receive blood. If blood flow through one artery is prevented by an occlusion or loss of a vessel, blood still goes to the tissue through an anastomosis, thus providing collateral circulation.

Portal systems

In several places throughout the body, there are also vessels that link one capillary bed to another. These are known as portal vessels. Such vessels have the histological structure of veins. The complex of two capillary beds and the intervening portal vessel is known as a portal system.

Muscles relaxed   Muscles contracted

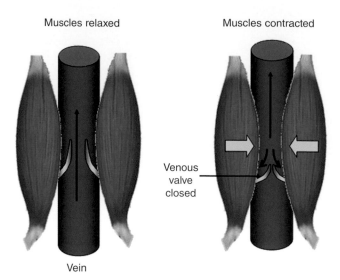

Venous
valve
closed

Vein

Fig. 13.20. Venous blood flow. Contraction of skeletal muscle and increased thoracic pressure due to respiration squeezes the veins, which causes the blood to move toward the heart. The blood is prevented from flowing backward, away from the heart, by one-way venous valves located in the veins.

One such portal system, called the hypophyseal portal system, consists of a capillary network in the median eminence supplied by the superior hypophyseal artery. This capillary network unites to form a series of vessels that spiral around the infundibulum and carry blood to a second capillary network located in the anterior pituitary.

A second example of a portal system is the hepatic portal system. The capillaries along the digestive system deliver blood into the inferior mesenteric vein, the splenic vein, and the superior mesenteric vein. These all deliver blood to the hepatic portal vein, which forms from a fusion of the superior mesenteric and splenic veins. The hepatic portal vein then carries blood to a capillary bed located in the liver. While carrying blood to the liver, the hepatic portal vein receives more blood from the gastric veins draining the stomach and the cystic vein coming from the gallbladder.

Capillary exchange

The purpose of the circulatory system is to deliver nutrients and remove wastes from tissues. This occurs through capillary exchange, in which substances move between the blood and interstitial fluid.

Diffusion

Capillary exchange generally occurs by simple diffusion, where chemicals move along their concentration gradient moving from an area of higher concentration to an area of lower concentration. O_2 and nutrients are generally in higher concentrations within the blood and therefore pass into the tissue; waste products are in higher concentration in the interstitial space and pass into the blood.

In all capillaries except sinusoids, the space between endothelial cells prevents the movement of plasma proteins from leaving the capillaries. In contrast, water-soluble chemicals, including glucose and amino acids, pass out of the capillaries through fenestrations of intercellular clefts. Lipid-soluble materials such as O_2, CO_2, and steroid hormones pass directly through the endothelial cell wall. In liver sinusoids, the gaps between the endothelial cells are large enough to allow proteins synthesized in the liver to enter the blood.

Bulk flow

The passive movement of large numbers of materials across a membrane is called bulk flow. Bulk flow moves from an area of higher pressure to an area of lower pressure. Diffusion accounts for most nutrient exchange across the capillary wall; bulk flow controls blood and interstitial fluid volume. The movement of fluid and solutes from capillaries into the interstitial space is called filtration, and the movement from interstitial fluid into the capillaries is called reabsorption.

Capillary hydrostatic pressure (HP_C) is the force exerted by blood against the capillary wall. This pressure tends to force fluid out of the capillary at the arteriole end of a capillary bed. HP_C is opposed by the interstitial fluid hydrostatic pressure (HP_{IF}), which pushes inward against the capillary. Therefore, the net hydrostatic pressure (Net HP) acting on a capillary is HP_C minus HP_{IF}. However, HP_{IF} is generally zero, so the effective hydrostatic pressure acting on a capillary is equal to HP_C. HP_C is larger at the arterial end of a capillary than at the venule end of the capillary.

HP_C is also opposed by the colloid osmotic pressure (OP_C), or oncotic pressure. This is the osmotic pressure inside the capillary caused by the presence of large plasma proteins that cannot leave the capillaries. The main protein responsible for OP_C is albumin. OP_C does not vary between the arterial and venule end of the capillary. Since the interstitial fluid has a few proteins, there is also an interstitial fluid osmotic pressure (OP_{IF}) opposing OP_C. OP_{IF} is generally only around 1 mm Hg.

Net filtration pressure (NFP), which is an interaction of hydrostatic and osmotic pressures, determines the direction of movement of fluids across the capillary wall (Fig. 13.21). NFP is calculated as follows:

$$NFP = (HP_C - HP_{IF}) - (OP_C - OP_{IF})$$

If we assume that at the arterial end of a capillary HP_C is 40 mm Hg, OP_C is 25 mm Hg, and OP_{IF} is 1 mm Hg, then:

$$NFP = (40 - 0) - (25 - 1) = 16 \text{ mm Hg}$$

If, at the venule end of the capillary, HP_C is 20 mm Hg, OP_C is 25 mm Hg, and OP_{IF} is 1 mm Hg, then:

$$NFP = (20 - 0) - (25 - 1) = -4 \text{ mm Hg}$$

Since HP_C varies along the capillary, there is a net movement of materials out of the capillary at the arterial end of the capillary and a net movement inward at the venule end. About 85% of the fluid filtered at the capillary is reabsorbed. The remaining fluid enters the lymphatic capillaries and eventually returns to the circulation at the subclavian vein.

Lack of reabsorption or an increase in filtration leads to edema, an abnormal increase in interstitial fluid volume. Lack of reabsorption can be caused by a decreased concentration of plasma proteins as is seen during liver disease, burns, malnutrition, or kidney disease. An increase in filtration can result from increased capillary pressure or damage to the endothelial wall caused by chemical, mechanical, or bacterial agents.

Factors affecting blood flow

Flow, pressure, and resistance

Blood flow (F) refers to the volume of blood flowing through a tissue during a given period of time. Total blood flow is equal to cardiac output. Blood flow is directly proportional to the difference in blood pressure (BP) between two points, and is inversely proportional to the resistance (R) to blood flow in the vessels:

$$F = \frac{\Delta BP}{R}$$

Since blood vessels have a great capacity to vasoconstrict and vasodilate, R has a greater affect on F than does BP. Since total blood flow is equal to cardiac output, CO equals $\Delta BP/R$.

Blood pressure

Blood flow occurs because of the pumping action of the heart. Blood pressure is the hydrostatic pressure exerted by the blood against the blood vessel wall. BP occurs because there is resistance to blood flow. BP is highest in the arteries, and decreases as blood moves through the circulatory system (Fig. 13.22).

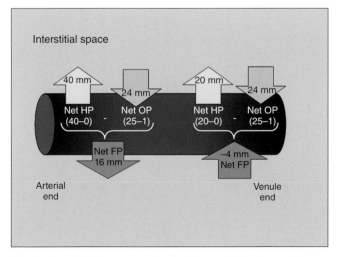

Fig. 13.21. Fluid flow across the capillary wall. At the arteriole end of a capillary, the hydrostatic pressure inside the capillary exceeds the oncotic pressure inside the capillary, which results in a net outward filtration pressure. In contrast, at the venule end of the capillary, the oncotic pressure inside the capillary exceeds the outwardly directed hydrostatic pressure, causing a net inwardly directed filtration pressure. The interstitial fluid that does not return to the capillary enters the lymphatic system.

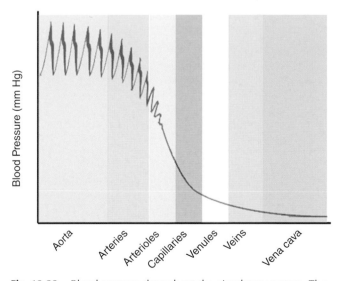

Fig. 13.22. Blood pressure throughout the circulatory system. The pulse pressure in the large arteries is substantial. As the blood moves through the circulatory system, pulse pressure declines. Although capillaries have a small cross-sectional area, blood pressure drops in the capillary bed due to the large numbers of capillaries. Blood pressure within the veins is low. (Modified from Marieb, 2004.)

BP is highest at the end of ventricular contraction, which is called systolic blood pressure. During diastole, the semilunar valves close, preventing blood from returning to the heart, and the elastic recoil in the large arteries maintains pressure that keeps blood flowing. At the end of diastole, the BP is at its lowest point, which is called diastolic blood pressure.

Pulse pressure is the difference between systolic and diastolic blood pressure. Mean arterial pressure (MAP) is the pressure that propels blood. Since the heart spends more time in diastole than systole, MAP is not simply the mean of diastolic and systolic blood pressure. Instead, MAP is equal to diastolic blood pressure plus one-third of pulse pressure:

$$MAP = Diastolic\ blood\ pressure + \frac{Pulse\ pressure}{3}$$

Resistance

Vascular resistance opposes blood flow, and is due to the friction between blood and the vessel walls. As shown in Figure 13.22, MAP and pulse pressure decline with increasing distance from the heart. This is due to the increased friction between the blood and vessel walls, and the decreasing elasticity of the vessel walls farther from the heart.

Vascular resistance is dependent on the size of the blood vessel lumen, blood viscosity, and total blood vessel length.

Blood vessel lumen

As lumen size decreases, resistance to blood flow increases. Resistance is inversely proportional to the fourth power of the lumen diameter. Therefore:

$$R \cong \frac{1}{d^4}$$

where d = lumen diameter. A small change in blood vessel diameter results in a large change in resistance. Decreasing the diameter of a vessel by one-half will increase resistance by 2^4, or sixteenfold. Therefore, vasodilation and vasoconstriction have a large affect on vascular resistance.

Blood viscosity

Blood viscosity is affected by the concentration of erythrocytes. Increasing the erythrocyte concentration, i.e., increasing the hematocrit, increases blood viscosity. This can be a result of dehydration or polycythemia. In contrast, decreased viscosity can result from hemorrhage or anemia.

Total blood vessel length

Resistance to blood flow is proportional to the blood vessel length. The longer the blood vessel, the greater the resistance. Hence, obesity in animals can result in hypertension due to increased length of blood vessels associated with adipose tissue.

Venous blood return

Blood pressure within the veins is relatively low due to the cumulative effects of peripheral resistance throughout the vascular system (Fig. 13.21). Therefore, there are other factors besides the heart that are important in venous circulation. First, the respiratory pump involves increases in abdominal pressure associated with inhalation. This increase in pressure squeezes venous blood toward the heart. As abdominal pressure is increasing, thoracic pressure is decreasing during inhalation, further allowing blood to enter the right atrium.

Second, there is a muscular pump that aids in venous return. As an animal moves, the skeletal muscle squeezes the veins, thus moving the blood toward the heart. As the muscles relax, the one-way valves in the veins prevent the backflow of blood.

Maintaining blood pressure

There are both short- and long-term mechanisms controlling blood pressure and blood flow. These mechanisms are responsible for controlling heart rate, stroke volume, systemic vascular resistance, and blood volume.

Neural regulation

The cardiovascular center is located in the medulla oblongata and is responsible for controlling heart rate and stroke volume. As discussed above, the cardiovascular center sends sympathetic signals via the cardiac accelerator nerve that increases heart rate and contractility. Conversely, parasympathetic signals from the cardiovascular center are carried via the vagus nerve and decrease heart rate and contractility. The cardiovascular center also sends signals to blood vessels via the vasomotor nerves, resulting in vasomotor tone, or a moderate amount of constriction within the vessels. The vasomotor tone can be altered by either vasoconstriction or vasodilation.

The cardiovascular center is involved in two reflexes controlling blood pressure: the baroreceptor reflex and chemoreceptor reflex.

Baroreceptor reflex

There are pressure-sensitive mechanoreceptors located in swellings within the internal carotid arteries, known as the carotid sinuses, the aortic arch, and the walls of most large arteries in the neck and thorax. In response to stretch, these receptors send signals resulting in inhibition of the cardiovascular center. This results in vasodilation and a decrease in blood pressure. Conversely, a sudden decrease in blood pressure results in stimulation of the cardiovascular center, a resulting vasoconstriction, and an increase in blood pressure.

This reflex is important in making rapid adjustments in blood pressure in response to acute changes. For example, as an animal stands, the pressure in the neck may decrease. The baroreceptor reflex quickly increases blood pressure to maintain adequate flow to the brain.

Chemoreceptor reflex

Chemoreceptors located in the carotid bodies and aortic bodies monitor blood O_2, CO_2, and H^+ concentrations. Hypoxia, acidosis, or hypercapnia (i.e., increased blood CO_2) stimulate the chemoreceptors. The resulting signals stimulate sympathetic output from the cardiovascular center, causing vasoconstriction and increased blood pressure.

Chemical regulation of blood pressure: Short-term control

There are several hormones and neurotransmitters that have significant affects on blood pressure. Some act directly on blood vessels, and others have differential affects on organs.

Renin-angiotensin-alsdosterone (RAA) system

A decrease in blood pressure or blood flow to the kidneys causes the juxtaglomerular cells of the kidneys to secrete renin. Renin acts on angiotensinogen produced in the liver to produce angiotensin I (ANG I). As ANG I travels through the lungs, it is converted to angiotensin II (ANG II), which raises blood pressure two ways (Fig. 13.23). First, it causes vasoconstriction, which increases vascular resistance, thereby increasing blood pressure. Second, it causes the release of aldosterone from the adrenal cortex. Aldosterone increases sodium and water reabsorption by the kidneys. This results in an increase in blood volume and thereby raises blood pressure.

Epinephrine and norepinephrine

Sympathetic stimulation causes the adrenal medulla to secrete both norepinephrine and epinephrine. These

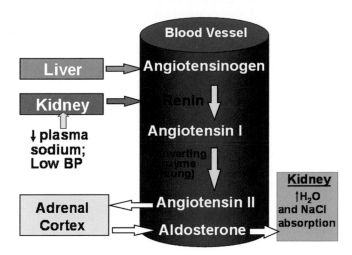

Fig. 13.23. Production and action of renin. Renin is produced by the juxtaglomerular cells in the kidney in response to low blood pressure. Renin converts angiotensinogen, produced by the liver, to angiotensin I, which is then converted to angiotensin II (ANG II) by a converting enzyme located in the lungs. ANG II acts on the adrenal cortex to cause the release of aldosterone, causing the kidneys to reabsorb Na^+, thus raising blood volume and blood pressure. ANG II also acts directly on blood vessels causing vasoconstriction.

neurohormones increase the rate and force of heart contractions, thereby increasing cardiac output. They also have a differential effect on various vascular beds, causing vasoconstriction in the skin and visceral organs, while causing vasodilation in skeletal muscle.

Antidiuretic hormone (ADH)

ADH is secreted from the posterior pituitary. It acts in the kidneys to increase water reabsorption, and it also acts directly on blood vessels to cause vasoconstriction. Both these effects cause an increase in blood pressure.

Atrial naturiuretic peptide (ANP)

ANP is released from the atria of the heart in response to high blood pressure, i.e., stretching of the atria. This hormone decreases sodium reabsorption from the kidneys, thereby decreasing water reabsorption from the kidneys. This results in decreased blood volume and blood pressure.

Endothelial-derived factors

Several chemicals affecting vasomotor tone are produced from the endothelial lining of blood vessels. Endothelin release is stimulated by angiotensin II, ADH, thrombin, cytokines, reactive oxygen species, and shearing forces acting on the vascular endothelium. Its release is inhibited by nitric oxide, prostacyclin, and ANP. Endothelin causes vasoconstriction (Fig. 13.24).

Endothelial cells also release a potent vasodilator called nitric oxide (NO). Originally called endothelial-derived relaxation factor, NO is a gas produced in response to high blood pressure, acetylcholine, and bradykinin. It diffuses to the neighboring smooth muscle cells where it causes the production of cGMP resulting in relaxation and vasodilation.

Inflammatory chemicals

Erythemia, or vasodilation, is associated with inflammation. A number of chemicals are involved in this response, including histamine, prostacyclin, and kinins. This response allows monocytes and neutrophils to leave the bloodstream and move toward the site of inflammation.

Renal regulation of blood pressure: Long-term control

Although most short-term blood pressure control mechanisms work by altering peripheral resistance, long-term renal control alters blood volume (Fig. 13.25). Blood volume has a direct affect on cardiac output, and therefore affects blood pressure. An increase in end diastolic volume increases cardiac output, thus increasing blood pressure.

Direct renal mechanism

An increase in blood pressure or blood volume causes an increased filtration rate in the kidney. As the filtra-

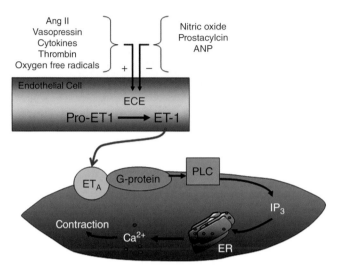

Fig. 13.24. Endothelin production and action. Endothelin is produced by endothelial cells lining the blood vessels. Various stimuli activate endothelin-converting enzyme (ECE), which converts Pro-endothelin-1(Pro-ET1) to endothelin-1 (ET-1). ET-1 diffuses to vascular smooth muscle cells and binds to the ET_A receptors. These receptors are coupled to a G-protein that activates phospholipase C (PLC), which results in the production of inositol triphosphate (IP_3). IP_3 causes the release of ET_A Ca^{2+} from the endoplasmic reticulum, which leads to smooth muscle contraction.

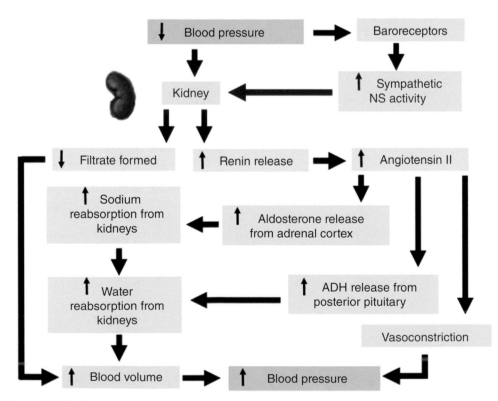

Fig. 13.25. Renal control of blood pressure.

tion rate exceeds the kidney tubules reabsorption rate, more urine is produced, resulting in increased fluid loss and decreased blood volume.

Indirect renal mechanism

If arterial blood pressure declines, the kidneys release the enzyme renin into the bloodstream. As shown in Figure 13.23, renin induces angiotensin II (ANG II) production. ANG II has three affects that increase blood pressure. First, it causes vasoconstriction. Second, it stimulates the adrenal cortex to secrete aldosterone, a hormone that stimulates sodium reabsorption from the kidney tubules. Third, ANG II stimulates ADH release from the posterior pituitary. ADH increases water reabsorption from the kidney tubules. Increased sodium and water reabsorption from the kidneys leads to increased blood volume and blood pressure.

Autoregulation of blood pressure

Local oxygen needs change throughout the body. In order to accommodate these local needs, capillary beds can alter their vasomotor tone in response to local physical and chemical factors.

Physical factors

Increased local temperature, such as occurs during inflammation or exercise, causes vasodilation. Decreased local temperature causes vasoconstriction. In addition, the smooth muscles in arteriole walls display myogenic responses, in which increased stretch causes enhanced contraction while decreased stretch caused relaxation. Such responses help regulate local blood flow as follows: If blood flow through an arteriole decreases, the arteriole wall is stretched less, resulting in smooth muscle relaxation and vasodilation. The vasodilation increases blood flow through the arteriole.

Chemical factors

Cells such as platelets, blood cells, smooth muscle, macrophages, and endothelial cells release a variety of chemicals that modify blood vessel diameter. Metabolically derived vasodilators include K^+, H^+, lactic acid, and ATP. Other tissue-synthesized vasodilators include nitric oxide (NO) produced by endothelial cells, histamine from mast cells, and monocytes and kinins produced during inflammation. Vasoconstrictors include thromboxane A2 and serotonin from platelets, superoxide radicals, and endothelins from endothelial cells.

Note that the systemic and pulmonary circulatory systems respond differently to changes in O_2 levels.

Systemic blood vessels dilate in response to low O_2, whereas pulmonary blood vessels constrict. Therefore, systemic vessels dilate in order to deliver more O_2 to needed areas while pulmonary vessels constrict so that blood is diverted from poorly ventilated alveoli.

Shock and homeostasis

Circulatory shock includes any condition in which blood vessels are unable to deliver adequate O_2 and nutrients to meet cellular needs. This results in hypoxia in the affected tissue, leading to a switch to anaerobic metabolism, lactic acid accumulation, and possibly tissue death.

Types of shock

The most common type of shock is hypovolemic shock resulting from massive blood loss. Blood loss can occur internally from the rupture of an artery, or externally from trauma. Excessive loss of body fluids such as occurs in profuse sweating, diarrhea, or vomiting can also cause hypovolemic shock. Treatment involves the restoration of fluids.

Cardiogenic shock occurs when the heart fails to adequately pump. This can be caused by a myocardial infarction, ischemia of the heart, heart valve problems, impaired contractility of the heart, or arrhythmias.

Vascular shock is a result of abnormal expansion of the vascular bed. Although there is no change in blood volume, there is a drastic drop in peripheral resistance leading to a drop in blood pressure. Causes can include anaphylactic shock from an allergic reaction or neurogenic shock resulting from head trauma damaging the cardiovascular center. Another cause can be septic shock resulting from bacterial toxins.

Circulatory routes

Pulmonary circulation

The pulmonary circulation functions to carry deoxygenated blood to the alveoli (air sacs) in the lungs where gas exchange occurs (Fig. 13.26). The blood picks up oxygen in exchange for carbon dioxide. The blood is pumped from the right ventricle into the pulmonary trunk, which then divides into the right and left pulmonary arteries. The pulmonary arteries divide into lobar arteries following the bronchi into the lungs. They then branch, eventually forming pulmonary capillaries in the air sacs. These capillary beds drain into the pulmonary veins. The pulmonary veins return to the left atria from which the blood enters the left ventricle and is then delivered to the body.

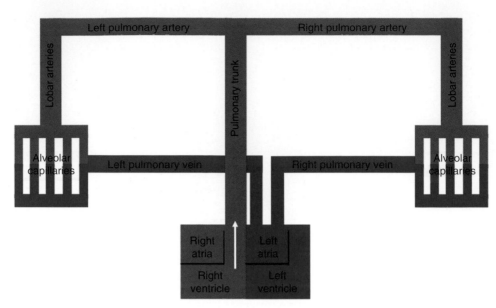

Fig. 13.26. Schematic diagram of pulmonary circulation. The pulmonary circulation carries deoxygenated blood to the lungs where the blood picks up oxygen in exchange for carbon dioxide. The blood returns to the left side of the heart where it enters the systemic circulation.

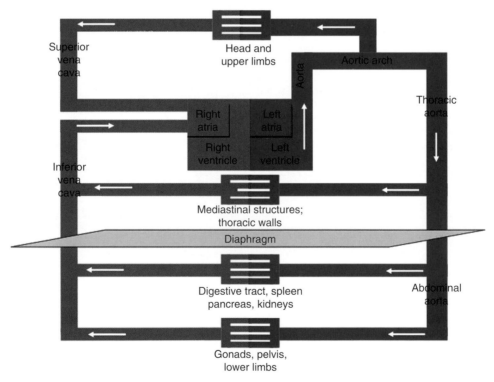

Fig. 13.27. Schematic diagram of systemic circulation. Blood delivered to the left side of the heart from the pulmonary circulation (pulmonary circulation has been omitted from this figure) leaves via the aorta to be circulated throughout the body. After passing through the capillary beds, the blood returns to the right side of the heart via the superior or inferior vena cava.

Systemic circulation

The systemic circulation includes vessels that deliver oxygenated blood from the left ventricle, throughout the body, and returns deoxygenated blood to the right atrium (Fig. 13.27). The systemic circulatory system includes vessels supplying the tissue needs of the lungs, as well as all the remaining tissues in the body. So, while the pulmonary circulatory system supplies blood only to the gas exchange portion of the lungs, the systemic circulation must supply blood to every tissue of the body. This is why the left ventricle has a thicker muscular wall than the right ventricle.

Systemic circulation begins with blood traveling through the aorta, and ends with the blood returning via the superior vena cava, inferior vena cava, or coronary sinus.

The aorta has four major divisions: the ascending aorta, arch of the aorta, thoracic aorta and abdominal aorta. The ascending aorta emerges from the left ventricle and runs posterior to the pulmonary trunk. It gives rise to two coronary arteries that supply the myocardium (Fig. 13.28). It then curves left, giving rise to the aortic arch. It then continues caudally running close to the vertebral bodies. As it courses caudally, it is called the thoracic aorta until it passes through the diaphragm becoming the abdominal aorta.

The aortic arch is a continuation of the ascending aorta. It gives rise to three major arteries: the brachiocephalic trunk, the left common carotid, and the left subclavian (Fig. 13.29). The brachiocephalic trunk gives rise to the right subclavian artery and right common carotid artery. These vessels provide the arterial supply to the head, neck, front limbs, and a portion of the thoracic spine (Fig. 13.30).

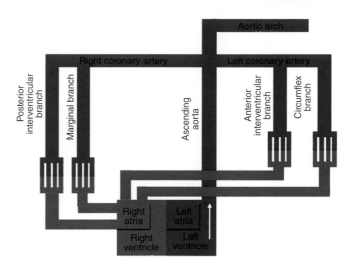

Fig. 13.28. Ascending aorta. The ascending aorta begins at the aortic valve and ascends dorsal to the aortic arch. It gives rise to vessels supplying the heart.

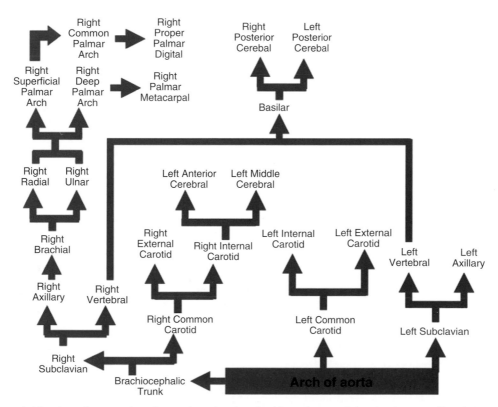

Fig. 13.29. Aortic arch. The thoracic aorta gives rise to visceral and parietal branches supplying the thorax wall and viscera (Fig. 13.30). The abdominal aorta supplies the abdominal walls and viscera. It ends in the right and left common iliac arteries supplying the pelvis and hindlimbs.

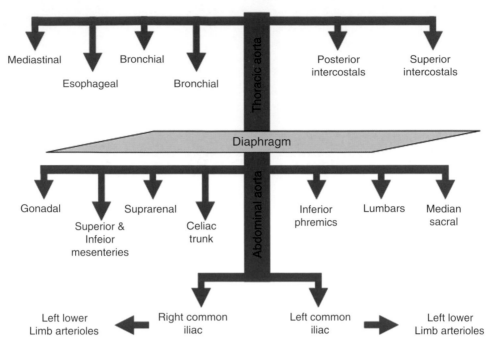

Fig. 13.30   Thoracic and abdominal aorta.

References

Constantinescu, G.M. 2001. Guide to Regional Ruminant Anatomy Based on the Dissection of the Goat. Iowa State Press, Ames, Iowa.

Constantinescu, G.M. 2002. Clinical Anatomy for Small Animal Practitioners. Iowa State Press, Ames, Iowa.

Constantinescu, G.M. and I.A. Constantinescu. 2004. Clinical Dissection Guide for Large Animals, Horse and Large Ruminants, 2nd edition. Iowa State Press, Ames, Iowa.

Marieb, E.N. 2004. Human Anatomy & Physiology, 6th ed. Pearson Education, Inc., San Francisco.

Swenson, J.J. and W.O. Reece. 1993. Duke's Physiology of Domestic Animals, 11th edition. Cornell University Press, Cornell University, Ithaca, New York.

Thrall, M.A., D.C. Baker, T.W. Campbell, D. DeNicola, M.J. Fettman, E.D. Lassen, A. Rebar, and G. Weiser. 2004. Veterinary Hematology and Clinical Chemistry. Lippincott Williams & Wilkins, Baltimore, Maryland.

Tortora, G.J. and S.R. Grabowski. 2003. Principles of Anatomy and Physiology, 10th edition. John Wiley & Sons, Inc., Hoboken, New Jersey.

14 Respiratory system

Contents

Introduction

As animals evolved from single-celled organisms to multilayered organisms, it became impossible for oxygen to diffuse effectively to every cell of the body. Therefore, animals evolved systems to deliver nutrients to every cell. The respiratory and circulatory system became the means by which nutrients are delivered to each cell and wastes are removed. The functions of the respiratory system include gas exchange, regulating blood pH, olfaction, filtering inspired air, producing sounds, and elimination of some water and heat via expired air.

The primary function of the respiratory system is the intake of oxygen and elimination of carbon dioxide from the body. The respiratory system consists of the nose, pharynx, larynx, trachea, bronchi, and lungs. Structurally, the respiratory system can be divided into the upper respiratory system, including the nose, pharynx, and associated structures, and the lower respiratory system, including the larynx, trachea, bronchi, and lungs. Functionally, it can also be divided into two sections: 1) the conducting portion consists of a series of connected tubes, both outside and within the lungs, that filters, warms, moistens, and conducts air to and from the lungs. This portion includes the nose, pharynx, larynx, trachea, bronchi, bronchioles, and terminal bronchioles; and 2) the respiratory portion is the site of gas exchange between the air and blood and consists of the respiratory bronchioles, alveolar ducts, alveolar sacs, and alveoli.

Functional anatomy—nose and paranasal sinuses

The nose is the externally visible portion of the respiratory system. It can be divided into an external and internal portion. The external nose consists of the bone, hyaline cartilage, muscle, skin, and mucous membrane protruding from the face. The immovable portion of the external nose consists of the rostral ends of the nasal bones and the incisive bones. The nasal cartilage extends rostrally from these bones.

The external nares (nostrils) are the external openings to the respiratory tract (Fig. 14.1). The philtrum is the area between the lips and nose. It is relatively deep in carnivores and small ruminants, but shallow or absent in the pig, ox, and horse. The pig possesses a rostral bone in the tip of its flattened, cylindrical-

shaped nose, apparently to assist in rooting. The lateral portion of the nose has sebaceous and sweat glands. The most rostral portion of the nose lacks sebaceous glands, except in the horse.

The nasal cavity extends from the external nares to the caudal nares, and it is separated from the mouth by the hard and soft palates (Fig. 14.2). The hard palate consists of the horizontal portions of the incisive, palatine, and maxillary bones; the soft palate is a musculomucosal extension of the hard palate dividing the rostral part of the pharynx into the oropharynx and nasopharynx.

The space inside the internal nose is the nasal cavity, which is divided into two halves by the median nasal septum. This septum is composed of the vomer, nasal, and ethmoid bones, and cartilage. The nasal cavity is divided into three sections. The vestibule is the most rostral portion located just inside the nostrils. The middle section is filled with the nasal conchae, which are scrolls of bone arising from the lateral wall, and covered with a mucous membrane (Fig. 14.2). Named superior to inferior, the three conchae are dorsal, ethmoidal, and ventral nasal concha. The areas between the conchae are called meatuses, and include the dorsal, middle, and ventral nasal meatus. The common nasal meatus is located between the median nasal septum and conchae, and it is continuous with the other nasal meatuses.

The caudal section of the nasal cavity contains many ethmoturbinates (chonchae of the ethmoid bone). The nasal cavity communicates with the paranasal sinuses, and posteriorly with the nasopharynx through two

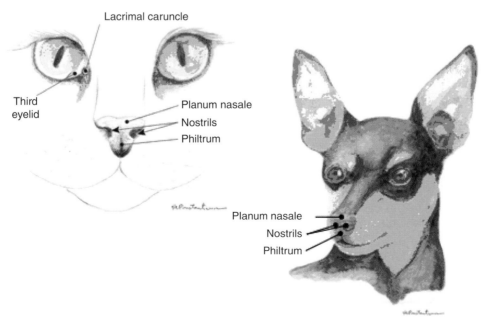

Fig. 14.1. External nose.

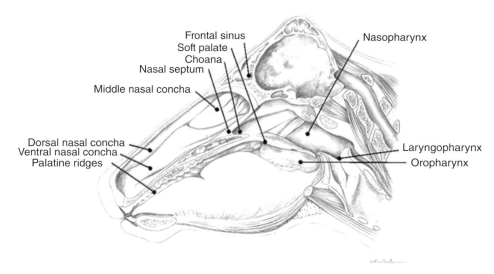

Fig. 14.2. Median aspect of head of large ruminant. The dorsal, ventral, and middle nasal concha are visible in the nasal cavity. They are located dorsal to the hard palate and are separated by dorsal, middle, and ventral nasal meatuses. Also shown are the oropharynx, nasopharynx, and laryngopharynx. (Reprinted from Constantinescu and Constantinescu, 2004. Used by permission of the publisher.)

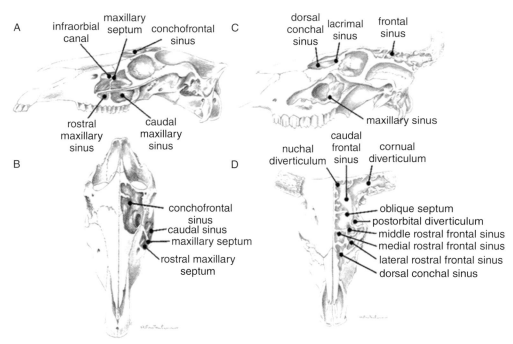

Fig. 14.3. Paranasal sinuses. A) Lateral aspect of horse. B) Frontal aspect of horse. C) Lateral aspect of large ruminant. D) Frontal aspect of large ruminant. (Reprinted from Constantinescu and Constantinescu, 2004. Used by permission of the publisher.)

openings called the internal nares, or choanae (Fig. 14.3). The paranasal sinuses are air-filled cavities within some bones of the skull. The major ones are the frontal and maxillary sinuses, but others may be present depending on the species. In horned cattle, the frontal sinus can extend into the horn as the cornual diverticulum.

Conducting pathway anatomy

Pharynx and nasopharynx

The pharynx connects the nasal cavity and mouth to the larynx and esophagus, respectively. Commonly called the throat, it directs food and air into the digestive and respiratory systems. The soft palate divides the rostral portion of the pharynx into the oropharynx and nasopharynx, and the common caudal portion is the laryngopharynx.

The nasopharynx is located dorsal to the soft palate extending from the internal nares to the laryngopharynx. The palatopharyngeal arches are found at the border of the nasopharynx and laryngopharynx. Since it is located above the mouth, it serves as a passageway only for air. When the animal swallows, the soft palate and uvula move superiorly closing off the nasopharynx and preventing food and water from entering the nasal cavity.

The pharyngotympanic, or auditory, tubes drain from the middle ear to the nasopharynx. It helps equalize the pressure within the middle ear with atmospheric pressure.

Oropharynx and laryngopharynx

The oropharynx lies ventral to the soft palate extending from the oral cavity to the base of the epiglottis. The palatoglossal arches lie at the border between the oral cavity and oropharynx. This is a common pathway for both swallowed food and inhaled air. The laryngopharynx also serves as a common pathway for food and air. It extends from the epiglottis to the larynx, the diverging point for the respiratory and digestive systems.

Larynx

The larynx connects the laryngopharynx with the trachea, and it contains the vocal cords. The two functions of the larynx are 1) provide a routing mechanism for air and food, and 2) make sounds. Superiorly, the larynx attaches to the hyoid bone. The larynx is formed by five mucous-covered cartilages including single epiglottic, thyroid, and cricoid cartilages, and paired arytenoid cartilages.

Box 14.1   Purring in cats

It is well known that cats purr while content, but they can also purr when injured and in pain. The mechanism of purring is not well understood. It was once thought that the purr was produced from blood surging through the inferior vena cava, but it is more widely believed that the intrinsic (internal) laryngeal muscles are the likely source for the purr. The laryngeal muscles are responsible for the opening and closing of the glottis (space between

---

the vocal chords), which results in a separation of the vocal chords and thus the purr sound. There is an absence of purring in a cat with laryngeal paralysis. Studies have shown that the movement of the laryngeal muscles is signaled from a unique "neural oscillator" in the cat's brain.

The epiglottic cartilage provides structure to the epiglottis, which closes the opening to the larynx during swallowing, thus preventing ingested materials from entering the lungs. The thyroid cartilage is the largest cartilage, and forms the "Adam's apple" in humans. The cricoid cartilage connects the thyroid cartilage and trachea. The arytenoid cartilages are paired and irregularly shaped. They have a ventral vocal process to which the vocal ligament (vocal cord) is attached. The glottis consists of the vocal ligaments and the slitlike gap between them, the glottic cleft.

Trachea and bronchi

The trachea, or windpipe, is a cylindrical tube extending from the larynx to the bifurcating right and left primary bronchi above the base of the heart. The cervical portion runs from the larynx to the thoracic inlet while the thoracic portion continues to the bifurcation of the primary bronchi. The thoracic inlet is formed by the first pair of ribs, the first thoracic vertebra, and the cranial parts of the sternum. The trachea consists of four layers: 1) mucosa, which is the deepest layer; 2) submucosa; 3) hyaline cartilage; and 4) adventitia, the most superficial layer composed of areolar connective tissue. The mucosa consists of pseudostratified ciliated columnar epithelium resting on the lamina propria containing elastic and reticular fibers.

The trachea contains a series of dorsally incomplete, C-shaped hyaline cartilage rings. These rings keep the trachea open. The trachea cartilages are united by the annular cartilage, thus making the trachea flexible (Fig. 14.4). The trachealis muscle is smooth muscle

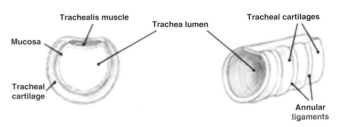

Fig. 14.4.   Trachea of the goat. A) Cross section of trachea. B) Annular ligaments. (Reprinted from Constantinescu, 2001. Used by permission of the publisher.)

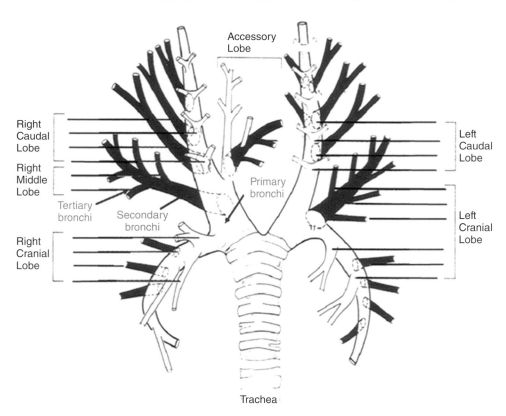

Fig. 14.5. The canine bronchial tree. (Reprinted from Constantinescu, 2002. Used by permission of the publisher.)

connecting the open, dorsal portion of the cartilaginous rings.

The trachea divides into the right and left primary, or principal, bronchi. Like the trachea, the primary bronchi contain incomplete cartilaginous rings and are lined with pseudostratified ciliated columnar epithelium.

Upon entering the lungs at the lung's hilus, the primary bronchi divide into the smaller secondary, or lobar, bronchi. These keep dividing into the following sequence of channels: tertiary, or segmental, bronchi → bronchioles → respiratory bronchioles → alveolar ducts → alveolar sac → alveoli (see Fig. 14.5; see also Fig. 14.7). This extensive branching of the respiratory channels is called the bronchial tree. The alveoli are thin-walled sacs where gas exchange occurs. Below the tertiary bronchi, the mucous membrane changes from ciliated cuboidal epithelium with no goblet cells to nonciliated simple cuboidal epithelium in the respiratory bronchioles.

Respiratory anatomy of the lungs and pleural membrane

The lungs are paired organs located within the thorax. In general, the left and right lungs have two and four lobes, respectively. The horse has three right lobes (Fig. 14.6). The cranial portion, or apex, of each lung is located in the thoracic inlet; the base is the caudal end of the lung resting on the diaphragm. The hilus of the lung is the medial area where the bronchi, blood vessels, and nerves enter the lungs. The cardiac notch is the indentation between the lobes where the heart makes contact with the lung.

The lungs are surrounded by a serous membrane called the pleural membrane. The superficial layer lining the thoracic cavity is the parietal pleura and the layer closely adhering to the lungs is the visceral pleura. The narrow parietal space between these two layers contains a small amount of pleural fluid that allows the two layers to slide over one another during breathing. Inflammation of the pleural membrane is called pleurisy. The mediastinum is the midline site formed where the two pleural membranes meet. It contains the heart, large vessels, esophagus, and other structures, and separates the two lungs from one another.

After the first breath, the lungs become less dense. This fact allows one to determine whether a newborn animal is stillborn. A sample of lung tissue can be placed in water to see whether it floats. If it floats, it indicates that the animal took at least one breath, and therefore was born alive.

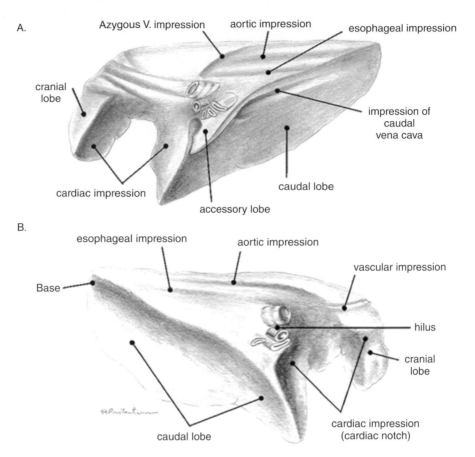

A.
Azygous V. impression   aortic impression   esophageal impression
cranial lobe
impression of caudal vena cava
cardiac impression
caudal lobe
accessory lobe

B.
esophageal impression   aortic impression
vascular impression
Base
hilus
cranial lobe
caudal lobe
cardiac impression (cardiac notch)

Fig. 14.6. Lungs of the horse. A) Medial aspect of left lung. B) Medial aspect of right lung. (Reprinted from Constanstinescu and Constantinescu, 2004. Used by permission of the publisher.)

The pressure inside the intrapleural space is negative. This negative pressure is vital for the expansion of the lungs. If an injury to the chest wall punctures the pleural membrane, it can allow air to enter the intrapleural space, resulting in a pneumothorax. Such an injury can be caused by a sharp object penetrating the chest cavity, or a traumatic blow such as being struck by a car. Because this allows the intrapleural pressure to equilibrate with atmospheric pressure, the lung on that side will collapse.

Alveoli

Surrounding the alveolar ducts are many alveoli and alveolar sacs. Within the alveolar sac are two or more alveoli, saclike outpouchings lined with simple squamous epithelium on a thin elastic basement membrane (Fig. 14.7). Alveoli walls contain predominantly type I alveolar cells, which are simple squamous epithelium and are the main site of gas exchange. They also contain type II alveolar (or septal) cells, alveolar macrophages, and fibroblasts that produce reticular and elastic fibers. Type II alveolar cells are cuboidal epithelial cells containing microvilli that secrete alveolar fluid containing surfactant. The alveolar macrophages are wandering phagocytes that remove debris from the lungs.

The respiratory membrane is where O_2 and CO_2 diffuse across the alveolar and capillary walls. It is a very thin membrane about 0.5 μm thick and consists of four layers.

1. A layer of type I and type II alveolar cells, and alveolar macrophages.
2. The epithelial basement membrane.
3. The capillary basement membrane.
4. The endothelial cells lining the capillary.

Blood supply to the lungs

The pulmonary and bronchial arteries supply blood to the lungs. The pulmonary artery carries deoxygenated blood through the pulmonary trunk and into the right and left pulmonary arteries. Oxygenated blood returns to the left atrium via the pulmonary veins. In most

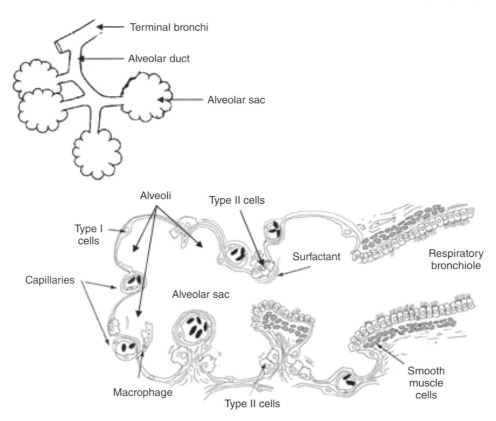

Fig. 14.7. Alveolar sacs and respiratory membrane. Within the alveolar sac are several alveoli. The alveoli contain type I alveolar cells that are the site of gas exchange. Type II alveolar cells produce surfactant. (Drawing modified from http://www.lab.toho-u.ac.jp/med/physi1/respi/respi4,5/respi4,5.html)

vessels, hypoxia causes dilation of blood vessels in order to increase O_2 delivery. However, in the pulmonary blood vessels, hypoxia causes vasoconstriction. This is called ventilation-perfusion coupling, which allows pulmonary blood to be diverted to well-ventilated areas.

Bronchial arteries arise from the aorta and deliver oxygen to the lungs. They mostly perfuse the bronchi and bronchioles. Their blood returns mainly via the pulmonary veins, but some returns via the superior vena cava.

During exercise, cardiac output can increase by as much as eightfold. During this time, blood flow to the lungs must increase in order to collect oxygen. Pulmonary blood vessels dilate. In the horse, pulmonary arterial pressure can be so high as to cause erythrocytes to leak from pulmonary capillaries, a condition called exercise-induced pulmonary hemorrhage. This is a significant problem in athletic horses.

Pulmonary ventilation

Respiration, the process of gas exchange, occurs in three steps:

1. Pulmonary ventilation, or breathing, is the mechanical movement of air into (inspiration) and out (expiration) of the lungs.
2. External respiration is the exchange of gases between the lungs and the pulmonary capillaries, which occurs across the respiratory membrane. The blood gains O_2 and loses CO_2.
3. Internal respiration is the exchange of gases between systemic capillaries and tissue. The blood gains CO_2 and loses O_2.

Pressure changes during respiration

Inspiration

Boyle's law states that at constant temperature and pressure, there is an inverse relationship between volume and pressure of a gas:

$$P_1V_1 = P_2V_2$$

where P is the pressure of the gas (ml of Hg), and V is the volume (cm^3). Therefore, the pressure inside a closed container will decrease as the volume of the container increases, and vice versa. When this law is applied to the lungs, we find that the pressure inside the lungs decreases as the volume of the lungs increases. Air moves into the lungs as a result of a decrease in air pressure within the lungs.

In most animals, inspiration is an active process. The main muscles responsible for quiet inhalation are the diaphragm and external intercostal muscles. The diaphragm is a dome-shaped muscle innervated by the phrenic nerves. As the diaphragm contracts, it increases the horizontal dimensions of the thoracic cavity, thus increasing the volume of the thorax. This causes the volume of the lungs to expand and thereby decreases the pressure inside the lungs. This results in inspiration.

Contraction of the external intercostal muscles causes the ribs to move cranially and ventrally, thus increasing the diameter of the thorax. This accounts for about 25% of the entry of air into the lungs.

In a horse at rest, the intrapleural pressure is negative, about 754 mmHg. As inspiration begins, this pressure drops to approximately 744 mmHg. Atmospheric pressure is 760 mmHg at sea level. As the volume of the thoracic cavity increases during inspiration, the parietal pleura is pulled outward, and the visceral pleura is pulled with it. As a result, the pressure inside the lungs, the alveolar pressure, decreases. Air then flows from an area of high pressure (the atmosphere) to an area of lower pressure (the alveoli).

As an animal increases the force of inspiration, additional muscles are engaged. These include the sterno-cleidomastoid muscles that move the sternum rostrally, the scalene muscles that pull the first two ribs forward, and the pectoralis minor muscles that pull several other ribs forward.

Expiration

Normal expiration is a passive process involving no active muscle contraction. Like inspiration, it is due to pressure gradients, but in an opposite direction. Because of the elastic recoil of the lungs and chest wall, there are two inwardly directed forces resulting in this recoil: 1) the elastic fibers that were stretched during inhalation, and 2) the inwardly directed force due to the surface tension arising from the alveolar fluid.

As the neural signals to the diaphragm cease, it relaxes and this dome-shaped muscle moves rostrally, thus decreasing the volume of the thoracic cavity. The external intercostals also relax, and allow the ribs to move dorsally and caudally, thus further decreasing the volume of the thoracic cavity. This decreases lung volume and causes alveolar pressure to increase approximately 2 mmHg above atmospheric pressure.

As a result, air flows out of the lungs to an area of lower pressure.

During forceful exhalation, the abdominal and internal intercostal muscles contract. This causes the ribs to move caudally and dorsally compressing the abdominal viscera and decreasing the thoracic volume. This increases pressure inside the thoracic cavity and forces air outward.

Other factors involved in pulmonary ventilation

Surface tension of alveolar fluid

Alveolar fluid coats the inside surface of the alveoli. Because of hydrogen bonding, this fluid has a surface tension. In a sphere such as that found in the alveoli, this surface tension produces an inwardly directed force causing the alveoli to assume the smallest possible diameter. In order to expand the lungs, this surface tension must be exceeded. This surface tension accounts for approximately two-thirds of the lung's elastic recoil.

Surfactant, produced by type II alveolar cells, is a complex of lipids and proteins that reduces the surface tension in much the same way the soap allows lipids to dissolve in aqueous solutions. Since surfactant is one of the last compounds produced during embryonic development, premature animals often have respiratory distress as a result of the underdeveloped respiratory system. In the case of sheep, surfactant is released into the alveolar spaces near the beginning of the fourth month of gestation. Its release correlates with a rise in plasma cortisol levels.

Box 14.2 Surfactant production in premature infants

Premature infants are at risk for respiratory distress syndrome. This is due to the lack of surfactant production, which does not line the alveolar walls till near parturition. The National Institute of Health recommends broad use of maternal glucocorticoid therapy to stimulate surfactant production in the fetus. In addition, surfactant replacement therapy is recommended in low birth weight immature infants. The preterm lamb is often used as a model for investigating the effects of glucocorticoids on surfactant production and its effects on postnatal development (see Ikegami et al., 1997).

Compliance of the lungs

The distensibility of the lungs is referred to as lung compliance. High lung compliance means that the lungs will expand easily. Lung compliance is related to 1) the distensibility of lung tissue and the thoracic cage, and 2) alveolar surface tension. Lung compliance is normally high due to the elasticity of the lung's tissue, and decreased alveolar surface tension from surfactant.

Compliance can be decreased by several factors: 1) scar tissue formed in the lungs as a result of certain diseases, 2) pulmonary edema resulting from accumulation of fluid in the lungs, 3) insufficiency of surfactant, and 4) decrease in the ability of the thoracic cage to expand.

Airway resistance

The flow of air into the lungs is inversely related to airway resistance:

$$F = \frac{\Delta P}{R}$$

where F is gas flow, P is pressure, and R is resistance. The walls of the airways into the alveoli, particularly the bronchioles, create resistance to airflow. The larger the diameter of the airway, the less the resistance to airflow. The diameter of the airways can be altered by the degree of contraction of the smooth muscle in these airways. Stimulation of the sympathetic nervous system causes relaxation of these walls, which allows air to more readily enter the lungs. Diseases or injuries to the airways can increase airway resistance.

During exercise, animals decrease the airway resistance by dilating the external nares and vasoconstriction of the vascular tissue in the nose. As exercise rate increases, cows and dogs breathe through their mouth in order to bypass the greater airway resistance associated with the nose. However, horses are considered obligate nose breathers and must rely on their ability to decrease airway resistance in order to increase airflow. One can watch the nostrils of a horse flare during exercise.

Box 14.3 Airway obstruction in short-nosed dogs

The term *brachycephalic*, or *brachiocephalic*, means short-nosed and refers to dogs with short muzzles, noses, and mouths. Brachycephalic airway obstruction syndrome (BAOS), also called brachycephalic airway disease (BAD) and brachycephalic airway syndrome (BAS), is an inherited condition in the Cavalier King Charles Spaniel, English bulldog, pug, Boston terrier, and Pekingese, in particular. The throat and breathing passages in brachycephalic dogs often are undersized or flattened.

The symptoms of this disorder typically include labored and constant open-mouthed breathing, noisy breathing, snuffling, snorting, excessive snoring, gagging, retching, exercise and/or heat intolerance, general lack of energy, and pale or bluish tongue and gums due to a lack of oxygen. Precautions should be taken to avoid overheating and excessive excitement and excessive exercise, which may cause increased panting. Excessive barking or panting may cause the throat to swell, which could result in a totally blocked airway. Most importantly, the owner should not let the dog get too hot, particularly in the summer months, and not allow the dog to become overweight, because obesity will exacerbate the respiratory difficulties. If severe, this disorder can result in death from such related causes as heatstroke.

Lung volumes and capacities

The respiratory capacities, or amount of air that moves in and out of the lungs, depends on the strength of inspirations and expirations. During normal, quiet breathing, the volume of air moving in and out of the lungs is called the tidal volume (TV). Only about 70% of tidal volume reaches the lungs. The remaining portion of the air is found in the airways including the nose, pharynx, larynx, trachea, bronchi, bronchioles, and terminal bronchioles. These airways are collectively called the anatomical dead space.

The minute volume (MV) is the volume of air inhaled and exhaled each minute, and is calculated as:

$$MV = TV \times \text{Respiration Rate}$$

The respiration rate varies by species (Table 14.1). Because of the anatomical dead space, not all of the minute volume is available for gas exchange. The alveolar ventilation rate (AVR) is that portion of the tidal volume that actually reaches the site of gas exchange.

$$\text{AVR} = \text{respiration rate} \times (\text{TV-dead space})$$
$$(ml/min) \quad (breaths/min) \quad (ml/breath)$$

If an animal inhales more forcefully, it can increase the volume of air entering the lungs above normal tidal volume (Fig. 14.8). The additional inhaled air is called the inspiratory reserve volume. Similarly, an animal can force more air out of its lungs than occurs during quiet respiration. This additional volume exhaled is called the expiratory reserve volume. Following a forced expiration, the air remaining in the lungs is the residual volume.

Table 14.1. Tidal volume and respiration rate.*

Species	Body Weight (kg)	Condition	Respiration Rate (Breaths/Minute)	Tidal Volume (ml/kg body weight)
Cat	3.7	Anesthetized	30	9.2
Holstein Cow	516	Standing	26	8.2
Jersey Cow	450	Standing	27	8.4
Dog	19	Anesthetized	13.6	10.7
	12.6	Anesthetized	21.0	11.4
Horse	486	Resting	10	15.4

*Data from Swenson and Reece (1993).

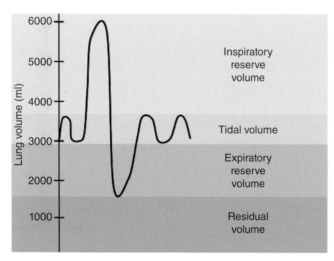

Fig. 14.8. Respiratory volumes and capacities. During quiet respiration, the volume of air inspired and expired is called the tidal volume. The additional air brought into the lungs during a forced inspiration is called the inspiratory reserve volume, and the additional air that can be expired during a forced expiration is called the expiratory reserve volume. The air remaining in the lungs after a forced expiration is called the residual volume.

Exchange of oxygen and carbon dioxide

Dalton's law and Henry's law

The exchange of oxygen and carbon dioxide between alveolar air and pulmonary blood is a passive process, which is explained by two gas laws. Dalton's law explains how gases move by diffusion based on pressure differences; Henry's law describes the diffusion of gas based on its solubility.

Dalton's law

Dalton's law states that each gas within a mixture exerts its own pressure independent of the other gases present. The pressure of an individual gas is called its partial pressure, designated P_x. The total pressure of a gas mixture is calculated by summing all its partial pressures. Atmospheric air is a combination of nitrogen (N_2), oxygen (O_2), carbon dioxide (CO_2), and water vapor.

At sea level, atmospheric pressure is 760 mmHg. Atmospheric air is 78.6% nitrogen, 20.9% oxygen, 0.04% carbon dioxide, 0.06% other gases, and varying water vapor, depending on the humidity. Therefore, atmospheric air can be computed as follows:

$$P_{N_2} = 760 \times 0.786 \text{ mmHg} = 597.4 \text{ mmHg}$$
$$P_{O_2} = 760 \times 0.209 \text{ mmHg} = 158.8 \text{ mmHg}$$
$$P_{H_2O} = 760 \times 0.004 \text{ mmHg} = 3.0 \text{ mmHg}$$
$$P_{CO_2} = 760 \times 0.0004 \text{ mmHg} = 0.3 \text{ mmHg}$$

$$P_{other\ gases} = 760 \times 0.006 \text{ mmHg} = \frac{0.5 \text{ mmHg}}{760 \text{ mmHg}}$$

Henry's law

Henry's law says that the quantity of a gas that will dissolve in a liquid is proportional to its partial pressure and its solubility coefficient. Therefore, gases will dissolve in body fluids more readily if they have a greater partial pressure and solubility coefficient. The solubility coefficient of CO_2 is 24 times higher than that of O_2. Therefore, CO_2 dissolves in blood more readily than O_2. In contrast, the solubility of nitrogen is very low, so even though atmospheric air has 79% N_2, it has very little effect on body functions.

External and internal respiration

External respiration, also called pulmonary gas exchange, is the diffusion of O_2 and CO_2 from the alveoli to pulmonary blood. Pulmonary blood is deoxygenated blood arriving from the right ventricle.

Blood circulating through the body picks up CO_2 and delivers O_2. As this blood travels through the pulmonary capillaries, CO_2 diffuses into the alveoli while O_2 diffuses from the alveoli to pulmonary blood. The exchange of these gases occurs independently and passively.

Pulmonary gas exchange is facilitated by a very thin respiratory membrane. In addition, there is a close association between the amount of gas reaching the alveoli, i.e., ventilation, and the blood flow through the pulmonary capillaries, i.e., perfusion. When ventilation becomes inadequate within alveoli, the P_{O_2} will decrease. This causes an autoregulatory response in which pulmonary arterioles constrict. Conversely, if P_{O_2} increases, the pulmonary arterioles dilate, allowing more blood to flow to those areas that can maximize gas exchange. Note that this is the opposite of what happens in systemic circulation, where a decrease in P_{O_2} results in vasodilation.

Internal respiration, or systemic gas exchange, occurs at the tissue level, where there is an exchange of O_2 and CO_2 between systemic capillaries and tissue. O_2 diffuses from the capillaries into the cells; CO_2 diffuses from the cells into the systemic capillaries.

Transport of oxygen and carbon dioxide

Hemoglobin and oxygen transport

Oxygen has a low solubility coefficient, so it does not readily dissolve in blood. Instead, over 98% of O_2 is bound to hemoglobin. The heme portion of hemoglobin contains four atoms of iron, each able to bind to one molecule of O_2.

Adult hemoglobin consists of two alpha and two beta chains. Fetal hemoglobin contains two alpha and two gamma chains. More than 400 different types of abnormal hemoglobin have been identified, but the most common associated with diseases in humans are the following:

- Hemoglobin S. This type of hemoglobin is present in sickle cell anemia.
- Hemoglobin C. This is another type of hemoglobin found in sickle cell anemia.
- Hemoglobin E. This type of hemoglobin is found in people of Southeast Asian descent.
- Hemoglobin D. This type of hemoglobin may be present with sickle cell anemia or thalassemia.
- Hemoglobin H (heavy hemoglobin). This type of hemoglobin may be present in certain types of thalassemia.

Box 14.4   Onion toxicity in cats and dogs

Allium species (meadow garlic, nodding onion, Pacific onion, and wild garlic) contain organosulfur compounds that can be very toxic when consumed by cats or dogs. These compounds can cause oxidative hemolysis, which results in cell lysis of erythrocytes. Consuming as little as 5 gm/kg or 15–30 g/kg of onions in cats and dogs, respectively, can cause this problem. Treatment includes inducing emesis in asymptomatic dogs and cats known to have ingested these products. If severely affected, a blood transfusion and supplemental oxygen may be necessary.

Oxygen bound to hemoglobin forms oxyhemoglobin. Hemoglobin that has released O_2 is called reduced hemoglobin, or deoxyhemoglobin. Because it picks up a H^+ ion after releasing O_2, reduced hemoglobin is abbreviated as HHb:

$$HHb + O_2 \rightleftarrows Hb\text{-}O_2 + H^+$$

Reduced   oxygen   oxyhemoglobin   hemoglobin

P_{O_2} is the most important factor controlling how much O_2 is bound to hemoglobin. When reduced hemoglobin is converted to oxyhemoglobin, it is fully saturated. When only a portion of hemoglobin exists as oxyhemoglobin, it is partially saturated. This can be graphically represented as an oxygen-hemoglobin dissociation curve (Fig. 14.9). At the level of the lungs,

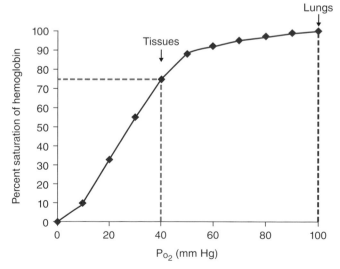

Fig. 14.9. Oxygen-hemoglobin dissociation curve. The saturation of hemoglobin is affected by changes in P_{O_2}. At the lungs, hemoglobin is 100% saturated. As the blood passes through tissue in which the P_{O_2} is lower, hemoglobin is able to rapidly unload O_2.

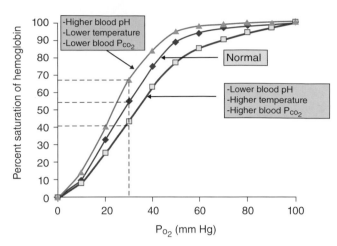

Fig. 14.10. Bohr effect. Increases in temperature, decreases in pH, or increases in blood P_{CO_2} shift the oxygen-hemoglobin dissociation curve to the right.

hemoglobin becomes fully saturated. As blood passes through tissue where the P_{O_2} drops to 40 mm Hg, hemoglobin unloads its oxygen and is only 75% saturated.

The oxygen-hemoglobin dissociation curve has a steep slope between 10 and 50 mm Hg P_{O_2}. When an animal is at rest, hemoglobin releases approximately only 25% of its oxygen. It maintains a reserve that is available when needed. If the animal begins vigorous exercise, hemoglobin is able to respond by releasing a greater amount of O_2.

Other factors affecting the oxygen-hemoglobin dissociation curve

Although the P_{O_2} is the most important factor affecting hemoglobin's affinity for oxygen, other factors can also influence this association. These factors can shift the oxygen-hemoglobin curve to either side of normal (Fig. 14.10):

1. pH of the blood. Increasing the acidity of blood, i.e., lowering the pH, lowers the affinity of hemoglobin for O_2. Therefore, as the metabolism of tissue increases, resulting in increased lactic and carbonic acid at the same P_{O_2}, hemoglobin releases more O_2 at that site. Mechanistically, this occurs because the binding of H^+ to hemoglobin causes a conformational change decreasing hemoglobin's O_2-carrying capacity. This shift of the curve to the right is termed the Bohr effect. The reverse reaction can also occur in which binding of O_2 to hemoglobin causes the liberation of H^+. Decreasing the acidity shifts the oxygen-hemoglobin dissociation curve to the left.

2. Temperature. An increase in temperature also shifts the oxygen-hemoglobin dissociation curve to the right. Like increased acidity, increased temperature is a by-product of increased metabolism. Increased metabolism requires additional O_2, so shifting this curve to the right provides necessary O_2.

3. BPG. An increase in the production of 2,3-bis-phosphoglycerate (BPG), formerly called diphosphoglycerate, also shifts the curve to the right, thus liberating more O_2. Increased production of BPG is also associated with increased metabolism.

4. P_{CO_2}. A decrease in pH acts similarly to an increase in P_{CO_2}. As shown below, CO_2 can react with water to form carbonic acid, which then dissociates to form bicarbonate and H^+. Thus, increased P_{CO_2} is associated with decreased pH.

$$CO_2 + H_2O \rightleftharpoons H_2CO_3 \rightleftharpoons HCO_3 + H^+$$

Hemoglobin–nitric oxide

Nitric oxide (NO), a gas, plays an important role in vasomotor tone. It is a potent vasodilator. Produced in lung and endothelial cells, NO can be carried by hemoglobin. The binding of O_2 to hemoglobin causes a change in the conformation of hemoglobin allowing NO to bind to the cysteine of hemoglobin. This protects NO from being broken down by the Fe in hemoglobin. As oxyhemoglobin releases its O_2, it simultaneously releases NO. NO dilates local blood vessels, thus further aiding in supplying O_2 to areas in need.

Carbon dioxide transport

Carbon dioxide is a waste product of metabolism. It is transported in the blood to the lungs in three forms:

1. Dissolved CO_2. Accounting for the smallest amount of transported CO_2, 7–10% is carried dissolved in the plasma.

2. Carbamino compounds. Approximately 20% of CO_2 is transported in the red blood cells attached to the amino acids of globin forming carbamino-hemoglobin. Since CO_2 is bound to globin, and not the heme molecule, the CO_2 does not compete with O_2 or NO transport:

Hb + CO_2	Hb-CO_2 $\longrightarrow$	
Hemoglobin	Carbon dioxide	Carbaminohemoglobin

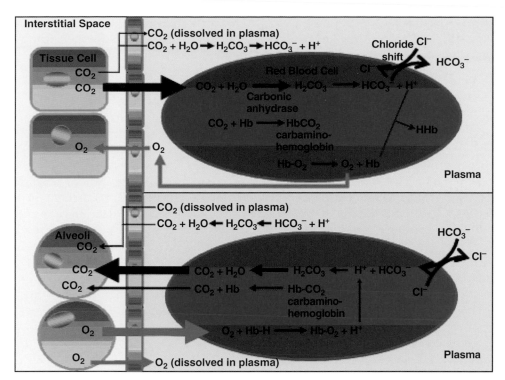

Fig. 14.11. Transport of O_2 and CO_2 in the blood. The top portion of the figure shows gas exchange at the tissue level, and the bottom portion is at the level of the lungs. As CO_2 is produced in the tissues, it diffuses into the red blood cells where it combines with water to form carbonic acid. As carbonic acid dissociates, the HCO_3^- that was formed diffuses out of the red blood cell and into the plasma in exchange for Cl^-, which moves into the RBC, a process called the chloride shift. Most (70%) of CO_2 is transported as HCO_3^-; the remainder is transported as either dissolved CO_2 (7%) or carbaminohemoglobin (22%).

The formation of carbaminohemaglobin is influenced by P_{CO_2} and the degree of oxygenation of hemoglobin. In the lungs where P_{CO_2} in alveolar air is low, carbon dioxide dissociates from hemoglobin and is exhaled. At the tissue level where P_{CO_2} is high, the formation of carbaminohemoglobin is favored since deoxygenated hemoglobin readily combines with CO_2.

3. Bicarbonate ions. Most carbon dioxide, about 70%, is transported in the blood as bicarbonate ions (HCO_3^-) (Fig. 14.11). As tissues produce CO_2, it diffuses into the systemic capillaries where most of it enters the red blood cells and, in the presence of carbonic anhydrase, it combines with water to produce carbonic acid. Carbonic acid dissociates to bicarbonate and hydrogen ions. The hydrogen ions bind to hemoglobin, causing the Bohr effect and enhancing the release of O_2. The HCO_3^- diffuses from the red blood cells into the plasma and is transported to the lungs. As HCO_3^- leaves the red blood cells, chloride ions (Cl^-) enter, a process called the chloride shift.

Control of respiration—neural mechanisms

The medullary rhythmicity area is located in the medullar oblongata, and it controls the basic respira-

tion rhythm. It consists of two areas, the inspiratory and expiratory areas, also called the dorsal respiratory group and ventral respiratory group, respectively. The inspiratory area sends signals to the diaphragm via the phrenic nerves and to the external intercostal muscles via the intercostal nerves. These signals cause muscle contraction resulting in inspirations. When these signals cease, inspiration is concluded, which allows the diaphragm and external intercostal muscles to passively relax, during which time the elastic recoil of the lungs and thoracic walls causes the volume of the thoracic cavity to decrease. Transection between the spinal cord and medulla oblongata stops breathing.

Although not active during quiet breathing, forceful expiration requires signals from the expiratory area that cause contraction of the internal intercostals and abdominal muscles. Contraction of these muscles further decreases the volume of the thoracic cavity, thus increasing exhalation.

Pneumotaxic and apneustic area

Located in the upper pons, the pneumotaxic area, also called the pontine respiratory group, sends inhibitory signals to the inspiratory area. These signals primarily function to prevent overfilling of the lungs. Conversely, the apneustic area located in the lower pons sends stimulatory signals to the inspiratory area that prolongs inspiration. The pneumotaxic area can override the apneustic area.

Chemoreceptors

The respiratory system functions to bring in O_2 and eliminate CO_2 from the body. This function is assisted by specialized receptors called chemoreceptors that monitor the levels of CO_2, O_2 and H^+, and then send such information to the respiratory center.

These chemoreceptors are located in several locations. There are central chemoreceptors found in the medulla oblongata that respond to changes in cerebrospinal fluid H^+ and P_{CO_2}. Peripheral chemoreceptors include the aortic bodies and carotid bodies whose removal eliminates a respiratory response to hypoxia. The aortic bodies are a cluster of chemoreceptors in the aortic arch; the carotid bodies are oval nodules in the wall of the left and right common carotid arteries, where they bifurcate into the internal and external carotid arteries. Axons from the chemoreceptors in the aortic bodies are part of the vagus nerve (cranial nerve X), whereas those of the carotid bodies project in the glossopharyngeal nerves (cranial nerve IX).

The levels of CO_2 and H^+ are highly correlated. Throughout the body, CO_2 is quickly converted to carbonic acid catalyzed by the enzyme carbonic anhydrase. Carbonic acid dissociates into HCO_3^- and H^+. Therefore, increases in CO_2 lead to increases in H^+ while decreases in CO_2 lead to decreases in H^+. As a result, P_{CO_2} has a large affect on respiration, whereas P_{O_2} affects respiration only if its levels change substantially.

Increases in arterial blood CO_2, called hypercapnia, cause an increase in H^+. This has a particularly large affect on central chemoreceptors since there is little protein within the cerebrospinal fluid to buffer the H^+. Activation of the central chemoreceptors causes increased respiration rate, possibly causing hyperventilation. Conversely, low arterial blood CO_2, called hypocapnia, inhibits respiration. Large drops in arterial PO_2 increase ventilation by stimulating peripheral chemoreceptors. An increase in plasma H^+ is also detected by the aortic and carotid bodies, which are highly responsive to changes in arterial H^+ concentration.

Pulmonary and airway receptors

Three types of sensory receptors have been identified in the lungs, including slowly adapting stretch receptors, irritant receptors, and unmyelinated C fibers. The stretch receptors increase their firing rate as the lungs and larger airways inflate.

Avian respiration

There are several differences between the avian and mammalian respiratory systems. Unlike mammals, bird lungs are inelastic and therefore do not change volume during respiration. In birds, the relative volume of the trachea is much larger, and therefore the bird must compensate for this large dead space. Rather than having alveoli, gas exchange in birds occurs in air capillaries. Furthermore, since birds lack a diaphragm, the movement of the ribs and the sternum are important in changing the abdominal pressure in order to move air in and out of the air sacs, another structure unique to birds.

Anatomy of the avian respiratory system

The avian respiratory system has a unique structure compared to other vertebrates (Fig. 14.12). The lungs do not expand; instead, air sacs act as bellows to move air in and out of the lungs. Gas exchange occurs in the lungs, but not the air sacs. Also, birds have no diaphragm, and the thoracic cavity is at atmospheric pressure instead of negative pressure as in mammals. Although birds have a larynx, sound is instead generated in the syrinx, which is composed of cartilage and vibrating soft tissue.

The avian lung is a rigid structure located in the thoracoabdominal cavity. The trachea extends from the larynx to the syrinx, and it is composed of complete tracheal cartilages. Tracheal volume in birds is about 4.5 times larger than in mammals since avian trachea are longer and wider, creating a larger dead space. Birds compensate by having a larger tidal volume and lower respiratory frequency.

Short primary bronchi extend from the syrinx to the lungs. The intrapulmonary primary bronchus travels through the lungs to the abdominal air sac at the caudal border of the lungs. Two groups of secondary bronchi exist. The cranial group includes 4–5 medioventral secondary bronchi originating from medioventral intrapulmonary bronchi; the caudal group includes 6–10 mediodorsal secondary bronchi. There is also a third group, which varies among species, consisting of lateroventral secondary bronchi. The primary and secondary bronchi do not participate in gas exchange.

The parabronchi, also called tertiary bronchi, originate from the secondary bronchi and are the site of gas exchange. There are two types of parabronchi. The

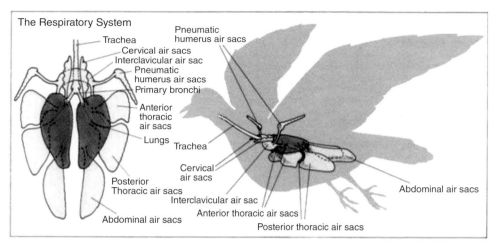

Fig. 14.12. Respiratory system in birds. (Figure from http://www.paulnoll.com/Oregon/Birds/Avian-Respiratory.html)

medioventral and mediodorsal secondary bronchi, also called paleopulmonic parabronchi, appear as parallel tubes extending from the secondary bronchi. Gas flow through the paleopulmonic parabronchi is unidirectional. There is also an irregular branching system of neopulmonic parabronchi through which gas flow is bidirectional. The lumen of the parabronchi is lined with smooth muscle surrounding the entrances to the atria that branch off and lead to infundibula, which give rise to air capillaries. The air capillaries intermesh with pulmonary blood capillaries, the site of gas exchange.

Air sacs

Air sacs are poorly vascularized, thin membranous structures connected to either the primary or secondary bronchi via ostia. Comprising most of the volume of the respiratory system, they do not participate in gas exchange, but function to move air through the lungs so that gas exchange can occur in the parabronchi. Air sacs can also extend into selected bones.

Birds possess nine air sacs; four are paired and one is unpaired (Fig. 14.12). The cranial group of air sacs consists of paired cervical and cranial thoracic air sacs and the unpaired clavicular air sac. The caudal group includes the paired caudal thoracic and paired abdominal air sacs.

Avian ventilation and gas exchange

Since birds do not have a diaphragm, they have a single thoracoabdominal cavity, which functionally behaves as a single compartment. During inspira-

tion, the sternum moves both cranially and ventrally as the coracoids and furcula (wishbone) simultaneously rotate forward at the shoulders (Fig. 14.13). The sternal ribs also move cranially, thus laterally expanding the sternal ribs and thoracoabdominal cavity. Both inspiration and expiration are active processes involving various muscles (Table 14.2). Therefore, in birds the volume of the respiratory system is half of end-inspiratory and end-expiratory volume when relaxed. This is in contrast to mammals, where during relaxation only the residual volume remains.

During inspiration, approximately half the tidal volume first enters the caudal air sacs and half enters the cranial air sacs. As the thoracic cavity expands during inspiration, the volume, and therefore pressure, inside the air sacs decreases. This causes air to move caudally through the intrapulmonary bronchus. About half of this air goes through the neopulmonic lung continuing directly to the caudal thoracic and abdominal air sacs. The other half goes into the mediodorsal secondary bronchi and into the paleopulmonic parabronchi, and then into the cranial group of air sacs (Fig. 14.14). During expiration, contraction of the expiratory muscles decreases the volume of the thoracoabdominal cavity causing air to flow out of the caudal thoracic and abdominal air sacs (Fig. 14.14). This gas passes through the neopulmonic lungs to the paleopulmonic lungs. Simultaneously, air leaves the cranial air sacs through the medioventral secondary bronchi flowing into the primary bronchus and the trachea to exit the body. Therefore, during quiet breathing, all air moves through the paleopulmonic parabronchi, and air passes through the paleopulmonic parabronchi in a caudal-to-cranial direction while traveling through the neopulmonary parabronchi bidirectionally.

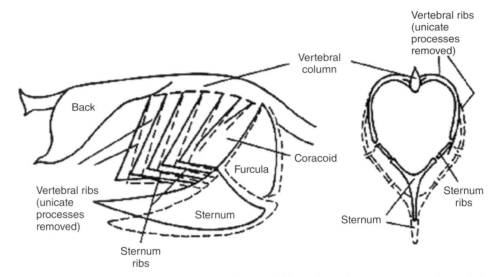

Fig. 14.13. Changes in the thoracic skeleton during respiration in birds. Solid lines show thoracic position at the end of expiration; dotted lines show position at the end of inspiration (Reprinted from Whittow, 2000. Used by permission of the publisher.)

Table 14.2. Muscles involved in respiration in birds.

Inspiration	Expiration
M. scalenus	Mm intercostals externi of fifth and sixth spaces
Mm intercostals externi (except in fifth and sixth spaces)	Mm intercostals interni of third to sixth spaces
M. intercostalis interni in second space	M. costosternalis pars minor
M. costosternalis pars major	M. obliquus externus abdominis
Mm. levatores costarum	M. obliquus internus abdominis
M. serratus profundus	M. transveresus abdominis
	M. rectus abdominis
	M. serratus superficialis, pars cranialis and caudalis
	M. costoseptalis

Gas exchange occurs between the air capillaries and blood capillaries. As shown in Figure 14.15, the flow of gas within the air capillaries is in the opposite direction as the flow of blood in the blood capillaries. Thus, this is a countercurrent system. As air moves through the parabronchus, CO_2 is added to the blood while O_2 is removed from the blood. The interaction between the respiratory system and cardiovascular system is shown in Figure 14.16.

Prehatching respiration in birds

Bird eggs contain all the nutrients necessary for embryonic development except oxygen. Oxygen passively diffuses into the egg through the pores found in the eggshell while carbon dioxide diffuses out of the same pores. A normal chicken egg contains approximately 10,000 pores. The number of these pores is important because the shell must allow adequate entry of oxygen to meet the embryo's needs while simultaneously preventing too much moisture loss, which would result in dehydration, or too little carbon dioxide loss, thus disrupting acid-base balance.

During the first 18 days of incubation, the prenatal period, the capillaries located in the chorioallantoic membrane, analogous to the mammalian placenta, function in gas exchange across the shell and its associated shell membranes. Such gas exchange is ample to meet the embryonic needs through 18 days of incubation. After this time, the embryo prepares for hatching. Simple diffusion across the shell is insufficient to meet the oxygen needs of the embryo.

On day 19 of incubation, the chick's beak penetrates the internal shell membrane, thus poking into the air cell located at the blunt end of the egg. This process, called internal pipping, allows the chick to begin pulmonary respiration using air located in the air cell. This time during which the embryo is breathing from the air cell is called the paranatal period. About 6 hr after internal pipping, the chick's beak penetrates the eggshell, which is called external pipping. The chick is now able to receive sufficient oxygen to complete the hatching process.

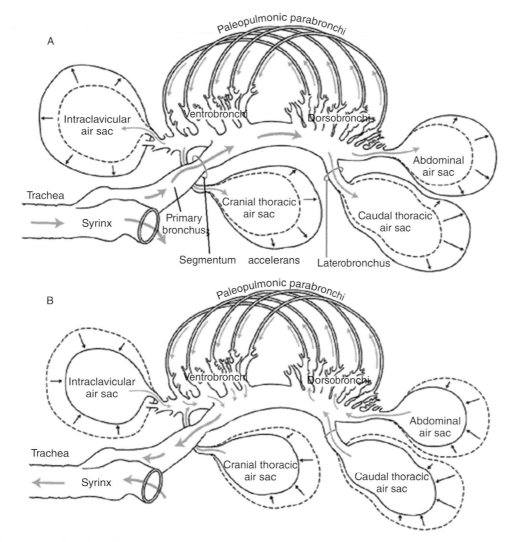

Fig. 14.14. Pathway of gas flow through avian pulmonary system during inspiration and expiration. A) Inspiration through the right paleopalmonic parabronchi; the neopulmonic parabronchi have been omitted for clarity. B) Expiration. (Used with permission from John W. Ludders and Michael Simmons, Cornell University, http://www.ivis.org/advances/Anesthesia_Gleed/ludders2/chapter_frm.asp)

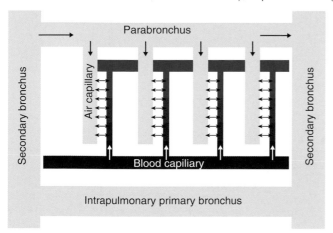

Fig. 14.15. Crosscurrent gas exchange in the avian lung. The parabronchi lie parallel to the intrapulmonary primary bronchus. Air capillaries branch perpendicular from the parabronchi. Gas exchange occurs between the air capillaries and blood capillaries, each of which flow in an opposite direction (Modified from Sturkie, 1986.)

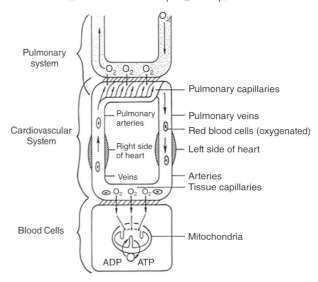

Fig. 14.16. Cooperation between respiratory and circulatory systems. Oxygen diffuses from the air capillaries to the pulmonary capillaries. It is then carried through the cardiovascular system and delivered to the tissues. (Reprinted from Sturkie, 1986. Used by permission of the publisher.)

Defense mechanisms of the respiratory system

While animals are grazing or playing outside, there is generally little particulate matter in the air. However, when animals are housed in confined areas or are being transported, exposure to particulate matter can increase dramatically. Such particulate matter can contain many harmful materials such as bacteria, viruses, and allergens. The respiratory system contains defense mechanisms to minimize the harmful effects from these materials.

Nonspecific defense mechanisms

Inhaled air can contain aerosols, airborne particles small enough to float in the air, and unwanted gasses. When airborne particles come in contact with the wall of the conducting airway or a respiratory unit they undergo a process of deposition, which prevents them from becoming airborne again. This can happen in one of four ways:

- Sedimentation, which is settlement by gravity, tends to occur in larger airways.
- Inertial impaction occurs when an airstream changes direction, especially in the nose but also in other large airways. This happens in places where there are bends in the large airways and airborne particles fail to make the turns.
- Interception applies mainly to irregular particles such as asbestos or fibrous dust, which, because of their shape, avoid sedimentation and inertial impaction. However, they are intercepted by collision with walls of bronchioles, especially at bifurcations or if the fibers are curved.
- Diffusion is when very small aerosol particles reach peripheral airways and alveoli and contact the epithelial surface and then move inward in the mucous membrane.

Most particles larger than 20 microns in diameter are filtered within the nose during breathing at rest. However, conditions that increase respiration rate or favor mouth breathing, (e.g., high ventilation rates and obstructive disease of the nasal airways) cause large particles to bypass this filter. Slow deep breathing favors the movement of particles deep into the lung; rapid shallow breathing favors deposition in the larger airways.

Particles trapped in the mucous lining of the respiratory tract are transported back toward the pharynx by the mucociliary escalator. The movement of the cilia pushes the mucous back toward the mouth, thus carrying unwanted particles out of the respiratory system. Allowing a horse to lower its head facilitates such movement and decreases the incidence of pneumonia by preventing the accumulation of bacteria in the lungs.

Specific defense mechanisms

The alveolar lining contains many macrophages. Alveolar macrophages are the cells within the lungs, such as phagocytose microbes and particulate matter, e.g., inhaled dust. Alveolar macrophages begin as monocytes produced in the bone marrow, and then they differentiate while in transit through the bloodstream where they leave the capillaries and enter the lungs.

Alveolar macrophages can function in two ways. They can either be fixed, in which case they are trapped within the connective tissue of the alveolar walls, or they can be free, in which they are mobile and can scavenge for particles that are trapped within the surfactant layer. These cells can leave the lungs by ascending in the layer of mucus on the "mucociliary escalator" to the larynx, or they can pass through the alveolar wall and pass into alveolar lymphatics.

Alveolar macrophages may phagocytize erythrocytes that have left the pulmonary capillaries as a result of pulmonary congestion. Such macrophages stain positively for iron in the altered pigment haemosiderin. These "heart failure" cells may be coughed up by the animal in its sputum.

Box 14.5 Chronic obstructive pulmonary disease

Chronic obstructive pulmonary disease (COPD) is the fourth leading cause of death in humans, and also occurs in animals. It is a lung disease that resembles human asthma. The condition is also known as heaves, recurrent airway obstruction, broken wind, emphysema, chronic bronchitis, or small airway disease.

Horses are more at risk for COPD if they spend their winters stabled and fed on hay. Small dust and fungal spores, particularly *Micropolyspora faeni* and *Aspergillus fumigatus*, enter the airways when the horse eats, causing irritation to the lungs and inflammation and narrowing of the airways.

Treatment first involves lifestyle changes in order to decrease the animal's exposure to allergens. If this proves ineffective, the animals may need to be given corticosteroids (prednisone, dexamethasone, triamcinolone) to suppress inflammation. Long-term use of corticosteroids can cause problems, particularly heart problems, immune suppression, and decreased ability to heal. The animals can also be given bronchodilators (clenbuterol, pirbuterol, albuterol) to help decrease smooth muscle contraction and reduce mucus production. Although oral administration is the easiest, the most effective treatment is to administer these drugs directly into the airways. This results in minimal systemic side effects, but it requires a special mask.

If the lung is injured by infectious agents, it can produce cytokines and chemokines which come from monocytes, injured epithelial or endothelial cells, or other cells involved in the inflammatory response. These compounds are involved in the inflammatory response.

References

Constantinescu, G.M. 2001. Guide to Regional Ruminant Anatomy Based on the Dissection of the Goat. Iowa State Press, Ames, Iowa.

Constantinescu, G.M. 2002. Clinical Anatomy for Small Animal Practitioners. Iowa State Press, Ames, Iowa.

Constantinescu, G.M. and I.A. Constantinescu. 2004. Clinical Dissection Guide for Large Animals, Horse and Large Ruminants, 2nd edition. Iowa State Press, Ames, Iowa.

Ikegami et al. 1997. Am J Respir Crit. Care Med. 156: 178–184.

Sturkie, P.D. 1986. Avian Physiology, 4th edition. Springer-Verlag, New York.

Swenson, J.J. and W.O. Reece. 1993. Duke's Physiology of Domestic Animals, 11th edition. Cornell University Press, Cornell University, Ithaca, New York.

Whittow, G.C. 2000. Sturkie's Avian Physiology, 5th edition. Academic Press, San Diego, California.

15 Immunity

Contents

Introduction

The capacity of animals to run from or disable potential predators is the essence of survival. Perhaps less apparent is the need to protect cells and tissues from attack by harmful agents—parasites, bacterial pathogens, toxins, or cells that have become cancerous.

Some everyday examples help us understand physiological processes involved in protection of animals from these various agents. Let's suppose that your puppy is playing in the yard and he is splashed by your little brother as your brother rides his bicycle through a puddle of debris from the gutter. Secretions from the puppy's eyes and mucus membranes of his nostrils act to flush material away to prevent the chance of infection. Similarly, his hair covering, eyelashes, and thick skin prevent bacteria and debris from the dirty water from gaining entrance. Even sebaceous secretions of his skin or ear canals can produce conditions that limit the potential growth of harmful bacteria. These are all examples of nonspecific defenses.

Let's suppose that your puppy simultaneously steps on a broken bottle as he runs through the puddle chasing your brother. He manages to soak the cut with dirty bacteria-filled water. However, fortunately for him, he has received a good supply of antibodies from his mother's colostrum. This means that he likely has specific antibodies in his bloodstream from his mother. This allows his fledgling immune system to recognize and ultimately kill bacteria present in the dirty water. This would be an example of specific but passive immunity. As the puppy grows and is exposed to various materials in his environment he will develop his own complement of specific antibodies and the cells necessary to regenerate additional supplies of specific antibodies. Thus, defense mechanisms are divided into nonspecific and specific divisions. The immune system primarily concerns specific protection.

The basis for specific immunity arose from observations in the late 1800s when scientists discovered that animals that had survived a bacterial infection had protective agents in their blood (now known to be immunoglobulins or antibodies) that defended the animals against a subsequent attack by the same pathogen. It was also shown that if antibody-containing serum from the surviving animals was given to animals that had not been exposed to the pathogen, these animals were also protected against attack. It was initially believed that production of antibodies was the only critical requirement for protection. However, in cases where transfer of antibody containing serum failed to provide protection, transfer of the donor's white blood cells often did provide protection. As experiments became more elaborate, it became clear that immunity involved both circulating agents as well as populations of white blood cells or leukocytes. Thus, the two overlapping arms of specific defense are humoral (blood-derived) immunity and cell-mediated immunity (Fig. 15.1).

One of the major types of white blood cells includes the lymphocytes. Furthermore, there are two broad classes of lymphocytes. When they are activated B lymphocytes, usually simply called B cells, they are induced to divide to generate clones of cells. You may have read or heard of polyclonal or monoclonal antibodies being used in scientific experiments or in treatments. Regardless, some of these clonal cells are retained in the body as memory B cells. Other B cells differentiate into plasma cells that synthesize and secrete large quantities of antibodies. The presence of the memory B cells explains the marked increase in antibody concentration (titer) when animals are exposed to the same pathogen or antigen a second time. Essentially, the pieces required for more antibody production are already in place. Cell-mediated immunity depends on T lymphocytes, which include several subclasses of cells (helper T cells, cytotoxic T cells, and suppressor T cells). Other cells critical to functioning of both branches of the immune system include the antigen-presenting cells (fixed and wandering macrophages) and neutrophils.

In reality the actions of the two divisions of the immune system are closely interwoven. But generally, humoral immunity is most effective against bacteria and their toxins or free viruses because antibody binding can directly inactivate these attackers, e.g., cause precipitation, agglutination, or mask surfaces, to make them susceptible to destruction by phagocytic cells or complement activation. Cell-mediated immunity is a better weapon against cellular targets; examples include cells that have been infected by viruses, parasites, or perhaps cancer cells.

In subsequent sections we will consider some of these elements of the immune system in more detail. But let's begin by considering defense attributes of the immune system and physiological systems generally. Defense of the internal environment centers on three main functions (Fig. 15.1):

- Destruction or neutralization of bacterial, viral, or parasitic pathogens
- Destruction of aged or damaged cells, i.e., consider the finite life of red blood cells

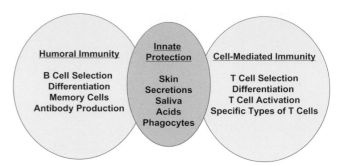

Fig. 15.1. Overview of defense mechanisms. Nonspecific or innate protection provides a first line of defense. The barrier derived from the epidermis of the skin or the stratified squamous epithelium of body openings and their secretions is a first line of protection. General effects of phagocytes, natural killer T cells, and antimicrobial proteins are also important. Humoral immunity involves activation of clones of B lymphocytes to produce memory B cells and daughter B cells that differentiate into plasma cells that synthesize and secrete large amounts of antibodies. Cell-mediated immunity depends on selection of clones of T lymphocytes by the action of antigen-presenting cells, which stimulate proliferation of the T cells. Subtypes of T cells (helper, cytoxic, and suppressor T cells) fine-tune cell-mediated immunity.

- Surveillance to detect and eliminate abnormal cells, cancerous, virally infected, etc.

Innate or nonspecific defenses

As the name suggests, nonspecific defenses do not distinguish one threat from another. The protection that is afforded is the same no matter what the circumstances. These measures include physical barriers, phagocytic cells, complement, general inflammatory response, and fever. The first line of defense against pathogens at first blush seems minor, but in reality the protective properties of the skin and the mucous membranes are substantial. Consider the physical barrier that intact skin provides, but problems that rapidly occur if there are cuts or open wounds. The stratified nature of the skin epithelium, presence of desmosomes to link the cells together, keratinized surface, and secretions of sebaceous and sweat glands are all highly protective. The importance of lanolin on the wool of sheep to provide protection from the elements is another example. Extend this to many animals, and the added physical protection provided by fur, hair, or wool becomes apparent. The acidity of skin secretions (pH 3 to 5) also inhibits bacterial growth. Move to the internal passageways of the respiratory, digestive, and urinary tracts. As you should recall, the more exterior portions of these tracts (oral cavity, esophagus, rectum, etc.) are also covered by stratified squamous epithelial cells. In more internal regions the epithelium is typically thinner and simple, but the cells are linked by tight junctions that increase the barrier function of the epithelium. In addition, specialized glands (goblet cells and various multicellular glands) provide mucus and specific proteins that act to coat and protect the internal surface. Saliva and lacrimal fluids of the eye contain the protein lysozyme and enzymes that can attack bacteria. In mammary secretions produced during the nonlactating or dry period, accumulation of the protein lactoferrin binds iron, which acts to impair growth of bacterial cells. The stomach mucosa with secretion of HCL and peptidases also kills many ingested microorganisms.

As a specific agricultural example, consider the importance of the epithelial layer of the teat end of the dairy cow in protection of the internal mammary gland from mastitis (inflammation of the mammary gland caused by invading microorganisms). The teat of the ruminant has a single opening called the streak canal that leads directly into a space within the teat called the teat cistern (see Chapter 18). This means that the structure of the streak canal is critical as the primary defensive barrier against mastitis. The lowest 2 cm of the streak canal is especially important because of the capacity of tissues in this region to act as a barrier to minimize milk leakage or entrance of environmental agents. Intuitively the diameter of the streak canal is positively related to the rate of milk flow but cows with the best balance of acceptable rates of milk flow and protection from bacterial invasion have the greatest longevity in the herd. Because the teat canal is lined with longitudinal folds, dilation of the streak canal during milk causes the epithelial lining to become flattened and thin during milking. This is analogous to the changes in transitional epithelium in the bladder. Regardless, this periodic stretch allows the keratin to spread over the surface to form a bactericidal barrier. With milking some of the keratin is flushed away during the periodic opening and closing of the teat canal, but fortunately it is constantly being renewed by the epithelium (Capuco et al., 1990). The keratin itself has antibacterial agents that inhibit the growth of pathogens. Some researchers also suggest that the minute areas of secretory tissue in the area of Furstenberg's rosette (near the opening of the teat cistern) secrete protein(s) with bactericidal effects, but others suggest the material is lipidlike and made by the epithelial cells secreting the keratin. Certainly the epithelial cells of the streak canal are constantly being renewed based on the appearance of mitotic cells in the basal layers of the epithelium (stratum germinativum). Passage of cannula through the teat canal or use of teat dilators scrapes away the keratin and can traumatize the epithelium. Experimentally, resistance to mastitis is markedly reduced if the keratin layer is removed. Studies in which pathogens were inoculated 3 mm into the streak canal caused infections in about one-third of treated glands. Inoculations 4 mm into the streak canal increased infection rates further, and inoculations 5 mm into the streak canal nearly always caused infection. This confirms the significance of this barrier function. Since pathogens, which cause mastitis, are not motile, to gain entrance into the parenchymal tissue they must be moved by physical forces from the outside of the teat through the streak canal, teat and gland cistern, and larger ducts to the alveoli. Other than during the period around milking the keratin of the streak canal makes an effective barrier. However, animals with inherently thin keratin or animals with damaged teat areas are susceptible to local colonization with microbes and are therefore at greater risk to infection. During milking itself, retrograde movement of milk due to vacuum fluctuations or vacuum slips with leakage of air around the teat cups, can allow bacteria laden droplets to pass the streak canal.

During machine milking, there are certainly dramatic effects on the teat and teat end. Given the rate of milk flow 7 to 8 m/s, it is reasonable to expect that resulting shear forces might remove some of the protective keratin. It is also probable that some milk constituents are absorbed into the keratin during the time of milking or from milk droplets remaining after milking. If milking removes substantial amounts of the keratin and if renewal is delayed or changes in composition favor the formation of bacterial colonies or adherence, this could have marked effects on the streak canal as the primary defense against mastitis.

Phagocytes are cells that engulf pathogens and cell debris. These include neutrophils and eosinophils that normally circulate in the blood and macrophages that typically reside within tissues. Some of these macrophages are considered fixed because they are permanent residents of a tissue. Examples include the Kupffer cells of the liver or the star-shaped dendritic cells of the skin. Other "free" macrophages are more mobile and can respond to problems throughout the body or act to patrol local tissue areas. An example of the latter is the alveolar macrophages of the lung, which patrol the internal surface of the alveoli. Monocytes in the bloodstream are converted into macrophages when they exit the circulation.

Macrophages (monocytes) and microphages (neutrophils, eosinophils) share the ability to migrate and squeeze between the endothelial cells of capillaries by a process called diapedesis. This process is typically initiated by injury to the endothelial cells and/or appearance of factors that act as attractants for the cells. This is called chemotaxis. The process begins with adhesion followed by the leukocytes forming a sort of pavement of cells lined up along the periphery of the capillary. With increased permeability or damage there is then an often rapid diapedesis of the cells

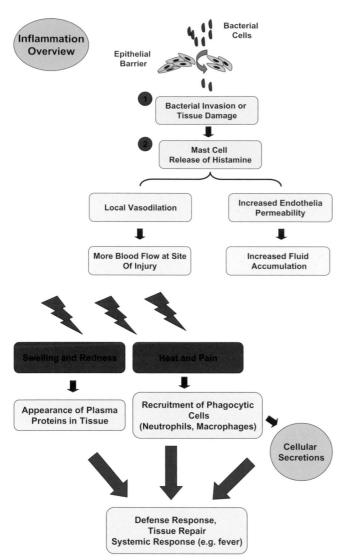

Fig. 15.2. Bacterial attack and inflammation response. Following penetration of the epithelial barrier by bacteria damage to tissues or release of bacterial products, the liberation of histamine, complement, and other molecules initiate a cascade of responses. Increased vasodilation, capillary permeability, and appearance of substances chemotactic to phagocytes produce rapid migration of these cells to the region. The four primary signs of acute inflammation are heat, redness, pain, and swelling.

between the endothelial cells to the region where the bacterial cells or toxins are located. Figure 15.2 illustrates general events that occur with an inflammatory response. Many of these effects are mediated by the release of chemical compounds produced by injured cells, proteins that appear in exudates from the circulation, and molecules released by stimulated platelets and phagocytes. The local response to infection is called inflammation, but depending on the particular circumstances, the physiological response can become more widespread. Fever, body temperature that is higher than normal, occurs in response to some micro-

organisms. For example, in dairy cattle, mastitis caused by Staph aureus species is typically localized, but mastitis caused by E. coli is characteristically associated with marked systemic effects well beyond appearance of abnormal milk, heat, and redness of the udder. Fever, lethargy, absence of appetite, and markedly reduced milk production are common. Neither is it uncommon for systemic problems to become so severe that physiological systems can fail and death occurs. With marked activation of leukocytes exposed to especially potent pathogens, pyrogens secreted by the leukocytes and toxins from the microorganisms act to reset the hypothalamic neurons responsible for homeostatic control of body temperature. Prolonged high fevers are dangerous because excess heat denatures enzymes. However, milder fever is beneficial because metabolic rates of tissues are increased, allowing for more rapid repair and healing.

When infection is severe, responses can be dramatic. The creamy or yellowish pus that fills infected tissue areas is a mixture of dead cells and tissue debris, as well as dead or dying microorganisms. If repair mechanisms do not clear the area of debris, these materials can become walled off by layers of collagen fibers and other extracellular matrix proteins, essentially scar tissue. This is a protective mechanism, e.g., isolation of the affected area, but this can also lead to creation of an abscess. In these cases it is often necessary to surgically drain the material before healing can take place. In some particularly difficult infections bacterial cells can be engulfed by macrophages but not destroyed. The macrophages with their now protected residents become encased in clusters or granulomas. Since the bacteria are not actually destroyed, if the granulomas are disrupted an active infection can resurface. This explains why the tuberculosis bacilli, which are resistant to digestion by macrophages and therefore protected from antibiotic treatment, can be so difficult to treat. It is believed that some mastitis-causing organisms behave in an analogous manner. Specifically, some organisms appear to find "protected" areas (likely walled off by connective tissue elements) so that they are safe from destruction. This could explain why some cases of mastitis are caused by the same organism repeatedly and/or some subclinical cases of mastitis.

Some of the important substances involved in inflammation and their effects are summarized in Table 15.1. Before we move to specific immunity, let's consider some of the effects of these molecules and related molecules involved in inflammation and chemical defenses. Some tissue proteins can inhibit or slow bacterial cell growth. For example, lactoferrin is a protein that is produced in secretions of the nonlactating mammary gland where it accumulates to a high concentration. This is important because it acts to bind

Table 15.1. Chemicals involved in inflammation.

Agent	Source	Reaction
Histamine	Basophils and mast cells; released after injury, in presence of microorganisms or secretions from neutrophils	Vasodilation of arterioles and better permeability of capillaries and formation of exudates
Prostaglandins	Fatty acid derived from arachidonic acid present in cell membranes of neutrophils, platelets, and other cells	Stimulate endothelial cells and leukocytes to secrete other inflammatory mediators
Kinins	Plasma kininogen appearing in interstitial fluid is cleaved by the enzyme kallikrein to produce active peptides	Effects similar to histamine but also induce chemotaxis of leukocytes and their activation
Complement	System of ~20 plasma proteins	When activated, provides a mechanism to inactivate bacteria (membrane attack complex) and target foreign debris for removal by phagocytes
Cytokines	Circulation, lymphocytes, macrophages, and other immune cells as well as fibroblasts	Examples include α, β, and γ interferons, at least 13 interleukins (IL- to IL-13), transforming growth factor β, macrophage, and others; all act to regulate immune function, inflammatory reactions, or healing

iron that is needed for bacterial cell growth. Histamine released by local mast cells at the site of an attack increases capillary permeability as well as vasodilation so that blood flow is increased. Mast cells also produce chemotaxins, which act as signals to induce the migration of phagocytic cells. Moreover, the binding of chemotaxins to receptors on the cell surface of macrophages increases Ca^{++} flow into the cells. The increase in Ca^{++} activates contractile elements in the cells that allow amoebalike movement of the cells along the gradient of chemotactic signals. In several instances, cascades of events enhance the inflammatory responses. As illustrated in Figure 15.3, kallikrein secreted from phagocytes cleaves inactive kinogens produced by the liver. These molecules appear in circulation and diffuse into inflamed areas because of increased vasodilation where they are converted into active kinins. Kinins subsequently stimulate several steps in complement activation, reinforce vascular bed changes initiated by histamine release, activate pain receptors, and serve as chemotaxins to produce even more leukocyte migration and more kinin production in a positive-feedback pattern of action. This enhances the opportunity to defeat the offending agent. The inflammatory reactions can be likened to an alarm response as a large mixture of chemicals is released into the extracellular fluids.

Macrophages are especially important because these cells (along with certain epithelial cells in mucosal membranes) express proteins on their surface called toll-like receptors (TLRs). To the present time more than 10 types of TLR have been identified. Each of the receptors recognizes a particular class of microbe based on the components of the bacterial cell wall.

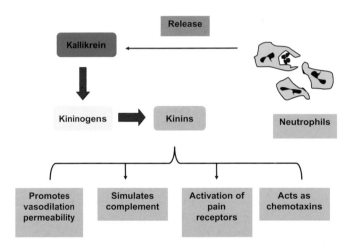

Fig. 15.3. Role of kallikrein in inflammation. Activated neutrophils release kallikrein, which acts enzymatically on kininogens to produce kinins. These kinins promote multiple reactions that ultimately aid the body to fight inflammation.

Activation of the TLR triggers the release of cytokines. Cytokine is a general term given to the many chemical messengers that regulate cells involved in immune responses. To give an idea of the complexity, more than 100 molecules (mostly proteins) have been classified as cytokines.

Most cytokines are of low molecular weight, soluble proteins produced following activation of a "sensing," cell, e.g., the macrophages with activated TLR described above. Cytokines are produced by nearly all cells involved in immunity, but the T cells are especially important. The activation of cytokine-producing cells triggers them to synthesize and secrete their particular class of cytokines. The cytokines then bind to specific cytokine receptors on other cells of the immune system and influence their activity in some manner. Actions of cytokines are described as multifaceted, redundant, and pleiotropic. The idea is that a specific cytokine is likely to impact multiple target cells, not just one type of cell. In addition, some cytokines are antagonistic so that one cytokine stimulates a particular action while another cytokine inhibits the same function. In other cases, cytokines act synergistically to produce a greater effect than either would have alone. These features mean that there are enormous opportunities for control and regulation of immune responses. Most of the cytokines act on leukocytes or the endothelial cells to affect inflammatory responses, but there are also overlaps between classic hormones and cytokine signaling pathways. For example, leukocytes and macrophages express prolactin receptors. It seems likely that in addition to its well-characterized actions in mammary development and reproduction, prolactin also acts as a cytokine in the immune system. Some features of a few selected cytokines are described below.

Tumor necrosis factor α (TNF-α) is the major cytokine involved in acute inflammation. It is primarily synthesized by monocytes, macrophages, and helper T cells. When produced in very large amounts it is believed to be the cause of systemic shock in severe reactions. It acts on the endothelial cells to stimulate inflammation and blood clotting. It also promotes endothelial cells to secrete selectins (adhesion molecules) that are important for diapedesis of leukocytes. Furthermore it triggers macrophages and endothelial cells to secrete chemokines. Chemokines also impact diapedesis, chemotaxis and additionally promote macrophages to secrete interleukins (see below). Finally, TNF-α is directly cytotoxic for some tumor cells, thus explaining its name.

The interleukins include a very large family of structurally similar cytokines. Interleukin 1 (IL-1) is especially significant. It has actions functionally similar to TNF-α (an example of some of the redundancy among cytokines). Common effects include induction of fever and sleep and stimulation of collagen synthesis as well as collagenase needed for tissue repair and remodeling. It also stimulates T and B lymphocytes to proliferate. IL-1 is also produced by monocytes, macrophages, dendritic cells, and a variety of other cells in the body.

Other interleukins include IL-2 that is secreted primarily by helper T cells to stimulate the proliferation of helper T cells and activate the natural killer T cells. It is also called T cell growth factor. IL-3 promotes hemopoiesis to generate precursors of lymphocytes and mast cells. IL-4, also produced by the helper T cells stimulates B cells and enhances antibody secretion by active plasma cells, especially secretion of IgE.

IL-5 behaves in a similar fashion but is more likely to promote plasma cells to secrete IgA type antibodies. It also acts as a chemoattractant for eosinophils. IL-6 has wide-ranging effects including promotion of differentiation of B cells into plasma cells and stimulation of the liver to secrete a mannose binding protein, which triggers complement protein binding to the surface of microorganisms that have mannose containing polysaccharides in their cell walls. IL-8 promotes angiogenesis, an action that is clearly important in repair of tissue damage. IL-10 acts to dampen or turn down immune responses, so it is important in overall regulation of immune function.

Transforming growth factor β (TGF-β) is also a suppressor of immune responses by its capacity to inhibit the proliferation and function of T cells and proliferation of B cells. Along with the other cytokines released, TGF-β is an important participant because of its role in several stages of wound healing. Vascular endothelial cells are early responders. There is enhanced secretion of adhesion molecules (VCAM-1, ELAM-1, ICAM-1) in the area of the endothelial cells, which gives a foundation for the anchoring of circulating leukocytes that express receptors (integrins, selectins, etc.) to recognize these adhesion factors and allow accumulation of the leukocytes, chemotactic attraction, and diapedesis. Indeed, TGF-β is a potent chemoattractant in its own right. Because of its effects on secretion of extracellular matrix proteins by stromal cells, (fibroblasts) it also promotes tissue repair. TGF-β is produced by T lymphocytes, macrophages, and other stromal tissue cells and appears in circulation in a latent form that is activated by tissue proteases.

The colony stimulating factors (CSF) are an additional group of proteins that impact immune function by their ability to induce production of colonies of the different leukocyte types in the bone marrow. Some specific CSF members include granulocyte macrophage colony stimulating factor (GM-CSF), granulocyte colony stimulating factor (G-CSF), and macrophage colony stimulating factor (M-CSF). Aside from effects on proliferation the CSFs also influence leukocyte function. For example, when GM-CSF binds to receptors on neutrophils, eosinophils, or monocytes, it activates the cells and also enhances survival of the cells. GM-CSF increases the capacity of these phagocytes to form pavements involved in diapedesis between endothelial cells and improves the ability of the cells to destroy engulfed bacterial cells. CSFs are produced mostly by T cells and macrophages.

A final group of cytokines to introduce are the interferons. As the name suggests these molecules were characterized by having an ability to interfere with something. In this case, it is the replication of viruses. As with other cytokines, there are multiple types of

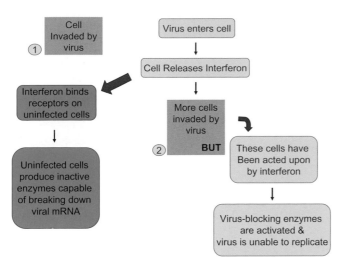

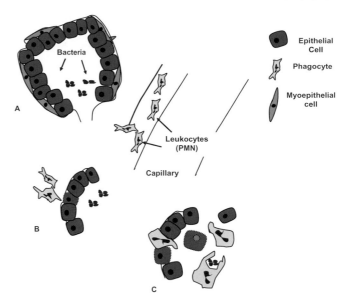

Fig. 15.4. Action of interferon. In step 1 a cell is invaded by a virus. In response, the infected cell produces and secretes interferon. The interferon binds to receptors on neighboring cells and induces the cells to produce inactive enzymes capable of breaking down viral mRNA. In step 2, a cell previously impacted by interferon is subsequently invaded by the virus. The virus-blocking enzymes are activated and viral replication in this cell is prevented.

Fig. 15.5. Leukocyte (PMN) response in the mammary gland. Chemotaxis causes PMNs to migrate from the capillaries and form a pavement along the basement membrane of the infected alveoli (A). Some groups of epithelial cells become damaged by the toxins or PMN activity and are sloughed into the alveolar spaces (damaged cells indicated by the broken cell membranes). Neutrophils and macrophages accumulate (B) where they engulf bacterial cells (C) and destroy them along with cell debris (Nickerson and Heald, 1981; Capuco et al., 1986).

interferons (α, β, and γ). In short, as illustrated in Figure 15.4, interferon provides some resistance to viral infections by interfering with the replication of the virus in neighboring potential host cells. In addition, interferon(s) enhance the phagocytic activity of macrophages and stimulate the secretion of antibodies by plasma cells. Furthermore, these molecules markedly improve the function of natural killer and cytotoxic T cells, which are important in the destruction of virus-infected and cancerous cells.

Figure 15.5 provides on overview of an essential aspect of inflammation, the migration of phagocytes to the affected area. In this example, the rapid response of neutrophils, sometimes called polymorphonuclear leukocytes (PMN, the lobed nucleus of these cells) into the mammary gland following an experimental insult, i.e., intramammary infusion of endotoxin is shown. Since the site of the inflammation is deep within the areas of the mammary gland that store milk, the phagocytes must move out of the capillaries (between the endothelial cells) but additionally pass the basement membrane and between the epithelial cells that compose the outer structure of the mammary alveoli. In these cases the phagocytes have responded to chemoattractant agents in milk that have diffused into surrounding interstitial fluids and local capillary beds.

As an example, the somatic cell count of raw milk is the most common dairy producer–related method to evaluate milk quality and udder health status of individual lactating cows. Leukocytes and a small percent-

age of epithelial cells normally occur in milk. This combination of cells is referred to as the milk somatic cell count (MSCC). The term *somatic*, which means body, alludes to the fact that these are normal body-derived cells. Most (~98%) of the cells are leukocytes and most of these are PMN. Milk from uninfected cows typically contains less than 200,000 cells per ml and it is not uncommon to find uninfected cows with MSCC of 50,000 cells or less. Milk samples with values greater than 400,000 cells per ml are likely from cows with inflammation, most likely caused by mastitis-producing organisms. These leukocytes enter the milk as a consequence of homing to the mammary gland from the bloodstream in response to chemicals released directly by bacterial cells or materials released by injured mammary cells. These chemicals induce chemotaxis, which initially recruits neutrophils, and thereafter macrophages (monocytes), into the udder. Since an increase in MSCC is closely correlated with intramammary infection, the MSCC is measured for milk samples collected as a part of routine monitoring of milk composition in many dairy herds. However, it is important to remember that, strictly speaking, bacteria-induced mastitis can be confirmed only by the isolation of pathogenic organisms in aseptically collected milk samples by approved bacteriological methods. Figure 15.6 shows the marked ability of PMN to

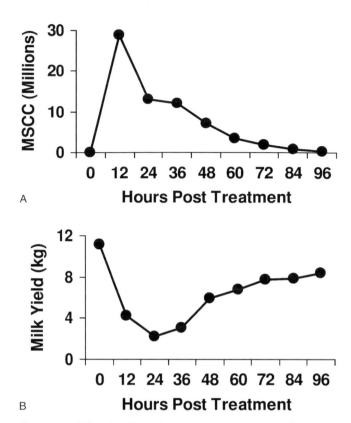

A

B

Fig. 15.6. Cell and milk production responses in cows. Changes in MSCC (Panel A) and milk production (Panel B) in cows given an intramammary infusion of bacterial endotoxin are shown. Note the marked increase and corresponding decrease in mammary function. Adapted from McFadden et al., 1988.

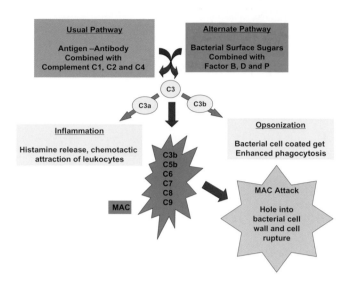

Fig. 15.7. Complement activation. In the classic activation pathway the binding of antibody to bacterial antigens induces complex formation with complement proteins C1, C2 and C4. Alternatively, plasma proteins (factors B, D, and P) can bind with surface polysaccharides in the cell wall of some bacteria and fungi. Regardless of the pathway, both converge with the activation of complement protein C3. This activation produces a cleavage reaction to yield C3a and C3b. When C3b binds to the bacterial cell surface, it initiates the recruitment of complement proteins C5b, C6, C7, C8, and C9 to produce the membrane attack complex (MAC). This complex penetrates the cell wall to create a hole or pore that leads to cell lysis. In addition, binding of C3b induces opsonization or coating of the bacterial cell, which enhances targeting by phagocytes for engulfment. Finally, presence of free C3a and C5a in the area promotes inflammation.

respond to an intramammary signal. In this case the mammary gland of the cow was infused with purified endotoxin diluted in sterile physiological saline. By the time of the next milking the MSCC has increased ~thirtyfold and there was a corresponding sharp decrease in milk production. However, after several days the cell response and milk production returned to normal. This is an experimental situation but it certainly demonstrates the dramatic response that phagocytic cells can make in response to stimulation.

Fortunately, most tissue regions have macrophages that are residents. For example, with a skin break these resident macrophages can begin phagocytizing microorganisms (assuming they are recognized as invaders) almost immediately. However, the number of cells is limited so that a full-blown response depends on chemotaxis to recruit additional phagocytes (more macrophages and neutrophils). It is important, of course, that these cells express the ability to recognize foreign material so that normal cells are not harmed. The tagging of materials to be engulfed is complex but when it comes to bacterial cells, the complement system is especially important. This is because the effects of activated complement can be very potent; second, presence of specific antibodies on the surface

of the bacterial cells (or other materials) acts to mark these invaders for destruction by phagocytes as well as attack by complement proteins.

The complement system, usually simply called "complement," is a complex of at least 20 proteins present in the circulation (originally produced by the liver). These proteins provide an important mechanism for the destruction of foreign substances because, when activated, they greatly enhance the inflammatory response; even more impressive, they can stimulate the direct destruction of bacteria and some other cells by causing the cells to rupture. Aside from direct effects on bacterial cells, activated complement also enhances inflammation in several ways.

- Stimulates release of histamine from mast cells
- Promotes vasodilation and thereby increased vascular permeability
- Activates kinins
- Coats the surface of microorganisms and act as opsonining agents

Thus, although complement is really nonspecific, it clearly enhances or "complements" the immune response. The effects of complement on bacterial cells are illustrated in Figure 15.7.

Specific immunity

Despite the impressive benefits of nonspecific defenses, this alone is not sufficient. Hallmarks of both cellular and humoral immunity include 1) specificity, 2) systemic rather than local responses, and 3) evidence of memory. Specificity indicates that the immune response is directed at a unique antigen. Systemic responsiveness refers to the notion that a response to attack can be mounted regardless of the point of entry. Memory indicates that the immune system is better prepared with a faster response when exposure to an antigen occurs a second time. This is the idea behind vaccinations. A vaccination is essentially the induction of a specific immune response and creation of immunological memory as a result of a planned exposure to the antigen in a manner that does not cause illness. For example, immunization with cell wall components or killed bacterial cells (incapable of causing disease) can nonetheless induce an immune response because of the foreign proteins or polysaccharides present in these preparations. If the animal is then exposed to live microorganisms, the animal can respond more quickly so that the chance of exhibiting the disease reduces or symptoms are milder and less severe compared with nonimmunized animals.

Let's first consider humoral or antibody-mediated immunity. However, it is worth remembering that the two divisions of the immune system (humoral and cell-mediated) do not function independently but rather together to enhance protection. As Figure 15.8 shows, it is also important to realize that immunity can be either passive or active. Clearly, the protection provided to the newborn calf (or puppy in our earlier example) by suckling colostrum from its mother is critical, but it is limited. The antibodies provided in the colostrum are only a stop gap measure until the calf or puppy is able to begin mounting its own immune responses with related immunological memory.

Antibody structure and function

There are five major classes of immunoglobulins: IgA, IgG, IgM, IgD, and IgE. IgG is the most abundant and diverse antibody in circulation. It accounts for ~80% of the total. It is primarily responsible for both primary and secondary antibody responses (increased blood titers) following immunization or other exposure to antigens. IgG also circulates as a monomer. IgA also appears as a monomer but is limited in the circulation. It occurs more frequently in secretions (saliva, sweat, intestine, etc.) associated with mucous membranes and epithelial surfaces. It also is most frequently secreted as a dimer with the two antibody molecules

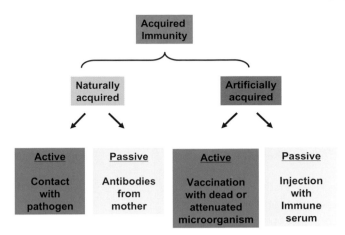

Fig. 15.8.   Types of acquired immunity. Both naturally and artificially acquired immunity can be very important, but only active immunity can establish immunological memory. Once antibodies from the mother or via injection are degraded, they can not be replaced by the animal.

joined by a third element called the secretory piece. IgM appears as a monomer and in groupings of five antibodies (pentamer) linked together. In the monomer form, the antibody is usually attached to the surface of B cells. During primary antibody responses the pentamer form of IgM is the first class of antibody released by the plasma cells. Since there is usually only a small amount of IgM free in the circulation, detection of an increase in the blood is diagnostically useful as an indicator of a current infection in an animal. IgD is nearly always attached to the surface of B cells where it functions as a receptor for the activation of the cells. IgE is secreted by plasma cells in the skin and mucosal membranes. When the IgE is bound to antigen, the stem region of the molecule reacts with mast cells and basophiles causing them to release histamine and other chemicals. Unfortunately, hyper- or inappropriate IgE-induced activation of these cells is involved in many allergic reactions. This explains the significance of antihistamine treatments to treat allergic reactions.

Whatever its specific class, each antibody molecule has a basic structure consisting of four protein chains linked by disulfide bonds. Two identical heavy chains of about 400 amino acids each make up the bulk of a structure that resembles the shape of the letter Y. Two additional identical protein chains (the light chains) essentially overlap the portions of the heavy chains in the arms of the Y and are joined by sulfide bonds. The heavy chains have a hingelike region near the top of the stem of the Y. The two ends at the top of the letter Y of the antibody molecule create the sites for binding of the antibody to its antigen. This means that the antibody is divalent; that is, one antibody molecule is

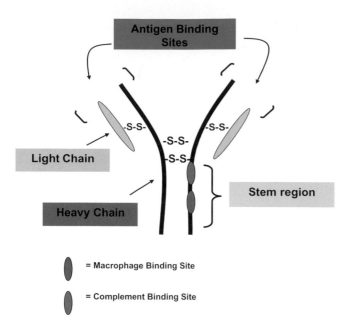

Fig. 15.9. Basic antibody structure. An antibody molecule consists of four protein chains, two heavy chains and two light chains. The portion of the heavy chain resembling the stem of the letter Y provides sites of activation of complement and interactions with macrophages. The combination of light and heavy chains at the ends of the arms of the Y creates two identical antigen-binding sites. Disulfide bonds are prominent in linking heavy and light chains together as well as at locations within the chains.

capable of binding two antigen molecules. The stem region of the molecule is significant because it contains sites for complement binding and for macrophage activation. These sites are important because the binding or fixing of the antibody allows the development of a cascade of reactions important in the immune attack. The structure of an antibody molecule is illustrated in Figure 15.9.

Although antibodies do not directly destroy pathogens, their binding to antigens on the surface of bacterial cells, for example, marks the cells for destruction. Antibody binding to toxins or foreign debris can also inactivate these agents by neutralization, precipitation, or, in the case of cell-associated antigens, agglutination. These reactions greatly enhance inflammation, and along with inflammation-induced chemotaxis recruits leukocytes that destroy bacterial cells by phagocytosis. Antibody binding also triggers complement fixation and exposes the macrophage-binding sites on the antibody molecule. The coating of foreign substances with antibodies is called opsonization.

Antigens are substances that can activate the immune system, thereby provoking an immune response. Most often these are large, complex molecules (typically proteins) that do not normally appear in the body. In other words, the immune system does

not recognize them as self. In the case of completely reactive or immunogenic antigens these molecules induce proliferation of specific lymphocytes and the synthesis and secretion of specific antibodies. In other cases many small peptides, nucleotides, are not immunogenic in themselves but when linked with other self proteins, the new combinations can produce a dramatic, even harmful, response. This is the basis of some allergenic responses. Researchers were able to take advantage of this property to create antibodies against normally nonresponsive molecules, i.e., steroid hormones to create many immunological-based assays, e.g., radioimmunoassay, enzyme-linked immunoassays (ELISA), and western blotting.

B cell selection and antibody secretion

When B cells are stimulated by antigens, a cascade is initiated so that antigen binding to surface receptors on a particular (naive or previously inactivated B cell) becomes activated to complete its differentiation cycle. This activation process, usually in combination with T cells, triggers clonal selection and expansion. The initial step induces B cell growth followed by rapid proliferation of an army or clone of identical daughter cells, all of which express receptors specific for the antigen that initiated the process. Since all of the cells are identical they form a group called a clone. In cases where a particular antigen leads to the production of a single clone of cells this would be called a monoclonal response. This situation is taken advantage of experimentally to produce highly specific monoclonal antibodies. More often in physiological situations several different families or clones of stimulated B cells are generated. Since each of the antibodies that are produced is likely to recognize different epitopes of the same antigen, these antibodies are referred to as polyclonal antibodies.

Most of the stimulated B cells are induced to become plasma cells. This is fortuitous because plasma cells have an extensive array of RER. Thus, the capacity of these plasma cells to synthesize and secrete antibody molecules (proteins) is very high. This is illustrated in Figure 15.10.

It is estimated that each plasma cell can secrete more than 2,000 antibody molecules per second. These antibodies have the same antigen-binding capacity as the receptor proteins on the surface of the B cells that first bound the antigen. Clonal B cells that are not activated to become plasma cells become long-lived memory cells. It is the presence of the memory B cells that explains the very rapid and sustained secretion of antibody that occurs when an animal is exposed to an antigen for a second time. This pattern of response is illustrated in Figure 15.11.

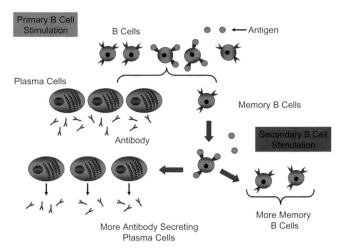

Fig. 15.10. Antigen stimulation of B cells. In the primary stimulation, antigen (green spheres) binds to receptors on the surface of selected B cells. This induces cell proliferation and production of clones of identical cells. Some of the cells enlarge into B lymphoblasts and then plasma cells that secrete antibodies specific to the antigen. Other clonal B cells remain as memory B cells. With a subsequent exposure to the antigen (weeks, months, or even years later), a second more rapid induction and secretion of antibody and generation of additional memory B cells occurs.

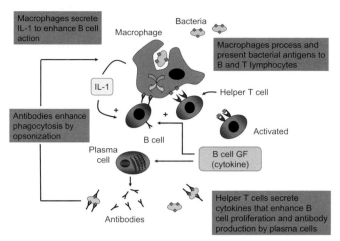

Fig. 15.12. Antigen process in macrophages. Bacterial cells are engulfed by macrophages and antigens are processed and expressed on the surface of the macrophage. Helper T cells associate with the macrophage and bind fragments of bacterial cell proteins "presented" by the macrophage. This activates the helper T cell so that it is stimulated to secrete cytokines, which stimulate proliferation of B cells and conversion into plasma cells that secrete antibodies specific to the bacterial antigen.

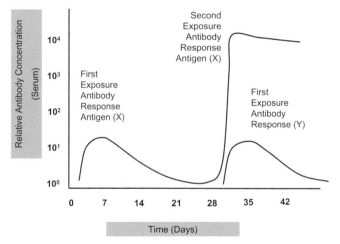

Fig. 15.11. Primary and secondary antibody responses. The blue line illustrates the relative antibody secretion response to immunization with antigen X. The initial response begins after several days, peaks at a relatively low level and declines markedly by 4 weeks. A second exposure to antigen X at this time elicits a rapid and relatively much greater response. Exposure to a second antigen Y at the same time has no effect on the response to antigen X, and the relative response to antigen Y is similar to the initial reaction noted to immunization with antigen X.

Cell-mediated immunity

Antibodies are extremely important, but it is also clear that effectiveness depends on the capacity of the antibodies to recognize specific pathogens. How are our

animals protected against viruses or infections from microorganisms that can "hide" from detection by antibodies? The T cells provide this added, more complex layer of protection. Two primary groups of T cells have been recognized based on the complexes of glycoproteins that are expressed on their cell surfaces. These are CD4 cells, also known as helper T cells (T_H), and a larger population, the CD8 cells that are mostly cytotoxic T cells (T_C). Some of the CD8-expressing T cells are also Suppressor (T_S) cells that act as modulators of cell-mediated immunity.

Although B cells and antibodies bind to and respond directly to antigens, T cells do not have this ability. Instead, the T cells can recognize and respond to pieces or fragments of protein antigens that have been processed by other cells of the immune system, the antigen-presenting cells (macrophages, neutrophils, dendritic cells of the skin, etc.). This process is illustrated in Figure 15.12.

Cytotoxic T cells (T_C), also called killer T cells, have the ability to attack and kill other cells directly. When activated, these cells migrate through the circulation and the lymphoid tissues seeking cells that express antigens for which the T_C cells have been sensitized. The primary targets of the cells are other cells that have been infected by viruses, but under some circumstances they can attack cells that are infected by bacteria or parasites. They can also act on cancer cells and are the primary cells involved in transplant rejection reactions.

Before the cells can respond, the T_C cells have to link or dock with potential targets by binding to the self-nonself complex on the cell surface. Briefly, the surface of all cells expresses a myriad of proteins. However, if the immune system has been appropriately programmed all of these self-antigens are not recognized as foreign by the particular animal but are strongly antigenic to other animals. This is the essence of blood transfusion or graft rejection between unrelated animals. Some of the major surface proteins are part of a group of glycoproteins called major histocompatibility complex or MCH proteins that are coded by MHC genes. Because there are virtually millions of possible combinations for the complex of genes that code for these proteins, except for identical twins, it is very unlikely that two animals would have expression patterns that would be the same. It is even more complex in that there are two major clusters of MHC proteins and genes. Class I MHC proteins are expressed on surfaces of essentially all cells, but class II MHC proteins appear only on certain cells of the immune system. Each MHC protein has a cleft or groove that displays a peptide. In normal cells the peptides that are displayed in this cleft are peptides that are derived from normal recycling of cellular proteins. When some cells become infected or are altered by cancer the MHC proteins can bind and display peptides derived from bacterial cells, viruses, or cancer-mediated processes. This then acts to mark the infected or cancerous cell as nonself thereby targeting it for close surveillance and possible attack by the T_C cells.

Essentially, the CD8 class of lymphocytes or T_C cells is activated when they dock with other cells that have processed antigens in combination with the class I MHC proteins that are not recognized as self. The example shown in Figure 15.13 illustrates the activation of T_C cells that have encountered a virus-infected cell and, as a consequence, a clone of activated T_C cells is produced. These cells can then detect and bind to other infected cells. The fundamental result is that this encounter induces the T_C cell to divide and produce clones of identical cells. Some of these new cytotoxic T cells become memory T cells; others are activated to seek out cells that exhibit the antigen/MHC on the cell surface that initiated the process in the beginning.

The actual mechanism for the T_C destruction of the "foreign" cell is complex and poorly understood, but several events occur at least in some cases. When binding between the cells occurs, the T_C cell releases granules that contain a protein called perforin, which inserts itself into the plasma membrane of the cell targeted for destruction. Especially in the presence of Ca^{++} the perforin molecules combine to create pores through the plasma membrane. This allows entrance

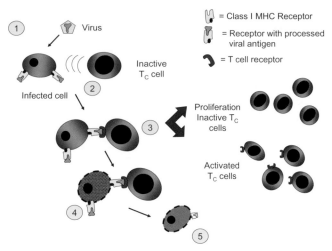

Fig. 15.13. Cytotoxic and helper T cells activation. Both T_C and T_H cells are stimulated to proliferate and produce clones when they associate with foreign antigens (1) that are in complexes with MHC proteins on cell surfaces. In this example, a competent T_C cell docks with a cell expressing a foreign viral antigen in combination with the cell's MHC proteins (2). Activation (3) induces proliferation leading to formation of more T_C cells (memory) as well as currently activated cells. When the activated T_C cells complexes with an infected cell (4), the infected cell is ultimately (5) destroyed. Activation of T_H cells would occur in a similar fashion except the complex would involve class II MHC proteins rather than class I MHC proteins.

of inactivated enzymes called granzymes, also contained in the vesicles released from the T cell, to enter the cytoplasm of the targeted cell. Once inside the target cell, like a miniature Trojan horse, the proteases are activated and the cellular machinery begins to degrade. In other cases, the T_C cells can produce the death of targeted cells by secretion of lymphotoxin, a protein that causes the fragmentation of the target cell's DNA. Other T_C cells release γ interferon, which activates macrophages in the area to killer status so that the death of the targeted cells is indirect. This is analogous to hiring a hit man to do the deed. Details of T_C attack are illustrated in Figure 15.14.

A final type of T cell to consider is the suppressor (T_S) cell. As the name suggests, these cells act to dampen the aggressive action of the T_C cells once the inflammation has subsided. In addition, it is believed that the T_S cells are important in minimizing autoimmune reactions, i.e., situations where the immune system can attack normal healthy cells. However, suppression does not occur immediately. In part this is because most of the activation that initiates the T cells to respond in the beginning increases the number of T_C and T_H cells to a much greater extent than for T_S cells. Table 15.2 summarizes the immune cells that participate in defense of tissues and cells.

Table 15.2. Immune cells involved in defense of tissues and cells.

Mast cells and basophils	Stimulate and coordinate inflammation by release of histamine, prostaglandins, and other cytokines
Neutrophils (PMN)	Aside from resident macrophages, these are the first of the phagocytes to arrive at a site of infection
Eosinophils	Important in phagocytosis of antigen-antibody complexes and in allergic responses
Macrophages	Both fixed and wandering essential active phagocytes
B-cells	Class of lymphocytes that, in response to antigen binding and interactions with helper T cells, proliferate to create clones of memory B cells as well as cells that differentiate into plasma cells
Plasma cells	Produce high levels of antibodies with specificity to the antigen responsible for initial stimulation; the cells are a further differentiation of B cells
Helper T cells (T_H)	Regulatory T cells that interact with antigen presented by APC stimulate the production of other cells (cytotoxic T cells and B cells)
Cytotoxic T cells (T_C)	Also referred to as cytolytic or killer T cells and are also activated by antigen presented by body cells; also recruited by helper T cells and are especially important in killing virus-infected cells and cancer cells
Suppressor T cells (T_S)	Inhibit the activity of B and T cells especially in later stages of infection
Memory cells	Daughter cells from previously activated B or T cells; *memory* refers to their capacity for rapid activation when exposed to the same antigen for a second time
Antigen-presenting cells (APC)	One of several cell types (macrophages, dendritic cells, activated B cells) that engulf antigen and then present the antigen or parts on their cell surfaces in combination with MCH proteins; this allows recognition by T cells, which express complementary receptors for the antigen; antigen presentation is very important

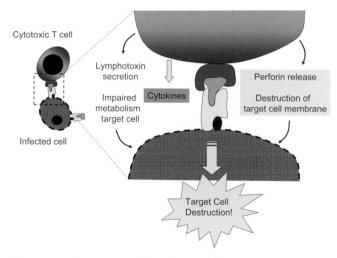

Fig. 15.14. Cytotoxic T cell attack. Once the T_C cell has encountered and responded to an infected cell, several different mechanisms can be induced to produce destruction of the target cell. Release of lymphotoxin can essentially poison the cell by disrupting its metabolism. Release of perforin can act to perforate and disrupt the plasma membrane of the cells. Granzymes released by T cell vesicles (granules) can degrade target cell proteins. Finally, some cytokines released act to promote apoptosis (programmed cell death in the target cell.

Avian versus mammalian systems

At a global level many aspects of immunology are similar between species—for example, the presence of humoral versus cellular immunity, significance of cir-

culating antibodies, impact of inflammation, and role of cell signaling in maturation of various classes of leukocytes. However, understanding of immune responses in avian species, especially chickens, is especially significant scientifically. In 1956, Glick et al. reported that the chicken bursa Fabricius (BF) was essential for development of humoral immunity. Bursectomized chickens had no antibody production responses when challenged.

The BF is an envagination of a portion of the cloaca. It contains 10 to 15 folds surrounding a lumen with tissue containing approximately 10,000 follicular structures. These follicles develop in part from stem cells that migrate from the yolk sac and embryonic liver to the BF. As development progresses, BF structures change from small buds to colonies of clonal B cells that proliferate and move to the outer regions of the BF. Complex gene rearrangements and gene conversion events ultimately create populations of potential B cells. Complicated regulation associated with cytokines specific to the bursa and cell interactions leave only about 5% of these cells to become fully functional B cells that are active in humoral immunity (Scott, 2004). Thus the identification of these cells as B lymphocytes reflects the fact that in birds these cells develop in the BF. It also distinguishes these lymphocytes from T cells, which are thymus-derived. Mammals do not have a structure equivalent to the BF. Consequently, the bone marrow serves as a site for B cell maturation.

As you might guess, B cell development occurs in progressive steps, but based primarily on mouse models, each stage depends on dramatic gene alterations. As discussed earlier, the antibody molecule is composed of two light (L) and two heavy (H) chains. Moreover, the genes directing the synthesis of these proteins are found in corresponding L and H chain loci. An H chain locus has three regions—V, D, and J—that recombine randomly as the cells mature. This creates unique variable domains in the immunoglobulin that can be made by each individual B cell. Similar rearrangements occur for L chain locus but there are just two regions (V and J). The following list briefly describes events during sequential developmental stages of B cell maturation:

1. Progenitor B cells start with germ cell H and L genes.
2. Early Pro-B cells activate D and J genes to rearrange H chains.
3. Late Pro-B cells begin V-DJ rearrangement of V, D, J on the H chains.
4. Large Pre-B cells evolve as the H chain is VDJ-rearranged, Germline L genes.
5. Small Pre-B cells undergo V-J rearrangement on the L chains.
6. In immature B cells the VJ are rearranged on L chains and the VDJ rearranged on H chains. This induces expression of IgM receptors.
7. Mature B cells begin to produce IgD.

If the B cell fails in any step of the maturation process, apoptosis leads to the death of the cell. Moreover, if the cell recognizes a self-antigen during the maturation process, the cell either become arrested or undergoes apoptosis. This probably explains why only a small percentage of precursor B cells survive to become part of the peripheral B cell pool.

References

Capuco, A., M.J. Paape, and S.C. Nickerson. 1986. In vitro study of polymorphonuclear leukocyte damage to mammary tissue of lactating cows. Am. J. Vet. Res. 47: 663–668.

Capuco, A.V., D.L. Wood, S.A. Bright, R.H. Miller, and J. Bitman. 1990. Regeneration of teat canal keratin in lactating dairy cows. J. Dairy Sci. 73: 1745–1750.

Glick, B., T.S. Chang, and R.G. Japp. 1956. The bursa of Fabricius and antibody production in the domestic fowl. Poultry Sci. 35: 224–225.

McFadden, T.B., R.M. Akers, and A.V. Capuco. 1988. Relationships of milk proteins in blood with somatic cell counts in milk of dairy cows. J. Dairy Sci. 71: 826–834.

Nickerson, S.C. and C.W. Heald. 1981. Histopathologic response of the bovine mammary gland to experimentally induced Staphylococcus aureus infection. Am. J. Vet. Res. 44: 1351–1555.

Nickerson, S.C. and J.W. Pankey. 1983. Cytological observations of the bovine teat end. Amer. J. Vet. Res. 44: 1433–1441.

Scott, T.R. 2004. Our current understanding of humoral immunity of poultry. Poultry Sci. 83: 574–579.

16 Urinary system

Contents

Anatomy of the urinary system

The urinary system is critical for homeostasis and performs many essential functions:

- Regulation of blood volume and blood pressure
- Control of blood concentrations of several ions (e.g., Na, K, Ca)
- Maintenance of blood pH via control of H^+ and HCO_3^- ion secretion
- Elimination of waste products and recovery of filtered nutrients

The urinary system is composed of the paired kidneys and ureters, urinary bladder, and urethra. Essentially dissolved materials in the liquid fraction of blood (plasma) are formed into a filtrate by the action of the kidneys. Once this filtrate is created, some additional materials are added (secretion) but others are recovered (reabsorption). The liquid that makes it through the microscopic tubular nephrons to the pelvis of the kidney and ultimately the urinary bladder exits the body as urine. Urine is typically slightly acidic (~pH 6.0) but its volume and composition varies depending on metabolism, diet, and the need to produce either dilute or concentrated urine to maintain extracellular fluid volume and osmolarity.

Let's now consider some of the detailed anatomy of this system, beginning with the kidneys. We'll use the ovine kidney to characterize some of the major features. In their normal position, retroperitoneal, the kidneys are positioned between the 12th thoracic and third lumbar vertebra. They are held in place by the peritoneum and are in contact with adjacent visceral tissue and surrounded by a layer of adipose tissue. The kidneys are generally well protected. The outermost renal fascia anchors the kidney to the peritoneum; the center layer of adipose tissue provides additional support and cushioning. The innermost connective tissue layer is the renal capsule that is closely attached to the outer surface of the kidney parenchymal tissue. The photograph provided in Figure 16.1 shows a bisected preserved sheep kidney. A portion of the thin but tough renal capsule is indicated. This specimen and companion drawing

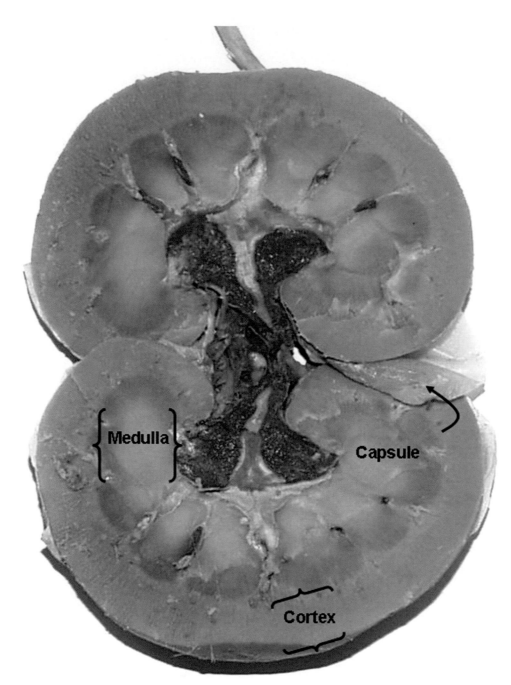

Fig. 16.1. Bisected preserved sheep kidney. Red latex fills much of the renal pelvis or hilus. The cortex is the outer rim of parenchymal tissue (brackets) and the medulla occurs in the region between the renal pelvis and cortex. A portion of the protective renal capsule is evident as a thin membranelike material.

illustrate major macroscopic features of the kidney. However, as we'll soon see, the ultimate work of filtration and reabsorption is done by complex multicellular tubules called nephrons that are evident only at a microscopic level. These functional units of the kidney are located in lobules within distinct zones or regions of the kidney that can be grossly distinguished.

The outermost region or zone, the cortex, lies over the inner region called the medulla and a central area called the renal pelvis or hilus of the kidney. This central area is the location for the entrance and exit of the renal vein and artery into the kidney as well as the origin of the ureter, which conducts urine to the bladder. The model illustrated in Figure 16.2 provides a three-dimensional representation of these structures. Figure 16.3 gives a "flow" diagram to link blood flow and corresponding urine production in the kidney. Briefly, the renal artery and vein branch at nearly right angles to supply each of the kidneys. As each of these vessels approaches the hilus it branches into smaller

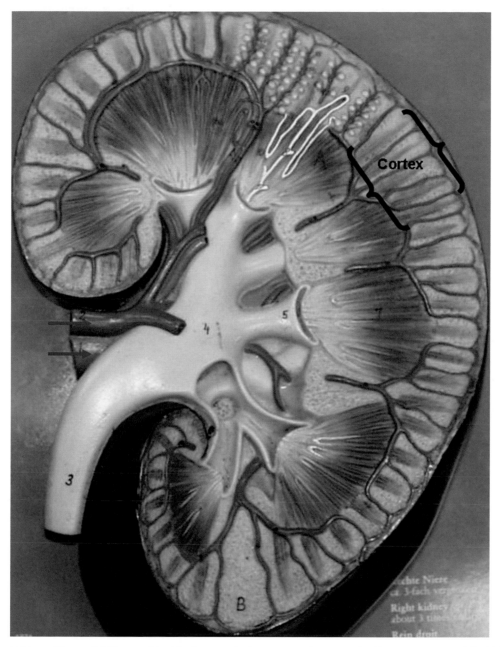

Fig. 16.2. Model of kidney. The model illustrated in this photograph demonstrates in greater detail gross anatomy of the kidney. The renal vein and artery (arrows) are evident in the region of the renal pelvis, as is the ureter (3). The funnellike structures that feed the exiting ureter are the major (closest to the ureter, 4) and minor calyces (5). These structures capture filtrate from the tips of the renal pyramids, as shown in the cutaway region. An example of a renal pyramid is illustrated by the dotted lines in Figures 16.1 and 16.2.

segmental arteries, named because they supply blood to sectors or segments of the mass of the kidney tissue. Each of the segmental arteries divides to create lobar arteries, which divide to yield interlobar arteries that pass between the pyramids of the medulla toward the kidney cortex.

Near the boundary between the cortex and medulla, the interlobar arteries branch into the arcuate arteries that arch (hence the name) over the bases of the medullary pyramids. Small interlobular arteries radiate outward to supply the tissue of the cortex. Most of the blood (~90%) that enters the kidney supplies the cortical tissue. Not surprisingly this is the region where the bulk of the nephrons are located. The veins trace essentially the same pathway in reverse (Fig. 16.4).

Among the domestic species, swine and large ruminants have kidneys that are described as multipyramidal or multilobar. In these cases a papilla (essentially the tip of the pyramid) projects into the space of a minor calyx; this is continuous with the ureters.

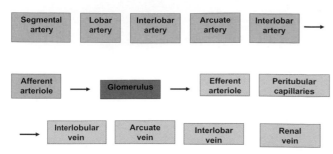

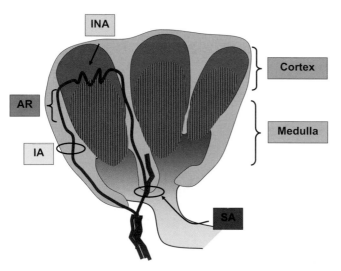

Fig. 16.3. Kidney blood flow. The group of progressive vessels (left to right) is the arterial branches (tan boxes) that ultimately supply the capillaries of the glomerulus where filtration takes place to supply fluid that enters the lumen of the nephron. Elements of the blood that are not filtered (cells and large proteins) and blood that is not subjected to filtration leaves the capillaries of the glomerulus and enters the venous circuit to exit the kidney via the renal vein (green boxes).

Fig. 16.4. Kidney blood supply. This stylized drawing illustrates some of the blood supply to kidney parenchymal tissue. Abbreviations include SA (segmental artery), IA (interlobar arteries), AR (arcuate arteries), and INA (interlobular arteries).

Unipyramidal or unilobar kidneys occur in most carnivores, small ruminants, and horses. The kidney consists of one lobe (cat, for example) that results from the fusion of several lobes during development. A single broad ridge or crest created by the fusion of the papillae is intimately associated with an expanded internal portion of the ureters, which spreads over the internal surface of the renal pelvis.

Under usual circumstances blood flow to the kidney is impressive, typically averaging 25% of cardiac output. As blood enters the renal artery, it progresses as outlined in Figure 16.3 and shown in Figure 16.4. The essential feature is that blood eventually passes into the tufts of capillaries that constitute the renal corpuscle (a surrounding structure called Bowman's capsule plus the tuft of capillaries), which is connected to the first segment of the nephron (proximal convoluted tubule).

Nephron structure

The function of the kidney is tied to the nephrons. Each nephron consists of the glomerulus (the tuft of blood vessels) and glomerular capsule (often called Bowman's capsule). This tuft or knot of capillaries has an afferent (toward) and efferent (away) arteriole. Blood that enters is subjected to filtration and osmotic pressures that act to force some of the liquid of the blood between the endothelial cells into the space surrounded by Bowman's capsule. Blood cells, larger molecules, and remaining liquid exit the tuft of capillaries via the efferent arteriole. Liquid that passes out of the capillaries into the space of Bowman's capsule enters into the first segment of the tubular portion of the nephron called the proximal convoluted tubule (PCT). This segment of the nephron gets its name because the tube is very highly coiled (convoluted) and it is the closest to the site of filtrate formation (proximal).

In sequence, the remaining parts of the nephron are the portion of the PCT leading to the thin or descending limb of the loop of Henle, ascending loop of Henle, distal convoluted tubule (DCT), and collecting duct (CD). The ends of the collecting ducts are located at the tips of the renal pyramids. This means that liquid that exits the nephrons at this point enters the ureter, passes to the bladder and is lost as urine. Nephrons occur in two classes. The majority class (cortical) is located primarily within the kidney cortex. However, so-called juxtamedullary nephrons are arranged near the boundary between the cortex and medulla so that the loop of Henle for these nephrons passes deep into the medullary region. As we'll soon see these nephrons play an especially important role in regulation of blood osmolarity. Figure 16.5 illustrates the orientation of nephrons within the kidney tissue.

In particular, notice that the branches from the arcuate arteries (paired artery and vein that arch over the boundary between the cortex and medulla) supply the interlobular arteries that ultimately supply the efferent arterioles of the glomerulus. These appear as circular white balls in the photograph. The two classes of nephrons (cortical) and the longer juxtamedullary nephrons are also illustrated in this photograph. The large branched structure in the center illustrates a CD, which, as the name suggests, collects effluent from the DCT of numerous nephrons as it traverses along the length of the renal pyramid. Further detail of the structure of the glomerulus and initial segment of the nephron is shown in Figure 16.6.

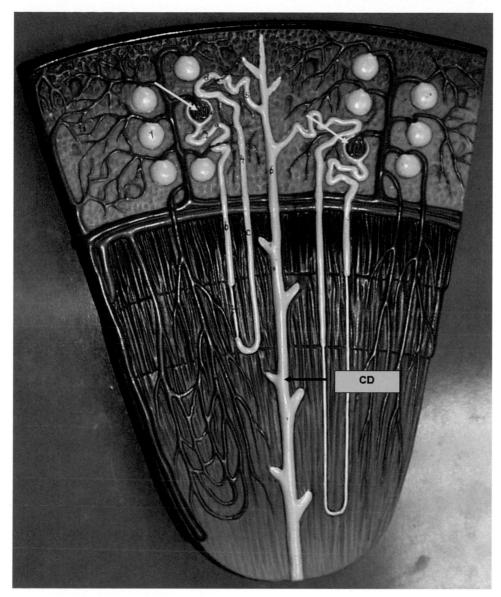

Fig. 16.5. Organization of nephrons. This photograph of a kidney model illustrates the orientation of microscopic structure within the tissue of a kidney pyramid. Numerous renal glomeruli (white globular structures) populate the renal cortex. Cross-sectioned glomeruli (yellow arrows) show the funnellike arrangement of the Bowman's capsule surrounding the tuft of capillaries and the afferent and efferent arterioles. The coiled tubule immediately exiting the glomerulus is the proximal convoluted tubule. Its path can be traced as it becomes the descending, and then ascending, loop of Henle. Once back in the region of the glomerulus the tubular nephron becomes the distal convoluted tubule before it joins the collecting duct (CD and arrow).

Figure 16.7 provides a drawing to illustrate the components of a nephron and associated blood supply to the glomerulus. The mammalian kidney is the best-understood osmoregulatory organ in the animal kingdom, thanks to extensive research over the past 40 years. Activities linked with the mammalian kidney include a number of functions that are tied with other organs in lower vertebrates—for example, the skin, bladder, and gills of fishes or the salt glands of many reptiles and birds. This perhaps explains the serious nature of kidney disease or defects in our animals.

In short, there is no substitute for a healthy well-functioning urinary system. As we have indicated in prior sections, structure and function are closely allied. The kidney and especially the elegant arrangement of the sections of the nephron, associated blood supply, and finally creation of a continuously maintained osmotic gradient within the tissue of the renal medulla are critical to kidney function. The nephron is a highly convoluted but nonetheless simple tube composed of a single layer of epithelial cells. The tube is essentially closed because of the tuft of capillaries and filtered

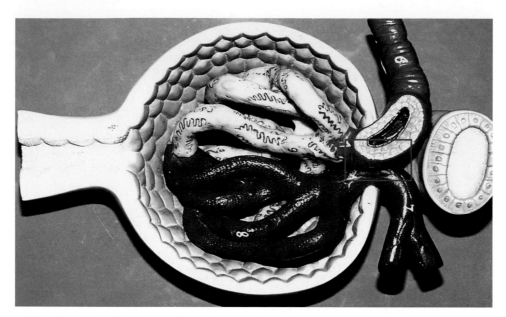

Fig. 16.6. Structure of the glomerulus. This photograph illustrates cellular structure associated with the glomerulus. The larger vessel on the upper right illustrates the afferent arteriole; the pale yellow covering on the surface of the vessel once it enters Bowman's capsule illustrates a layer of cells called podocytes that support the endothelial cells of the afferent capillary bed. These cells aid in regulation of the filtration process as discussed below. The other half of the tuft of vessels demonstrates the efferent vessels leading to the efferent arteriole. The pale blue layer of cells inside the Bowman's capsule represents the simple squamous epithelial cells that line its internal surface. To the left these cells give rise to simple cuboidal epithelial cells that constitute the internal lining of the proximal convoluted tubule (CT). The structure on the extreme right illustrates a cross section of the distal CT. The boxed area represents cells of the wall of the afferent arteriole and adjoining distal CT that comprise a structure called the juxtaglomerular apparatus or JGA. As discussed in the text the JGA is important in sensing decreases in blood pressure that lead to homeostatic events to restore pressure to normal.

fluid as it leaves the Bowman's capsule, but it is open at its distal end as it joins the collecting ducts that ultimately empty into the renal pelvis. We will explore these relationships by discussing in some detail the cellular structure of different epithelial cells located along the course of the nephron. To help you understand the role of the kidney in long-term control of blood pressure, blood flow, and stimulation of erythrocyte production, we will describe the importance of a specialized cluster of modified distal convoluted cells called the macula densa and the juxtaglomerular cells of the wall of the afferent arteriole, which together make up the juxtaglomerular apparatus. In addition, we'll consider the significance of the network of peritubular capillaries that intertwine around the loop of Henle and the curved course of blood flow that mirrors the hairpin bend in the loop of Henle called the vasa recta.

Mechanisms of urine formation

Remember, there are three critical processes that contribute to control the volume and composition of urine: 1) filtration of the blood plasma to create ultrafiltrate within the lumen of Bowman's capsule, 2) tubular reabsorption of water and most of the salts of

the ultrafiltrate, and 3) tubular secretion, much of which occurs via active transport. Let's begin by considering factors that control the creation of filtrate.

As you might guess one of the factors that directly impacts the rate of filtration is the blood pressure supplying the glomerulus, just as the rate of water flow through a sprinkler increases as the water faucet is opened (Fig. 16.8). Indeed, one of the symptoms of high blood pressure is more frequent urination. The data plotted demonstrates the dramatic nature of this response.

Factors affecting filtration

Other forces within Bowman's capsule also influence the rate of filtrate formation. Once filtration has started and fluid begins to collect, the fluid-filled space produces hydrostatic pressure against the endothelial cell from outside the capillaries. You can imagine this as the difference between filling an empty water bucket with a hose compared with pushing the hose to the bottom of a barrel that is already filled. The water coming from the hose is counteracted by the force of the water already in the container. In addition, the osmotic properties of the blood and newly created filtrate impact the rate of water movement across the

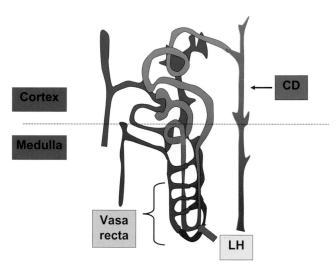

Fig. 16.7. Nephron diagram. This simplified diagram illustrates key aspects of a juxtaglomerular nephron. While in reality the convoluted tubules are more extensive, relative orientation is maintained. Notice that the branches of the efferent arteriole that supplies the region surrounding the convoluted tubules give rise to the network vessels surrounding the loop of Henle (LH) and the vasa recta, which allows blood from the region of the convoluted tubules to flow around the loop of Henle but in the opposite direction of fluid flow within the tubule. This is important because the countercurrent flow allows a steep osmotic gradient that is created by the action of cells of the loop of Henle to be maintained within the surrounding interstitial space. In practical terms this means that fluid that then passes up the ascending loop of Henle into the distal convoluted tubule and into the collecting duct transits down the collecting duct (CD) and through this surrounding osmotic gradient. Controlling the degree of permeability of the collecting duct to water allows either dilute (water is not recovered from the fluid entering the collecting duct) or concentrated urine (water follows osmotic forces and leaves the collecting duct lumen) to be produced.

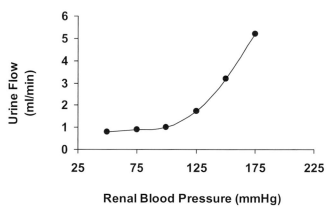

Fig. 16.8. Urine formation and blood pressure. The relationship between renal blood pressure and rate of urine formation is evident.

capillary cells. This means that despite a typical hydrostatic pressure of about 55 mmHg at the level of the afferent arteriole, the combination of competing forces produces a net filtration force of about +10 mmHg. Regardless of this seemingly small pressure differen-

tial, because of the very large number of glomeruli in each kidney, i.e., typically 2–4 million (depending on the species), this produces an enormous degree of filtration. For a 70 kg primate the average glomerular filtration rate (GFR) is 125 ml per min. As a crude estimate let's assume that blood volume equals 10% of body weight and that the blood is 50% plasma. This results in a blood volume of 7 kg. Let's further estimate that as 1 kg = 1 L. This then would yield a blood volume of 7 l or 3.5 l of blood plasma. Since the plasma is mostly water, at a normal rate of GFR it would take only 28 min for the entire plasma volume to be filtered. In other words, without mechanisms to minimize urine production the entire plasma volume would be lost in about 30 min. This staggering calculation highlights not only the degree of filtration but also the significance of the actions of the kidney to recover the majority of filtered water and important nutrients.

In addition to the hydrostatic pressure within the glomerulus, these capillaries also are structurally designed to maximize bulk fluid flow. Specifically, they are fenestrated. Compared with capillaries in other regions of the body the endothelial cells contain numerous large pores so that permeability is about 100 times greater than for other capillary beds. Despite the benefit of enhanced fluid filtration, it is also important that large macromolecules within the blood are not filtered. Thus the basement membrane surrounding the endothelial cells contains collagen and numerous negatively charged glycoproteins. This acts to repel albumin and other serum proteins. There are also specialized cells called podocytes that cover the outer surface of the endothelial cells. The podocytes send out numerous pseudopodia, which create processes called pedicels that interdigitate to create filtration slits. Filtrate driven by hydrostatic pressure passes through the pores of the endothelial cells, through the basement membrane, and then through these filtration slits. These three layers effectively act as a kind of molecular sieve so that small molecules and water readily pass into the lumen of Bowman's capsule but essentially all proteins are excluded from filtrate based on charge and/or molecular size. There is bulk flow of water through the glomerulus so that small dissolved ions, sugars, amino acids, urea, and most other small molecules enter the filtrate. Table 16.1 illustrates the relationship between molecular weight and transfer of several common blood components into kidney filtrate.

Proximal convoluted tubule

The composition of the filtrate is similar to that of blood plasma with the exception of the protein content,

Table 16.1. Relationship between molecular weight and properties of selected substances and urinary filtration.

Substance	Molecular Weight	Radius (nm)	Blood/Filtrate Ratio
Water	18	0.11	1.0
Glucose	180	0.36	1.0
Sucrose	342	0.44	1.0
Insulin	5,500	1.48	0.98
Ova albumin	43,500	2.85	0.22
Hemoglobin	68,000	3.25	0.03
Serum albumin	69,000	3.55	<0.01

Adapted from *Eckert Animal Physiology, Edition 5*.

Table 16.2. Features of three major classes of ATPase pumps.

Property	H^+ F-ATP Synthase	H^+ V-ATPase	Na^+/K^+ P-ATPase
Location	Mitochondria	Plasma membranes (apical)	Plasma membranes (basolateral)
Function	ATP synthesis	Acidification, gradient energy formation	Gradient energy formation
Action	Uses H^+ gradient to power ATP synthase	Uses ATP to create H^+ gradient	Uses ATP to create gradients for H^+, Na^+, K^+ and Ca^{2+}
Inhibitors	Azide	Bafilomycin	Ouabain

but the composition of urine is very different; thus it is apparent that both the volume and composition of the filtrate is markedly altered as it passes through the segments of the nephron. Essentially the kidneys filter blood plasma and then reabsorb needed materials from the ultrafiltrate. In fact, nearly all of the water and the majority of critical nutrients are recovered before the fluid reaches the end of the proximal convoluted tubules. The activity of the cells of the proximal convoluted tubule is reflected by the structure of the cells. Specifically, these cuboidal epithelial cells have plentiful mitochondria and RER as well as numerous apical microvilli. These attributes provide for synthesis of abundant amounts of ATP, much of which is needed to power active transport mechanisms to recover important nutrients that should not appear in urine. In short, ATP is expended either directly or indirectly in transferring ions (and other molecules) across the epithelium against a concentration gradient. Ionic gradients that are developed depend on the activity of three classes of ATPases or protein pumps. ATPases were discussed generally in Chapter 3. In reality these are quite complex components of cell membranes in many organisms. They are composed of membrane domains as well as catalytic and regulatory subunits located on the cytoplasmic face of the membrane. For example, protons (H^+) from electron transport in the mitochondria pass through the F-ATPase system that powers ATP synthesis within the internal membranes of the mitochondria. The proton V-ATPase pump utilizes the hydrolysis of ATP

to transport protons out of the cell or across membranes to generate an electrochemical gradient. These gradients then can serve many functions—for example, by acting via cotransport to direct movement of ions through specific channels, via symporters or antiporters as described in earlier chapters. V-ATPase pumps have a phosphorylated intermediate form of the transport protein. This feature is important because it adds an element of control to the activity of the pump. In other words, changes in molecules (hormone receptors, for example) that impact the degree of phosphorylation of this intermediate protein have a direct impact on the functionality of the transporter. Three subclasses of this type of ATPase pump includes the Na^+/K^+ P-ATPase discussed in relation to nerve function, the Ca^{2+} P-ATPase pump that is involved in muscle contraction, and the H^+/K^+ pump that is involved in acidification of gastric juices as well as kidney cell activity. Table 16.2 provides a summary of some of the features of these pumps.

So how are these pumps specifically involved in kidney function? The Na^+/K^+ P-ATPase pumps located on the basolateral membranes of the tubular epithelial cells regulate intracellular sodium levels and thereby cell volume by moving sodium out of the cell into extracellular fluid. If the cell also has K^+ channels in the apical membrane, K^+ ions will be excreted into the extracellular fluid as long as the electrochemical gradient is maintained in the appropriate direction (Fig. 16.9). If there are K^+ channels in the basolateral membrane, then there will be K^+ movement between intra-

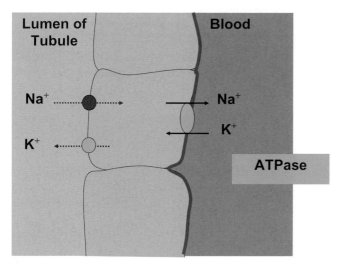

Fig. 16.9. Distal tubule ion transport. In the distal convoluted tubule and collecting duct of the nephron, the cells secrete K⁺ into the filtrate. Na⁺/K⁺ ATPase pumps in the basolateral membrane actively transport K⁺ into the cell where it then passes down its concentration gradient and exits from the apical end of the cell into the lumen. This allows the recovery of Na⁺ essentially in exchange for elimination of K⁺.

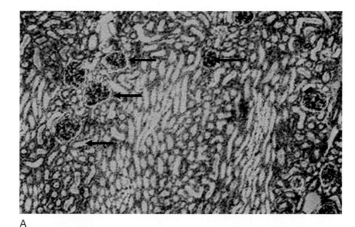

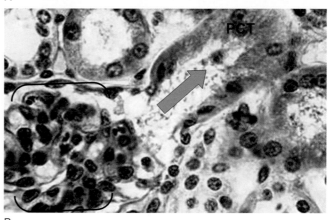

Fig. 16.10. Nephron histology. The Panel A gives a low-power survey image of the tissue from the cortex of the kidney. The larger rounded structures (arrows) are the renal corpuscles. The other abundant circular profiles are cross-sectioned areas of various segments of nephrons. Most of the profiles would be either proximal or distal convoluted tubules. The Panel B shows some of the detail of a renal corpuscle (outlined by the brackets). Ultrafiltrate flows from this structure into the proximal convoluted tubule (PCT). In this case by chance a portion of the tubule that drains this renal corpuscle has been sectioned. The large arrow indicates the direction of flow.

and extracellular compartments that is driven by the Na⁺/K⁺ ATPase pump. These mechanisms are involved in the overall secretion of K⁺ and recovery of Na⁺ by the cells of the nephron.

Although it is critical that appropriate quantities of sodium and potassium be recovered from kidney filtrate to maintain the osmolarity of body fluids, the Na⁺/K⁺ ATPase pumps either directly or indirectly support the movement of many substances. For example, if the apical membrane of the tubular cells contains a Na⁺/glucose or Na⁺/2Cl⁻/K⁺ symporters, the activity of these pumps can control the uptake of glucose, K⁺, or Cl⁻. This is just what selectively happens within specific sections of the nephron. If the Na⁺/2Cl⁻/K⁺ pump is located in the basolateral membrane of the cell, its activity can drive the uptake of Cl⁻ from the extracellular fluid (to be secreted into the filtrate). Specifically, the presence of chloride channels or pores in the apical membrane of the cell allows the passage of higher concentrations of chloride out of the cell and into the filtrate.

Figure 16.10 illustrates the histological appearance of a renal corpuscle as well as several cross-sectioned profiles of parts of a nephron. At first it may seem confusing. The larger rounded structures are the renal corpuscles, and the various tubules are sections through proximal or distal convoluted tubules, perhaps an ascending or descending loop of Henle or collecting ducts. Other tubelike structures include the network of peritubular capillaries. Remember the name of the beginning and ending section of the

nephron: convoluted tubule. Because of its highly coiled, curving structure a given histological section from the kidney might well exhibit many profiles of the same tubular structure as it is cut at various places. However, there are distinct structural features that allow the identification of proximal versus convoluted tubules, or differences between loops of Henle and collecting ducts for that matter. One simple feature that allows a quick orientation is the presence of renal corpuscles. If these structures are present, the tissue section was taken within the cortex or the tissue included the boundary between the cortex and medulla. The appearance of long parallel arrays of simple tubes is a major indication that the tissue section was prepared from a sample collected deeper into the renal medulla, perhaps near the apex of a

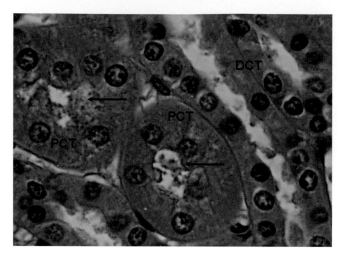

Fig. 16.11. Proximal and distal tubules. This image taken from the renal cortex shows profiles of proximal (PCT) and distal convoluted tubules (DCT). In both cases the cells are cuboidal, but cells of the PCT are larger and have evidence of stained material along the apical cell surface, evidence of abundant microvilli (arrows).

renal pyramid. These tubules likely represent the walls of the ascending or descending loops of Henle of the juxtamedullary nephrons, peritubular capillaries, or numerous collecting ducts.

As filtrate enters the PCT, forces begin the recovery of important nutrients, ions, and water. Because of these activities the structure of the cells of PCT and DCT are distinct. As shown in Figure 16.11 epithelial cells of both PCT and DCT are cuboidal, but the cells of the PCT typically have abundant microvilli and mitochondria. In paraffin sections of fixed kidney tissue, the lumenal spaces of the PCT sometimes appear as if the apical ends of the cells are painted. This color and thickness is an indication of stain accumulation on the proteins that coat the microvilli.

The remarkable capacity of the nephron to recover important nutrients is illustrated in Figure 16.12. Under normal circumstances, nearly all of the glucose and amino acids are recovered from the filtrate before it reaches the loop of Henle. The significance of measuring of inulin and hippuric acid to understanding kidney function is also indicated. Table 16.3 summarizes major functions associated with each of the segments of the nephron.

In addition to the recovery of dissolved substances, the rate of fluid flow also is dramatically reduced as each of the progressive segments of the nephron is traversed. As indicated earlier, the capacity to regulate the volume of urine produced is critical. As shown in Table 16.4, despite an average rate of filtrate formation of ~125 ml/min in a 70 kg primate, urine production is typically only about 1 ml per min. Just how this regulation takes place will be discussed in subsequent sections.

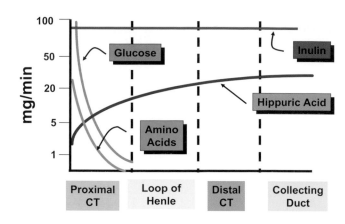

Nephron Region

Fig. 16.12. Flow of selected materials. This diagram illustrates the dramatic rate of removal of amino acids and glucose from the ultrafiltrate formed in the glomerulus. By the time fluid enters the loop of Henle, essentially all of the amino acids and glucose have been recovered in normal circumstances. When animals are given inulin or hippuric acid, the rate of appearance of these substances can be used to monitor kidney health. For example, inulin that enters the filtrate remains; it is neither reabsorbed nor is any transported from the peritubular blood (no secretion). This gives a measure of the glomerular filtration rate or GFR. Hippuric acid is not recovered, but in addition all of it in the blood that enters the glomerulus is transported into the filtrate (100% secretion). Thus evaluation of hippuric acid concentrations provides a measure of plasma flow rate to the kidney.

Table 16.3. Summary of functions of nephron regions

Region	Function
Glomerulus	Creation of filtrate from blood
Proximal convoluted tubule	Major area for reabsorption of filtrated water and solutes, obligatory water reabsorption
Thin descending limbs of loops of Henle	Maintenance of hypertonicity of medullary tissue via countercurrent system
Thick ascending limbs of loops of Henle	Na$^+$, K$^+$, Cl$^-$ reabsorption creation of osmotic gradient in medullary tissue
Distal convoluted tubule	NaCl reabsorption, facilitative water resorption
Collecting ducts	Final control of excretion of electrolytes and water, regulation of acid-base balance

Table 16.4. Rate of fluid flow in regions of the nephron.

Region	Rate of Flow (ml/min)	Percent
Glomerulus	124	100
Loop of Henle	50	40
Distal CT	25	20
Collecting duct	12	9
Renal pelvis	1	0.8

Countercurrent mechanisms and medullary osmotic gradient

The mammalian kidney has a remarkable ability to regulate the concentration of urine to maintain the water content of the body so that the osmolarity of body fluids remains within very narrow boundaries. For most animals there is a very real danger of desiccation, so the kidney is designed to reabsorb nearly all of the water that is filtered. However, if necessary the kidney is also capable of responding to produce very hypotonic urine to eliminate water. For example, consider that a 10 kg dog likely produces more than 50 l of glomerular filtrate per day but only 0.2 to 0.25 l of urine. If the dog is water deprived it can produce a very low volume of urine whose osmolarity is 10 times as great as blood plasma or with water loading urine with an osmolarity of only 100 mosm/l. How does the kidney manage these remarkable shifts?

The answer to this question is reflected in the complex but elegant structure of the nephron, variable function of cells within different nephron segments, and a unique arrangement of blood vessels within the tissue surrounding the nephrons. Three key elements are involved in determining whether concentrated or dilute urine will be produced. First there is the presence of an osmotic gradient that is generated and maintained in the tissue surrounding the juxtaglomerular nephrons whose loops of Henle dip from the cortex of the kidney, deep into the medulla. Second, the fluid of the tubule becomes progressively dilute as it passes through the loop of Henle into the distal convoluted tubule. Third, the permeability of the collecting duct cells to water can be directly regulated by the action of antidiuretic hormone (ADH). As the dilute filtrate fluid passes from the distal convoluted into the collecting ducts, it again traverses from the region of the cortex down through the renal medullary tissue to the apex of the renal pyramids for release. As illustrated in Figure 16.13, the osmolarity of the tissue fluid becomes progressively greater, ~1,200 mosm/l near the lower regions of the medulla, so that given the opportunity to respond to the osmotic pressure, water will pass across the cells of the collecting ducts into the interstitial fluid and be recovered in surrounding capillaries. However, this does not occur automatically. In the absence of sufficient secretion of ADH the water is retained within the tubular fluid and a more copious and dilute urine is produced. Water recovery or excretion within this region of the nephron is sometimes referred to as facultative reabsorption. That is, water recovery does not occur unless ADH is secreted to facilitate this process. This is contrasted with the reabsorption of water that happens within the PCT. In these areas of the nephron, the cells are always permeable to water. This means, for example, when sodium

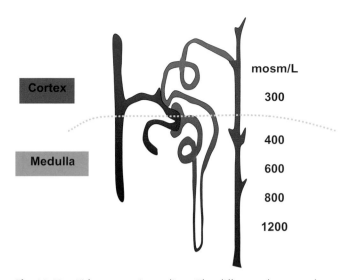

Fig. 16.13. Kidney osmotic gradient. The difference between the osmolarity of interstitial fluid in the cortex compared with the medulla is dramatic. The development and maintenance of this gradient is important; it allows the production of either dilute or concentrated urine.

is reabsorbed from the tubular fluid the osmotic difference that is created allows water to follow. Thus, water reabsorption in these regions is referred to as obligatory transport. Since the tubule is permeable to water, the removal of sodium or other solutes creates an osmotic drive that water is "obligated" to follow. Figure 16.14 illustrates factors that create and help maintain the interstitial osmotic gradient.

The vasa recta, the network of capillaries that follow the course of the loop of Henle, is also essential in maintenance of the osmotic gradient. This is because this arrangement acts as a countercurrent exchange mechanism to minimize alterations in the concentrations of solutes within the interstitial fluid. Essentially, this allows the recycling of salt. Without this arrangement, if ordinary vessels paralleled the loop of Henle the medullary gradient would quickly be dissipated. Specifically, as large amounts of Na^+ were absorbed, water would follow and the gradient would essentially be flushed away. In contrast, the vasa recta functions to minimize disruption. First, these capillaries get only about 10% of the blood flow. This acts to make blood flow relatively slow in comparison with other capillaries. In addition, throughout the course of the vessels the cells are freely permeable to both water and sodium. Consequently, the blood makes passive exchanges with the tubular fluid to maintain equilibrium with the surrounding interstitial fluid. For example, as the blood flows toward the apex of the renal pyramid, it loses water and gains salt because of the increasing osmolarity. In other words, the blood becomes hypertonic. However, after the vessels bend in the region of the hairpin loop the process is reversed.

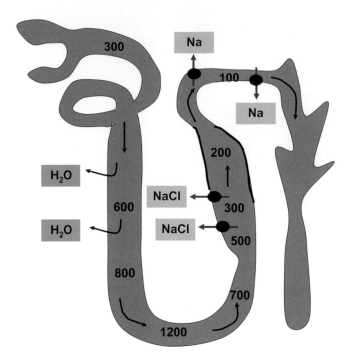

Fig. 16.14.   Role of loop of Henle. The thin limbs of the loops of Henle and the DCT generate and maintain the osmotic gradient between the cortex and medulla. The osmolarity of the tubule fluid leaving the PCT is about 300 mosm/L. It becomes progressively more concentrated so that osmolarity increases as water leaves in response to the tonicity of the surrounding fluids. This is because the descending limb is permeable to water but not sodium. After the hairpin turn the fluid becomes progressively more dilute because the cells are impermeable to water but not to sodium. The differences in permeability of the descending and ascending limbs and the countercurrent flow act to create and maintain the interstitial tissue osmotic gradient. In the upper regions of the ascending loop (indicated by the thick lines) the cells are impermeable to water, but active transport of sodium (chlorine follows via electrochemical attraction), indicated by the black circles and arrows, occurs. This creates dilute tubular fluid (~100 mosm/L) as the fluid enters the collecting ducts. As indicated, the permeability of the collecting ducts to water is controlled by secretion of ADH. Control of permeability allows either diluted (low ADH secretion) or concentrated urine (high ADH secretion) to be created as needed to maintain homeostasis.

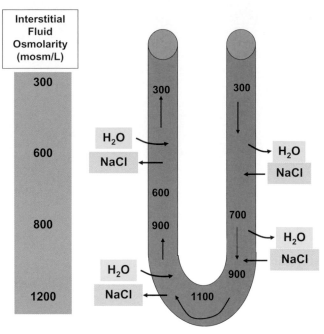

Fig. 16.15.   Countercurrent exchange in the vasa recta. The vessels of the vasa recta follow the curved course of the loop of Henle. Since the cells are freely permeable to both sodium and water, osmolarity of the blood (values with in the vessel) can reach equilibrium with the surrounding interstitial fluid during transit. However, the blood has essentially the same osmolarity when it enters and leaves the system. These transient shifts allow the osmotic gradient in the surrounding interstitial fluid to be maintained.

As the blood leaves the medulla and enters the cortex the osmolarity is essentially the same as when it entered the descending side of the system. These countercurrent exchanges protect the osmotic gradient that is created by the selective actions of the descending and ascending limbs of the loop of Henle. Figure 16.15 illustrates the idea of a countercurrent system generally and of the vasa recta specifically.

Although the structure-function relationships among parts of the nephron explain much of the action of the kidney with respect to the capacity of the kidney to control production of either dilute or concentrated urine, what are the factors that determine which type of urine should be produced? To understand this regulation we need to appreciate the fact that the kidney—specifically specialized cells within the glomerulus,

afferent arteriole, and distal convoluted tubule—is important in the long-term chronic control of blood pressure. A second key element is the fact that maintenance of blood and interstitial fluid osmolarity, while sensed by cells of the hypothalamus, requires changes in kidney function to effect homeostatic control of body fluid osmolarity.

We begin by considering the role of sodium chloride. More than 90% of the osmotic activity of extracellular fluid is directly related to concentrations of NaCl, especially Na. In most situations reabsorption or movement of salt across an epithelial or cell membrane also results in the movement of water because of osmosis. Thus, the amount of salt in the body is a very important determinant of extracellular fluid volume and consequently blood volume and blood pressure. In short, all things being equal, reabsorption of more sodium from the glomerular filtrate of the kidney leads to greater reabsorption of water. Thus there is a direct relationship between kidney function and control of blood pressure via control of extracellular fluid volume. Certainly something so important as control of blood pressure (volume) and osmolarity cannot be left to chance. The first component involved is the renin-angiotensin system.

Figure 16.16 shows cells that make up the juxtaglomerular apparatus (JGA). The JGA is a combination of the cells of the wall of the afferent arteriole and a

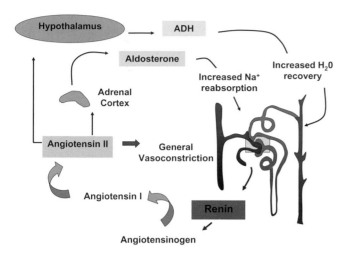

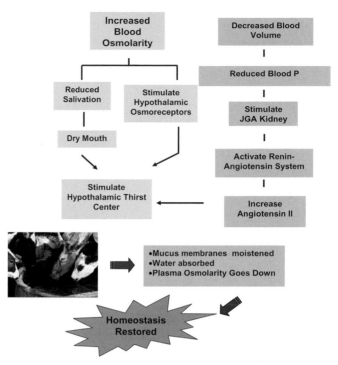

Fig. 16.16. Renin-angiotensin system. The secretory cells of the juxtaglomerular apparatus (JGA) indicated in the boxed area release renin in response to low blood pressure in the afferent arteriole and/or low sodium in distal CT. In a cascade of reactions, renin first promotes the cleavage of the serum protein angiotensinogen (synthesized in the liver). This action produces angiotensin I, which is modified by angiotensinogen converting enzyme (ACE) by removal of 2 additional amino acids to form the 8 amino acid peptide, angiotensin II, as the blood passes through the lungs. Angiotensin II has two major actions. First, it stimulates a general vasoconstriction, which increases blood pressure rather quickly; second, it promotes secretion of aldosterone from the adrenal cortex. As described previously, aldosterone promotes increased reabsorption of sodium, which leads to increased water recovery, increased extracellular fluid volume, and ultimately increased blood volume and therefore increased blood pressure. Finally, increased angiotensin II also increases synthesis of antidiuretic hormone in the hypothalamus. ADH increases water permeability of the collecting ducts to also increase blood volume and pressure.

Fig. 16.17. Thirst reactions. In addition to the kidney control of urine production, drinking must also be regulated. Multiple elements (dry mouth, reduced blood osmolarity, and increased blood angiotensin II) act via osmoreceptors in the hypothalamus to elicit the sensation of thirst that leads to drinking. Ingestion of water moistens mucus membranes and absorption increases osmolarity of fluid, bathing osmolarity-sensitive cells in the hypothalamus, reducing the sensation of thirst, and along with kidney action restoring homeostasis.

segment of the distal convoluted tubule. Secretory cells within the JGA respond to decreases in blood pressure and/or very low concentrations of Na within the fluid of the distal CT by secreting the enzyme renin. Renin acts to restore blood pressure in two ways. Most rapidly, as outlined in Figure 16.16, the increased blood renin causes an increase in the blood concentration of angiotensin II. This agent has two actions to help restore blood pressure; first it causes a generalized vasoconstriction of capillary sphincters throughout the body. This acts to reduce blood flow through many capillary beds, which increases vessel resistance and thereby increases venous return to the heart. The increased volume produces increased cardiac output and therefore an increase in blood pressure. In addition, angiotensin II also promotes the secretion of the steroid hormone aldosterone from the adrenal cortex. Aldosterone acts to promote increased reabsorption of Na from the distal CT. As indicated previously, enhanced recovery of Na within this region of the nephron leads to simultaneous reabsorption of water. The reabsorbed water enters the capillaries and consequently the vascular system, which also increases blood pressure. Furthermore, the angiotensin II also

promotes the secretion of ADH. This is called the renin-angiotensin system.

The mechanism aldosterone uses to increase sodium reabsorption in the distal CT is not fully understood. Like other steroid hormones, aldosterone diffuses across the membrane of its target cells and binds to receptors in the cytoplasm. These activated receptor-hormone complexes migrate to the nucleus ultimately to produce transcription of specific genes. These newly minted proteins are responsible for the effects of aldosterone. However, three detailed mechanisms have been proposed to explain the increased sodium reabsorption.

First, the sodium pump hypothesis suggests that the activity of the Na^+/K^+ pumps in the basolateral membrane is simply stimulated. Second, the metabolic hypothesis suggests that aldosterone increases production of ATP, perhaps due to enhanced fatty acid oxidation, and that making more ATP available simply powers the Na^+/K^+ membranes pumps more effectively. A third hypothesis is that aldosterone increases the synthesis of sodium channel proteins that are deposited in the apical membranes of the cells. Furthermore, animals are stimulated by thirst to increase water intake, as illustrated by Figure 16.17.

There are also elements to "adjust" the activity of the renin-angiotensin system to prevent extremes. For example, atrial natriuretic peptide (ANP) is released by cells in the atrium of the heart in response to increased venous blood pressure. ANP acts to increase urine production and sodium excretion by inhibiting the release of ADH and renin and thus secretion of aldosterone by the adrenal gland.

Renal clearance

Data illustrated in Figure 16.12 shows absorption and secretion patterns for some selected substances as these materials pass through regions of the nephrons. Measuring changes in the concentrations of two of these substances, inulin and hippuric acid are very valuable as tools to evaluate kidney function. Specifically, to really evaluate how effectively plasma is cleared or cleaned of unwanted waste products, two variables related to kidney action must be measured. First, we need a measure of the rate of blood or plasma flow to the kidneys and second, we need a measure of how much of the blood plasma is filtered. You might recall from our description of blood flow to the renal glomerulus that blood enters via the afferent arteriole, some fluid is lost to create the ultrafiltrate that enters the lumen of the nephrons, and the remainder exits via the efferent arteriole.

Inulin, a sugar that is isolated from the tubers of dahlias, is filtered from the blood but it is neither reabsorbed from the filtrate nor is any additional inulin secreted into the lumen of the nephrons. For this reason measuring the concentrations of inulin in samples from the renal vein and artery following injection into systemic circulation gives a measure of the volume of blood plasma that is filtered by the kidney. This is called the glomerular filtration rate (GFR). This determination of the GFR is based on the idea of clearance, specifically the rate at which the plasma is cleared or cleaned of a given substance. The clearance rate (RC) is determined by the rate of elimination divided by the plasma concentration as shown in this equation:

$$RC_x = \frac{U_x V}{P_x}$$

where RC_x is the volume of plasma cleared of substance x per unit time, U_x is the urine concentration of substance X, V is the volume of urine collected divided by the time period of the collection, and P_x is the plasma concentration of X. GFR is considered the best single parameter for assessing overall renal function because its value is directly related to the functional mass of kidney tissue. In veterinary practice, measure-

ment of blood levels of urea nitrogen (BUN) and creatine concentration are often used as screening tools to detect renal dysfunction. Unfortunately, values typically rise markedly only when 75% or more of the nephrons no longer function.

The total clearance of a particular substance is the sum of the rates of filtration and secretion with the rates of reabsorption subtracted. To determine the filtration rate accurately the effects of secretion and reabsorption have to be taken into account. In the case of inulin, since it is freely filtered but is neither secreted nor reabsorbed and is not produced in animals, it is ideal for calculating GFR. Indeed, the equation for calculation of inulin clearance is in effect an equation for calculation of GFR as shown below, where *GFR* is in ml per min, C_{inulin} is the rate of clearance of inulin from the plasma in ml per min, U_{inulin} is the inulin concentration in a urine sample collected over a period of time T in minutes; *V* is the volume of urine collected over time T; and P_{inulin} is the average plasma inulin concentration during time T:

$$GFR = \frac{C_{inulin} = U_{inulin} V}{P_{inulin}}$$

Again, since infused inulin (typically a standard dose to achieve an initial concentration of ~1 mg/ml of plasma or 3,000 mg/m^2 body surface area) is eliminated only in the urine, its clearance rate value is equal to the GFR. Measured values for inulin in man are U = 125 mg/ml, V = 1 ml/min, and P = 1 mg/ml. Thus, the calculated value for RC for inulin = (125 × 1)/1 = 125 ml/min. This means that in 1 min the kidneys have removed or cleared the amount of inulin that would have been in 125 ml of blood plasma. Typical values for healthy cats, for example, average about 2.7 ml/min/kg or ~12 ml/min for a typical adult cat. Figure 16.18 illustrates the relationship between BUN and GFR in a population of cats. In this case, GFR was estimated from the clearance of injected inulin. It was also found that the serum inulin value after a single time period (180 min) corresponded well with more extensive blood sampling. In practical terms, this would minimize stress associated with multiple sampling. Since some of the animals in this trial were suspected of being in early stages of renal disease, it is also apparent that several of the cats with elevated serum creatine levels have correspondingly reduced GFR values. This supports the predictions of impaired kidney function.

Although the standard method to calculate GFR is by measuring the clearance rate of inulin from the blood, GFR can be estimated by measuring other endogenous substances. In clinical veterinary situations it can be done by measuring the clearance of creatine. Creatine is a by-product of muscle metabo-

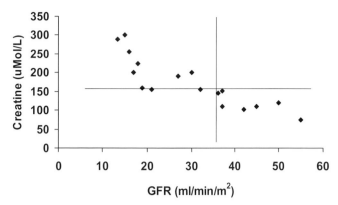

Fig. 16.18. Relationship between GFR and serum creatine. The vertical line indicates the lower value for GFR that is still considered normal. The horizontal line indicates a normal upper limit for serum creatine. Animals in the upper-left quadrant of the graph have higher than normal serum creatine concentrations and correspondingly reduced kidney function, as evidenced from the reduced GFR. Adapted from Haller et al. (2003).

lism that is handled by the kidney (at least in the dog) much like inulin. That is, it is freely filtered, is not reabsorbed, and is not secreted into the tubular lumen. This, however, may not be true in all species. For example, in some animals about 10% of the creatine in urine occurs because of secretion. In practical terms, the usual procedure is to collect the urine that is produced over 24 h (either catheterization or collection in a metabolic cage). The volume produced is recorded and the creatine concentration measured. The concentration of creatine in blood collected at the start and end of the collection period is typically measured and averaged to provide a measure of plasma concentration. These values are used in the clearance equation to give an estimate of GFR. When many different animals are evaluated, it is better to express the GFR on a body weight or body surface basis (ml per min per kg or ml per min per sq m) to account for the large variation between species. Note the example given in Figure 16.18.

Hippuric acid is useful because it is filtered as it passes into the glomerulus. Moreover, the remaining portion that passes out of the efferent arteriole is secreted into the tubular fluid. Thus, all of the material that is in the blood plasma that enters the kidney appears in the filtrate and ends up in urine. This property allows a calculation of plasma flow to the kidney. This can be very useful to evaluate kidney as well as cardiovascular health.

If less of a substance appears in the urine than was initially produced at the time of filtration, some reabsorption of the substance must have occurred in the tubule. In a human, the GFR averages 125 ml

per min (mostly water) but urine production is only about 1 ml per min. Clearly, most of the water is recovered. For important nutrients (Fig. 16.12), reabsorption is essentially complete in most circumstances. For example, consider glucose: Unless blood concentrations are abnormally elevated all of the filtered glucose is recovered so that the clearance is zero. There is, however, a maximum rate at which glucose can be recovered from the filtrate. In humans, for example, the transport maximum (Tmax) is about 320 mg/min. As long as plasma glucose remains below about 1.8 mg/ml (180 mg/dL), all of the glucose appearing in the filtrate is recovered. At about 300 mg/dL of plasma, the transport mechanism becomes completely saturated so that glucose is lost in the urine. Exact transport values likely differ between species but the idea remains the same. Specifically, elevated blood glucose occurs with diabetes so that appearance of glucose in the urine is an initial indication of diabetes in both humans and other animals.

Kidney excretion of wastes and control of pH

As we learned in earlier sections, maintenance of blood and extracellular fluid pH within relatively narrow boundaries is critical for homeostasis. Movement of carbon dioxide from tissues and the bicarbonate buffering system of blood is a critical component in maintenance of pH. Clearly, the ratio of ventilation rate to the rate of CO_2 production determines the body concentration of CO_2. Changes in ventilation rate therefore have an important role in modulation of pH, especially in the short term. However, the capacity to regulate excretion of CO_2 via the lungs and excretion of acid via the kidneys combine to provide long-term control of blood and extracellular fluid pH. In particular, the excretion of acid or H^+ ions in the urine is an important aspect of maintaining the plasma bicarbonate (HCO_3^-) concentration in mammals. It is worth remembering that normal digestive and metabolic processes produces large quantities of acids that must be buffered and/or excreted.

At this point a brief reminder of some pH and buffering fundamentals are in order. Since all functional proteins (enzymes, receptors, etc.) are influenced by pH, it follows that acid-base balance is critical for homeostasis. When the pH rises above the optimal value (~7.4 for most animals), the situation is referred to as alkalosis if pH drops below pH 7.35; this is known as acidosis. Because in a chemical sense a pH of 7.0 is neutral, a pH of 7.35 is not, chemically speaking, acidic, but the hydrogen ion concentration is higher than optimal for the animal. So for most animals any arterial pH between pH 7.35 and 7.0 is deemed physiological acidosis.

Although all animals ingest small amounts of acidic substances, most H$^+$ ions are derived as by-products of metabolism. Consider the breakdown of amino acids from proteins or fatty acids from triglycerides or the buildup of lactic acid. Concentrations of H$^+$ in blood and consequently extracellular fluids are controlled by 1) buffer systems, 2) respiratory centers in the brain stem, and 3) the kidneys. The chemical buffers act virtually instantaneously to prevent dramatic swings in pH. Changes in respiration rate and depth of respiration begin to compensate for either acidosis or alkalosis within a matter of minutes. The kidneys have very potent effects, but these changes require hours or perhaps days before they are fully effective.

The chemical buffers act by converting either strong acids or bases into weaker acids or bases. The point to remember is that strong acids or bases dissociate rapidly and completely, so the change in free H$^+$ ion concentration can be dramatic. Weaker acids or bases dissociate less effectively, so changes in H$^+$ ion or OH$^-$ concentration is reduced. Important buffer systems in the body include the bicarbonate buffer system, phosphate buffer system, and protein buffer system.

The respiratory system regulation of H$^+$ ion concentration evolves around the elimination of carbon dioxide generated by cellular respiration. Briefly, CO$_2$ that enters the circulation combines with water to create carbonic acid. It then dissociates to produce H$^+$ and bicarbonate ion:

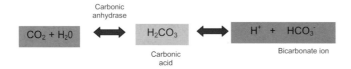

Most of the CO$_2$ that enters blood through the capillary beds in transit for exhalation in the lungs also passes through the red blood cells. Much of the H$^+$ that is liberated from carbonic acid in the creation of bicarbonate ion is captured by oxygen-depleted hemoglobin (Hb). CO$_2$ is also carried by depleted hemoglobin (carbamino hemoglobin). Bicarbonate ions diffuse out of the red blood cells in exchange for chloride ions from the plasma. The situation is essentially reversed as the blood gets to the lungs. Oxygen entering the red cells displaces the protons from the Hb, and CO$_2$ enters the plasma. Carbonic anhydrase in the membrane of the endothelial cells also converts some of the bicarbonate into CO$_2$.

The various chemical acid-base buffer systems in the body are essentially pairs of molecules that act to resist changes in H$^+$ concentration when a strong acid or base is added to the system. Recall that the three systems are the bicarbonate, phosphate, and protein buffer systems. The idea of protein buffering was illustrated by the capacity of Hb to capture protons coming from carbonic acid production. The bicarbonate buffer system is especially important in the extracellular fluid compartments and is a mixture of carbonic acid (H$_2$CO$_3$) and its sodium salt (NaHCO$_3$). In this combination, if a strong acid (HCl) is added, bicarbonate ions of the salt act as a weak base to capture much of the H$^+$ produced from the dissociation of HCl. This produces more of the weaker carbonic acid. Again, since it is a weak acid it dissociates only modestly, so the pH of the solution is lowered much less than would have been expected. In a similar way, if a strong base (NaOH) were added, more of the carbonic acid reacts with the NaOH to produce more of the weak base (sodium bicarbonate) and water. The net result is that the pH of the solution rises only modestly:

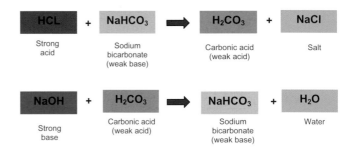

The phosphate buffer system operates in a similar fashion. Its components are the sodium salts of dihydrogen phosphate (H$_2$PO$_4^-$) and monohydrogen phosphate (HPO$_4^{2-}$). NaH$_2$PO$_4$ acts as a weak acid; Na$_2$HPO$_4$ acts as a weak base. The phosphate buffer system is only in low concentrations in the extracellular fluids but it is an important buffer in urine and within intracellular compartments where phosphate concentrations are typically higher. As illustrated below, hydrogen ions from strong acids are captured by converting a weak base to a weak acid and strong base countered by conversion of a weak acid to a weak base:

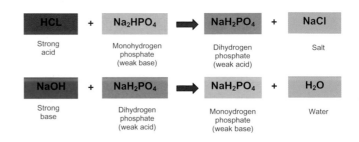

Proteins located in the blood plasma and intracellular proteins are also critically important buffering elements (protein buffering system). Because of their abundance, proteins account for most of the buffering capacity of the body. As we discussed in early chapters, proteins are chains of amino acids. Some of the amino acids have reactive or free carboxyl residues (so-called organic acid groups [–COOH]), which dissociate to release H^+ ions when the pH begins to rise. Other amino acids have reactive groups that can act as bases to accept protons. For example, an exposed NH_2 group can bind a hydrogen ion to become NH_3^+. This action effectively removes free hydrogen ions, which prevents the solution surrounding the protein from becoming too acidic. The same proteins can function in a reversible manner either as acids or bases, depending on the pH of their environment. Molecules with this capacity are called amphoteric molecules.

These buffer systems can effectively capture excess hydroxyl or hydrogen ions in the short term, but they cannot eliminate excess acids or bases from the body. The lungs can dispose of carbonic acid by exhalation of CO_2, but the kidneys are critical in eliminating most of the other acids produced by metabolic activity. These include things like phosphoric, uric, and lactic acid. Calling these metabolic or fixed acids is sometimes done to make a distinction between carbonic acid derived from CO_2 and these other "metabolic" acids. For example, acidosis that is caused by the accumulation of these metabolic acids is sometimes called metabolic acidosis to distinguish it from acidosis that can be caused by a failure of the lungs to eliminate sufficient CO_2. This failure can produce an accumulation of carbonic acid, thus an acidosis referred to as respiratory acidosis. Clearly, both types of acidosis depend on alterations in metabolism, but sources of the problem can be distinguished.

The kidneys then are critical for long-term regulation of body pH because of their ability to compensate for acid-base imbalances caused by changes in diet or disease. One of the most important aspects is the capacity of the kidney to either conserve (reabsorb) or produce new bicarbonate ions as well as the ability to excrete bicarbonate ions if required. The concentration of HCO_3^- in the plasma of most mammals is about 25×10^{-3} M/l and H^+ ion concentration about 40×10^{-9} M/l. Since the composition of the filtrate that enters the nephrons is about the same, there are relatively large amounts of bicarbonate but much less hydrogen ion. However, urine has a pH of about 6.0 with a minimal amount of bicarbonate ions. As we discussed, metabolic processes demand that excess acid produced from catabolic events must be excreted. So how is this accomplished? The goal is to add excess H^+ to the filtrate to be lost in urine with little bicarbonate. If you consider the operation of the bicarbonate-carbonic acid buffer system described earlier, losing an HCO_3^- from the system pushes the equation to the right and effectively increases H^+ ion concentration. In the opposite manner, the creation or reabsorption of HCO_3^- from the kidney filtrate is the same as losing H^+ as the equation is pushed to the left. To summarize, to reabsorb bicarbonate, H^+ ions are secreted, but when excess HCO_3^- is excreted, H^+ is retained.

Let's first consider the events that allow for excretion of H^+ into the filtrate (remember this is in addition to H^+ that was initially filtered—you might also recall that urine is typically slightly acidic, ~6 compared with blood plasma). Hydrogen ion excretion occurs primarily within the PCT as well as the so-called type A cells of the collecting ducts. The hydrogen ions to be secreted arise from the dissociation of carbonic acid. However, as in the red blood cells the carbonic acid is produced within the tubular epithelial cells from the diffusion of CO_2 from the peritubular capillaries and the action of carbonic anhydrase, which combines water and CO_2 to produce carbonic acid. As each H^+ ion is excreted an Na^+ ion is reabsorbed. This maintains the electrochemical balance across the tubular cells. In general, the rate of H^+ excretion varies with changes in the CO_2 content of the peritubular blood. Since blood CO_2 is directly related to blood pH, these systems can respond to adjust to either rising or falling pH. High CO_2 (corresponding with low pH) would lead to a larger diffusion gradient for movement of CO_2 from the peritubular blood into the tubular cells. This would be followed by increased production of carbonic acid, its dissociation, and therefore excretion of more H^+. Some of this excreted H^+ can combine with urinary bicarbonate ions (HCO_3^-) to produce CO_2 and water. Some of this urinary filtrate CO_2 can also enter the tubular cells and promote further excretion of H^+. A reduction in blood CO_2 would produce the opposite effect.

The type A cells are located primarily in the DCT and CD and serve as acid-secreting cells. Specifically these cells have a proton pump in the apical membrane and a chloride-bicarbonate exchange system in the basolateral membrane. The cells also have high concentrations of carbonic anhydrase, which serves to combine CO_2 and H_2O, making protons and bicarbonate ions available. The H^+ ions are moved across the apical membrane (facing the filtrate), and the bicarbonate ions transported across the basolateral membrane into the surrounding interstitial fluid. The H^+ ions that are secreted can react with bicarbonate ions in the filtrate to create carbon dioxide and water, which can diffuse back into the cell. The net result of this process is that activated type A cells can produce

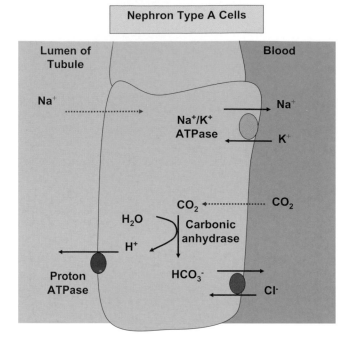

Nephron Type A Cells

Lumen of
Tubule

Blood

Na$^+$

Na$^+$

Na$^+$/K$^+$
ATPase

K$^+$

CO$_2$

CO$_2$

H$_2$O

Carbonic
anhydrase

H$^+$

HCO$_3^-$

Proton
ATPase

Cl$^-$

Fig. 16.19. Acid-secreting type A cells. A-type cells pump protons into the filtrate of the nephron by action of an apical H$^+$ ATPase. This acidifies the filtrate so that the potential favors reabsorption of Na$^+$ ions. The intracellular Na$^+$ concentration is reduced by the activity of a basolateral Na$^-$/K$^+$ ATPase pump.

a positive uptake of bicarbonate into the blood through the recycling of CO_2 while adding protons to the filtrate. Thus type A cells are acid-secreting cells (Fig. 16.19).

The activity of the A-type cells and therefore the degree of acid secretion can be regulated. For example, in periods of acidosis the activity of the cells is stimulated. This is believed to involve direct changes in the proton ATPase activity (increases synthesis of transporter proteins and/or activity) as well as increased activity or synthesis of the basolateral membrane bicarbonate-chloride exchange proteins. In this way increases in blood bicarbonate would serve to counter the acidosis. For example, aldosterone is known to stimulate the activity of the proton ATPases.

As H$^+$ secretion by the tubular cells continues, the pH of the filtrate drops and consequently continued secretion is against an increasing concentration gradient. The ability to secrete more protons decreases with decreasing pH (higher H+ concentration) until at a pH of about 4.5 acid secretion stops. However, more protons can be secreted if needed if the acidic filtrate can be buffered. Depending on conditions, bicarbonate, phosphates, and ammonia can accomplish this mission. Hydrogen ions can react with bicarbonate

to form carbon dioxide and water, with HPO_4^{2-} to produce $H_2PO_4^-$, or with NH_3 (ammonia) to produce ammonium ions (NH_4^+). Thus the kidney has three systems (bicarbonate, phosphate, and ammonia) to act as buffering agents. The cells of the nephron are nearly impermeable to both ammonium ions and phosphates so that these agents effectively capture excess hydrogen ions for excretion from the body. The phosphates that appear in the filtrate are derived when filtration of the blood takes place in the glomerulus; ammonia on the other hand diffuses from the blood into the tubular cells where it gets converted into the less toxic ammonium ion. The availability of phosphate for buffering is dependent on the diet.

Under acidosis conditions, plasma bicarbonate concentrations can fall so that the buffering capacity of the renal filtrate is also reduced. When this occurs ammonia can become a major pathway for elimination of excess acid. Specifically, ammonia is synthesized in the tubular cells by the enzymatic deamination of amino acids. The amino acid glutamine is especially important in this process. Ammonia is formed routinely in hepatic cells, but it is rapidly converted to less toxic urea and glutamine. Effectively ammonia is carried to the kidney cells in the form of glutamine, where its deamination produces ammonia. In its nonpolar, unionized form (NH_3) it readily diffuses across the cells into the filtrate to combine with H$^+$ to yield the highly polar ammonium ion (NH_4^+). Because of its polarity it is essentially trapped in the filtrate so that it is excreted in the urine. This pathway therefore allows for the excretion of excess nitrogen as well as excess hydrogen ions.

Bicarbonate ions are also plainly critical in the bicarbonate buffer system. If this reserve of base is to be maintained, the kidneys must not only act to counter rising H$^+$ concentrations by excreting more H$^+$, they must also either recover HCO_3^- ions that have been filtered or secreted or create additional bicarbonate ions. This involves a convoluted process because the tubule cells are nearly impermeable to HCO_3^- ions present in the filtrate. A second cell, the B-type cell, functions as a base-secreting cell (Fig. 16.20). These cells are arranged so that they express a proton ATPase transporter in the basolateral membrane and a chloride-bicarbonate exchange protein in the apical membrane. These cells also have carbonic anhydrase. The result is that bicarbonate is secreted into the filtrate while protons are recovered.

Excretion of nitrogenous wastes

Although we have touched on the relationship between urinary excretion of ammonia and control of pH, it is

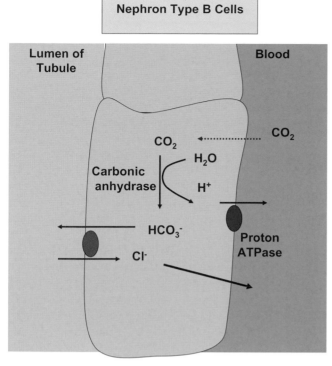

Fig. 16.20. Base-secreting type B cells. B-type cells use the proton ATPase proteins in the basolateral membrane to pump protons into the blood in concert with recovery of chloride ions.

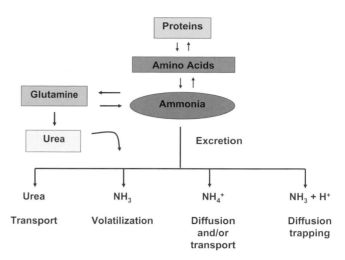

Fig. 16.21. Nitrogen excretion. Ammonia accumulates in tissue from the catabolism of proteins. It is either directly excreted or, as in most mammals, it is converted into less toxic urea or uric acid for elimination from the body.

worth considering this important topic in a broader context. When amino acids are catabolized to be used as energy sources or for use as carbon skeletons to synthesize other building blocks, the amino groups ($-NH_2$) are removed (deamination reaction). In other cases the amino group is salvaged for rebuilding nonessential amino acids. However, if the amino group is not transferred in this fashion, it must be eliminated from the body to prevent the buildup of toxic waste. Excessive ammonia can cause convulsions, coma, and subsequently death. This also explains the importance in removal of wastes from animal bedding and housing facilities. Animals excrete most of the excess nitrogen in the form of ammonia, urea, or uric acid. These associations with protein catabolism are outlined in Figure 16.21.

Ammonia is much more toxic than either urea or uric acid, so concentrations must be kept low. Since ammonia is freely diffusible, keeping concentrations low (to allow movements down a concentration gradient) requires large amounts of water. It is estimated that 0.5 liters of water is necessary to excrete 1 g of nitrogen waste in the form of ammonia. Nonetheless, some animals do excrete their nitrogenous waste primarily as ammonia. These animals are called ammo-

notelic. Many fishes and aquatic invertebrates are ammonotelic. There are also some animals (snails and crabs) that excrete ammonia into the air as a volatile gas.

Urea is much less toxic than ammonia, and in addition only about 10% as much water is required to excrete 1 g of nitrogenous waste as urea compared with ammonia. On the other hand there is an energy cost since ATP is required for urea synthesis. Ureotelic animals excrete most of their nitrogenous waste as urea. Two primary pathways are used for urea formation. Most animals generate urea largely in the liver via the ornithine-urea cycle, as illustrated in Figure 16.22.

Uricotelic animals, which include birds and reptiles, excrete nitrogenous wastes as uric acid or the closely related compound guanine. Both of these molecules have the advantage of carrying away four nitrogen atoms in each molecule. The nitrogen groups in uric acid are derived from the breakdown of glycine, aspartate, or glutamine. These animals lack the enzyme uricase and so cannot break down uric acid. This means that the poorly soluble uric acid precipitates and is excreted as a semisolid material. For example, the whitish-colored material in chicken manure is largely uric acid. An advantage is that relatively little water is required for excretion.

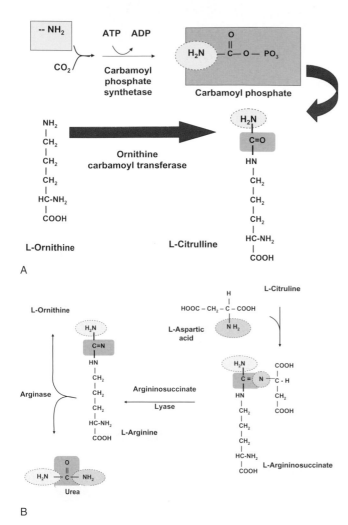

Fig. 16.22. The ornithine-urea cycle.

Comparative urinary physiology and function

Although we have focused on the mammalian system to describe and illustrate the anatomy and physiology of the urinary system, some appreciation of the diversity in other animals is important. For this we will describe some aspects of avian urinary physiology and anatomy. This is because of the importance of various domestic species—chickens, turkeys, ducks, geese, etc.—in production agriculture and because of many other birds utilized as pets. It is evident that birds, like all animals, must regulate water and electrolyte balance to maintain osmoregulation for homeostasis. Some reflection illustrates marked variation not just between mammals and birds but also between various bird species that occupy an enormous range of environmental niches. For example, consider marine birds that depend on seawater to provide their needs. Some wild birds can routinely obtain the water they need through their food or production of metabolic

water. The majority, however, depend on drinking to supply requirements. Consequently, just as in mammals, osmoregulation ultimately involves interactions between multiple organs and organ systems. This includes the kidneys, intestinal tract, skin, respiratory system, and salt glands (for birds that possess these structures. For our discussion, we will focus on kidneys and the cloaca.

Avian urinary organs consist of the paired kidneys and ureters, which carry urine to the urodeum of the cloaca. As a reminder, the major segments of the avian digestive tract include esophagus, proventriculus and gizzard, small intestine, cecum, and rectum. The rectum (also referred to as the colon in birds) is relatively short and serves to link the ileum of the small intestine with the coprodeal compartment of the cloaca. The cloaca acts as a common pathway for digestive wastes, excretory material, and reproductive activity. It has three chambers: coprodeum, urodeum, and proctodeum. The cranial coprodeum empties into the rectum. The middle urodeum is separated from the other two compartments by folds that serve to isolate this chamber. The urinary and reproduction tracts empty into the urodeum. Birds do not have urinary bladders.

The avian kidney is typically elongated and divided into anterior, middle, and posterior regions. Within each region there are cone-shaped subunits with a cortex and medulla called medullary cones. The medullary cone and region of associated cortex that is drained create a kidney lobule. Compared with a typical mammalian kidney, avian nephrons are very heterogeneous. Smaller nephrons, usually positioned near the surface of lobules, have simple (modestly coiled) glomeruli, and they lack loops of Henle (LLN, loopless nephrons). These were traditionally called reptilian-type (RT) nephrons because they resemble nephrons found in reptiles. Deeper in the lobules, the nephrons exhibit the loop of Henle (LN, looped nephrons). This appearance is typical of mammals—thus, the older name of mammalianlike (MT) nephrons. There are also variations in structure between the LN and LLN nephrons that are called transitional nephrons (TN). On average, about 20% of nephrons are classified as LN or MT. Regardless, both classes of nephrons empty in a regular pattern into common collecting ducts. The collecting ducts combine and descend to the end of the medullary cone where a single large collecting duct empties into the ureter. Since the tissue of the cloaca, like the large intestine, has substantial resorption capacity much of the water can ultimately be recovered.

Like the mammalian system, the avian kidney has a countercurrent multiplier arrangement where the loops of Henle parallel the collecting ducts (LN). This means that birds are capable of producing urine that is hyperosmotic to blood plasma. For example, water-deprived birds can produce urine that is approximately 2 times more concentrated than plasma. However, some mammals can produce urine that is 20 to 25 times more concentrated. This likely reflects the differences in nephron morphology described above.

Avian nitrogen excretion

Urates, ammonia, urea, and creatinine all contribute to nitrogen excretion in the urine of birds. However, based on experiments with domestic chicken, whether fed or fasted or provided low- or high-protein diets, urates constitute 55 to 84% of total nitrogen excretion. Indeed, urates are the major waste product of nitrogen-containing metabolites excreted by the urinary system of birds and most reptiles and amphibians. Secretion of urates or uricotelism is an important adaptation to allow animals with no ability of concentrate (i.e., greater osmolarity than blood plasma) urine (reptiles and amphibians) or limited capacity (birds) to survive and prosper in arid habitats. Alterations in ammonia excretion are also closely related to acid/base homeostasis.

Urate circulating in avian blood is believed to be mostly unbound and therefore available to be filtered by the glomeruli. However, given the plasma concentration and rate of filtration, clearance of urate exceeds that of inulin. It is clear that 90% or more of urinary urate comes from tubular excretion. Most urate is derived from liver metabolism of purine. Uric acid is relatively inert and markedly less toxic than ammonia or urea. After secretion or filtration the fate of uric acid varies. In an acidic environment uric acid is poorly soluble but with a typical urinary pH of 6–7 most of the uric acid exists as monobasic urate. Urate also forms salts with sodium or potassium. This is important because of the abundance of these ions in urine. Sodium and potassium urate are also much more soluble (6.8 and 12.1 mmol/liter, respectively) than uric acid (0.38 mmol/liter). However, this still does not account for the high concentrations of urate typical of avian urine. Urates can exist in supersaturated solutions because of their ability to form colloidal suspensions and to combine with mucopolysaccharides and glyoproteins, especially in the distal convoluted tubules. This is believed to minimize formation of uric acid crystals, thereby promoting the passage of urates through the nephrons and into urine. In addition, precipitated but suspended spheres of urate trap Na and K so that these ions are not free in solution; thus, these trapped ions do not impact urine osmolarity. This likely is a mechanism to enhance secretion of these ions despite the relatively small proportion of LN nephrons in the avian kidney.

Avian salt glands

For many terrestrial animals, sodium is not easy to obtain. Most fresh water is low in minerals and most plants are low in sodium. This explains why herbivores like sheep, cows, and deer, use natural salt licks or mineral rich soil. Most of these animals also have high blood levels of aldosterone, the steroid hormone important to enhance renal reabsorption of sodium to minimize losses. For marine animals excessive sodium intake is a serious issue. Yet many species of marine and shore birds can drink seawater as their only source of water for indefinite periods of time. Given the relative inability of birds to concentrate their urine, compared with most mammals, how is this possible? The answer is that there is a nonrenal pathway.

Suborbital or salt glands exist evidently in nearly all birds but are fully functional primarily in marine birds and in species that depend on hypersaline food and water. These glands are best described in the domestic duck. In fact, when ducklings never before exposed to excessive salt become osmotically stressed, the salt glands quickly begin to secrete a hypertonic sodium chloride solution, and within 48 hours cells per gland increase two- and threefold and the secretory cells become fully differentiated and active.

The glands are paired and located in depressions either in or above the orbit of the eye. The glands are also distinct from lacrimal glands. Structurally, they are composed of lobes that exhibit closed secretory units (tubuloacinar gland structures) that drain into central canals. Blood flow runs countercurrent to the direction of flow of the secretions, and the central canals coalesce into common ducts that drain into the nasal cavity. Each gland has a medial and lateral duct that receives branches from groupings of lobes or lobules. Salt gland secretions either drip or are shaken from the beak. Stimulation of secretion depends on nervous input via cranial nerve VII (glossopharyngeal) and postganglionic fibers that release acetylcholine and vasoactive intestinal peptide (VIP). Both central and peripheral receptors are thought to be involved in initial stimulation of nerve impulses. Osmoreceptors in the area of the third ventricle appear especially sensitive to increases in Na^+ concentration. Other receptors located around the heart and larger arteries respond by initiating impulses to the central nervous system via the vagus (X cranial nerve).

Salt gland secretions, as you would guess from the name, are nearly all NaCl with small amounts of K^+, Ca^{++}, HCO_3^-, and Mg^{++}. It is important to remember that just as in mammals, interactions and integration between multiple systems is required for osmotic regulation. Nonetheless, the salt glands represent a critical adaptation in these animals. For example, when the salt glands are stimulated by salt feeding or dehydration, 75% or more of Na$^+$ excretion occurs via salt gland secretion and more than 30% of K$^+$ elimination.

References

Banks, W.J. 1983. Applied Veterinary Histology. Williams and Wilkins, Baltimore/London.

Goldstein, D.L. and E.J. Braun. 1989. Structure and concentrating ability in the avian kidney. Am. J. Physiol. Regulat. Integrat. Comp. Physiol. 256: 501–509.

Haller, M., K. Rohner, W. Muller, F. Reutter, H. Binder, W. Estelberger, and P. Arnold. 2003. Single-injection inulin clearance for routine measurement of glomerular filtration rate in cats. J. Fel. Med. Surg. 5: 175–181.

Hildebrandt, J. 2001. Coping with excess salt: Adaptive functions of extrarenal osmoregulatory organs in vertebrates. Zool. 104: 209–220.

Hughes, M.R. 2003. Regulation of salt gland, gut and kidney interactions. Compar. Biochem. Physiol. Part A 136: 507–524.

Randall, D., W. Burggen, and K. French. 2002. Eckert Animal Physiology. W.H. Freeman and Company, New York.

Whittow, G.C., ed. 2000. Sturkie's Avian Physiology, 5th edition. Academic Press, San Diego, California.

17

Digestive system

Contents

Digestive system overview

All animals need a supply of nutrients and oxygen that are obtained via the digestive system and respiratory system, respectively. The digestive system consists of the digestive tract, also called the gastrointestinal or alimentary tract, and its accessory organs. The accessory organs include the teeth, tongue, salivary glands, liver, pancreas, and gallbladder.

The digestive tract is a muscular tube running through the body extending from the mouth to the anus. Contents within the digestive tract are considered outside the body, so in addition to digesting and absorbing nutrients, the digestive tract must act as a barrier blocking the entry of pathogenic organisms.

Functions of the digestive tract

The digestive tract has eight functions:

1. Ingestion. This is the active process of bringing material into the oral cavity.
2. Propulsion. Ingested materials are moved through the digestive tract by swallowing and peristalsis (*peri* = around + *stalsis* = constriction), which involves alternating waves of contraction and relaxation of muscles along the digestive tract wall (Fig. 17.1), and is the major propulsive mechanism moving food through the tract.
3. Mechanical processing. Material entering the digestive tract is physically reduced in size. This begins in the oral cavity where food is crushed

A.

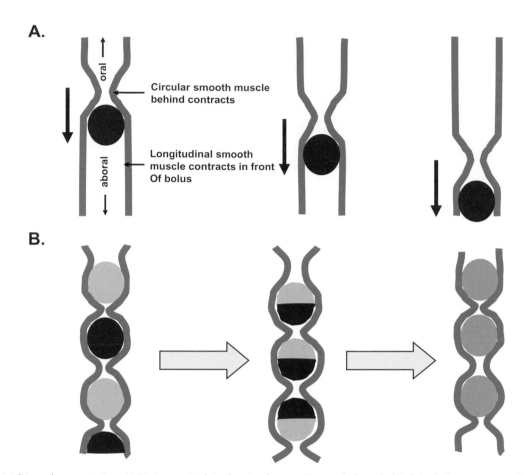

oral

Circular smooth muscle
behind contracts

Longitudinal smooth
muscle contracts in front
Of bolus

aboral

B.

Fig. 17.1.   Peristalsis and segmentation. A) During peristalsis, the circular smooth muscle layer behind the bolus contracts while that in front of the bolus relaxes. Conversely, the longitudinal smooth muscle layer behind the bolus relaxes while that in front of the bolus contracts. This increases the diameter of the lumen in front of the bolus while constricting the diameter of the lumen behind the bolus. This results in propulsion of the bolus down the digestive tract. B) During segmentation, nonadjacent sections of the digestive tract contract and relax, resulting in mixing of the contents.

and sheared before being propelled along the digestive tract. The reduction in size of ingested material increases its surface area, thereby facilitating enzymatic digestion. In the case of ruminant animals, food materials are also moved from the stomach back to the mouth for further reduction in particle size. Food is also churned along the digestive tract by segmental contractions (Fig. 17.1), which further mix the contents with digestive juices, but do not advance their movement.

4.   Digestion. Following reduction in size, ingested nutrients are chemically broken down into particles small enough for absorption. Although simple molecules such as monosaccharides and amino acids can be absorbed without further reduction in size, macromolecules such as protein, DNA, polysaccharides, and triglycerides must first be reduced into smaller molecules. Specific enzymes complete such reduction.

5.   Secretion. Water, mucous, acids, enzymes, buffers, and salts are released into the lumen of the digestive tract along its length. Secretions come from epithelial cells and glandular organs.

6.   Absorption. Along the length of the digestive tract, nutrients including organic substrates, electrolytes, vitamins, and water pass from the lumen into the body. In addition to absorbing ingested nutrients, the digestive tract must absorb secreted water, salts, and other secreted material. Failure of such absorption will result in dehydration.

7.   Excretion. The digestive tract is a site of elimination of waste products. Such waste products can be eliminated via either defecation or egestion.

8.   Immunity. The digestive tract must provide a substantial barrier to prevent the entry of pathogens into the body. The digestive tract acts not only as a physical barrier, but also has an innate immune system.

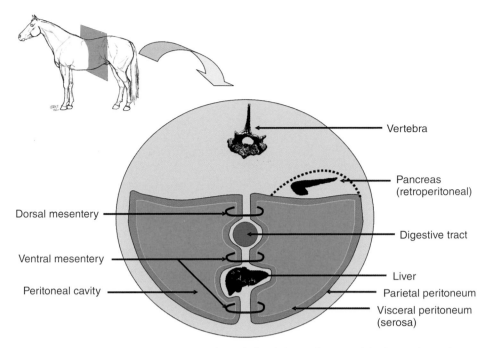

Vertebra

Pancreas
(retroperitoneal)

Dorsal mesentery

Digestive tract

Ventral mesentery

Liver

Peritoneal cavity

Parietal peritoneum

Visceral peritoneum
(serosa)

Fig. 17.2. Peritoneum and peritoneal cavity. The cross section through the abdominal cavity of the horse shows the visceral and parietal peritoneum, and the dorsal and ventral mesentery. Although not shown, the peritoneal cavity is filled with organs. Note that some organs, such as the pancreas, are located in a retroperitoneal position, or outside the peritoneal cavity.

Peritoneal cavity

The peritoneal cavity is formed from a serous membrane, called the peritoneum, which lines the abdominopelvic cavity, forming the largest serous membrane in the body (Fig. 17.2). It consists of a layer of simple squamous epithelium, the mesothelium, with an underlying connective tissue layer. The peritoneal membrane has a serosa, or visceral layer, that covers the organs in the peritoneal cavity, and a parietal peritoneum that lines the inner surface of the body wall.

The peritoneal membrane produces peritoneal fluid providing lubrication between the serosa and parietal layers, called the peritoneal cavity, thus reducing friction and irritation. Diseases of the liver, kidney, and heart can cause increases in this fluid production producing an abdominal swelling called ascites. Accumulation of this fluid can distort the internal organs, causing pain and discomfort.

Mesenteries

The mesentery consists of two layers of serous membranes fused back to back, and suspends portions of the digestive tract from the body wall. The mesenteries have three functions: 1) provide a route for blood vessels, lymphatic vessels, and nerves to travel to the digestive system; 2) hold organs in place; and 3) store lipid.

During embryonic development, the digestive organs are suspended from the body wall by the dorsal and ventral mesentery. The ventral mesentery largely disappears except on the ventral surface of the stomach, between the stomach and liver and between the liver and the ventral abdominal wall. The mesenteries are named for the organs they supply (e.g., mesoduodenum, mesoileum, mesocolon).

The omentum refers to those portions of the mesentery connecting the stomach to the abdominal organs or abdominal wall. In animals with simple stomachs, such as carnivores, pigs, and horses, the greater omentum connects the greater curvature of the stomach to the dorsal abdominal wall (Fig. 17.3). It folds over itself forming deep and superficial layers (i.e., four layers). It normally contains considerable adipose tissue. The lesser omentum connects the lesser curvature of the stomach and initial segment of the duodenum with the liver. The falciform ligament attaches the liver to the ventral midline while the hepatoduodenal ligament connects the liver to the proximal duodenum.

In ruminants, the superficial and deep portions of the greater omentum attach to the left side of the rumen and the right side of the rumen, respectively. They tract toward the right side of the animal attaching to the intestine and then to the right abdominal wall. Although most abdominal organs are located within the peritoneum, some are located between the posterior parietal peritoneum and the posterior

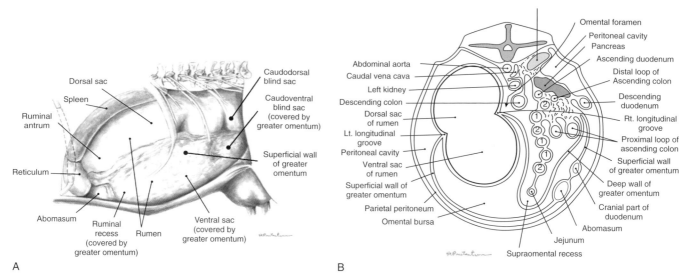

Fig. 17.3. Arrangement of mesenteries in ruminants. A) In this view of the left side of a large ruminant, the greater omentum is visible. B) A cross section of the flank of a large ruminant showing greater omentum and peritoneum. (Reprinted from Constantinescu and Constantinescu, 2004. Used by permission of the publisher.)

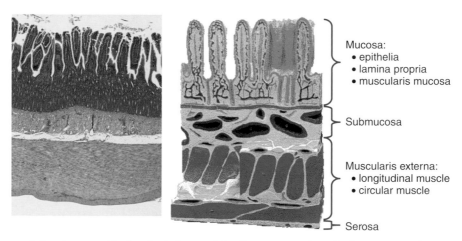

Fig. 17.4. Basic structure of digestive tract. The four basic layers of the digestive tract, from the lumen outward, are the mucosa, submucosa, muscularis externa, and serosa.

abdominal wall, and are thus outside this cavity and are said to be retroperitoneal (*retro* = behind). These organs include the kidneys, adrenal glands, ureters, duodenum, ascending colon, descending colon, and pancreas. Those organs whose mesenteries remain inside the peritoneal cavity are called intraperitoneal or peritoneal organs.

Blood supply of the digestive organs

The splanchnic circulation serves the digestive organs and hepatic portal system. The arteries of this system include the hepatic, splenic, and left gastric branches of the celiac trunk serving the spleen, liver, and stomach, respectively, and the mesenteric arteries serving the small and large intestines. At rest, the splanchnic circulation receives approximately 25% of the cardiac output.

Histology of the digestive tract

The digestive tract includes four major layers (Fig. 17.4). Listed from the lumen outward, they are 1) the mucosa, 2) the submucosa, 3) the muscularis externa, and 4) the serosa. These layers vary somewhat according to region of the digestive tract, so the following description applies to the small intestine.

Mucosa

The mucosa layer is a mucous membrane lining the inside of the digestive tract. It consists of three sub-layers including a layer of epithelial tissue in direct contact with the contents of the digestive tract, the lamina propria, and the muscularis mucosae.

Within the oral cavity, pharynx, esophagus, and anal canal, the epithelial tissue is stratified squamous epithelium that performs a protective function. The remainder of the tract is mostly simple columnar epithelium and mucous-producing goblet cells. Shortly after birth, the simple columnar epithelial cells develop tight junctions, thus forming a barrier between the lumen contents and the body. Prior to the formation of these tight junctions, an animal is able to absorb antibodies found in the colostrum until the epithelial cells undergo closure, or until the development of tight junctions. Closure generally occurs within a couple days after birth. Also found scattered among the epithelial cells are endocrine cells, collectively called enterendocrine cells, which secrete hormones coordinating digestive functions.

The epithelial cells have a life span of approximately 2–3 days in the esophagus and up to 6 days in the large intestine. These cells are always being sloughed off, and they are continually replaced.

The lamina propria, consisting of areolar connective tissue, binds the epithelial cells to the muscularis mucosae. This layer also contains blood vessels, sensory neurons, lymphatic vessels, smooth muscle cells, and lymphatic nodules that are part of the mucosa-associated lymphatic system (MALT). The MALT is present along the digestive tract and contains cells of the immune system. The appendix and tonsils are part of the MALT.

The muscularis mucosa is a thin layer of smooth muscle fibers. This layer helps create folds in the stomach and small intestine, thus increasing their surface area.

Submucosa

The submucosa consists of dense irregular connective tissue and contains large blood vessels, lymphatic vessels, and—in some regions—exocrine glands secreting buffers and enzymes into the lumen.

Muscularis externa

Within the oral cavity, pharynx, and parts of the esophagus, depending on the species, this layer contains skeletal muscle that controls swallowing. The external anal sphincter also generally contains skeletal muscle permitting voluntary control of defecation. Along the remainder of the digestive tract, the muscularis externa generally consists of two layers of smooth muscle: an inner layer of circular smooth muscle fibers and an outer layer of longitudinal smooth muscle fibers. These layers control peristalsis and segmental contractions.

Serosa

Most portions of the digestive tract lie within the peritoneal cavity. The outermost portions, or superficial layer, of the digestive tract is lined with the adventitia. As the digestive tract passes through the diaphragm and enters the peritoneal cavity, this layer is composed of the visceral portion of the peritoneum, also called the serosa. There is no serosa around the oral cavity, pharynx, esophagus or rectum. Instead there is a layer of collagen fibers attaching the digestive tract to surrounding structures.

Enteric nervous system

The digestive tract has its own nervous system, called the enteric (*enteric* = gut) nervous system, sometimes called the "brain of the gut." It is composed mostly of two large plexuses: the submucosal plexus and myenteric plexus. If the digestive tract is deinnervated, it will begin to function near normally due to the sensory and motor neurons in the enteric nervous system.

The submucosal plexus, or Meissner's plexus, is located within the submucosal layer. It includes sensory and motor neurons, and postganglionic fibers of both the sympathetic and parasympathetic nervous system. It regulates the activity of glands and smooth muscle in the mucosa.

The myenteric plexus, or plexus of Auerbach, is located between the two layers of smooth muscle fibers in the muscularis externa. These neurons coordinate the frequency and strength of digestive tract motility. Therefore, this plexus controls patterns of peristalsis and segmentation through automatic local reflex arcs.

The enteric nervous system also communicates with the central nervous system via afferent visceral fibers of the sympathetic and parasympathetic branches of the autonomic nervous system. The autonomic nervous system also exerts extrinsic control over the functions of the digestive tract. Parasympathetic input generally enhances digestive functions, whereas sympathetic input inhibits these functions.

Table 17.1.   Length and capacity of the parts of the digestive tract.

Species	Part of Digestive Tract	Relative Length of Intestines (%)	Average Length (m)	Relative Capacity (%)	Absolute Capacity (L)
Cat	Stomach			69.5	0.34
	Small intestine	83	1.72	14.6	0.11
	Cecum			15.9	
	Large intestine	17	0.35		0.12
Chicken	Small intestine	79	1.08		
	Cecum	9	0.13		
	Large intestine	5	0.68		
Dog	Stomach			62.3	4.33
	Small intestine	85	4.14	23.3	0.09
	Cecum	2	0.08	1.3	0.09
	Large intestine	13	0.60	13.1	0.91
Horse	Stomach			8.5	17.96
	Small intestine	75	22.44	30.2	63.82
	Cecum	4	1.00	15.9	33.54
	Large intestine	21	6.47	38.4	81.25
Pig	Stomach			29.2	8.00
	Small intestine	78	18.29	33.5	9.20
	Cecum	1	0.23	5.6	1.55
	Large intestine	21	4.99	31.7	8.70
Sheep and goats	Rumen			52.9	23.40
	Reticulum			4.5	2.00
	Omasum			2.0	0.90
	Abomasum			7.5	3.30
	Small intestine	80	26.2	20.4	9.00
	Cecum	1	0.36	2.3	1.00
	Large intestine	19	6.17	10.4	4.60

Adapted from Swenson and Reece, 1993.

Functional anatomy of the digestive system

The digestive system shows great variation among species (Table 17.1). These variations in structure are necessary depending on whether the animal is a carnivore (meat-eating), herbivore (plant-eating) or omnivore (meat- and plant-eating). A rabbit is a typical nonruminant example; its stomach and small intestine are relatively small, whereas the cecum is well developed in order to allow for microbial digestion. Nonruminant herbivores typically have a well-developed cecum since this is the primary site of cellulose digestion. Ruminants have a complex stomach that accommodates microbial digestion, a proportionately long small intestine and a large colon. Carnivores, such as dogs and cats, have a short small intestine, poorly developed cecum, and average colon. The pig, which is an omnivore, has an intermediate size colon since this is a major site of microbial digestion.

Further evolutionary adaptations have occurred in the stomach and gastrointestinal tract of animals to accommodate differing methods of digesting carbohydrates. As a result, animals can be classified into four groups as follows. The first group includes animals with a simple stomach, such as humans, pigs, dogs and cats. The second group is foregut fermenters, which includes cattle, sheep, and goats. These animals have a ruminant stomach in which they can ferment nondigestible carbohydrates. The third group consists of hindgut fermenters such as horses, rabbits, guinea pigs, etc. These animals rely on fermentation that occurs in the cecum. The final group consists of birds in which various adaptations have occurred to both store and grind various foodstuffs.

Mouth

The mouth is the space extending from the lips or beak to the pharynx and it is bounded laterally by the cheeks. It is also called the oral cavity, or buccal cavity, and is where food first enters the digestive tract. The mouth is lined with stratified squamous epithelium, which protects against friction. For further protection,

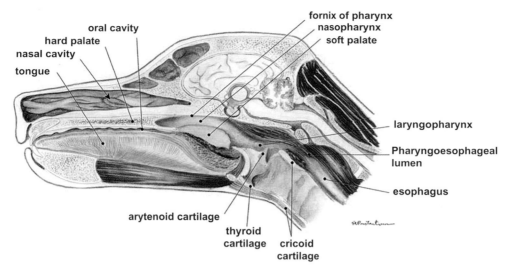

Fig. 17.5. Oral cavity. The hard and soft palate of the mouth is visible in the median section through the head of a dog. (Reprinted from Constantinescu, 2002. Used by permission of the publisher.)

the epithelium of the gums, hard palate, and dorsum of the tongue are slightly keratinized.

Lips, cheeks, and gums

The lips and cheeks contain skeletal muscle covered by skin. The orbicularis oris muscle forms the lips. The lips possess long, tactile hair, and regular hair. The median cleft of the upper lip in carnivores and small ruminants is called the philtrum.

The cheeks form the caudolateral wall of the oral cavity. The gums, or gingivae, enclose the necks of the teeth. The oral cavity is divided into the vestibule and oral cavity proper. The vestibule (porch) is the recess bounded internally by the gums and teeth and externally by the lips and cheeks. The oral cavity proper lies within the teeth and gums.

The palate is the roof of the oral cavity and oropharynx, and it separates the respiratory and digestive passages within the head (Fig. 17.5). It consists of a rostral bony part called the hard palate and a caudal musculomembranous portion called the soft palate. The horse is unable to voluntarily raise its soft palate, and therefore breathes through its nose. The hard palate is formed by the palatine, maxillary, and incisive bones. It forms a hard surface against which the tongue can press food.

The soft palate divides the rostral region of the pharynx into the oral and nasal portions. Projecting downward from the soft palate is the fingerlike uvula. The soft palate closes the nasopharynx as the animal swallows. Birds, unlike mammals, lack a soft palate. The oral and pharyngeal cavities are combined and referred to as the oropharynx.

Tongue

The tongue is the muscular organ filling most of the oral cavity. It is composed of interlacing bundles of skeletal muscle fibers, and it is involved in gripping, repositioning food, mixing food with saliva, and forming the compact mass of food called a bolus.

The tongue has intrinsic and extrinsic muscles. The intrinsic muscles, confined to the tongue and not attached to bone, run in several directions allowing the tongue to change shape as necessary for prehension, moving food, and making sounds. The extrinsic muscles attach the tongue to bones of the skull and the soft palate. They allow the tongue to protrude, retract and move side to side. The lingual frenulum attaches the tongue to the floor of the mouth.

The superior surface of the tongue has many papillae that are named for their shape. Filiform papillae are thorn-shaped, giving the tongue roughness and thus aiding in licking and manipulating food. They have a mechanical function. In the ox and cat, they are heavily cornified. Fungiform papillae are mushroom-shaped, scattered among the more numerous filiform papillae, have taste buds, and are thus mechanical and gustatory (Fig. 17.6). Foliate papillae have a series of leaf-shaped ridges, are located on the lateral borders of the tongue, and have a gustatory function. They are absent in the ox. Vallate, or circumvallate, papillae are the largest and least numerous. They are located in a V-shaped row near the back of the tongue. They resemble the fungiform papillae, but are circled by a cleft containing taste buds. Marginal taste buds are found along the edge of the rostral portion of the tongue of newborn dogs, but they disappear when puppies switch to solid food.

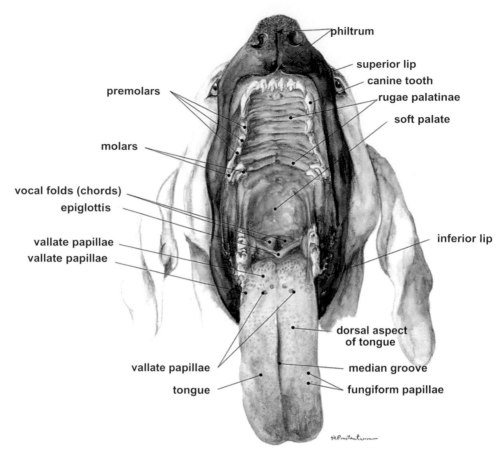

Fig. 17.6. Tongue of the dog. The vallate and fungiform papillae are shown on the tongue of the dog. (Reprinted from Constantinescu, 2002. Used by permission of the publisher.)

Salivary glands and saliva

Salivary glands are extramural glands (glands outside the wall of the digestive system) that are associated with the oral cavity. The secretions of the salivary glands can be serous, mucous, or mixed. Serous cells produce a watery secretion containing enzymes, ions, and a small amount of mucin, whereas mucous cells produce a viscous, stringy secretion called mucous. Minor salivary glands are located within the wall of the oral cavity and oral pharynx, and have short ducts. They are named for their location (labial, buccal, palatal). They are mixed glands, meaning they have mucous and serous secretions.

The major salivary glands are located some distance from the oral cavity, and require ducts to carry their secretions. The parotid salivary gland is located below the ear (auricular) cartilage, between the masseter muscle and skin (Fig. 17.7). The parotid duct parallels the zygomatic arch and opens into the buccal vestibule. It produces a predominantly serous secretion. The mandibular (submandibular, submaxillary) salivary gland is located caudal to the angle of the jaw, and is a mixed gland. The mandibular duct runs ros-

trally along with the sublingual duct, medial to the mandible, and opens near the sublingual caruncle. The sublingual salivary gland is under the tongue and secretes mostly mucous.

Saliva consists of water (97 to 99.5%), and is therefore hypoosmotic. Electrolytes in the saliva include sodium, potassium, chloride, bicarbonate, and phosphate. It tends to be slightly acidic, (pH 6.75–7.00). Saliva has several functions:

1. Solubilizes food. Dissolves foods so they can be tasted and digestive reactions can occur.
2. Provides alkaline buffering and fluid. Bicarbonate and phosphate in the saliva can neutralize acidic feedstuffs. As discussed below, the addition of alkaline fluid via the saliva is particularly important in ruminants.
3. Removes wastes. Metabolic waste products such as urea and uric acid are excreted in the saliva.
4. Lubricates and binds. The mucous in the saliva helps bind masticated food so that it can be formed into a bolus. In addition, saliva coats the oral cavity and esophagus, thus protecting the mucosa of the oral cavity and esophagus.

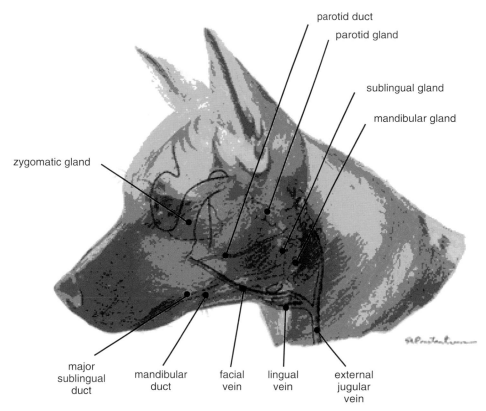

Fig. 17.7. Salivary glands. The major salivary glands are shown in the dog. (Drawings from Constantinescu, 2002, and Constantinescu and Constantinescu, 2004.)

5. Initiates starch digestion. Salivary amylase begins starch digestion.
6. Assists oral hygiene. Lysozyme, found in saliva, is a bacteriostatic enzyme that lyses bacteria, thus protecting the mouth. IgA attaches to microbes, thus decreasing their ability to penetrate the epithelium. Cyanide, found in saliva, acts as a bacteriocide and a cyanide compound while defensins act as cytokines to attract lymphoctyes and neutrophils that protect against microbes.
7. Enables evaporative cooling. This is particularly important in dogs, which have very poorly developed sweat glands. However, it is also used by cats that preen themselves and avian species that display gular flutter (very rapid, but shallow, respiration).

In nonruminants, as the secretion of saliva increases the concentration of Na^+, bicarbonate, and Cl^- increase while K^+ decreases. In ruminants, as saliva production increases, the levels of Na^+ and PO_4^- in the saliva decrease while that of bicarbonate, Cl^-, and K^+ increase.

Salivary glands continuously secrete saliva, thus keeping the oral cavity moist. However, presence of food increases salivation due to parasympathetic nervous system stimulation. Chemoreceptors and mechanoreceptors send signals to the superior and inferior salivatory nuclei in the brain stem. Parasympathetic impulses travel via the facial nerve (cranial nerve VII) and glossopharyngeal nerve (cranial nerve IX) to stimulate salivation.

The sight, smell, sound, or thought of food can also stimulate saliva production. This was evidenced when Pavlov trained dogs to salivate at the sound of a bell. Such salivation helps initiate digestion as soon as food enters the oral cavity.

The saliva in ruminants is isotonic, containing high concentrations of bicarbonate and phosphate, and a high pH. This saliva acts to buffer the acids produced during fermentation in the rumen. An adult cow can produce as much as 100 to 200 l of saliva daily.

Teeth

The teeth, or dentes, are accessory digestive organs. They are located in the sockets of the alveolar processes of the mandible and maxillae. Domestic animals have two types of teeth: low-crowned (brachydont) and high-crowned (hypsodont). All domestic species have two sets of teeth, deciduous and permanent. Deciduous teeth are smaller and fewer in number.

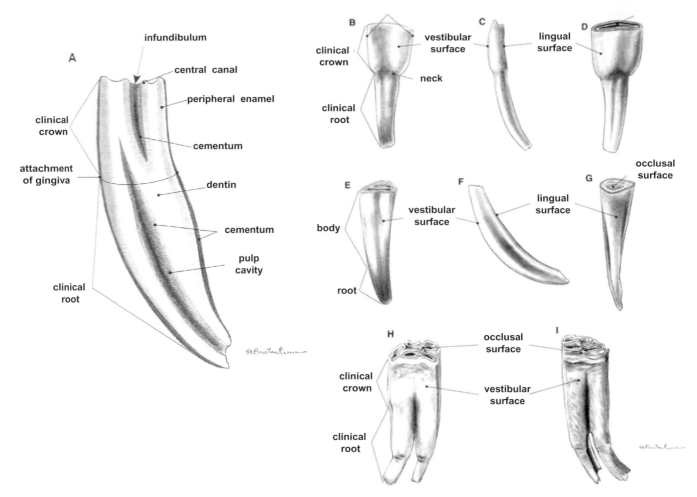

Fig. 17.8. Teeth of the horse. Vertical section of a permanent incisor (A). Vestibular surface (B), left side (C), and lingual surface (D) of the first right-lower deciduous incisor. Vestibular surface (E), left side (F), and lingual surface (G) of first right-lower permanent incisor. Third right-lower permanent premolar (H) and second left-lower permanent molar (I). (Reprinted from Constantinescu and Constantinescu, 2004. Used by permission of the publisher.)

Low-crowned teeth are simple teeth, as found in man, carnivores, pigs, ruminant incisors, and horse deciduous incisors. They consist of a crown, neck, and root. The crown is the part projecting above the gum line, and is covered with enamel. The neck is the constriction between the crown and root, and it is located at the gum line. The root is the part below the gum line. High-crowned teeth, which have no distinct neck, are found in all permanent horse teeth, ruminant cheek teeth (i.e., premolars and molars), and the tusks of pigs.

Teeth are composed of three layers: cementum, enamel, and dentin (Fig. 17.8). Cementum, a thin, bonelike covering is found on the entire tooth of high-crowned teeth, but only on the root of low-crowned teeth. It attaches the root to the periodontal ligament. Enamel, the hardest substance in the body (consisting of 95% calcium salts by dry weight) covers the crown of low-crowned teeth and the body (portion of tooth below crown in high-crowned teeth) and crown of

high-crowned teeth. The enamel protects the dentin from acids. Dentin, which makes up the bulk of the tooth, is similar to bone only harder because it has a higher content of calcium salts.

The dentin surrounds a cavity. Within the crown, this cavity is the pulp cavity, and it is filled with pulp, a connective tissue containing blood vessels, nerves, and lymphatic vessels. Narrow extensions of the pulp cavity project into the roots, and are called the root canals.

Teeth are divided into groups according to their location and function. Incisors are located in the rostral portion of the mouth (Fig. 17.9). The upper incisors are embedded in the incisive bone and the lower incisors in the incisive part of the mandible. The canine is the large tooth between the incisors and cheek teeth. Cheek teeth are those teeth caudal to the canine and incisors in the maxillary. They include the premolars located in the rostral cheek area and molars located caudal to the premolars. Cheek teeth function in

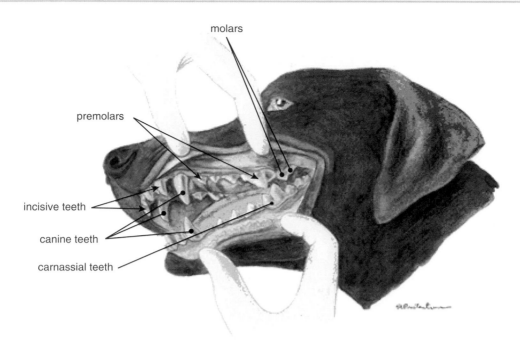

molars

premolars

incisive teeth

canine teeth

carnassial teeth

Fig. 17.9. Teeth of the dog. (Reprinted from Constantinescu, 2002. Used by permission of the publisher.)

Table 17.2. Number of teeth.

Species	Deciduous	Permanent
Cat	2 (I 3/3 C 1/1 P 3/2) = 26	2 (I 3/3 C 1/1 P 3/2 M 1/1) = 30
Dog	2(I 3/3 C 1/1 P 3/3) = 28	2 (I 3/3 C 1/1 P 4/4 M 2/3) = 42
Horse	2(I 3/3 C 0/0 P 3/3) = 24	2(I 3/3 C 1(0)/1(0) P 3(4)/3 M 3/3) = 36–42
Pig	2(I 3/3 C 1/1 P 3/3) = 28	2 (I 3/3 C 1/1 P 4/4 M 3/3) = 44
Ruminant	2(I 0/4 P 3/3) = 20	2(I 0/4 P 3/3 M 3/3) = 32

Due to bilateral symmetry, only half the teeth are numbered within the parentheses of the shorthand representation. The numerator represents the teeth in the upper jaw and the denominator represents the teeth in the lower jaw. The number in the parentheses must be multiplied by 2 to get the total number of teeth. I = Incisors; C = Canine; P = premolars; M = molars.

grinding while incisors are merely for shearing and biting.

Pigs have 44 teeth; other domestic species have fewer due to a decreased number of cheek teeth (Table 17.2). Ruminants lack upper incisors and canines, which are replaced by a dental pad. They also lack the 1st upper and lower premolar, giving them 32 permanent teeth. Dogs are missing the upper 3rd molars, and therefore have 42 teeth. Brachiocephalic breeds (those dogs that have shortened noses and very prominent eyes due to shallow orbit) may be missing additional teeth. Horses are usually missing the 1st upper premolar and always missing the lower 1st premolar. Mares often have smaller canines that may not erupt. As a result, horses may possess 36 to 42 permanent teeth. Various terms used when discussing teeth are shown in Table 17.3.

The eruption and wear of the lower incisors can be used to estimate a horse's age (Fig. 17.10). If no permanent incisors are present, the horse is probably under 2-1/2 years old. Deciduous teeth are characterized by a distinct neck, and are smaller and usually lack longitudinal ridges seen in permanent teeth. The incisors erupt at the following times: I1, 2-1/2 years; I2, 3-1/2 years; and I3, 4-1/2 years. If all incisors have erupted, and I3 is worn such that a little dentin is seen, the horse is approximately 5 years old. Disappearance of the cup from the respective lower incisors can indicate age as follows: I1, 6 years old; I2, 7 years old; and I3, 8 years old. Disappearance of the cup from the upper incisors can indicate age as follows: I1, 9 years old; I2, 10 years old; I3, 11 years old.

Pharynx

The pharynx is the common passageway for food and air. As food first passes from the mouth, it enters the pharynx. It extends from the internal nares to the esophagus. It connects the nasal and oral cavities with

Table 17.3. Nomenclature for teeth.

Term	Meaning
Floating	The filing off of sharp edges (points) of the horse's cheek teeth
Needle teeth	The pig's deciduous third incisors and canines; they are often nipped off in newborn pigs to benefit the sow suckling
Parrot mouth	Seen in a horse when the mandible is shortened
Scissor mouth	Seen in a horse when an oblique angle to the incisors forms on the occlusal surface due to uneven wear
Shear mouth	Seen in a horse in which there is a narrow lower dental arch requiring frequent floating
Sow mouth	Seen in a horse when the mandible is elongated
Tusks	The canine teeth of the pig; the lower tusks are larger than the upper
Wolf teeth	The horse's rudimentary upper first premolars, which are usually absent

the trachea and esophagus, respectively. The soft palate divides the rostral portion of the pharynx into the oropharynx and nasopharynx, and the caudal-most portion of the pharynx is called the laryngopharynx (Fig. 17.11). The nasopharynx is located dorsal to the soft palate extending from the caudal nares to the laryngopharynx with the caudal edge of the soft palate and palatopharyngeal arches separating it from the laryngopharynx. The oropharynx lies ventral to the soft palate. The laryngopharynx is where air crosses to the larynx and food and water crosses to the esophagus. It is located between the base of the epiglottis and esophageal entrance.

The tonsils are an aggregation of lymphatic tissue in the mucosa of the pharynx. They are named for their location (i.e., palatine, pharyngeal, or tubal, which are found around the auditory tube). They help protect the pharyngeal opening against microorganisms and toxic substances. In birds, there is no sharp distinction between the pharynx and mouth.

Swallowing

The act of swallowing, or deglutition, moves food from the mouth, through the pharynx to the esophagus, so that it can be transported to the stomach. Saliva and mucus facilitate this movement. Swallowing involves three stages:

1. Voluntary stage. Bolus moved into the oropharynx.

2. Pharyngeal stage. Bolus moves involuntarily through the pharynx to the esophagus.
3. Esophageal stage. Bolus moves involuntarily through the esophagus to the stomach.

The tongue, after forming a bolus, propels it from the oral cavity to the oropharynx (Fig. 17.12). This is carried out by skeletal muscle fibers, and is thus the voluntary stage. The presence of a bolus in the oropharynx initiates the pharyngeal stage in which impulses are carried to the deglutition center in the medullar oblongata and lower pons of the brain stem. Motor signals from these centers close off the nasopharynx, and cause the larynx to move forward and upward, allowing the epiglottis to move backward and downward sealing off the rima glottides, the opening in the larynx. After the bolus travels from the laryngopharynx to the esophagus, the respiratory passageways reopen.

Esophagus

The esophagus is a collapsible muscular tube lying behind the trachea. It extends from the laryngopharynx, passes through the mediastinum, pierces the diaphragm at the esophageal hiatus, and ends at the superior portion of the stomach. A hiatal hernia occurs when a part of the stomach protrudes through the diaphragm at the esophageal hiatus.

In many species of birds, the upper portion of the esophagus is expanded to form the crop. The crop stores food and, in some species (i.e., pigeons), produces a secretion called crop milk that is used to feed the young.

Histology of the esophagus

The esophagus has four layers, as described previously in this chapter. The outermost layer is the adventitia rather than the serosa since the areolar connective tissue is not covered by mesothelium, and the connective tissue merges with structures in the mediastinum, thus attaching the esophagus to surrounding structures. The muscularis externa layer varies in the proportion of skeletal and smooth muscle, depending on the species. The esophagus of birds consists entirely of smooth muscle; that of cats, dogs, pigs, and ruminants consists mostly of smooth muscle, with a small portion of skeletal muscle just as the esophagus nears the stomach.

Stomach

The stomach is located at the inferior end of the esophagus and cranial portion of the abdominal cavity. It is found left of the median plane. It has four functions:

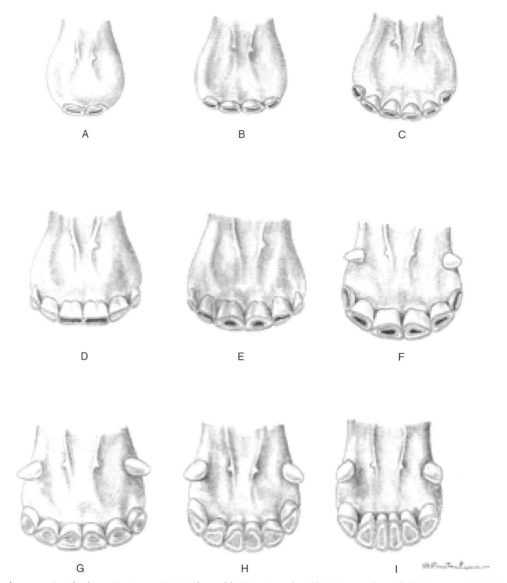

Fig. 17.10.   Aging horses using the lower incisors. A) 4–7 days old. B) 3–5 weeks old. C) 7 months old. D) 3 years old. E) 4 years old. F) 5 years old. G) 10 years old. H) 15 years old. I) 20 years old. (Reprinted from Constantinescu and Constantinescu, 2004. Used by permission of the publisher.)

1) storage of ingested food, 2) mechanical breakdown of ingested food, 3) disruption of chemical bonds of food through the action of acids and enzymes, and 4) production of the intrinsic factor required for vitamin B_{12} absorption from the small intestine. Monogastric animals have a single, simple stomach, and ruminants have a complex stomach consisting of four chambers. The true stomach is the area that produces hydrochloric acid.

Anatomy of the monogastric stomach

In monogastric animals, the stomach appears as a J-shaped structure. Its concave lateral surface is the greater curvature, and the smaller concave medial surface is the lesser curvature. The greater and lesser omentum attach to the greater and lesser curvature, respectively.

In addition to the circular and longitudinal smooth muscle layers found along the remainder of the digestive tract, the muscularis externa of the stomach has an additional inner oblique or transverse layer. This extra layer of muscle helps strengthen the stomach wall and assist with mixing the chyme (kīm), the partially digested food, with enzymes and acid. As food is ingested, the muscles of the stomach relax to accommodate the increased volume of food. While relaxed, prominent folds called rugae are visible on the stomach mucosa. As the stomach expands, the rugae spread or flatten out.

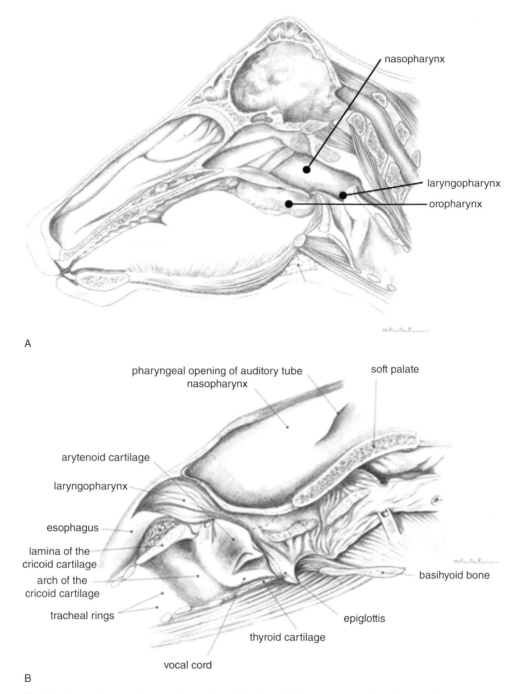

Fig. 17.11. Upper digestive tract of horse. A) A median section of the head of the horse showing the nasopharynx, oropharynx, and laryngopharynx. B) An expanded drawing of the pharynx and larynx. (Reprinted from Constantinescu, 2004. Used by permission of the publisher.)

The stomach is typically divided into four regions (Fig. 17.13):

1. Cardia. The cardia is the smallest region, and is found at the junction between the stomach and esophagus. It is located near the heart, and thus is the "cardia" region. This region contains numerous mucous glands that help protect the esophagus from the acids and enzymes of the stomach.

2. Fundus. The fundus lies superior to the junction between the cardia region, acting as a blind-ended sac.

3. Body. The body, the largest region, is located between the fundus and the pylorus. The body functions as a mixing tank for the stomach, and it is the site where most acid and enzyme secretion occurs.

4. Pyloric region. The pyloric region is the caudal-most portion of the stomach. It consists of the

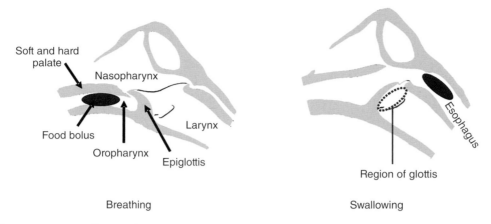

Breathing   Swallowing

Fig. 17.12. Swallowing. During swallowing, the tongue forces the bolus into the oropharynx, thus raising the soft palate and closing off the nasopharynx. Then, the larynx rises allowing the epiglottis to cover the glottis, directing the bolus to the esophagus while preventing its entry into the larynx. Once in the esophagus, the bolus is moved to the stomach by peristaltic waves. (Figure modified from Pasquini et al., 1995.)

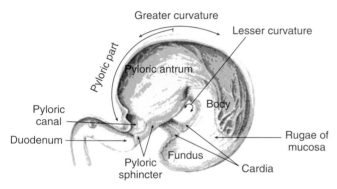

Fig. 17.13. Stomach of the horse. (Reprinted from Budras et al., 2003.)

pyloric antrum (*antrum* = cave) connected to the body. The pyloric antrum narrows to the pyloric canal, which connects to the pylorus. The pylorus is separated from the duodenum by the pyloric sphincter. The pyloric sphincter consists of modified smooth muscle that acts as a valve controlling the flow of chyme exiting the stomach.

The stomach is innervated by fibers from the autonomic nervous system. Sympathetic fibers originate from the thoracic splanchnic nerves and carry signals to the celiac plexus. Parasympathetic fibers are supplied by the vagus nerve (cranial nerve X). The arterial supply comes from branches of the gastric and splenic arteries; the veins are part of the hepatic portal system.

Histology of the monogastric stomach

The stomach is lined with simple columnar epithelium with goblet cells. The many goblet cells produce a layer of mucous protecting the mucosal surface of

the stomach. Gastric pits, or shallow depressions, are visible on the mucosal surface. The walls of the gastric pits are formed mainly from goblet cells. Gastric pits open into gastric glands (Fig. 17.14). The gastric glands are composed of different cells depending on the stomach region. The cardia and pyloric regions contain primarily mucus-secreting cells, and the glands in the pyloric antrum produce mucus and hormones including gastrin. In the fundus, the glands produce the majority of the stomach secretions, including acid. There are four cell types in gastric glands.

1. Mucous neck cells. Found in the upper, or neck, region of a gastric gland, they produce a more acidic mucus than goblet cells.
2. Parietal cells. Found in the middle region, they secrete hydrochloric acid (HCl) and intrinsic factor. Intrinsic factor is a glycoprotein necessary for absorption of vitamin B_{12} in the small intestine. These cells are shaped like pitchforks with three prongs, each covered extensively with microvilli, thus increasing their surface area for secretion. The HCl decreases the pH of the stomach to 1.5–3.5. This low pH has several functions: 1) it is necessary for the function of pepsin, 2) it provides a harsh environment for bacteria ingested with food, 3) it denatures proteins and inactivates enzymes in food, and 4) it breaks down cell walls of plant material and connective tissue in meat.
3. Chief cells. These cells produce pepsinogen, the inactive form of pepsin, and an enzyme that digests proteins. When pepsinogen is first released, it interacts with HCl and converts it to its active form, pepsin. Once activated, pepsin can convert other molecules of pepsinogen to pepsin. Chief cells also secrete minor amounts of lipases.

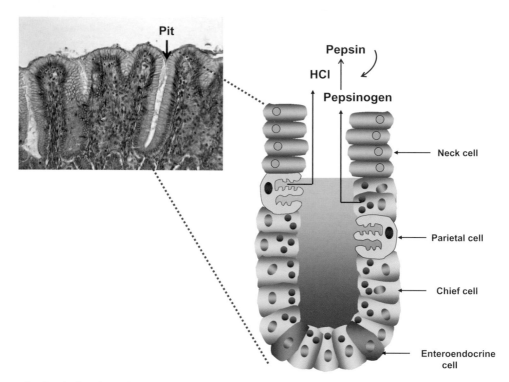

Fig. 17.14. Gastric glands. The histological section of a gastric gland shows the gastric pit, the entrance to the gastric gland. Within the gland are neck cells that secrete mucous, parietal cells that secrete HCl, chief cells that secrete pepsinogen, and enteroendocrine cells that secrete hormones. G cells, which secrete gastrin, are an example of enteroendocrine cells. Once released into the stomach lumen, pepsinogen is converted to pepsin by the action of HCl and pepsin.

4. Enteroendocrine cells. These cells produce a variety of hormones or hormonelike products that are released into the lamina propria. Products include gastrin, histamine, endorphins, serotonin, cholecystokinin, and somatostatin.

The mucosa of the stomach must provide a substantial barrier against the harsh environment found in the stomach. The concentration of H^+ is 10,000 times that found in blood. Pepsin, if not contained, can digest the lining of the stomach. The mucosal barrier of the stomach contains a thick, bicarbonate-rich mucus lining. In addition, the epithelial cells are connected by tight junctions to prevent the leakage of luminal contents to deeper gastric layers. Finally, the epithelial cells are replaced every 3 to 6 days by division of undifferentiated stem cells found in the gastric pits.

Gastric secretions

Pepsin is not produced within the chief cells because this would cause the self-digestion of the cells. Instead, chief cells produce the zymogen (i.e., the precursor form of an enzyme) pepsinogen, which is activated when it enters the stomach lumen and comes in contact with HCl (Fig. 17.14). Once activated, pepsin can activate other pepsinogen molecules.

Protein digestion is initiated in the stomach via the action of pepsin, the only enzyme found in the stomach of adult animals. Dietary proteins are denatured by HCl secreted by the parietal cells. However, HCl is not produced within the parietal cells because it would destroy the cell. Both H^+ and Cl^- are independently transported from the parietal cells into the stomach lumen (Fig. 17.15). Hydrogen ions are generated from the dissociation of carbonic acid that is produced by the enzyme carbonic anhydrase acting upon CO_2 and H_2O. Hydrogen ions are then transported into the stomach lumen in exchange for K^+. Chloride ions enter the parietal cell in exchange for bicarbonate ions. The chloride ions then travel down their concentration gradient and enter the stomach lumen. Once in the lumen, hydrogen and chloride ions combine, producing HCl. Since the pH of the lumen can be as low as 1.5–2.0, this can represent nearly a millionfold (6 log units) increase in hydrogen ion concentration. When parietal cells are producing considerable HCl, a significant amount of bicarbonate enters the blood, thus increasing the pH in what is called the alkaline tide.

Parietal cells respond to many signals. Located on their surface are receptors for histamine, acetylcholine (ACh), and gastrin (Fig. 17.16). Histamine comes from mast cells located in the lamina propria, ACh from postganglionic parasympathetic fibers, and gastrin

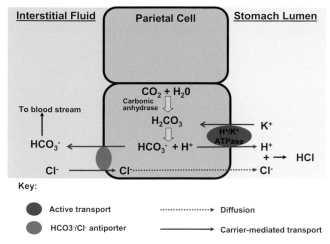

Fig. 17.15. Secretion of HCl by the stomach. Carbonic acid is produced within the parietal cells by the action of carbonic anhydrase. After dissociation, the bicarbonate ions are transported into the intestinal fluid, whereas the hydrogen ion is actively transported into the stomach. Chloride ions enter the cell in exchange for HCO_3^-, and then move down their concentration gradient and into the stomach lumen where they combine with hydrogen ions forming HCl.

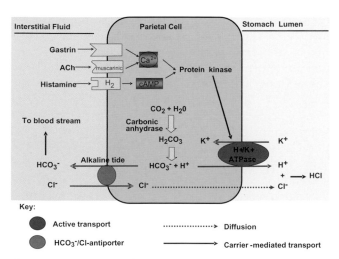

Fig. 17.16. Regulation of HCl secretion from parietal cells. Parietal cells have receptor sites for histamine, gastrin, and acetylcholine (ACh). Histamine binds to H_2 receptors while ACh acts at muscarinic receptors. Stimulation of these receptors by the appropriate ligand initiates a second-messenger system that results in increased HCl secretion into the stomach lumen.

from G cells. Histamine acts at H_2 receptors, whereas ACh acts at muscarinic receptors. Stimulation of these receptors results in stimulation of protein kinase, which then stimulates the H^+/K^+ ATPase, thus increasing HCl secretion by parietal cells.

Endocrine cells located in pyloric glands produce at least seven hormones. The major hormone, gastrin, is secreted by G cells found most abundantly in the

gastric pits of the pyloric antrum. Gastrin stimulates secretion of both parietal and chief cells, and causes contractions of the gastric wall, thus mixing luminal contents. Pyloric glands also contain D cells that secrete somatostatin. Somatostatin, which is released into the interstitial fluid bathing the G cells, inhibits gastrin release. This inhibition can be overridden by other neural and hormonal stimuli such as ACh and histamine.

Gastric motility

With the arrival of food, the stomach can stretch to accommodate this increased volume without an increase in luminal pressure. This reflexive relaxation is mediated by the vagus nerve. In addition, the stomach can actively dilate in a process called adaptive relaxation, which appears mediated by the release of nitric oxide freed by local neurons. In addition to the propulsion of food into the duodenum, the stomach churns and mixes food within its lumen.

Peristalsis in the stomach begins near the cardiac sphincter with gentle ripplelike movements toward the pyloric sphincter. The peristaltic waves strengthen as they move toward the pylorus. The pyloric sphincter, acting sort of like a dam, allows only liquids and small particles to pass over its opening. Heavier particles settle below the level of the sphincter and thus do not pass through. As the peristaltic wave nears the pyloric sphincter, a small amount of chyme is squirted through the sphincter before the peristaltic wave closes the sphincter, causing the remainder of the material to be propelled backward into the pylorus and further churned. Such an action further breaks down the particle size of the ingesta.

The peristaltic rhythm is controlled by the spontaneous activity of pacemaker cells located in the longitudinal smooth muscle layer. These noncontractile cells called interstitial cells of Cahal located near the cardiac sphincter depolarize and repolarize approximately three times per minute producing slow waves, or the basic electrical rhythm. These slow waves migrate throughout the stomach via the gap junctions that electrically couple smooth muscle cells. Slow waves establish the maximum rate of smooth muscle contraction by producing subthreshold depolarizations on which depolarizations resulting in contractions are superimposed (Fig. 17.17).

Vomiting and egestion

Presence of irritants or toxins in the stomach can stimulate vomiting, or emesis. Sensory impulses sent to the emetic center in the medullar initiate a motor response that causes the diaphragm and abdominal wall muscle to contract, increasing intraabdominal

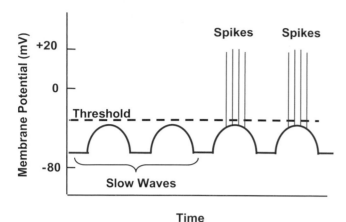

Fig. 17.17. Slow waves. Slow, rhythmic depolarizations and repolarizations, called slow waves or basic electrical rhythm, are initiated by the interstitial cells of Cahal. They establish the background rhythm for peristalsis, which involves spikes superimposed on the slow waves resulting in depolarizations above threshold that cause smooth muscle contractions.

pressure. As the pressure increases, the cardiac sphincter relaxes, the soft palate rises to close off the nasopharynx, and the stomach contents are forced upward through the esophagus, pharynx, and mouth. Excessive vomiting can cause metabolic alkalosis, dehydration, and electrolyte imbalances.

Egestion is a process unique to birds. During egestion, nondigestible materials such as bone, fur, or feathers are orally eliminated from the digestive tract. Approximately 12 min prior to egestion, gizzard contractions increase resulting in the compaction of this undigestible material into a pellet. Seconds before egestion, the pellet is moved orad by esophageal antiperistalis. This process does not use abdominal or duodenal muscles.

Regulation of gastric secretions and emptying

Gastric secretions are controlled by neural and hormonal mechanisms. The nervous control includes both long and short nerve reflexes involving the vagus nerve. Stimulation of the vagus nerve (i.e., parasympathetic nervous system) increases secretory activity of the stomach. In contrast, sympathetic stimulation inhibits stomach secretion.

Gastric secretions are controlled at three levels, including the central nervous system, stomach, and small intestine. Controls from these three sites are the cephalic phase, gastric phase, and intestinal phase of gastric secretion, respectively (Fig. 17.18). These control mechanisms can either increase or decrease gastric secretions.

Cephalic phase

The cephalic phase causes an increase in gastric secretions prior to the arrival of food. This stage is controlled by the central nervous system, and it prepares the stomach for the arrival of food. The sight, smell, and taste of food stimulate the parasympathetic nervous system to send signals via the vagus nerve that synapse on the submucosal plexus located in the wall of the stomach. This stimulates the postganglionic parasympathetic fibers innervating mucous cells, chief cells, parietal cells, and G cells in the stomach, thus increasing gastric secretions. This phase is short, lasting minutes. Emotional responses associated with activation of the fight-or-flight response decrease gastric secretions and gastric motility.

Gastric phase

Beginning with the arrival of food in the stomach, this phase further stimulates gastric secretion and motility. This phase accounts for about two-thirds of gastric secretions. Stimuli for the gastric phase include distention of the stomach, an increase in gastric pH, and the presence of undigested food, especially proteins and peptides. The arrival of protein in the stomach increases the pH since proteins act as buffers. Activation of stretch receptors sends signals to the myenteric plexus (short loop reflex) and the medulla via the vagus (long loop reflex). These reflexes result in the release of acetylcholine, which stimulates gastric secretions. Chemical stimuli, such as partially digested proteins and increasing pH, also directly activate G cells to secrete gastrin, which strongly stimulates HCl but also has a weaker effect of increasing pepsinogen secretion. A decrease in the luminal pH below 2 inhibits gastrin secretion. Finally, local release of histamine in the lamina propria, presumably from mast cells, also stimulates parietal cells to secrete HCl. Therefore, there are three chemicals that can stimulate parietal cells to release HCl.

Intestinal phase

Involving neural and hormonal signals, this phase functions to decrease gastric motility. Stimulation of chemoreceptors and stretch receptors triggers the enterogastric reflex. This reflex inhibits gastrin production and gastric motility, and stimulates contraction of the pyloric sphincter, thus slowing gastric emptying into the duodenum. The enterogastric reflex has three components: 1) inhibition of vagal nuclei in the medulla, 2) inhibition of local reflexes, and 3) sympathetic stimulation of the pyloric sphincter causing it to tighten. The enterogastrone reflex is a hormonal reflex. The arrival of lipids (especially medium- and

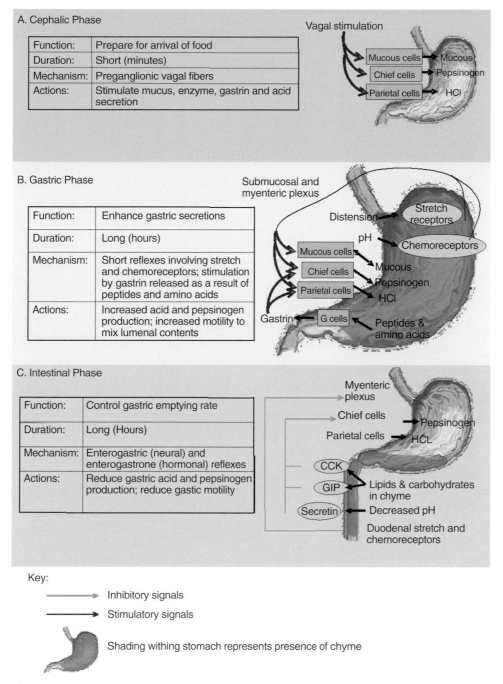

A. Cephalic Phase

Function:	Prepare for arrival of food
Duration:	Short (minutes)
Mechanism:	Preganglionic vagal fibers
Actions:	Stimulate mucus, enzyme, gastrin and acid secretion

Vagal stimulation

Mucous cells → Mucous
Chief cells → Pepsinogen
Parietal cells → HCl

B. Gastric Phase

Function:	Enhance gastric secretions
Duration:	Long (hours)
Mechanism:	Short reflexes involving stretch and chemoreceptors; stimulation by gastrin released as a result of peptides and amino acids
Actions:	Increased acid and pepsinogen production; increased motility to mix lumenal contents

Submucosal and myenteric plexus

Distension → Stretch receptors
pH → Chemoreceptors
Mucous cells → Mucous
Chief cells → Pepsinogen
Parietal cells → HCl
Gastrin ← G cells → Peptides & amino acids

C. Intestinal Phase

Function:	Control gastric emptying rate
Duration:	Long (Hours)
Mechanism:	Enterogastric (neural) and enterogastrone (hormonal) reflexes
Actions:	Reduce gastric acid and pepsinogen production; reduce gastic motility

Myenteric plexus
Chief cells → Pepsinogen
Parietal cells → HCL
CCK
GIP ← Lipids & carbohydrates in chyme
Secretin ← Decreased pH
Duodenal stretch and chemoreceptors

Key:

———▶ Inhibitory signals

━━━▶ Stimulatory signals

Shading withing stomach represents presence of chyme

Fig. 17.18. Phases of gastric secretion. (Figure modified from Martini, 2004.)

long-chain fatty acids) and amino acids (especially tryptophan) cause the release of cholecystokinin, or CCK, and gastric inhibitory peptide (GIP). CCK inhibits gastric secretion of acid and enzymes while GIP inhibits gastric secretions as well as gastric motility. These reflexes act to prevent the excessive decrease in pH of the small intestine, as well as slow up gut motility in order to facilitate digestion and absorption from the small intestine, particularly in response to lipids. A decrease in duodenal pH below 4.5 also stimulates

secretin release by enteroendocrine cells in the duodenum. Secretin further inhibits gastric HCl and pepsinogen release in the stomach. A summary of these intestinal inhibitory effects on motility is shown in Figure 17.19.

In addition to these inhibitory effects occurring during the intestinal phase, there is an excitatory component. The presence of partially digested proteins in the duodenum stimulates G cells in the duodenal wall to release gastrin that circulates to the stomach to

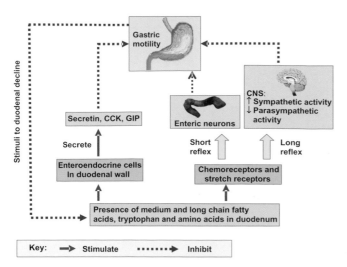

Key: ⟶ Stimulate   ┈┈┈▶ Inhibit

Fig. 17.19. Neural and hormonal inhibition of gastric emptying. Inhibitory signals originating in the duodenum slow gastric emptying allowing the duodenum time to buffer the acid and absorb nutrients.

facilitate enzyme secretion. This gastrin is referred to as intestinal (enteric) gastrin. The excitatory phase is short because it is overridden by the inhibitory intestinal phase mechanisms described in the preceding paragraph.

Anatomy of the stomach of ruminants

Ruminants are those animals that ruminate (i.e., chew their cud). They have a specially modified stomach that consists of three, nonsecretory forestomachs and a secretory "true" stomach. The forestomachs include the reticulum, rumen, and omasum; the true stomach is the abomasum (Fig. 17.20). The forestomachs serve as a large fermentation chamber where microbial digestion occurs, allowing the ruminant to digest feedstuffs not available to nonruminants. The fermentation end products, such as volatile fatty acids, are absorbed and used as metabolic substrates.

The esophagus connects with the reticulum at the cardiac opening (Fig. 17.20). The reticulum is separated from the heart by only the diaphragm. As a result, any hardware such as nails or wire entering the reticulum can puncture the pleural and pericardial spaces, or the liver (hardware disease). Often a magnet is placed in the reticulum to attract hardware and prevent its migration to the remainder of the stomach.

The lining of the reticulum has a honeycomb arrangement of ridges (Fig. 17.21). The reticulum is separated from the rumen by the ruminoreticular fold, or groove. While this separates the two chambers, there remains an opening connecting the two. Therefore, the rumen and reticulum act as a functional unit,

the reticulorumen, which is lined with keratinized, stratified squamous epithelium.

In young animals, the reticuloomasal fold (Fig. 17.22), sometimes called the reticular groove, prevents food from entering the rumen and instead directs it to the omasum. Since the milk ingested during suckling does not require fermentation, it is shunted directly to the abomasum through the omasal canal. This groove closes as a result of a reflex initiated by stimulation of receptors in the mouth and pharynx. This reflex diminishes with age, thus attenuating the reticular groove.

The rumen, sometimes called the "pouch," occupies almost the entire left side of the abdominal cavity. The rumen is divided into a ventral and dorsal sac by the cranial and caudal pillars as well as by the right and left longitudinal pillars (Fig. 17.23). The dorsal sac is further divided into the cranial sac found between the ruminoreticular fold and cranial pillar, the dorsal sac, and a caudodorsal blind sac. The luminal surface of the rumen is lined with papillae to increase its surface area.

The omasum is kidney-shaped, and lies to the right of the ruminoreticulum and is located between the rumen-reticulum and abomasum. Its lining consists of many leaflike folds, or plies, attached to the greater curvature with their free edges extending into the omasal canal. It is therefore sometimes called the "book stomach" since its interior looks like pages of a book. The leaves have small papillae, thus further increasing the surface area. Food enters the omasum via the reticuloomasal orifice and exits to the abomasum via the omasoabomasal orifice.

The abomasum consists of two glandular regions equivalent to the fundus and pyloric region of the monogastric stomach. The cardiac region is confined to the area adjacent to the omasoabomasal orifice. The interior of the abomasum has about 12 rugae (folds) that spiral over the fundus and body, but are absent from the pylorus. A constriction in the pylorus separates this region from the duodenum.

The ruminant stomach provides several advantages compared to the monogastric stomach: 1) it allows animals to use feedstuffs too fibrous for monogastrics, 2) cellulose can be broken down and used by ruminants, 3) it allows the use of nonprotein nitrogen sources (urea and uric acid), which are converted by the rumenal microbes to high-value organic nitrogen compounds, and 4) it provides B complex vitamins due to the action of microbes as long as cobalt is present in the diet. However, there are also disadvantages associated with ruminant digest: 1) animals must spend a considerable part of each day ruminating (chewing), 2) a large amount of alkaline saliva is necessary, 3) considerable amounts of volatile acids are released into the environment.

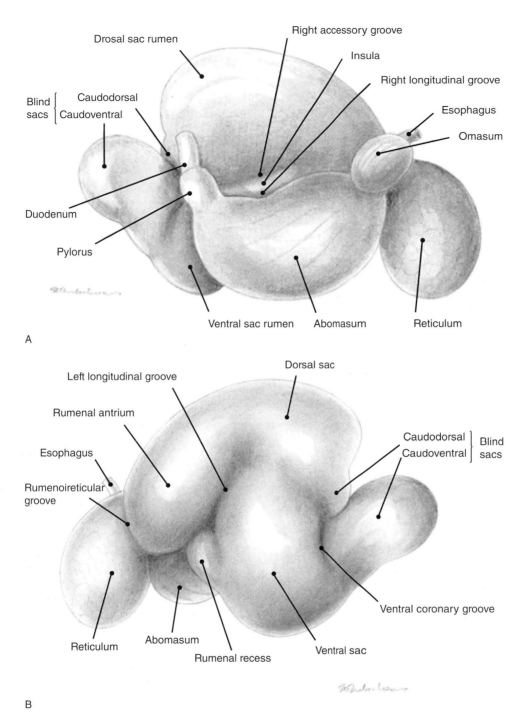

Fig. 17.20. Ruminant stomach. The right (A) and left (B) aspect of the stomach of the goat. (Reprinted from Constantinescu, 2001. Used by permission of the publisher.)

Motility of the ruminant stomach

The mixing, or A, sequence spreads across the reticulorumen in a "Z" pattern. It begins with a double contraction in the reticulum that proceeds across the dorsal rumen to the caudodorsal area. The contraction then propagates through the ventral region of the rumen. This sequence provides extensive mixing of the rumen contents, which disrupts the layering of luminal contents that would allow gas to collect at the top, with coarse solids floating on the surface and finer particles suspended below. Soil and sand gathers in the ventral region. See Figure 17.24 for further explanation of this mixing sequence.

With fermentation comes the production of gas, which must be removed from the animal. The B, or

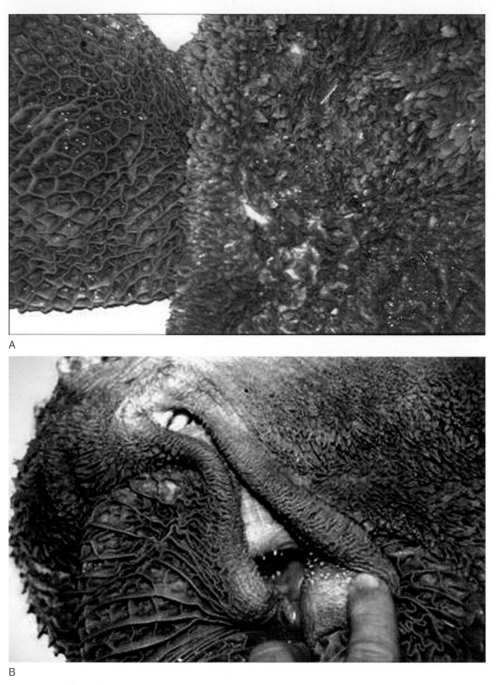

Fig. 17.21.   Inside of ruminant stomach. A) The inside of the reticulum (honeycomb) and rumen. Note the hardware found in the rumen that was ingested as the animal grazed. B) The reticuloomasal fold (reticular groove). C) The many plies shown in the omasum.

eructation, sequence moves gas from the rumen toward the oral cavity (Fig. 17.24). This sequence allows the formation of a gas bubble, which is eventually forcibly ejected into the esophagus by contraction of the ventral rumen. Excess accumulation of gas in the reticulum and rumen leads to bloat.

While grazing, ruminant animals quickly move feed into the rumen before it is completely masticated. This feed is then returned to the oral cavity through a process called rumination. Rumination is a series of

coordinated events involving the respiratory muscles, larynx, pharynx, esophagus, oral cavity, and reticulum. At the height of a single contraction of the reticulum, the animal inhales while the glottis is closed so that air cannot flow into the lungs. This generates great negative pressure in the thorax. The transfer of this negative pressure to the esophagus allows a bolus of reticular contents to move through the cardia and, by a process of reverse peristalsis, to move into the oral cavity. Immediately, there is a swallowing event

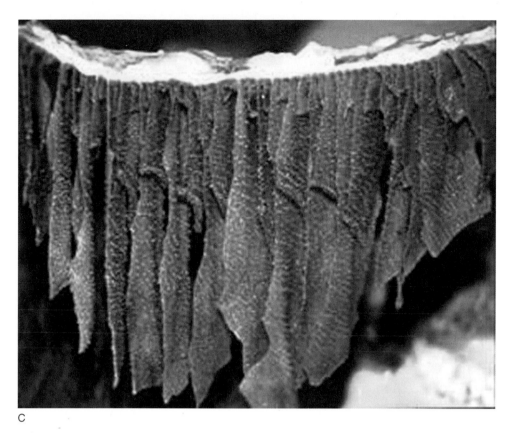

C

Fig. 17.21. *Continued*

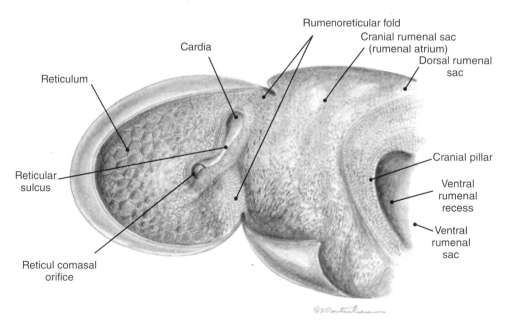

Fig. 17.22. Internal configuration of the reticulum and rumenal atrium of the goat. (Reprinted from Constantinescu, 2001. Used by permission of the publisher.)

that carries the liquid portion of the bolus back to the rumen. The remaining residue is chewed, saliva is added, and it is again swallowed. Time spent ruminating varies with the diet. A cow consuming a coarse hay diet will spend approximately 8 h/day.

Rumenal microbial fermentation

Fermentation involves the anaerobic action of bacteria and protozoa with bacteria accounting for about 80% of rumen metabolism. Primary bacteria are those that

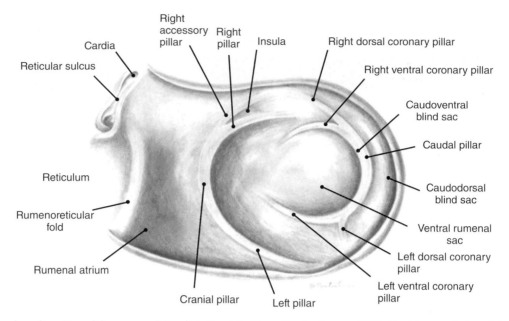

Fig. 17.23. Internal configuration of the rumen of the goat. (Reprinted from Constantinescu, 2001. Used by permission of the publisher.)

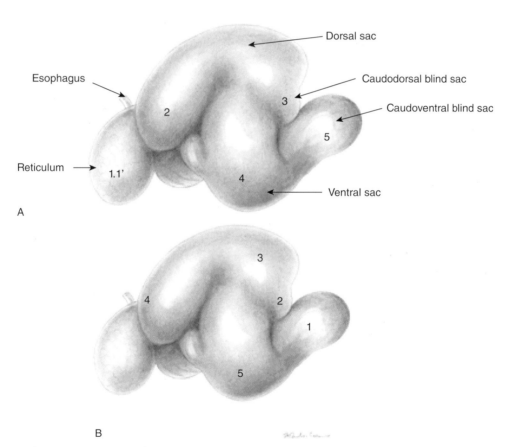

Fig. 17.24. Mixing and eructation sequence of rumen motility. A) The mixing, or A, sequence, begins in the reticulum in a biphasic, or double, contraction (1, 1'). The contraction is next seen in the rumen in the following sequence: Anterior dorsal sac (2), caudal region (3), ventral rumen (4), and finally in the caudoventral sac (5). B) The eructation sequence allows elimination of gas produced by fermentation. The sequence begins in the caudodorsal blind sac (1) and proceeds to the craniodorsal blind sac (2) and dorsal sac area (3), the cardia (4), and then the ventral rumen (5) (Reprinted from Constantinescu, 2001. Used by permission of the publisher.)

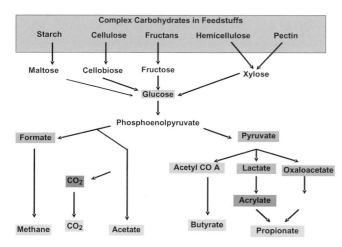

Fig. 17.25. Rumenal carbohydrate fermentation. Complex carbohydrates are fermented by microorganisms within the rumen. Those compounds displayed in blue do not accumulate; those shown in green are the end products.

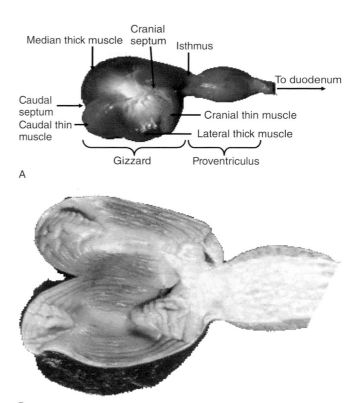

Fig. 17.26. Avian stomach. A) The avian stomach has two chambers. The gizzard is the most orad and is the muscular, nonglandular portion. The proventriculus is the glandular portion. B) The inside aspect of the gizzard and proventriculus.

break down the dietary constituents; secondary bacteria further break down the end products of the primary bacteria. Secondary bacteria include those that produce propionate from lactate, and methane-producing bacteria. The protozoa consume rumenal bacteria, plant starch granules, and perhaps linoleic and linolenic acids.

Rumenal carbohydrate digestion

Products of the bacteria and protozoa carbohydrate digestion include short-chain volatile fatty acids (VFA), carbon dioxide, and methane (Fig. 17.25). The major VFAs are acetic, propionic, and butyric acids, which are produced in the following proportions: 60–70% acetic acid, 15–20% propionic acid, and 10–15% butyric acid. The percentage of propionic acid increases when the animal is fed concentrates with soluble sugars or starch. The rumen epithelium can absorb glucose and volatile fatty acids.

Rumenal protein digestion

Rumen microorganisms hydrolyze dietary proteins to peptides and amino acids. In addition, these microorganisms can make amino acids from nonprotein nitrogen sources such as uric acid, urea, and ammonia. As a result, as much as 50% of the diet of ruminant animals can include poultry waste since the rumenal bacteria will convert the uric acid into amino acids. These amino acids are then absorbed and used by the animal.

Rumenal lipid digestion

Triglycerides are hydrolyzed by rumenal bacteria yielding glycerol and fatty acids. The glycerol is generally metabolized to propionic acid while the fatty acids pass to the duodenum where they are absorbed.

Anatomy of the stomach of birds

In mammals, the stomach is a single chamber. Birds have a two-chambered stomach, including the proventriculus (pars glandularis) and gizzard (pars muscularis) (Fig. 17.26). The proventriculus is the glandular, or true stomach, and is located orad to the gizzard.

The interior of the gizzard is lined with a cuticle, occasionally called koilin, produced by the mucosal glands. The cuticle protects the gizzard from acid and proteolytic enzymes secreted from the proventriculus, as well as abrasion from grinding of hard feedstuffs. The gizzard consists of two pairs of opposing circular muscles called thick and thin pairs. Alternating contraction of these muscles results in a grinding motion much like placing a large nut in one's palm and trying

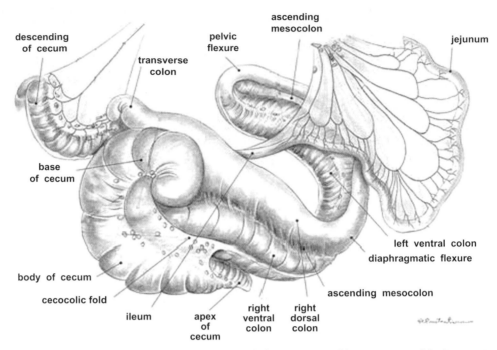

Fig. 17.27. Horse intestinal tract. A) The small intestine, beginning with the jejunum, and large intestine of the horse. (Figure from Constantinescu and Constantinescu, 2004.)

to crack it open while squeezing and twisting the hands.

Small intestine

The small intestine is the area where most digestion and 90% of absorption occur. Digestion occurs with the aid of accessory organs that produce necessary enzymes, buffers, and other secretions.

Anatomy of the small intestine

The small intestine extends from the pylorus to the large intestine and is divided into three sections: 1) duodenum, 2) jejunum, and 3) ileum. The duodenum is the first section past the stomach, and is largely a retroperitoneal organ. It is the area where the chyme from the stomach is mixed with the secretions from the pancreas and liver. The duodenum has a descending and ascending segment separated by the caudal flexure (Figs. 17.27, 17.28).

The pancreatic and bile ducts empty into the descending duodenum. The bile and pancreatic ducts combine at a point in the wall of the duodenum called the hepatopancreatic ampulla, which opens into the duodenum via the duodenal papilla. The entry of fluid into the duodenum is controlled by the hepatopancreatic sphincter, or sphincter of Oddi (Fig. 17.29).

The longest part of the small intestine, the jejunum runs ventrally and caudally within the abdomen, forming many loops and coils. This is the site of the bulk of chemical digestion and absorption.

The ileum is the short, terminal segment of the small intestine. On gross examination, it is indistinguishable from the jejunum. In birds, the ileum is generally separated from the jejunum at the yolk stalk (diverticulum vitellinum), formally called Meckel's diverticulum. The ilium ends at the ileocecal valve, a sphincter controlling the movement of digesta from the ileum into the cecum.

An extensive mesentery attaches the jejunum and ileum to the dorsal abdominal wall. Blood vessels, lymphatics, and nerves reach the small intestine through the mesentery. The blood supply is from the cranial and caudal mesenteric artery (Fig. 17.30). The venous blood from the small intestine drains into the hepatic portal vein that runs to the liver.

Histology of the small intestine

The interior of the small intestine contains transverse folds called plicae, or plicae circulares (Fig. 17.31). Although the rugae of the stomach are transient depending on the stretch in the lumen, the plicae are permanent. They increase the surface area.

The mucosa has fingerlike projections called intestinal villi. The villi are covered with simple columnar epitheliums that have microvilli on their surface. The

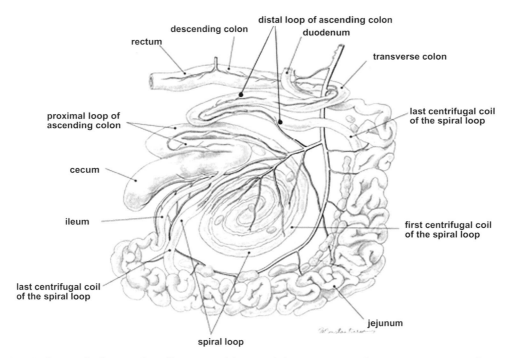

Fig. 17.28. Goat intestinal tract. The large and small intestine of the goat, left aspect. (Figure from Constantinescu and Constantinescu, 2004. Used by permission of the publisher.)

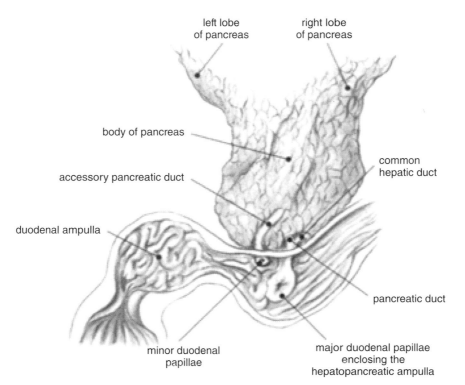

Fig. 17.29. Bile and pancreatic ducts of the horse. The hepatopancreatic sphincter, or sphincter of Oddi, is found surrounding the hepatopancreatic ampulla. (Figures from Constantinescu and Constantinescu, 2004. Used by permission of the publisher.)

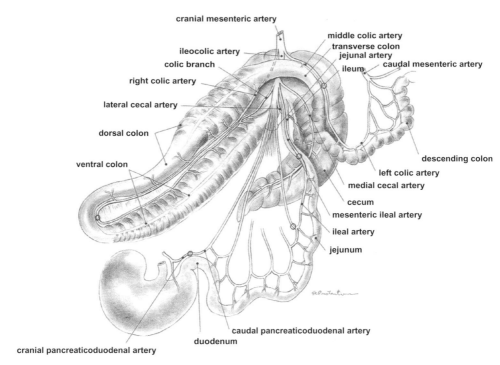

Fig. 17.30. Blood supply to the intestines of the horse. (Figures from Constantinescu and Constantinescu, 2004. Used by permission of the publisher.)

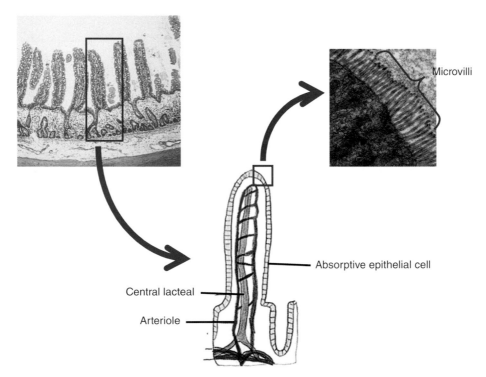

Fig. 17.31. Intestinal wall. Histological section of the wall of the small intestine showing with and microvilli.

microvilli make up the brush border. As discussed below, enzymes are embedded in the walls of the plasma membranes of the microvilli. These enzymes are involved in mucosal digestion of carbohydrates and proteins. The combination of plicae, villi, and brush border increase the surface area of the small intestine approximately 600-fold.

The lamina propria within each villi has an extensive network of capillaries originating in the submucosa. These capillaries carry absorbed nutrients to the liver. In addition, there is a lymphatic capillary called a lacteal, or central lacteal, which transports materials not entering the blood capillaries. The lacteals carry lipid-protein mixtures called chylomicrons to the thoracic ducts where they enter the venous blood supply at the left subclavian vein.

Contraction of smooth muscle located in the muscularis mucosa allows the intestinal villi to move back and forth. Such movement assists in moving the liquefied intestinal contents into contact with the mucosa aiding in digestion and absorption. Such movement also assists with squeezing the lymph along the lacteal and out the villi.

Goblet cells are located between the columnar epithelial cells lining the villi. These cells secrete mucous into the lumen. At the base of each villi are entrances to intestinal glands, or crypts of Lieberkuhn. These glands secrete a watery mucous-containing intestinal juice that assists with absorption of nutrients. The stimulus for secretion is distension or irritation of the intestinal mucosa. Located at the base of each gland are stem cells that produce new epithelial cells that migrate up the villi. These cells replace cells sloughed off near the villi tips and constantly replace brush-border enzymes. Also located within the crypts are Paneth cells, which secrete lysozyme and are part of the immune system.

The submucosa consists of areolar connective tissue. It contains aggregates of lymphatic tissue called Peyer's patches that become more numerous toward the end of the small intestine. These function to prevent bacteria from entering the bloodstream. Also in the submucosa are duodenal glands, sometimes called submucosal glands or Brunner's glands. These glands produce large amounts of alkaline mucous to protect the epithelium from the acidic chyme arriving from the stomach.

The duodenum has a bilayered muscularis externa containing circular and longitudinal smooth muscle. Since the bulk of the duodenum is retroperitoneal, it is lined with an adventitia. When located within the peritoneal cavity, the external surface is covered with the peritoneum. The serosal layer of the peritoneum lines the intestinal surface, and the visceral portion lines the peritoneal cavity.

Intestinal juices and brush-border enzymes

Intestinal juices are secreted from the mucosal lining of the small intestine. They contain water and mucous, and are slightly alkaline (pH 7.6). This liquid aids in absorption of substances from the digestive tract lumen. Also embedded in the microvilli of the absorptive epithelial cells lining the small intestine are enzymes called brush-border enzymes. These enzymes include the carbohydrate-digesting enzymes α-dextrinase, maltase, sucrase and lactase, the protein-digesting enzymes aminopeptidase and dipeptidase, and nucleotide-digesting enzymes nucleosidases and phosphatases, as well as enterokinase, the enzyme that activates trypsinogen.

Mechanical digestion and motility in the small intestine

Small intestine motility is regulated mainly by the enteric reflex responding to the presence of materials in the intestinal lumen. There are two types of movements within the small intestine: segmentation and peristalsis. Segmental contractions are a nonpropagating type of movement that results in churning and mixing of the luminal contents with digestive juices (Fig. 17.1). Segmental contractions, the prominent motility pattern in the small intestine, consist of oscillating ringlike contractions separated by relaxed areas containing a bolus of chyme. The constant formation and then relaxation of these contractual rings along the length of the small intestine results in a mixing action, as if kneading dough, thus forcing the chyme to move from a previously relaxed area into a previously contracted area.

The segmental contractions are initiated by intrinsic pacemaker cells located in the longitudinal smooth muscle layer. The pacemaker cells produce a basic electrical rhythm similar to the slow waves discussed in the stomach. Various factors can change the resting potential of this basic electrical rhythm, moving it either closer or farther away from the threshold. Parasympathetic stimulation enhances, and sympathetic stimulation reduces, segmental contractions. The presence of ingesta in the duodenum moves the resting potential toward threshold, thus allowing segmental contractions to increase. Segmental contractions are simultaneously increased in the ileum, even though ingesta is not present. This latter effect is caused by gastrin produced in response to food in the stomach (gastroileal reflex).

Late in the intestinal phase, when most nutrients have been absorbed, segmental contractions are replaced by peristaltic contractions. Peristaltic contractions propel chyme along the length of the digestive tract. Peristalsis in the small intestine is controlled by the migrating myoelectric complex (MMC), which is a type of slow wave characterized by three phases. Phase 1 involves quiescence, Phase 2 has irregularly spaced spike activity superimposed on slow waves, and Phase 3 is characterized by high-amplitude, regular spike activity superimposed on slow waves. The MMC begins near the caudal end of the stomach and pushes contents along a short segment of the small intestine before decaying. MMCs slowly migrate down the small intestine. These complexes

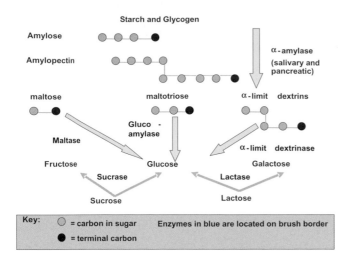

Fig. 17.32. Carbohydrate digestion in the small intestine. Lumenal digestion of carbohydrates results in the production of maltose, maltotriose and α-dextrins. Mucosal digestion is then completed by the brush-border enzymes. The shaded circles represent the monosaccharides found in the polysaccharides.

strengthen as nutrients and water are absorbed, thereby decreasing the distension of the wall of the small intestine.

The MMC is thought to serve a "housekeeping" role by sweeping residual undigested material through the digestive tract. In dogs and man, the cycle recurs every 1.5 to 2 hours. The MMC is thought to be controlled from the central nervous system and may be initiated in part by motilin. The growling sound that is occasionally heard from the gastrointestinal tract is caused by the MMC. Ingesting food will switch this pattern to the quieter segmental contractions.

Birds display a unique type of intestinal motility involving intestinal refluxes. This motility involves the reflux of intestinal contents into the proventriculus.

Chemical digestion in the small intestine

Some starch digestion occurs in the mouth by the action of salivary amylase. In the stomach, some chemical protein digestion occurs as pepsin converts proteins to peptides. However, most chemical digestion occurs within the small intestine.

Carbohydrate digestion

Since food remains in the mouth only a short time, little starch is totally digested. Instead, pancreatic amylase completes this process. Starch and glycogen are acted upon by salivary and pancreatic amylase to form maltose, maltotriose, and α-dextrins (Fig. 17.32, Table 17.4). This is the lumenal phase of carbohy-

drate digestion since it occurs within the lumen. The smaller di- and trisaccharides then move into contact with the brush border where mucosal digestion by brush-border enzymes digests these sugars to monosaccharides.

Protein digestion

Chemical digestion of protein begins in the stomach by the action of pepsin. Pepsin, which works optimally at a pH of 1.5–2.5, cleaves bonds involving tyrosine and phenylalanine. Pepsin digests approximately 10–15% of dietary protein before being inactivated in the lumen of the small intestine.

Once in the small intestine, trypsin and chymotrypsin secreted by the pancreas break down proteins into peptides. Carboxypeptidase and aminopeptidase, both brush-border enzymes, cleave one amino acid at a time from the carboxyl and amino end of a polypeptide, respectively, while the other brush-border enzymes aminopeptidase and dipeptidase further cleave the proteins.

Lipid digestion

Triglycerides are the most abundant lipid in the diet. Triglycerides and phospholipids are digested by lipases. Although most lipid digestion occurs in the small intestine, lingual and gastric lipases begin the process. Bile salts assist in emulsifying dietary lipids within the aqueous environment found in the small intestine lumen. During this emulsification process, large lipid masses are dispersed into small droplets in which the polar portion (ionized) of the lipids face the outside of the droplet while the nonpolar (hydrophobic) portions face the inside of the droplet. This increase in surface area produced by reducing the droplet size allows the water-soluble pancreatic lipase to act more efficiently. Pancreatic lipase cleaves off two fatty acids from triglycerides producing two free fatty acids and monoglyceride (Fig. 17.33).

Nucleic acid digestion

DNA and RNA are part of ingested foods. Pancreatic nucleases digest these molecules to their nucleotide monomers. The nucleotides are then acted upon by brush-border nucleosidases and phosphatases that release free bases, pentose sugars, and phosphate ions.

Absorption in the small intestine

Having decreased the size of the particles through mechanical and chemical digestion, nutrients are now

Table 17.4. Digestive enzymes.

Enzyme	Source	Substrate	Products
Saliva			
Salivary amylase	Salivary glands	Starch and glycogen	Maltose (disaccharide), maltotriose (trisaccharide), and α-dextrins
Lingual lipase	Gland in the tongue	Triglycerides and other lipids	Fatty acids and diglycerides
Gastric secretions			
Pepsin	Chief cells	Proteins	Peptides
Gastric lipase	Chief cells	Short-chain triglycerides	Fatty acids and monoglycerides, α-dextrins
Pancreatic Secretions			
Trypsin	Pancreatic acinar cells	Proteins, chymotrypsinogen, procarboxypeptidase	Peptides
Chymotrypsin	Pancreatic acinar cells	Proteins	Peptides
Elastase	Pancreatic acinar cells	Proteins	Peptides
Carboxypeptidase	Pancreatic acinar cells	Terminal amino acid at carboxyl end of peptides	Peptides and amino acids
Pancreatic lipase	Pancreatic acinar cells	Triglycerides	Fatty acids and monoglycerides
Ribonuclease	Pancreatic acinar cells	Ribonucleic acid	Nucleotides
Deoxyribonuclease	Pancreatic acinar cells	Deoxyribonucleic acid	Nucleotides
Brush Border Enzymes			
α-dextrinase	Plasma membrane of microvilli	α-dextrins	Glucose
Maltase	Plasma membrane of microvilli	Maltose	Glucose
Sucrase	Plasma membrane of microvilli	Sucrose	Glucose and fructose
Lactase	Plasma membrane of microvilli	Lactose	Glucose and galactose
Enterokinase	Plasma membrane of microvilli	Trypsinogen	Trypsin
Aminopeptidase	Plasma membrane of microvilli	Terminal amino acid at amino end of proteins	Peptides and amino acids
Dipeptidase	Plasma membrane of microvilli	Dipeptides	Amino acids
Nucleosidases	Plasma membrane ot microvilli	Nucleotides	Nitogenous bases, pentoses, and phosphates
Phosphatases	Plasma membrane of microvilli	Nucleotides	phosphate ions

in a form suitable for absorption. Absorption is the process whereby compounds and ions move through the epithelial cells lining the mucosa and pass into the bloodstream or lymphatic system.

About 90% of absorption occurs within the small intestine, with the rest occurring in the stomach and large intestine. Absorption occurs via diffusion, facilitated diffusion, osmosis, and active transport (Fig. 17.34).

Absorption of monosaccharides

The result of lumenal and mucosal digestion of carbohydrates is the production of monosaccharides, the only form of carbohydrates absorbed. Fructose, a monosaccharide found in fruits, is absorbed by facilitated diffusion, and therefore can only move down its concentration gradient.

Glucose and galactose are absorbed via secondary active transport. These latter two sugars are cotransported across the apical epithelial membrane along with two molecules of Na^+. Since Na^+ and the sugars are moving in the same direction, this is a symporter. All three binding sites must be occupied for transport to occur. While transport across the apical membrane is passive, the driving force for this movement is derived from the Na^+-K^+-ATPase that actively transports Na^+ out of the cell at the basolateral membrane and into the interstitial space. The active transport of Na^+ out of the cell produces a lower concentration of

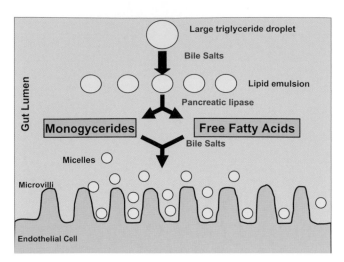

Fig. 17.33. Lipid digestion in the small intestine. Lumenal digestion of lipids results in the production of monoglycerides and free fatty acids. With the help of bile salts, these then form water-soluble micelles that can move toward the microvilli located on the epithelial cells lining the villi of the small intestine.

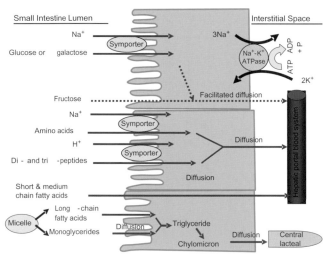

Fig. 17.34. Absorption of nutrients in the small intestine. Carbohydrates, amino acids and peptides are absorbed by secondary active transport systems. As Na^+ is actively pumped out of the epithelial cells and into the interstitial space, this creates a Na^+ concentration gradient in which there is a higher concentration in the small intestine lumen than within the epithelial cell. As Na^+ enters the epithelial cells moving down its concentration gradient, it carries glucose, galactose, or amino acids with it. Peptides enter epithelial cells via a H^+ symporter. Long-chain fatty acids and monoglycerides enter epithelial cells and are reesterified into triglycerides. These are packaged into chylomicrons and transported into the central lacteals, and eventually into the subclavian vein.

Na^+ inside the cell than that found in the small intestine lumen. Glucose, galactose, and Na^+ can therefore move down their concentration gradient from the intestinal lumen into the epithelial cells. Once inside the cell, the sugars move out of the cell at the basolateral membrane by facilitated diffusion, and into the hepatic portal vein.

Absorption of amino acids, dipeptides, and tripeptides

Although it was once believed that only amino acids are absorbed, it is now well established that di- and tripeptides are also actively absorbed in the small intestine. Some amino acids enter the epithelial cells by a secondary active transport system similar to that described for glucose and galactose. There are some amino acids that utilize a sodium-independent cotransporter in which the amino acids enter along with H^+ instead of Na^+. In this case, H^+ is pumped into the intestinal lumen in exchange for Na^+. The Na^+ is then pumped out of the cell by the Na^+-K^+-ATPase on the basolateral membrane. This creates a concentration gradient for H^+, which is now in high concentrations within the lumen. As H^+ enters the epithelial cells, selected amino acids are cotransported. Peptides are absorbed via this sodium-independent cotransporter. Once inside the epithelial cell, the peptides are hydrolyzed to single amino acids, which then move by diffusion into the hepatic portal vein.

Absorption of lipids

Since lipids are not water soluble, lipid absorption and transport within the body pose unique challenges compared to carbohydrate and protein absorption. Within the small intestine lumen, triglycerides are broken down into fatty acids and monoglycerides. The bile salts within the gut lumen help emulsify the lipids by forming water-soluble particles, which helps the lipids migrate within the aqueous chyme found in the gut. Since lipids are fat soluble, once the micelles come in contact with the lumen wall, the monoglycerides and free fatty acids can cross the epithelial membrane by simple diffusion. The bile salts that helped form the micelles continue to form new micelles down the length of the small intestine. Upon reaching the ileum, the bile salts are reabsorbed via active transport and recycled. This allows a small amount of bile salts to assist with the absorption of large amounts of lipids.

Once inside the epithelial cells lining the gut, the short-chain fatty acids, those having fewer than 12 carbons, pass into the hepatic portal system similarly to amino acids and monosaccharides. The remaining triglycerides and monoglycerides are resynthesized into triglycerides (Fig. 17.35). These triglycerides combine with cholesterol and proteins formed in the rough endoplasmic reticulum to form droplets called chylomicrons. The phospholipids and cholesterol are oriented in the chylomicrons so that their hydrophobic ends face the interior of the droplet and their hydrophilic ends face the surface, thus making these

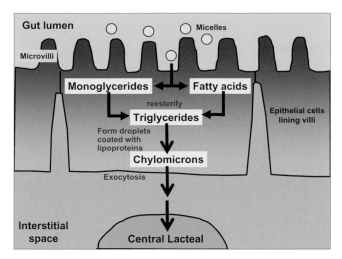

Fig. 17.35. Transport of lipids through the enterocytes. As the micelles produced in the lumen of the small intestine come in contact with the microvilli on the enterocytes lining the villi, the monoglycerides and fatty acids passively pass into the enterocytes. Inside the enterocytes, then reesterify forming triglycerides. These form droplets that are then coated with lipoproteins, thus forming chylomicrons. The chylomicrons pass through the basal surface of the enterocytes into the interstitial space and then enter the central lacteal found in each villi.

droplets water soluble. The proteins found on the chylomicron surface stabilize the structure.

The chylomicrons are secreted by a process of exocytosis into the interstitial fluid of the villus. In mammals, these chylomicrons then enter the central lacteal, which is part of the lympathic system, and are carried to thoracic ducts where they merge with the venous blood supply at the left subclavian vein. In birds, reesterified lipids are packaged into portomicrons. After leaving the enterocytes, portomicrons pass directly into the hepatic portal blood supply and are carried directly to the liver.

Although fat absorption into the epithelial cells is a passive process, it still requires energy. Bile salts are actively secreted by the liver, and the reesterification of monoglycerides and fatty acids into triglycerides requires energy.

Accessory organs

Pancreas

Chyme passes from the stomach to the small intestine. The chemical digestive processes that occur within the small intestine depend upon accessory organs, including the pancreas, liver, and gallbladder.

The pancreas is a V-shaped retroperitoneal organ lying posterior to the greater curvature of the stomach. It is composed of two lobes joined by a body. The body

is the middle portion of the pancreas and is in contact with the pyloric part of the stomach. The right lobe is in the mesoduodenum next to the descending duodenum, and the left lobe lies in the greater omentum. The pancreatic duct (Wirsung's duct) opens with the common bile duct on the major duodenal papilla. There are also accessory pancreatic ducts opening on the minor duodenal papilla. Pigs have only accessory ducts, whereas small ruminants have only pancreatic ducts.

The pancreas has both endocrine and exocrine functions. Its endocrine function includes the synthesis and release of insulin and glucagons, which is discussed in Chapter 12. Its exocrine function is to release enzymes involved in the digestion of all nutrients, including carbohydrates, lipids, proteins, and nucleic acids.

Histology of the pancreas

The pancreas is composed of small clusters of glandular epithelium. Approximately 99% of these cells are arranged in clusters called acini composed of secretory cells surrounding ducts, and are involved in the exocrine portion. These cells have an extensive endoplasmic reticulum and dark-staining zymogen granules. The remaining 1% of the cells are scattered among the acini and are called pancreatic islets (islets of Langerhans) involved in the endocrine function. They secrete glucagons, insulin, somatostatin, and pancreateic polypeptide.

Composition and function of pancreatic juice

Pancreatic juice is a clear, colorless liquid. Containing mostly water, it also has salts, sodium bicarbonate, and enzymes. Sodium bicarbonate serves as a buffer to neutralize stomach acid within the small intestine, thus stopping the action of gastric pepsin. Neutralizing gastric acid also allows pancreatic enzymes to function. Pancreatic enzymes include the carbohydrate-digesting enzyme pancreatic amylase; several protein-digesting enzymes, including trypsin, chymotrypsin, carboxypeptidase, and elastase; the triglyceride-digesting enzyme pancreatic lipase; and the nucleic acid–digesting enzymes ribonuclease and deoxyribonuclease.

These protein-digesting enzymes are produced within the pancreas in an inactive form so that they do not digest the pancreas. Pancreatic acinar cells secrete a protein called trypsin inhibitor that prevents the activation of trypsinogen (Fig. 17.36). Upon entering the duodenal lumen, trypsinogen is acted upon by the brush-border enzyme enterokinase, which splits off a small part of the trypsinogen molecule, thus activating it. Trypsin then activates the remaining zymogens chymotrypsinogen, procarboxypeptidase, and proelastase producing the respective active enzymes.

Regulation of pancreatic secretions

Similar to gastric secretions, pancreatic secretions are controlled by both neural and hormonal mechanisms:

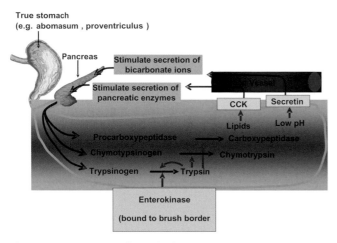

Fig. 17.36. Activation of protein-digesting enzymes. Trypsinogen is secreted into the small intestine lumen where it is converted to trypsin by the enzyme enterokinase found on the brush border. Trypsin then activates the other pancreatic zymogens including chymotrypsinogen and procarboxypeptidase.

1. During the cephalic and gastric phases of gastric secretion, parasympathetic signals carried via the vagus nerve (cranial nerve X) increase secretion of pancreatic enzymes.
2. Partially digested lipids and proteins within the duodenal lumen stimulate the secretion of CCK from enteroendocrine cells in the duodenal wall. CCK stimulates the secretion of pancreatic enzymes.
3. Decreased pH in the duodenal lumen stimulates the release of secretin from enteroendocrine cells in the duonenal wall. Secretin stimulates release of bicarbonate ions from the pancreas.

Liver and gallbladder

The liver and gallbladder are accessory organs of the digestive system. The liver is the largest gland of the body. It resides just under the diaphragm mostly in the right hypochondriac and epigastric region, although it can extend to the left hypochondriac and umbilical regions (Fig. 17.37). The liver receives blood from the intestines and the general circulation. The gallbladder, which stores bile, is a thin-walled muscular green sac found on the ventral surface of the liver. Water is absorbed, thus concentrating the bile as much as tenfold. Bile formed in the bile canaliculi moves

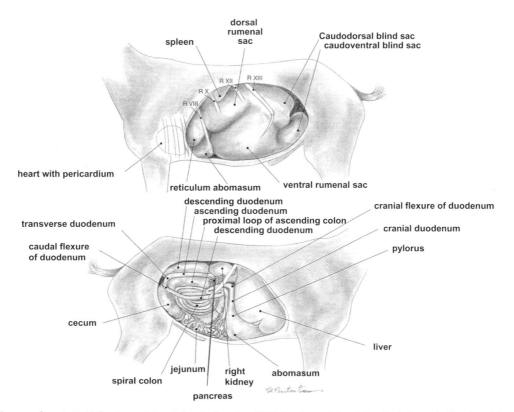

Fig. 17.37. Abdomen of goat. A) Right view of the abdominal cavity. B) Right view of the abdominal visceral. (Reprinted from Constantinescu, 2001. Used by permission of the publisher.)

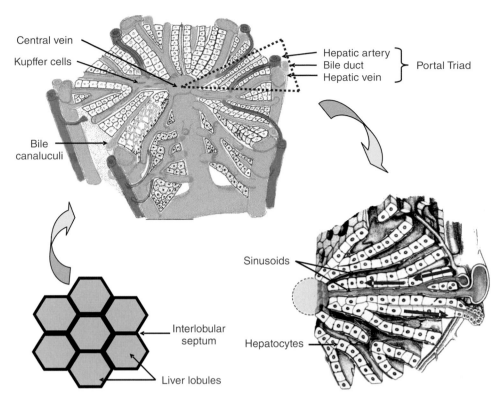

Fig. 17.38. Liver lobules. The functional unit of the liver is the lobule. Lobules are hexagonal in shape, and are separated by the interlobular septum as shown in the lower left hand corner. The portal triad consists of the portal arteriole and venule that bring blood to the liver sinusoids, and the bile duct that collects bile from the bile canaliculi. Liver macrophages, called Kupffer cells, are also found in the sinusoids. Blood from the portal artery and portal vein flow into the sinusoids and towards the central vein. Material filters through the hepatic plates into the bile canaliculi and then flows into the bile ducts (3-D sinusoid modified from http://www.ener-chi.com/d_liv.htm).

into the bile ducts, which fuse to form the common hepatic duct.

Deep fissures divide the liver into four lobes. The right lobe is the largest, and is separated from the left lobe by a deep fissure. The quadrate lobe is located between the right and left lobes and ventral to the liver porta, or hilus, the area where blood vessels and nerves enter the organ on the visceral surface. The caudate lobe is located dorsal to the porta.

The liver is covered with visceral peritoneum that closely adheres to its surface. There are also several attachments holding the liver in place. The falciform ligament connects the ventral liver to the sternal part of the diaphragm and ventral abdomen. The round ligament located on the free border of the falciform ligament is a vestige of the umbilical vein. The right and left triangular ligaments attach the liver to the right and left crus of the diaphragm, respectively. In addition, the lesser omentum extends from the liver porta to the lesser curvature of the stomach. The hepatic artery, hepatic portal vein, and other structures enter the liver at the porta, having traveled through the lesser omentum.

Histology of the liver

Each lobe of the liver has approximately 100,000 liver lobules, the functional unit of the liver (Fig. 17.38). Lobules are approximately hexagonal in shape and are separated from each other by an interlobular septum. The cells of the liver, hepatocytes, are arranged in plates that radiate longitudinally outward from the central vein like the spokes of a wheel.

At each corner of the hexagonal lobule is a portal triad consisting of a branch of the hepatic artery, a branch of the hepatic vein, and a bile duct. Instead of capillaries, between the hepatic plates are cavities called sinusoids. They resemble fenestrated capillaries except that they have spaces between adjacent endothelial cells and the basal lamina is thinner or absent. The sinusoids allow even large plasma proteins to pass out of the bloodstream and into the spaces surrounding the hepatocytes. In addition to the endothelial cells lining the sinusoids, there are also star-shaped fixed macrophages called Kupffer cells that are confined to the liver. They phagocytize pathogens, cell debris, and damage red and white blood cells.

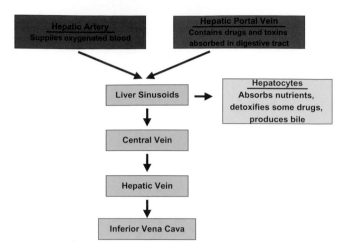

Fig. 17.39.   Blood flow through the liver lobule.

Bile is secreted by hepatocytes and enters the bile canaliculi, which are narrow intercellular canals between the hepatocytes. The bile empties into the bile ducts located at the periphery of the lobules. Bile ducts merge to form the right and left hepatic duct, which then unite to form the common hepatic duct that travels toward the duodenum. Before entering the duodenum, the cystic duct from the gallbladder fuses with the common hepatic duct to form the common bile duct. Note that the horse does not have a gallbladder.

Blood supply of the liver

As stated above, the liver receives oxygenated blood from the hepatic artery and also receives deoxygenated blood from the hepatic portal vein that contains nutrients, drugs, and toxins from the digestive tract. Branches from both of these arteries enter the liver sinusoids where the hepatocytes remove some nutrients and toxins. As the blood passes through the sinusoids, metabolites from the hepatocytes are secreted into the blood. This blood then passes to the central vein and then into the hepatic vein (Fig. 17.39).

Histology of the gallbladder

The mucosa of the gallbladder is lined with simple columnar epithelium. The surface has rugae similar to that found in the stomach. The middle layer of the gallbladder consists of smooth muscle that allows for expulsion of the bile into the small intestine. The outer layer of the gallbladder is the visceral peritoneum.

Bile composition and function

Bile consists of water, bile salts, bile acids, cholesterol, the phospholipid lecithin, bile pigments, and ions. The

bile salts include sodium and potassium salts of bile acids, mostly cholic acids and chenodeoxycholic acid. These salts assist in emulsification of lipids within the small intestine lumen. This decreases the surface area to volume ratio of the lipids, thus increasing the efficiency of pancreatic lipase as it digests triglycerides. Bile salts, free fatty acids, and lecithin combine to form micelles within the small intestine lumen. The polar ends of the molecules are arranged to the outside of the micelle, and the nonpolar portions face the inside of the micelle. Cholesterol and fat-soluble vitamins are packaged inside the micelle.

As aged red blood cells are phagocytized, iron, globin, and bilirubin are liberated. Bilirubin is the main waste product of heme breakdown. The globin and iron are recycled, but bilirubin is absorbed from the blood by the hepatocytes and excreted into the bile conjugated to glucuronic acid. When in the small intestine, it is metabolized by bacteria. Stercobilin, one of its breakdown products, gives feces their dark brown color. Most bile salts are reabsorbed via active transport in the ileum whereupon they enter the hepatic portal blood and return to the liver.

Regulation of bile secretion

In those animals that have a gallbladder, bile is stored between meals. The sphincter of the hepatopancreatic ampulla (sphincter of Oddi) restricts the entrance to the duodenum. There are neural and hormonal stimuli that can stimulate bile secretion:

1. Parasympathetic signals traveling along the vagus nerve can stimulate bile production by the liver.
2. Fatty acids, particularly medium- and long-chain, and amino acids in the chyme cause duodenal enteroendocrine cells to secrete CCK. CCK causes the smooth muscle cells of the gallbladder to contract, and bile is squeezed into the cystic duct and through the common bile duct. CCK also relaxes the sphincter of the hepatopancreatic ampulla. The action of hormones controlling digestion is summarized in Table 17.5.

Functions of the liver

The liver is a vital organ. It performs many functions:

1. Carbohydrate metabolism. The liver plays a vital role in maintaining blood glucose levels. When blood glucose levels are high, the liver converts glucose to glycogen (glycogenesis) and triglycerides so that energy can be stored until needed. When blood glucose levels drop, the liver can break down glycogen to glucose (glycogenolysis) and release the glucose into the bloodstream. In

Table 17.5. Hormones controlling digestion.

Table 17.5. Hormones controlling digestion.

Hormone	Site of Secretion	Stimulus for Secretion	Actions
Gastrin	Enteroendocrine G cells located in pyloric antrum mucosa; also secreted from duodenal mucosa	Stomach distention, partially digested protein, high pH in the stomach	Increases secretion of gastric juice; increases gastric motility; stimulates growth of gastric mucosa; constricts lower esophageal sphincter while relaxing ileocecal sphincter
Secretin	Enteroendocrine S cells in duodenal mucosa	Acidic pH in duodenal lumen	Stimulates pancreatic secretion rich in bicarbonate ions
Cholecystokinin (CCK)	Enteroendocrine CCK cells in duodenal mucosa	Partially digested proteins, medium- and long-chain fatty acids in duodenum	Stimulates pancreatic secretion rich in enzymes; causes bile ejection from the gallbladder while opening hepatopancreatic ampulla; inhibits food intake acting peripherally and within the central nervous system

addition, the liver can convert certain amino acids to glucose (gluconeogenesis), as well as lactic acid to glucose.

2. Lipid metabolism. Hepatocytes can store triglycerides as well as use fatty acids to synthesize ATP. In addition, hepatocytes synthesize lipoproteins that carry fatty acids, triglycerides, and cholesterol throughout the body. Cholesterol can be synthesized in the liver, and cholesterol is used to make bile salts.

3. Protein metabolism. Hepatocytes remove the amino group (deamination) of amino acids so they can be used for ATP synthesis. Hepatocytes also synthesize carbohydrates and fats from certain amino acids. Hepatocytes can synthesize various plasma proteins such as albumin, prothrombin, fibrinogen, and alpha and beta globulins (needed for hemoglobin synthesis).

4. Removal of waste products. The liver detoxifies substances such as alcohol and antibiotics, and can alter and excrete steroid hormones. The liver is an important site of detoxification of ammonia, which is converted to the less toxic urea, which is excreted in the urine. The waste product of red blood cell destruction, bilirubin is eliminated via the bile.

5. Synthesis of bile salts. The bile salts necessary for lipid emulsification within the small intestine are synthesized in the liver.

6. Storage. The liver is the primary storage site of fat-soluble vitamins (A, D, E, and K), as well as vitamin B_{12}. Glycogen and certain minerals (Fe and Cu) are also stored in the liver.

7. Phagocytosis. Kupffer cells destroy aged blood cells and microbes that may have entered via the hepatic portal blood.

8. Activation of vitamin D. The liver combines with the skin and kidneys to synthesize the active form of vitamin D.

Large intestine

The terminal portion of the digestive tract is the large intestine. It extends from the end of the ilium to the anus. The primary functions of the large intestine are electrolyte and water absorption, microbial digestion and vitamin production, formation of feces, and expulsion of feces. These functions require considerable time, so transit time through the large intestine is slow.

Anatomy of the large intestine

The large intestine is divided into the cecum, colon, rectum, and anal canal. The ileum attaches to the large intestine at the ileocecal valve (sphincter), which controls the movement of chyme into the large intestine.

The cecum is a blind diverticulum that extends off of the colon at the ileocecal valve (Fig. 17.40). It is located on the right side of the abdomen, except in the pig where it is located on the left. In those animals that are hindgut fermenters (e.g., the horse), the cecum is a major site of digestion. Extending from the cecum is another twisted, coiled blind pouch called the appendix, or vermiform appendix.

The colon consists of three segments called the ascending, transverse, and descending colon. The ascending colon ascends on the right side of the abdomen until it reaches the inferior surface of the liver. It then turns sharply to the left at the right colic (hepatic) flexure, continuing as the transverse

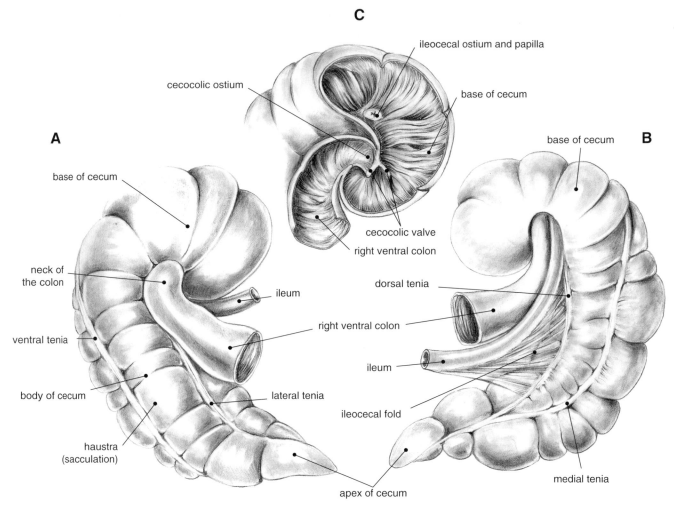

Fig. 17.40. Cecum of the horse. A) Right aspect. B) Left aspect. C) Communications of the cecum. (Figure from Constantinescu and Constantinescu, 2004. Used by permission of the publisher.)

colon. Upon reaching the left side of the abdomen near the spleen, it again abruptly bends at the left colic (splenic) flexure and passes inferiorly as the descending colon to the level of the iliac crest. From this point, the sigmoid colon projects medially to the midline, terminating as the rectum. The rectum extends from the large intestine to the anal canal. The digestive tract terminates at the anal canal, which has an exterior opening called the anus.

Histology of the large intestine

Unlike the small intestine, the mucosal lining of the large intestine lacks villi and plicae (circular folds). Since almost no chemical digestion occurs in the large intestine, the lining also lacks cells that secrete digestive enzymes. The colon is lined with simple columnar epithelium and mucous-secreting goblet cells. The anal canal is lined with stratified squamous epithelium that merges with the skin surrounding the anus.

Unique to the large intestine, portions of the longitudinal smooth muscle found in the muscularis externa layer are thicker, forming three visible longitudinal bands called the teniae coli. The areas between the teniae coli are thinner or lack longitudinal muscle. Tonic contractions of the teniae coli result in a series of pouchlike expansions along the length of the colon called haustra (sing. = haustrum). The outermost layer of the large intestine is the visceral peritoneum. Small fat-filled pouches of visceral peritoneum called epiploic appendages are attached to the teniae coli.

Mechanical digestion in the large intestine

The ileocecal valve controls the movement of chyme into the large intestine. Normally closed, the gastroileal reflex initiated immediately after a meal opens this valve so that peristalsis allows chyme to move from the ileum into the large intestine. Gastrin also relaxes this valve.

Haustra churning is characterized by the slow filling of a haustrum until it is distended, at which time its walls contract, squeezing the contents into the next haustrum. Peristalsis also occurs along the large intestine, although at a slower rate than in the small intestine. Finally, mass peristalis occurs when a strong peristaltic wave begins near the middle of the transverse colon and quickly forces the contents to the rectum. Such movement normally occurs near the beginning or end of a meal.

Chemical digestion in the large intestine

Although no chemical digestion occurs in the large intestine, considerable fermentation takes place, especially in those animals that are hindgut fermenters. Microbes ferment any remaining carbohydrates releasing hydrogen, carbon dioxide, and methane. These gases lead to flatulence in the large intestine. Amino acids are converted to indole, skatole, hydrogen sulfide, and fatty acids. Indoles and skatole are eliminated in the feces, contributing to its odor, while some of the remaining products are absorbed and transported to the liver. The microbes synthesize B vitamins and vitamin K, which are also absorbed by the large intestine.

References

Budras, K-D., W.O. Sack, and S. Rock. 2003. Anatomy of the Horse. An Illustrated Text. Schlütersche GmbH & Co., Hannover, Germany.

Constantinescu, G.M. 2001. Guide to Regional Ruminant Anatomy Based on the Dissection of the Goat. Iowa State Press, Ames, Iowa.

Constantinescu, G.M. 2002. Clinical Anatomy for Small Animal Practitioners. Iowa State Press, Ames, Iowa.

Constantinescu, G.M. and I.A. Constantinescu. 2004. Clinical Dissection Guide for Large Animals. Iowa State Press, Ames, Iowa.

Martini, F.H. 2004. Fundamentals of Anatomy and Physiology, 6th edition. Benjamin Cummings, San Francisco.

Pasquini, C., T. Spurgeon, and S. Pasquini. 1995. Anatomy of Domestic Animals, 8th Edition. SUDZ Publishing, Pilot Point, Texas.

Swenson, J.J. and W.O. Reece. 1993. Duke's Physiology of Domestic Animals, 11th edition. Cornell University Press, Cornell University, Ithaca, New York.

18 Lactation and animal agriculture

Contents

Introduction

In biology, students learn early in their schooling that the presence of mammary glands distinguishes mammals from other animals. With a few exceptions, e.g., bottle-fed human infants or dairy calves that were weaned early, lactation is critical for survival of the neonate and ultimately reproductive success. Regardless of the specific arrangement or number of mammary glands, milk synthesis and secretion requires development of a functionally mature mammary gland. In reproductively competent mammals the mature mammary gland consists of a teat or nipple, associated ducts that provide passage of milk to the outside, and alveoli composed of secretory epithelial cells and supporting tissues. The epithelial cells are arranged to form the internal lining of the spherical alveoli and these epithelial cells synthesize and secrete milk. Secretions are stored within the internal space of the hollow alveoli and larger ducts between suckling episodes (see Figure 18.6, later in this chapter). Milk is a complex fluid. Consequently, understanding lactation requires multiple disciplines: histology and cytology,

biochemistry, endocrinology, cardiovascular physiology, and metabolism, to name a few. In addition the fully functioning mammary gland places striking demands on the physiology of the lactating mother.

Development of the mammary gland during gestation and subsequent differentiation of alveolar cells to allow onset of milk synthesis and secretion in correspondence with parturition is a biological marvel. Mammary secretions first appear as colostrum and subsequently as mature milk and provide the neonate with a spectrum of all the nutrients necessary for good health and early development. Milk of all mammals contains variable amounts of proteins, carbohydrates, and fats suspended in an aqueous medium. Although there are species differences in milk composition, having the birth of the neonate and functionality of the mammary gland coincide is critical. Among scientists, study of lactation and mammary development provides a rich resource for cell biologists, endocrinologists, nutritionists, cancer researchers, dairy specialists, and others. The goal of this chapter is to provide an overview of mammary development and function.

Table 18.1.   Variation in location, number, and nipple openings of mammary glands of selected species.

Order	Common Name	Position of Glands			Total	Openings Per Teat
		Thor	Ing	Ab		
Marsupialia	Red kangaroo		4		4	15
Marsupialia	Opossum		13		13	8
Carnivora	House cat	2	6		8	3–7
Carnivora	Domestic dog	2	6	2	10	8–14
Rodentia	House mouse	4	2	4	10	1
Rodentia	Norway rat	4	4	4	12	1
Lagomorpha	Rabbit	4	4	2	10	8–10
Cetacea	Whale			2	2	1
Proboscidea	Elephant	2			2	10–11
Perissodactyla	Horse			2	2	2
Artiodactyla	Cattle			4	4	1
Artiodactyla	Sheep			2	2	1
Artiodactyla	Goat			2	2	1
Artiodactyla	Pig	4	6	2	12	2
Primate	Man	2			2	15–25

Given the variety of mammals and the environmental niches occupied, it is no surprise that there is much variation in number of mammary glands, location, and composition of secretions. Unlike common dairy species (cows, goats, or sheep) aquatic mammals, especially those in cold environments, also produce milk very high in lipid content with little or no lactose. Milk fat provides the suckling young the opportunity to rapidly produce a layer of insulating fat for protection from the cold and to provide a source of metabolically derived water. This illustrates the relevance of lactation to provide a strategy for survival of offspring and reproductive success for mammals in multiple niches.

For the placental mammals, the number of mammary glands varies markedly between classes and species (Table 18.1). However, among those studied (only about 10% of all mammals) each mammary gland has a teat or nipple. For example, lactation is not common in males, but development of small amounts of mammary tissue and limited secretion occurs. Lactation in males has been reported to occur spontaneously in humans most likely associated with pituitary dysfunction. However, anecdotal tales of "witch's milk" in male and female infants are not rare. Apparently, normal lactation has been reported in male wild fruit bats. Likely, the first reported lactation in a male ruminant was when Aristotle noted in his *Historia Animalium* that "a he-goat was milked by his dugs (teats) to such effect that cheese was made of the product." These examples, illustrate how little is known about mammary development and lactation in many mammals.

Herds of Holstein cows' routinely average 305-day yields of 13,000 kg of milk, and individual cows produce much more milk. Such prodigious production of milk requires massive mammary glands and careful attention to the feeding and management of these impressive animals. Regardless of the rate of milk production, all milk is produced by the epithelial cells of the mammary alveolus. Consequently, to appreciate milk secretion it is essential to understand the structure and function of the mammary gland. We'll begin by describing the ontogeny of mammary development, followed by a description of physiological processes that allow final structural development of the mammary alveoli and onset of functional differentiation of the secretory epithelial cells.

Overview of mammary development

Although the evolutionary origins are unclear, the mammary epithelium arises from the germinal ectoderm and the primitive mammary buds. The first indication is a slight thickening of the ventrolateral ectoderm in the embryo at about the time that limb buds begin to lengthen. This thickened tissue is variously referred to as the mammary band, streak, or line. The cells within the mammary line condense or coalesce to form mammary buds. Each mammary bud gives rise to each of the individual mammary glands. In ruminants, the mammary buds are closely grouped so that the developing mammary glands are oriented in an udder, e.g., two glands in goats and sheep but four in cattle. In the bovine, the mammary buds appear

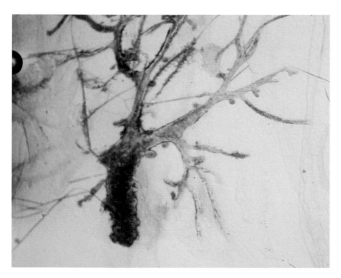

Fig. 18.1. Rudimentary mammary gland of the 1-week-old mouse. The nipple and primary mammary sprout are oriented at the lower portion of the figure. Other secondary sprouts radiate as if they were bare tree branches into the surrounding fat pad.

at about day 40 of gestation. By day 80 the teat and primary sprout form. The primary sprout gives rise to the teat cistern. Secondary sprouts occur by day 90 and by day 100 the primary and secondary spouts are canalized. At birth, the teat, teat cistern, and gland cistern are formed. In most species, mammary structure at birth is similarly rudimentary.

Figure 18.1 illustrates the epithelial portion of the mammary gland of a mouse at 1 week old. Mice of course do not have a teat or gland cistern but the structure of the nipple and branches from a number of secondary sprouts are evident. For mammals without the mammary glands arranged into an udder, a teat or gland cistern is absent but there is a nipple and a cluster of primary and secondary sprouts for each gland. Further growth of secondary sprouts yields the major ducts that drain groups of alveoli (lobules) in the mature gland. Development of the alveoli is usually restricted to pregnancy.

The mammary gland is one of only a few tissues in mammals, which repeatedly undergo growth, functional differentiation, and regression. This is one of the reasons for great interest in study of the mammary gland. The term *mammogenesis* refers to the development of mammary gland parenchymal structures. In usual circumstances, studies of mammogenesis are focused on the very large changes in the mammary gland, which begin around the time of puberty or, more likely, during pregnancy. However, the foundation for the dramatic mammogenesis during these stages begins when the animal is an early fetus. Fundamentally, mammary development can be developmentally considered a joining of the epithelial ectoderm and the underlying mesoderm.

Across species, there are dramatic differences in milk composition. Milk from Holstein cows (the source of the majority of milk for human consumption in Western societies) has about 3.2% protein, 3.4% fat, and 4.6% lactose. In contrast, hooded seals produce milk with about 6.0% protein, 50% fat, and virtually no carbohydrate. Much of this variation reflects evolution-induced responses, which provide the best stratagem for offspring survival. Because the seal pups are born on potentially unstable pack ice, they must rapidly gain sufficient strength and insulation to survive. In fact, mothers suckle their pups for only 4 days during this period but pups can double their 20 kg birth weight. Although the hood seal has the shortest lactation of any known mammal, the high-fat milk provides the pup with the energy and metabolic water necessary for an abrupt introduction into a polar environment.

Prepubertal and postpubertal mammary development

Generally, little or no true lobulo-alveolar development occurs before conception. This period is associated with creation of a framework to allow proliferation of the secretory alveolar cells needed for lactation. The period is generally considered a time during which the duct system is extended and growth of the adipose and connective tissue increases. Ductular growth is limited for dogs, cats, and rabbits but more extensive for rats, mice, the rhesus monkey, cattle, and sheep.

Since it is expected that most organs in growing animals would also grow in concert with the rate of overall body growth, the regulated, cyclic development of the mammary gland can be difficult to study under these conditions. One approach is to evaluate mammary development in terms of relative growth and to ask whether growth of the mammary gland fits the law of simple allometry: $y = bx^\alpha$. A usual approach is to log transform variables associated with body and tissue growth and use linear regression analysis to calculate the equilibrium constant (α), which relates the difference in growth rate of the organ under study to the growth of the body as a whole. Simple body weight or body weight$^{2/3}$ (to approximate surface area) is usually used as the independent variable in these analyses. The dependent variable (mammary gland area, mammary gland weight, DNA content, weight of parenchymal mass) serves as an index of the growth of the mammary gland. When $\alpha = 1$, growth is said to be isometric. If $\alpha > 1$, the growth rate is positively allometric (simple allometry), but an $\alpha < 1$ indicates growth rate of the organ is negatively allometric (enantiometry).

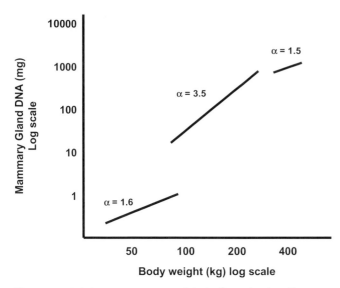

Fig. 18.2. Relative mammary growth in heifers. The data illustrate the relationship between mammary DNA and body weight in Holstein heifers. Segments illustrate periods from birth to 2, 3 to 9, and 10 to 12 months of age. Redrawn from Sinha and Tucker, 1969.

Data for rodents, cattle, and sheep demonstrate that from birth until before puberty, the mammary gland grows only somewhat faster than the rest of the body. Thereafter the rate of mammary gland growth becomes markedly allometric, usually through the first few estrus cycles. Growth then reverts to a period of isometric growth that also waxes and wanes during the course of the estrus cycle. As demonstrated for heifers, the classic study by Sinha and Tucker (1969) shows that positive allometric begins at about 3 months of age and continues until about 9 months of age. Specifically, when mammary development was expressed as the log of mammary DNA and body growth as the log of body weight, the equilibrium constant (α) averaged 1.6 in the period from birth to 2 months, 3.5 from 3 to 9 months, and 1.5 between 10 and 12 months of ages (Fig. 18.2). These data indicate that the mammary gland grows somewhat faster than the body during the early postpartum period but dramatically faster between 3 and 9 months of age.

Although the absolute amount of mammary growth during the period prior to conception is only a fraction of the mature mammary gland late in gestation, there is compelling evidence that alterations in mammary growth during the peripubertal period can affect subsequent mammary function. For example, rapid prepubertal weight gain inhibits subsequent mammary parenchyma tissue growth and can reduce subsequent milk production (Sejrsen and Purup 1997). Not surprisingly, very few cattle studies have considered changes in mammary development in the period shortly after parturition. While minor in terms of

absolute mass, our observations of mammary glands of Holstein calves between 1 and 3 months of age (Akers, unpublished data) suggest that parenchymal tissue per gland increases approximately sixtyfold in only a few weeks. It is intriguing to consider that growth during even this very early postnatal period may also be critical to the success of lactation.

Figure 18.3 illustrates various stages of mammary development using the mouse mammary gland as an example. Small rodents are especially useful for this purpose because an entire mammary gland can be removed, spread onto a microscope slide, fixed, defatted, and stained. Observing structural differences in mammary glands from various physiological stages quickly illustrates the dramatic changes in the development of the mammary epithelium as the gland prepares for the onset of lactation. However, a word of caution is advised. Although the fundamental developmental processes are similar in rodents and other species, there are clearly substantial differences in the tissue composition of the mammary gland in rodents compared with other species as well as differences in the pattern of ductular development.

Compared with the rodent pattern of development where the end buds allow for filling of the entire mammary fat pad during the prepubertal period (Fig. 18.3), the developmental pattern in the ruminants is more compact. Specifically in rodents as the epithelial ducts develop, they are surrounded by stromal cells and the stromal tissue contains a sea of adipocytes. A higher-power view (Fig. 18.4B) of a similar area from the mammary gland of a prepubertal heifer, illustrates several epithelial structures, which radiate from a mammary duct. Pre- and postpuberty cross-sectioned ducts often demonstrate a scalloped appearance, suggesting a complex tubular structure. Indeed, recent three-dimensional computer animations prepared from serial sections of prepubertal bovine mammary parenchymal tissue elegantly confirm this tissue architecture (Capuco et al., 2002). This suggests that in the ruminant, in contrast with rodents, the gland is not filled with elongated ducts during the prepubertal period waiting for subsequent development of side branches. To use a plant analogy, in the peripubertal rodent, widely spaced mammary ducts fill the mammary fat pad like the bare branches of a tree. In the peripubertal ruminant, closely packed ducts radiate from the gland cistern in broccoli-like fashion, but the ducts generally fill only a fraction of the mammary fat pad.

As the gland continues to develop, the relative tissue area occupied by the epithelium increases at the expense of the surrounding stromal tissue. This is especially evident with the growth of alveoli during gestation. It is also evident that much of the tissue area in histological sections of mammary tissue taken from

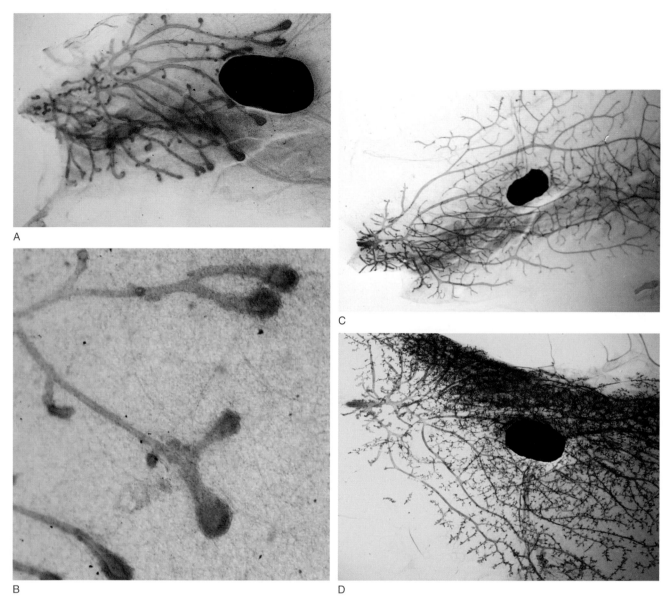

Fig. 18.3. Physiological stages and mammary development. These images illustrate a series of whole mounts prepared from an inguinal mammary gland of mice at various stages of development from the prepubertal period into lactation. Panel A shows the gland of a 4-week-old mouse. Ducts have elongated from the region of the primary sprout and nipple (left) to just beyond the lymph node. This progressive growth depends on the highly mitogenic end buds, which appear as enlargements at the ends of the ducts. Panel B shows enlarged end buds. Panel C shows a gland from a mouse at about 40 days of age. The mammary fat pad is largely filled with mammary ducts, but notice that the end buds have now regressed. Panel D shows the mammary gland of a mouse after the onset of estrus cycles. The number of branches has increased and alveolar buds have begun to appear. Panel E shows enlarged alveolar buds. Panel F provides an image of just a portion of the mammary gland on day 12 of gestation. Alveoli are now beginning to develop, and the gland becomes thickened so that images of tissue structure are possible only at the thinner margins of the gland. Panel G provides an enlargement of an area of developing alveoli. Panel H shows the margin of the mammary gland on day 4 of lactation. Because of the marked increase in alveolar growth and accumulation of secretions, the rounded structure of clusters of lobules and alveoli are evident at the thinner margins of the whole mount.

cows in late gestation and lactation is also occupied by lumenal space. This does not mean that there is necessarily a loss of stroma cells as the gland develops, but rather that there is a dramatic rearrangement of cells and tissue elements so that that the stromal cells are less evident. As gestation advances, clusters of alveolar structures appear as scattered, round islands,

until late in gestation when histological fields are filled with closely packed alveoli. Under normal circumstances, true alveoli are not formed until conception. Variation among species reflects the number of estrus cycles that occur prior to conception. Using cattle as an example, in the early stages of pregnancy the duct system continues to develop with appearance of a

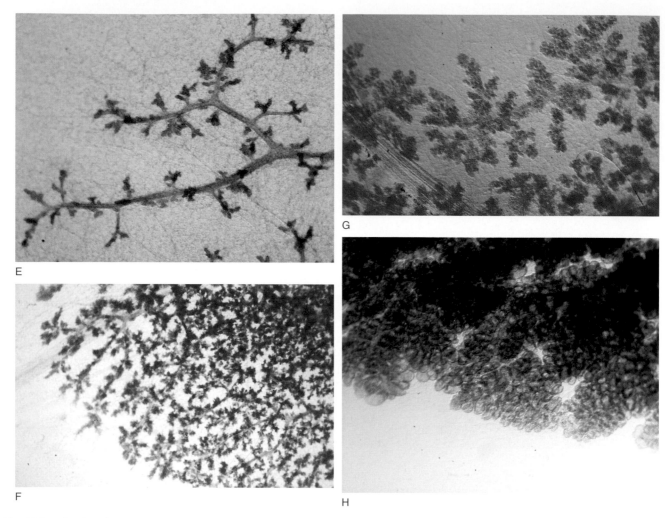

Fig. 18.3.   *Continued*

rudimentary lobulo-alveolar system by about 5 months of gestation.

Mammary development during pregnancy

It is estimated that 94% of mammary development for the hamster takes place as pregnancy advances. Estimates for other species range from 78% for the mouse and sheep to 66% in rabbits and 60% for rats. By far the greatest promoter of natural mammary growth or mammogenesis is pregnancy and associated hormonal and physiological changes. With influence of pregnancy, mammary growth is reinitiated after reversion to isometric growth following puberty. This growth can be described by an exponential equation with the following form:

$$Y = a^{bt}$$

where Y = mammary size, t = day of gestation, and the terms a and b are constants. Such equations have been developed to model mammary growth in cows, goats and guinea pigs. The term a is mammary gland mass or size at the beginning of gestation, and the term b is the first-order rate constant. The time necessary for the mammary gland to double is equal to $\ln 2/b$ (Sheffield, 1988).

Measurement of mammary DNA or weight of dissected parenchymal tissue is useful to quantify rates of mammary growth, but these techniques do not distinguish differences among cell types. Problems of trying to distinguish between stromal and parenchymal tissue are especially difficult in rodents. For example, both wet weight and defatted dry weight of the inguinal mammary glands of rats are reported to vary from 50 to 120% during pregnancy, but total mammary DNA changes 200 to 300%. Since total DNA is a reflection of cell number, changes in weight alone underestimate cellular development. Table 18.2 illustrates changes in mammary development of ewes during gestation. Changes in weight, total DNA, or % epithelium show a marked increase in parenchymal

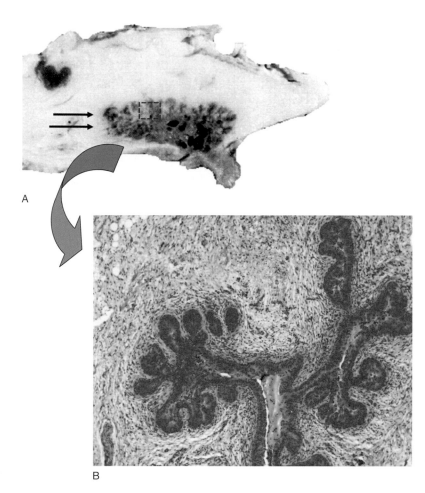

A

B

Fig. 18.4. Ruminant mammary development. Panel A illustrates a midsaggital section through the udder of a prepubertal ewe lamb. Note the dark, dense tissue near the center of the image above the teat (arrows). Panel B is a histological section of mammary parenchymal taken from a region similar to this dense region of parenchymal tissue shown in panel A.

Table 18.2. Effect of gestation on mammary growth, histology, and epithelial cell labeling index in ewes.

	Day of Gestation			
Measurement	Day 50	Day 80	Day 115	Day 140
Trimmed udder weight (g)	304 ± 43	253 ± 30	557 ± 29	1050 ± 188
Total DNA (mg)	94 ± 4	57 ± 14	1304 ± 152	2324 ± 321
% Epithelium	14.2 ± 0.3	19.2 ± 2.1	41.2 ± 2.3	40.3 ± 1.8
% Stroma	85.8 ± 0.3	77.8 ± 3.2	35.7 ± 6.5	20.7 ± 3.0
% Lumen	NP	1.0 ± 0.2	23.1 ± 4.3	39.0 ± 2.9
Alveolar cell no.	NP	NP	36.4 ± 3.8	36.6 ± 1.4
Labeling index	0.16 ± 0.03	1.0 ± 0.2	3.6 ± 1.7	1.0 ± 0.4

NP indicates not present; specifically, alveoli appeared between days 80 and 115 of gestation. Labeling index indicates the percentage of epithelial cell nuclei that incorporated tritiated thymidine following a 1 hr incubation of tissue explants. Data adapted from Smith et al., 1987.

tissue between day 80 and 115 of gestation. However, between day 115 and 140, quantitative histology (% epithelial area) alone suggests there is no continued parenchymal development. This is clearly not the case since both tissue weight and total DNA doubles. Lack of change in epithelial area between day 115 and 140 is a reflection that alveoli are present and at these stages of gestation, but an increase in lumen and decrease in stromal tissue area reflect accumulation of some secretions and compression of stromal tissue

between alveoli. In addition to the appearance of alveoli during gestation, the cells undergo a progressive structural and biochemical maturation as parturition approaches. The increase in DNA labeling index on day 115 reflects the rapid growth during this period.

Mammary growth as measured by total DNA continues during the early days of lactation in rats, rabbits, guinea pigs, and mice. In the rat, for example, as much as 26% of the total mammary growth occurs during lactation. In the mouse there is a transient surge in mammary cell proliferation 2 to 3 days postpartum. In fact it is reported that the cell population doubles between the last day of gestation and day 5 of lactation. The guinea pig is especially interesting in that there is little change in total mammary DNA during gestation but a dramatic increase within 2 days of the birth of the pups. However, if suckling is not permitted in these species the increased growth just after parturition is prevented. This suggests that signals associated with suckling or milking are important for growth, especially in early lactation. Regardless, it seems clear that once lactation is established, the rate of mammary cell proliferation is markedly lower than during other stages of mammary development. However, recent reports show that several weeks of "extra" milking stimulation within the first 2 months of lactation in dairy cows increase subsequent milk production when milking frequency is returned to normal. Mechanisms for the effect are unknown, but the fact that it continues after treatment supports the idea that it may involve recruitment of additional well-differentiated cells. This might reflect overt proliferation of additional secretory cells or perhaps enhanced functional differentiation in a population of preexisting nonsecretory cells (Bar-Peled et al., 1995). This effect contrasts with the galactopoietic of treatment of cows with bovine somatotropin (bST) in that milk production is dramatically increased during the period of treatment but returns to control levels when treatment is discontinued. This pattern of response has been interpreted to indicate that bST alters metabolism rather than cell proliferation. This is clearly an area of intense research interest.

In dairy species, it is usually concluded that there is normally little mammary growth during established lactation. However, comprehensive data for early lactation is lacking. The concentration of DNA in mammary parenchyma is relatively unchanged in early lactation in sheep, goats, or cows, but it is risky to interpret this as a lack of mammary growth since it does not evaluate the entire mammary gland. Total parenchymal DNA doubles between 2 weeks before and after parturition (27.9 versus 46.0 g) but these data do not determine whether the growth occurs before or after parturition. Rates of thymidine incorporation are very low for mammary tissue taken from lactating ruminants, but mitotic cells are sometimes observed.

In lactating goats, unilateral inhibition of secretion in one gland of goats results in a compensatory increase in milk production of the other gland. There are also reports of increased milk production in cows by uninfected quarters among cows with mastitis. The relative contributions of hypertrophy and hyperplasia for this effect are unknown. However, in lactating beef cows, covering one-half of the udder to prevent sucking

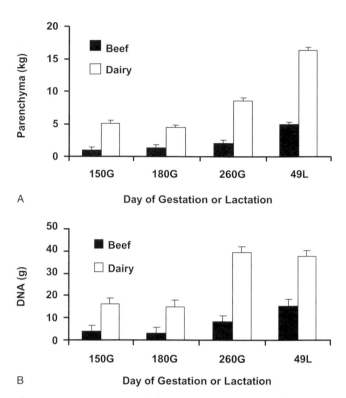

Fig. 18.5. Mammary growth during gestation in cattle. Chart A illustrates the growth of the mammary tissue of beef and dairy heifers during pregnancy and lactation based on weights of parenchymal tissue dissected from udder slices obtained at slaughter. Chart B provides similar data, except growth is reflected by changes in total parenchymal tissue DNA. Both measures demonstrate a consistent advantage for the Holstein, compared with Hereford, heifers. However, the increased weight of parenchymal mass between day 260 prepartum and day 49 of lactation for Holsteins is not reflected in DNA. This suggests that much of the increase in Holsteins reflects onset of milk secretion. Figure adapted from Keys et al., 1989.

increased thymidine incorporation in lactating mammary glands compared with control glands of cows, which continued suckling in all glands. Morphologically, lactating tissue from control and compensatory treatment cows was indistinguishable and the tissue did not appear consistently different between zones within lactating quarters. About 40% of the parenchymal tissue consisted of closely packed alveoli. In some areas the secretory cells appeared highly differentiated similar to cells from dairy cows. Remaining parenchymal tissue contained alveoli more widely scattered in the stromal matrix, and the cells were less well differentiated. Labeled cells were observed in both regions but appeared more frequently in the less well-differentiated tissue (Akers et al., 1990).

Figure 18.5 shows changes in the growth of mammary parenchymal of beef and dairy heifers during pregnancy and into lactation. Comparisons between Panels A and B illustrate that those measures of udder parenchymal mass alone can be misleading.

Table 18.3.   Mammary parenchymal growth in heifers and ewes.

Measure	Stage of Development				
	Prepuberty	Postpuberty	Mid Gest	Late Gest	Lactation
Heifers					
DNA (g)	1.1	2.6	16.3	39.3	38.8
Wt. (g)	495	957	5,110	8,560	16,350
Ewes					
DNA (g)	0.02	0.09	1.3	2.3	2.6
Wt. (g)	15	78	557	1057	1340

Data adapted from Smith et al., 1989; Keys et al., 1989; McFadden et al., 1988; Sejrsen et al., 1982, 1986.

Specifically, based on udder parenchymal mass there is marked growth of parenchymal tissue between day 260 and day 49 of lactation in both Holsteins and Herefords (Fig. 18.5A). In contrast, when udder growth is evaluated based on parenchymal DNA (Fig. 18.5B), marked differences between breeds remain, but little change occurs between day 260 of gestation and day 49 of lactation in Holsteins. This is likely explained by the increased accumulation of secretions in the Holstein heifers compared with the Hereford heifers. When lactation performance is considered, it is clear that differences in milk production (3.5 versus 20.3 kg/d) are explained by both changes in udder parenchymal tissue mass and function. For example, total RNA as well as RNA/DNA ratio is greater in Holstein than Hereford heifers. Interestingly, ability of mammary explants from lactating animals to secrete α-lactalbumin (a specific milk protein) in culture closely mirrored (57 versus 289 ng per mg of tissue per 24 h) the corresponding 5.8 fold difference in daily milk production. The relative failure of cytological differentiation (Akers et al., 2006) in mammary tissue of beef compared with dairy heifers is puzzling since milking stimulation and management was identical between breeds in this study. Is it possible that selection for increased milk production (in dairy cattle) has allowed for the maximization of differentiation signals during the critical periparturient period?

Realization in the early 1960s that the DNA content of cells is essentially constant (with the exception of the generally small proportion of cells that are undergoing DNA synthesis in preparation for cell division at a given moment) ushered in a host of studies to estimate mammary cell number based on total DNA content. This method is especially valuable when combined with careful dissection of the mammary gland to distinguish the parenchymal portion from the stromal tissue of the mammary gland. Even with careful dissection of the mammary gland to remove apparent connective tissue, there are clearly nonglandular cellular elements, i.e., blood vessels, lymphatic vessels, nerves, fibroblasts, adipocytes, and white blood cells, which contribute to the DNA content of the parenchymal tissue compartment. Regardless, classic studies in a variety of lactating species give direct evidence that the number of mammary epithelial cells is proportional to milk production. Indeed, the correlation between total parenchymal DNA and milk production averages about 0.85. Consequently, any activity that reduces the number or function of the mammary alveoli will also reduce milk production (Tucker, 1981; 1987).

In addition to the nonsecreting epithelial cells and various stromal cells, extracellular secretions, i.e., proteins and proteoglycans that surround the mammary ducts and alveoli are also critical for development. Collagen is the major extracellular protein component of the mammary stromal tissue. Moreover, the amino acid hydroxyproline is a specific and major component of collagen. Thus, assay of tissue content of hydroxyproline provides a quantitative measure of stromal tissue. When coupled with measurement of fat the relative amounts of connective tissue associated with the parenchymal tissue can be estimated.

Data in Tables 18.2 and 18.3 illustrate the dramatic changes in mammary growth from birth to lactation in Holstein heifers and crossbred ewes. Measured as trimmed udder weight or parenchymal DNA, mammary growth is greatest during gestation. However, relative lack of change in DNA from late gestation into lactation compared with trimmed udder weight suggests that DNA is a better measure of cell growth, since increased weight may be accumulated secretions.

Measurement of parenchymal tissue RNA and/or protein indicates synthetic capacity and is useful to evaluate the fully developed mammary gland. The reason for this is simple. As the secretory cells differentiate in concert with parturition, there is a marked increase in the presence of rough endoplasmic reticulum and corresponding production of mRNA for specific milk proteins. Consequently, onset of milk synthesis and secretion corresponds with a marked increase in the mammary tissue RNA. On a per cell basis, increased synthetic capacity can be evaluated by comparing the ratio of RNA/DNA in mammary parenchymal tissue. Late in gestation after alveoli have formed, but before the onset of copious milk synthesis and secretion, this ratio is generally about 1. During established lactation the RNA content of the secretory cells increases dramatically so that this ratio more than doubles. Changes in parenchymal tissue protein follow a similar pattern; however, care must be taken to account for the milk protein, which may be trapped in the tissue. Finally, any of these measures are more useful if they can be applied on a whole mammary gland basis. For rodents or other animals, in which an entire mammary gland (or parenchymal tissue) can be isolated and sampled, these measures can be related to milk production.

Alveolar cell differentiation and lactogenesis

A common biological theme is that structure follows function. The structural differentiation of the alveolar cells around the time of parturition illustrates this principle. As parturition approaches, these cells become polarized, with appearance of abundant arrays of RER, numerous mitochondria, and competent tight junctions just as full-scale milk synthesis and secretion is initiated. This process is called lactogenesis. Two events are critical. The structural differentiation of the alveolar epithelial cells allows for packaging of milk components for secretion while biochemical differentiation allows for synthesis of milk constituents. We will review some of the structural changes now.

The mammary gland begins to reach its mature structural state late in gestation. That is, alveoli and mammary ducts are in place. Indeed, soon after the alveoli are formed some accumulation of secretions begins. For example, in cows during first gestation small but variable volumes of secretions can be expressed from the mammary gland several months prior to parturition. Prepartum milking of dairy heifers is sometimes initiated during the month before parturition as a management technique to relieve intramammary pressure. Irrespective of prepartum milking, secretions obtained prior to calving are generally high in protein and low in lactose compared with normal milk but with relatively small concentrations of specific milk proteins. Because extensive removal of mammary secretions prior to calving can alter the course of mammary development, i.e., premature mammary cell differentiation, it is recommended that prepartum milking, once initiated, should continue until onset of normal milking at calving.

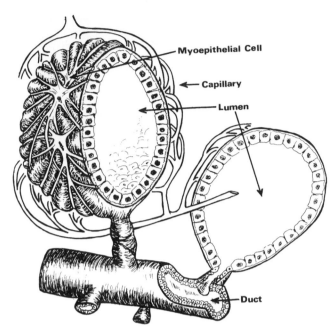

Fig. 18.6. Mammary alveolus. This diagram illustrates the three-dimensional structure of the mammary alveolus. The hollow center of the alveolus allows a space for the accumulation of milk components that have been synthesized and secreted by the secretory cells that compose the internal wall of the structure. The outside of the alveolus has a network of myoepithelial cells that contract in response to release of oxytocin at the time of milking. This forces stored milk into the terminal duct, which exits the lumen of the alveolus. The milk progresses through larger ducts to be emptied at the nipple or teat end. This figure was taken from Larson, 1985.

High concentrations of protein in secretions obtained prepartum in cows reflect the accumulation of immunoglobulins transferred into secretions from the blood stream. As the alveolar cells differentiate, accumulation of immunoglobulins is reduced. However, the accumulated immunoglobulins in the secretions obtained with the first milking or suckling postpartum, i.e., colostrum, provide passive immunity to the offspring. This is critical for those species that lack immunoglobulin transfer to the fetus in utero. With the onset of regular milking or suckling, the composition of mammary secretions progressively changes to reflect normal milk composition.

Figure 18.6 illustrates the major structure of a mammary alveolus; Figures 18.7 and 18.8 illustrate the dramatic change in alveolar cell structure that accompanies lactogenesis. Much of this change is coordinated by alterations in circulating hormones and changes in hormone signaling on mammary target cells.

Ultrastructure of the mammary epithelium during lactation has now been documented in many species. The percentages of various cellular organelles within the cytoplasm of alveolar secretory cells from lactating

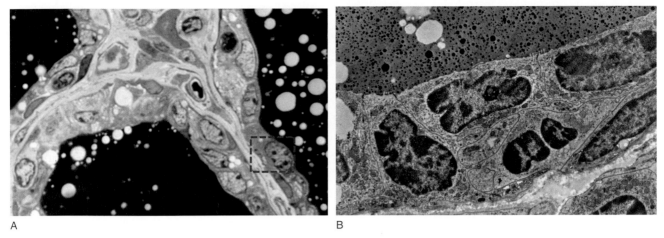

Fig. 18.7. Prepartum alveolar structure. Panel A illustrates a portion of three different alveoli from the mammary gland of a cow about 2 weeks prior to calving. This light microscope image demonstrates the relative lack of differentiation of the epithelial cells. However, the luminal spaces are darkly stained because of accumulation primarily of colostrum. Panel B illustrates the ultrastructure of cells similar to those outlined in the dashed box in Panel A. Notice that most of the cell area is occupied by the cell nucleus. Structurally, these cells are poorly differentiated.

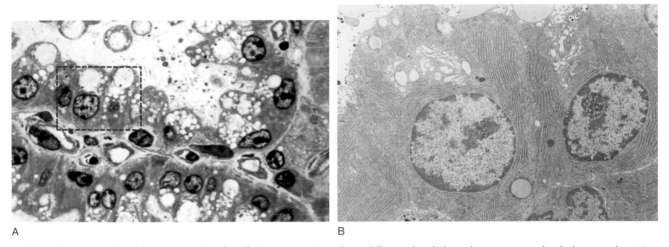

Fig. 18.8. Postpartum alveolar structures. Panel A illustrates a portion of two different alveoli from the mammary gland of a cow about 2 weeks after calving. This light microscope image demonstrates very well-differentiated epithelial cells. The nuclei are generally rounded and basally displaced in the cell. There is also abundant RER indicated by the staining of the basolateral area near the nucleus. The apical ends of the cells have a lacy appearance because of the abundance of Golgi, secretory vesicles, and lipid droplets. Panel B illustrates the ultrastructure of cells similar to those outlined in the dashed box in Panel A. Notice the rounded nuclei, numerous arrays of RER and Golgi.

rats and cows are illustrated in Table 18.4. This generally uniform structure includes basal and paranuclear cytoplasm occupied by parallel arrays of rough endoplasmic reticulum (RER). The supranuclear Golgi apparatus typically consists of stacks of smooth membranes whose terminal cisternae release casein and lactose containing secretory vesicles. Lipid droplets and secretory vesicles seemingly fill the apical ends of the cells and microtubules are most frequently observed oriented perpendicular with respect to the apical plasma membrane. Mitochondria and free ribosomes are abundant throughout the basal-lateral cytoplasm. The basal plasma membrane is often thrown into complex folds, believed to indicate active

Table 18.4. Ultrastructural analysis of cytoplasmic organelles in well-differentiated mammary epithelia from lactating rats and dairy cows.

Cytological Parameter	Rats	Cows
RER[a]	14.7	16.1
Golgi	20.9	18.8
Lipid	1.4	4.7
Mitochondria	7.1	6.3
Nucleus	21.7	22.0
Other	34.2	31.1

[a] Rough Endoplasmic Reticulum.
Data are expressed as mean percentage cytoplasm occupied by each cytoplasmic component. Data adapted from Nickerson and Akers, 1984.

pinocytosis. Myoepithelial cells frequently occur interspersed between the basal plasma membrane and the basal lamina that forms a loose barrier between the simple cuboidal epithelial cells and the underlying stromal tissues. It is now apparent that parenchymal tissue from glands of high-yielding animals has an abundance of structurally highly differentiated polarized alveolar cells.

Hormonal control of lactogenesis and lactation

The endocrine system, perhaps more than any other physiological system, plays a central role in all aspects of mammary development (mammogenesis), onset of lactation (lactogenesis), and maintenance of milk secretion (galactopoiesis). Lactogenesis is frequently described as a two-stage process. Stage I consists of limited structural and functional differentiation of the secretory epithelium during the last third of pregnancy. Stage II involves completion of cellular differentiation during the immediate periparturient period coinciding with onset of copious milk synthesis and secretion. During lactation, the secretory cells synthesize and secrete copious amounts of carbohydrate, protein, and lipid. Production of this complex mixture of nutrients depends on coordination between biochemical pathways to supply metabolic intermediates and secretory pathways for secretion. For example, the disaccharide lactose is the predominate milk sugar. The enzyme complex necessary for lactose synthesis, membrane-bound galactosyltransferase, and the whey protein α-lactalbumin, combines in the Golgi apparatus to form lactose synthetase, which links glucose and galactose producing lactose. Activation of the α-lactalbumin gene and synthesis of α-lactalbumin is most closely associated with stage II of lactogenesis.

Experiments beginning in the 1920s (Stricker and Grueter, 1928) showed that milk secretion could be induced in virgin rabbits by injecting a pituitary extract. In 1933, Riddle, Bates, and Dykshorn purified the protein responsible for the milk secretion response observed by Stricker and Grueter, they named it prolactin (Prl). Even now, the widely touted and utilized galactopoietic effect of somatotropin to increase milk production in lactating dairy cows had its foundation in studies by Asimov and Krouze in the 1930s. They showed that injections of pituitary extracts consistently increased milk production in lactating cows. Scientists describing and quantifying the potent effects of the pregnancy on mammary growth and changes in the mammary gland at puberty spurred others to isolate and identify the steroid hormones estrogen and progesterone. Advances in purification techniques

and understanding of steroid hormone chemistry allowed further studies leading to the production of these steroids for widespread animal testing.

Although the existence of mammogenic and lactogenic substances from the pituitary had long been known, the efforts of C. H. Li and colleagues in the 1940s to purify larger quantities of Prl and growth hormone (GH) were essential. Soon thereafter, specific roles for these hormones in the regulation of mammogenesis in rodents were delineated in classic ablation replacement experiments (Lyons et al., 1958; Nandi, 1958). In an extensive series of studies, triply operated (adrenalectomized, ovariectomized, and hypophysectomized) rats and mice were treated with various combinations of purified hormones to see whether normal mammary development could be restored. Injections of estrogen and GH together caused proliferation of mammary ducts. However, treatment with estrogen, progesterone, Prl, and GH were needed for lobulo-alveolar development. The maximum ductular and lobulo-alveolar development, although still less than that in pregnancy, was obtained in animals also given glucocorticoids. For some strains of mice, GH and Prl were both capable of stimulating lobulo-alveolar development.

British researchers, focused on efforts to improve and maintain milk supplies during World War II, initiated many endocrine studies on mammary development and function in dairy animals (Cowie et al., 1980). For example, the effects of estrogen and progesterone on mammogenesis were extensively evaluated in attempts to induce lactation in nonpregnant animals. Although difficulties with needed surgeries and expense continues to limit use of ablation replacement experiments to study mammary development and function in cattle, Cowie (1969) studied hypophysectomized-ovariectomized goats and showed that mammary development comparable to midgestation could be obtained in animals treated with a combination of estrogen, progesterone, Prl, GH, and ACTH. Such experiments served to confirm that at least general effects attributed to these hormones on mammary development in rodents, applied to mammary development in dairy animals.

Although it should be clear that mammogenesis involves more than increased secretion of estrogen and progesterone, which occurs during pregnancy, this is nonetheless critical. During the estrus cycle, estrogen concentrations increase as a consequence of follicle growth, but with the appearance of the dominant follicle and ovulation concentrations of estrogen decline and progesterone concentrations increase. Since estrogen and progesterone are both important for final duct growth and lobulo-alveolar development, the lack of a sustained simultaneous increase of both steroids during the estrus cycle likely explains the lack of marked parenchymal tissue development at this time. Furthermore, few of the studied species show evidence of lobulo-alveolar development prior to conception. With conception, the corpus luteum is maintained, and along with increasing production by the placenta in many species, blood concentrations of progesterone are elevated throughout gestation. Concentrations of estradiol are higher (relative to the estrus cycle) with a gradual increase during gestation until a more dramatic increase during the final few weeks before birth. Consequently, concentrations of estrogen and progesterone are both simultaneously elevated during much of gestation, especially so during the later portion of gestation. This is believed to be responsible for much of the mammary growth during gestation. Prl and possible prolactinlike activity associated with secretion of placental lactogen is also important in mammogenesis in some ruminants (sheep and goats). In cattle, Prl is most likely a permissive agent for the mammogenic effects of the steroids and other growth factors. There are no specific changes in secretion of Prl in cattle associated with mammogenesis and lobulo-alveolar formation during pregnancy.

An interesting accidental discovery reported by Smith and Schanbacher (1973) created a flurry of activity on hormonal induction of lactation in cattle. These researchers were studying the effects of steroids on secretion of immunoglobulins into mammary secretions of nonlactating cows, i.e., animals that had failed to conceive. They observed that injections of estradiol-17-β and progesterone for only 7 days, at doses that mimicked blood concentrations in animals near calving, caused the udders of some of the animals to "bag up." When these animals were milked, the initial colostrumlike secretions rapidly gave way to secretion of milk. As reviewed (Akers, 1985), subsequent studies showed that lactation could be induced in about 70%

of these nonpregnant cows and that milk yields for the successful animals averaged 70% of normal. Others found positive correlations between the success of induced lactations and concentrations of Prl as well as improved yields when cows were also given drugs to induce Prl secretion. Also, greater milk yields measured for cows induced into lactation during the spring and summer was attributed to higher concentrations of Prl in serum compared with cows treated during winter months.

Although changes in blood concentrations of mammogenic hormones are important in explaining changes in mammary growth, changes in tissue sensitivity and availability of biologically active hormones are also important. In circulation, the steroid hormones are bound to transport proteins. Even in tissues, the steroids can become sequestered with cellular lipids and therefore effectively unavailable (Capuco et al., 1982). This effect coupled with a decrease in progesterone receptor concentration and a change in isoforms of the receptor explains the disappearance of the negative effect of progesterone on lactogenesis at the time of parturition in cattle. This illustrates the concept that the biological effectiveness of circulating hormones may change independent of the total blood concentration of the hormone. In addition, changes in expression, synthesis, or availability of hormone receptors in target cells also clearly impact biological response. While there is little data for expression of estrogen or progesterone receptors in bovine mammary tissue during mammogenesis, data from assay of ovine mammary tissue shows that expression of the progesterone receptor occurs in close correspondence with appearance of lobulo-alveolar development (Table 18.2). Serum concentrations of progesterone are consistently elevated during gestation, with higher concentrations in later stages of gestation and in ewes with more than one fetus. Table 18.5 illustrates

Table 18.5. Effect of stage of gestation upon serum concentrations of mammogenic hormones mammary tissue receptor concentration.

Measurement	Day of Gestation			
Hormone binding	50 (n = 3)	80 (n = 4)	115 (n = 3)	140 (n = 4)
Progesterone (fmol/mg cytosolic protein)	125 ± 53	149 ± 26	656 ± 216	57 ± 22
Prolactin (fmol/mg microsomal protein) Hormone concentration	7.2 ± 2.1	5.2 ± 1.9	32 ± 3.6	22.2 ± 2.9
Progesterone (ng/ml)	3.6 ± 1.3	5.6 ± 1.0	29.9 ± 8.6	14.8 ± 0.7
Prolactin (ng/ml)	58 ± 10	24 ± 4	31 ± 8	134 ± 26
Growth hormone (ng/ml)	2.4 ± 0.4	4.4 ± 1.4	8.1 ± 1.3	15 ± 6.0

Data adapted from Smith et al., 1987, 1989.

changes in serum concentrations of some important mammogenic hormones during gestation as well as mammary tissue receptor concentration.

As its name might suggest, Prl has undoubtedly been the most intensely studied hormone related to lactation and mammary growth. Despite understanding that the presence of the pituitary is essential for normal mammary development, whether Prl or GH is predominating in mammogenesis is not clear. The answer to this question is likely species dependent.

In addition to the ovary and corpus luteum, the placenta produces estrogen, progesterone, and a prolactinlike hormone called placental lactogen (PL). PL was first recognized by its Prl-like biological effects. However, the PLs of many species have both GH and Prl-like activities. For example, Prl and nonprimate GH molecules interact only with their specific receptors, called lactogenic and somatogenic, respectively. Human GH, in contrast, recognizes both receptor classes. This coincidentally probably explains the inappropriate breast development sometimes observed in human males with pituitary tumors that overproduce GH. Both ovine and bovine PL behave like human GH; they compete for both somatogenic and lactogenic receptors. This explains some of the names associated with these proteins isolated from the placenta, i.e., chorionic somatomammotropin or chorionic mammotropin. Although PL is implicated in preparation for the mammary gland for lactation, stimulation of steroidogenesis, fetal growth, and alteration of maternal metabolism, direct evidence for effects in cattle are lacking. The best evidence for a role for Pl in mammogenesis is in rodents and in sheep and goats.

In contrast with a role for Prl in mammogenesis, there is no doubt about the importance of Prl in lacto-genesis. Some of the best evidence for the importance of increased periparturient secretion of Prl in stage II lactogenesis has come from experiments in which the administration of a dopamine agonist was used to inhibit Prl secretion and correspondingly impair lactation. In ruminants where postpartum milking continues, administration of the dopamine agonist α-bromoergocryptine (CB154) reduced basal prolactin concentration about 80% and prevented the usual periparturient rise as well as the milking induced Prl rise during the first week postpartum. Milk production was reduced 45% during the first 10 days postpartum. Lost milk production was associated with reduced synthesis of α-lactalbumin, lactose, and fatty acids, as well as impaired structural differentiation of the mammary secretory cells. Selected effects are summarized in Table 18.6. Cows treated with exogenous Prl in addition to the agonist (to replace the periparturient surge in prolactin) showed no loss of milk production or negative effects on milk component biosynthesis or alveolar cell differentiation. The effect of Prl suppression and replacement during the periparturient period on milk production in multiparous cows is shown in Figure 18.9. Clearly, Prl is important in mammary cell differentiation and lactogenesis (Akers et al., 1981).

Aside from circumstantial evidence related to changes in circulating hormone concentrations, there is a marked increase in numbers of mammary cell receptors for Prl, IGF-I, and cortisol during late gestation. Progesterone receptor concentration is also correspondingly reduced with the onset of lactation. Thus, simultaneous, coordinated changes in circulating hormones and receptors serve to regulate the timing of lactogenesis. It is believed that high concentrations of progesterone during most of gestation act to inhibit the onset of lactation. Near the time of par-

Table 18.6. Changes in lactose synthesis, α-lactalbumin, RNA and DNA in mammary gland of cows before and after parturition and with treatment with CB154 to suppress Prl secretion.

	Treatment			
	Prepartum	*Postpartum*	*CB154*	*CB154 + Prl*
Lactose synthesis (μg/h/100mg)	39 ± 63	552 ± 70	327 ± 63	628 ± 81
α-Lactalbumin (μg/mg/cytosol protein)	1.7 ± 0.4	5.4 ± 0.4	2.8 ± 0.4	6.8 ± 0.5
RNA (g)	23.6 ± 2.1	87.2 ± 16.8	56.0 ± 7.9	91.5 ± 12.8
DNA (g)	27.9 ± 2.9	46.0 ± 3.8	40.1 ± 3.8	42.2 ± 3.8

Control animals were killed 10 days before or after parturition. CB154 was administered for 12 days prior to expected parturition through parturition. Animals given Prl were infused continuously for 6 days immediately before parturition. Data adapted from Akers et al., 1981.

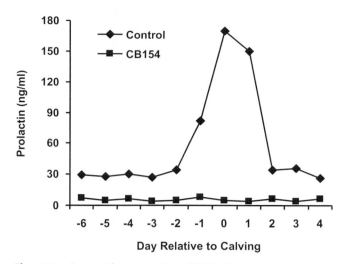

Fig. 18.9. Serum Prl in cows given CB154. Cows were administered daily injections of ergrocryptine (CB154) during the periparturient period. Both basal concentrations and the surge in Prl, which accompanies parturition, were blocked. Data adapted from Akers et al. 1981.

turition, progesterone concentrations begin to wane and estrogen concentrations increase. Removal of the negative effects of progesterone along with the positive effects of Prl and glucocorticoids set the stage for the onset of copious milk production (stage II of lactogenesis).

Data from culture experiments also support a role of these hormones in lactogenesis. For example, additions of estradiol or cortisol markedly enhance Prl-induced secretion of α-lactalbumin (a specific milk protein) by mammary explants taken from pregnant cows. Mammary explants from estrogen-primed or pregnant mice also require insulin, cortisol, and Prl for the accumulation of casein and α-lactalbumin. However, some caution is advised with wholesale extrapolation of results from culture experiments to the intact animal as well as uncritical extrapolation between species. For example, induction of the various milk proteins in culture does not necessarily reflect the timing of events in vivo. Neither do existing culture methods allow consistent synthesis and secretion of milk lipids. Finally, hormone concentrations employed may not accurately reflect the situation at the level of the mammary cell in the animal. Culture systems by their very nature represent relatively uncomplicated regulation compared with the intact animal. Nonetheless, results shown in Figure 18.10 illustrate the positive effects of Prl, cortisol, and estradiol on synthesis and secretion of α-lactalbumin by explants of bovine mammary tissue.

Application of molecular techniques to mammary gland biology has solidified knowledge that Prl

and glucocorticoids are the primary stimulators of mammary cell differentiation. Both Prl and glucocorticoid response elements are found within the promoter regions of the genes for several mammary-specific milk proteins. Induction of both mRNA and specific milk proteins in the presence of Prl or glucocorticoids in isolated mammary epithelial cells confirms the importance of these hormones in lactogenesis and provide details for mechanisms of action of these hormones in control of milk protein gene expression (Rosen et al., 1999; Akers, 2006).

The term *galactopoiesis* was originally coined to describe the enhancement of an established lactation. With this strict definition, only exogenous GH (bST) and thyroid hormone are undisputed galactopoietic hormones in dairy animals. Responses also suggest that these hormones are endogenously rate limiting. However, more generally, galactopoiesis can also be described as the maintenance of lactation. In this sense, a larger number of hormones and growth factors are candidates as galactopoietic agents. Continued secretion of galactopoietic hormones, growth factors, and regular milk removal are essential for regulation and maintenance of lactation following lactogenesis.

The pituitary gland and its hormones are essential integrators of the endocrine regulation of milk secretion. This is dramatically shown by the loss of milk production in hypophysectomized lactating goats. However, milk yield can be fully restored to prehypophysectomy levels by the combined administration of Prl, GH, glucocorticoids, and triiodothyronine (T_3) (see Fig. 18.11). Although species differences exist, endocrine organ ablation/replacement studies show that Prl, GH, glucocorticoids, and thyroid hormones are typically required for the full maintenance of lactation (Topper and Freeman, 1980). This does not mean that additional hormones and growth factors (humoral and local, identified and unidentified) might not also be important or mediate effects of these hormones.

Secretion of oxytocin at milking or suckling is necessary in most species for efficient removal of accumulated milk, and in some species it is essential to obtain any milk at all. The importance of regular milk removal to prevent mammary involution has been known for many years, but it has also long been hypothesized that the secretion of galactopoietic hormones with milking or sucking was also important. Secretion of Prl and oxytocin as well as related secretions of norepinephrine or epinephrine, which can impact the secretion (or action) of oxytocin, are most often associated with hormone secretion at milking and effects on milk synthesis. However, glucocorticoids are also secreted in response to milking or suckling, as is GH in some species.

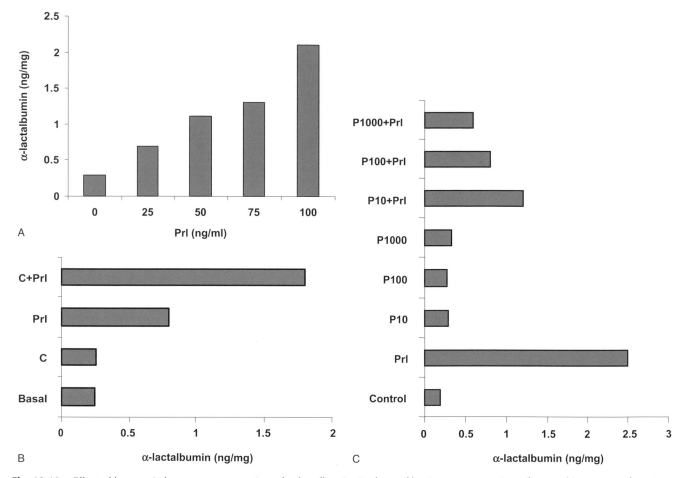

Fig. 18.10. Effect of lactogenic hormones on secretion of α-lactalbumin. Explants of bovine mammary tissue from multiparous, nonlactating, pregnant cows were incubated with various combinations of hormones. Panel A demonstrates a concentration-dependent increase in α-lactalbumin in response to addition of bovine Prl. Panel B shoes the additive effect of cortisol on Prl-induced α-lactalbumin secretion. Panel C demonstrates a concentration-dependent inhibitory effect of progesterone (P) on Prl stimulation of α-lactalbumin secretion. Data adapted from Goodman et al., 1983.

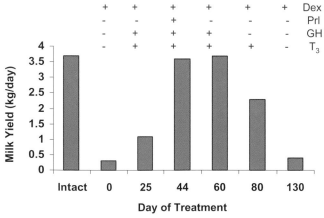

Fig. 18.11. Milk yield after hypophysectomy.
A lactating goat was hypophysectomized and administered hormone replacement. Milk production averaged 3.7 kg per day prior to surgery (intact). After treatment for 2 months with dexamethasone (Dex, a synthetic glucocorticoid) yields were as indicated at time zero. Milk production is depicted per addition or removal of hormone treatment as indicated. Adapted from Cowie, 1969.

Milk synthesis and secretion

The mammary gland is an unusual exocrine gland in several respects. The product is a very complex mixture, which depends on apocrine and meocrine modes of secretion. Other components are derived by passage of soluble molecules across (transcellular) and sometimes between (paracellular) cells. Physically, milk is a complex solution of salts, carbohydrates, miscellaneous compounds with dispersed proteins and protein aggregates, casein micelles, and fat globules. Milk osmolarity generally equals blood (~300 mosm) and has a pH between 6.2 and 7.0. Bovine and human milk have an average pH of 6.6 and 7.0, respectively.

Once initiated milk secretion continues more or less continuously throughout lactation. This secretion mixture includes membrane-bound lipid droplets, casein micelles, and an aqueous phase usually containing lactose, minerals, other proteins, and a variety of other soluble components. Milk is stored within the lumen of the alveoli and ductular system until it is

Table 18.7. Gross milk composition of various species.

Species	Percentage by Weight					
	Water	Fat	Casein	Whey	Lactose	Ash
Human (Homo sapiens)	87.1	4.5	0.4	0.5	7.1	0.2
Cow (Bos Taurus)	87.3	3.9	2.6	0.6	4.6	0.7
Sheep (Ovis aries)	82.0	7.2	3.9	0.7	4.8	0.9
Goat (Capra hircus)	86.7	4.5	2.6	0.6	4.3	0.8
Horse (Equus caballus)	88.8	1.9	1.3	1.2	6.2	0.5
Pig (Sus scrofa)	81.2	6.8	2.8	2.0	5.5	1.0
Dog (Canis familiaris)	76.4	10.7	5.1	2.3	3.3	1.2
Cat (Felis catus)	–	4.8	3.7	3.3	4.8	1.0
Rat (Rattus norvegicus)	79.0	10.3	6.4	2.0	2.6	1.3
Mouse (Mus musculus)	73.6	13.1	7.0	2.0	3.0	1.3
Blue whale (Balenopteridae musculus)	45.5	39.4	7.2	3.7	0.4	1.4

Data adapted from Oftendal, 1984, 1997; Jenness, 1985.

removed by the milking machine or the suckling offspring. Suckling intervals vary widely between mammals, ranging from minutes to hours in cattle, to once daily in rabbits, to once every 2 days in tree shrews, or only once a week in some seals. Moreover, although there are species-specific changes in milk composition with stage of lactation, milk composition for most of lactation is generally only moderately affected by environmental or nutritional changes, despite the often-dramatic changes in milk volume. Function of the mammary gland during established lactation is closely linked with a number of hormones, growth factors, and local tissue regulators, but it is difficult to ascribe a specific transport activity to a particular molecule or to determine whether effects are direct or indirect.

Across species, there are dramatic differences in milk composition. Milk from Holstein cows (the source of the majority of milk for human consumption in Western societies) has about 3.2% protein, 3.4% fat, and 4.6% lactose. In contrast, hooded seals produce milk with about 6.0% protein, 50% fat, and virtually no carbohydrate. Table 18.7 provides milk composition data for some selected species.

Along with mammary cell–specific constituents milk contains a myriad of minor components. Many of these molecules are important nutrients or regulators of the neonate (growth factors, water, and ions) but other components may include drugs or other xenobiotic substances transported from the circulation. Molecules are transported into the milk by several possible routes. Mammary epithelial cells are able to maintain substantial gradients for Na^+, K^+, and Cl^- ions across the cell membrane. During established lactation there are also gradients between milk and plasma. These ions are important to maintain normal electrical gradients across the alveolar cell membranes but they also are critical in regulation of milk osmolar-

ity, especially for those species with low lactose production. Concentrations of Na^+ inside (~43 nM) the cells are typically lower than outside (150 nM) but the gradient for K^+ is the opposite (143 nM inside compared with 4.5 nM). These differentials are maintained by the action of Na^+ K^+ ATPase pumps in the basolateral membranes. The apical plasma membrane is permeable to both ions so that the distribution of these ions into milk is controlled by the electrical potential across the apical plasma membrane. Milk is electrically positive with respect to the cell, so that the concentrations of Na^+ and K^+ are lower in milk than in the cells, but the ratio K^+/Na^+ ratio (~3 : 1) is similar. Concentration of Cl^- is higher inside the cells than the equilibrium distribution would suggest, so membrane pumps in the basolateral and apical membranes act to sequester Cl^-. It is easy to imagine that this balance of ions between milk and blood is readily compromised if the leakiness of the tight junctions is altered (Stelwagen, 2001).

As dietitians and nutritionists frequently note, milk is a rich source of calcium, with total concentrations equaling 100 nM or more. With the onset of lactation the mammary gland extracts large quantities of calcium to supply the developing neonate. Indeed, for high-producing dairy cows this demand can lead to metabolic periparturient paresis unless animals are carefully managed. The calcium in the milk exists as free calcium, casein-bound calcium, or calcium associated with various inorganic anions, e.g., citrate and phosphate. There is little movement of calcium from milk to blood, which suggests that calcium cannot pass across the apical plasma membrane. Given that most of the calcium is associated with the casein micelles, the Golgi vesicle route of secretion is the predominating pathway. However, since all of the milk calcium is derived from the circulation, there must be differences in transport between basolateral and apical membranes. Mammary cells maintain a low intracellular free calcium concentration in spite of the marked accumulation of calcium in milk. This is important because changes in free calcium concentration are closely linked with several hormone and growth factor–signaling pathways. One idea is that the rate of calcium influx into the cell is matched by a corresponding uptake of calcium by cellular organelles. The presence of an ATP-dependent calcium pump on Golgi membranes has been demonstrated. Calcium uptake by mammary cells is also likely hormonally regulated since parathyroid hormone–related protein and $1,25\text{-}(OH)_2$ vitamin D_3 stimulates the uptake of calcium in cultured mammary tissue.

Lactation curves

Once initiated, lactation depends on regular suckling or milking of the mammary gland to maintain the lactation. Although the time required for regression varies markedly between species, i.e., days for rodents versus weeks for ruminants, without milk removal the alveolar structure is eventually degraded, alveolar cells de-differentiate and many cells undergo apoptosis. Without the stimulus of another gestation, the gland progressively reverts to a structure similar to that of the mature virgin. However, in dairy cows milk production increases with each successive lactation. This suggests cumulative mammary growth with each lactation cycle. Normal husbandry dictates that dairy cows are rebred soon after the onset of lactation and milked for much of the concurrent pregnancy. Consequently, during the later part of lactation the cow has dual functions of growth of the developing calf and continued lactation. Compared with wild ruminants or beef cows the period between consecutive lactations is relatively short. Consequently there is less opportunity for mammary regression or involution. Second, hormonal and metabolic changes associated with late gestation and preparation for parturition is conducive for mammary development. This means that the time course of mammary involution is impacted by concurrent gestation.

Although early sections provide an overview of mammary development, the somewhat unique anatomy of the udder deserves special attention. In the cow and other ruminants, the mammary glands are clustered together into groups of two (goats or sheep) or four (cattle) mammary glands to create the udder. This arrangement provides a practical advantage. Since the mammary glands and teats are close together, the portion of the milking machine attached to the animal (teat cups and teat cluster) can be relatively compact. For those not familiar with milking and management of modern dairy cows, the udder of

a lactating Holstein cow, for example, can be massive. It is not unusual for a single cow to yield 30 kg or more of milk at a single milking. Combined with the mass of the udder tissues this means that the connective tissues of the mammary glands have to support as much as 70 kg of tissue and stored milk just before milking. Given the dorsal inguinal orientation of the udder, this is no trivial matter. Support is provided by strong flat suspensory ligaments, which are attached to the pelvic bone and to the strong tendons of the abdominal muscles in the pelvic area.

The udder is divided into two distinct halves, separated by the medial or median suspensory ligament, which provides most of the strength to hold the udder attached to the dorsal body wall. Fibers of the lateral ligaments are continuous with the medial ligament but spread over either side of the udder so that it appears to be held in a sling of connective tissue. The medial ligament is somewhat elastic, but the lateral ligaments are not. As the milk accumulates in the udder, the normally vertical orientation of the teats is lost as teats progressively protrude laterally. As animals age, excessive degradation of the fibers of the medial suspensory ligament can reduce its support capacity so that the udder becomes pendulous irrespective of time relative to milking. This can lead to difficulty with milking, i.e., problems maintaining attachment of teat cups as well as problems with teat injury and increased mastitis risk. Figure 18.12 illustrates the appearance and strength of the medial and lateral ligaments. The mammary glands of the udder are directly connected to the abdominal cavity only via passage through the inguinal canals. These are paired narrow oblique passages through the abdominal wall on either side of the midline, just above the udder. These canals allow passage of blood and lymph vessels and nerves to the udder.

Compared with most other mammary glands, those of animals with udders also have relatively large nipples or teats. Specifically, the teat of the ruminant has a single opening called the streak canal that leads directly into a space within the teat called the teat cistern. The structure of the streak canal is considered further with respect to its roll as the primary defensive barrier against mastitis. The space of the teat cistern would typically hold only a few ml of milk. Near the base of the teat there is an annular fold of tissue, which separates the teat cistern from the gland cistern. The gland cistern is roughly the size of an orange and holds ~200 ml of milk. The gland cistern has many irregularly shaped cavities, which accommodate the endings of large intralobular ducts, which drain milk from the secretory tissue. Except for the terminal ducts that are directly adjacent to the alveoli, ducts are lined with at least two layers of nonsecretory epithelial cells. It is estimated that 40–60% of the milk is stored in the

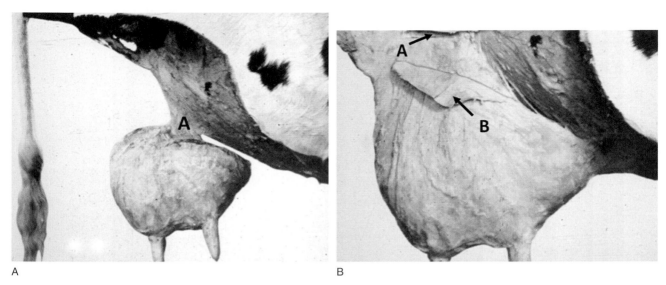

A   B

Fig. 18.12. Medial and lateral suspensory ligaments. Panel A shows the dissected udder of a cow supported by only the medial suspensory ligament. Panel B shows a portion of the lateral suspensory ligament dissected as a flap of tissue, the upper section (A, with arrow) and the lower section (B, with arrow). Adapted from Swett et al., 1942.

lumenal spaces of the ducts or cisterns. Above the gland cistern the tissue is progressively more dense and compact because of the relative lack of very large ducts and the closely arranged lobules.

It has long been assumed that milk is prevented from escaping from the teat by the action of bands of sphincterlike smooth muscle cells in the teat meatus surrounding the streak canal. However, recent studies suggest that most of these smooth muscle cell elements are located some distance from the streak canal and that they are more likely involved in rhythmic contractions of the teat. Thus, closure of the teat canal depends on passive elastic elements in the region surrounding the streak canal. A more recent suggestion is for a multispiraled, netlike combination of elastic fibers and associated smooth muscle cells, which produce a spiraling of the internal epithelial folds of the streak canal to affect closure. Regardless of the exact mechanism, the internal structure of the streak canal and its surface secretions prevent milk leakage and act as a barrier. Although milking ease and milk speed are important factors in the economics of a dairy operation, selection of cows with wide, short teat canals may well speed the milking process at the expense of increased risk of mastitis.

The skin of the teat is hairless but tough and resistant to tears or punctures. Histologically, it is a stratified squamous epithelium that extends over the teat end and into the teat opening for the length of the streak canal. However, relative lack of insulation seems to make the teats susceptible to cold weather problems. The washing of udders and teats in preparation for milking and movement of cows into freezing temperatures and winds before drying likely

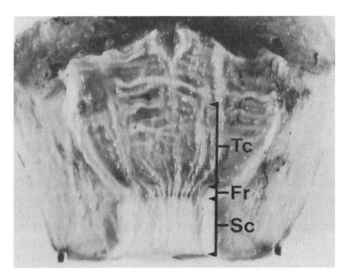

Fig. 18.13. Internal structure of the cow's teat. Areas illustrated include the streak canal (SC), Furstenberg's rosette (Fr), and the teat cistern (Tc). Adapted from Nickerson and Pankey, 1983.

amplify teat injury problems. Between the outside skin of the teat and internal surface of the streak canal or teat cistern the stromal tissue contains a network of blood vessels, lymphatic vessels, smooth muscle cells, and nerves. This extensive blood supply is important in maintenance of normal tissue temperature and especially so during severely cold temperatures. Because mechanical milking can retard blood flow in the teat, produce vascular congestion, or cause swelling of the stromal tissue, this likely acerbates problems with teat skin injury in cold weather.

The streak canal ranges from 7–16 mm in length with a mean diameter of 0.82 mm (Fig. 18.13). The

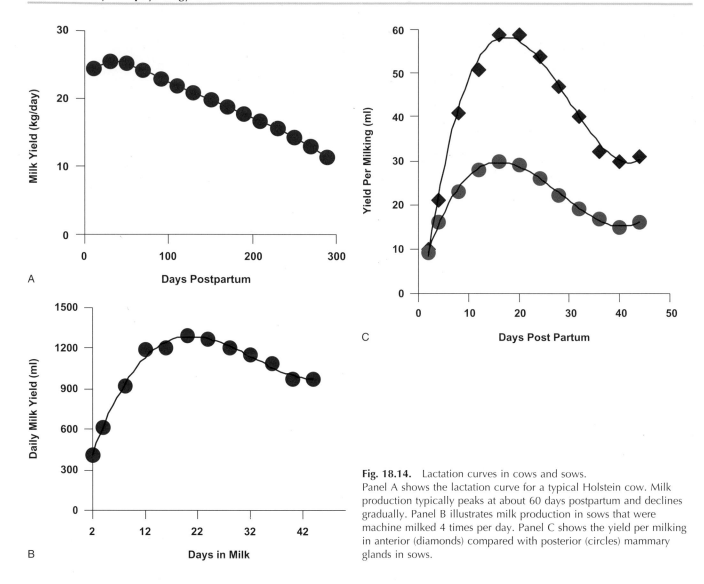

Fig. 18.14. Lactation curves in cows and sows.
Panel A shows the lactation curve for a typical Holstein cow. Milk production typically peaks at about 60 days postpartum and declines gradually. Panel B illustrates milk production in sows that were machine milked 4 times per day. Panel C shows the yield per milking in anterior (diamonds) compared with posterior (circles) mammary glands in sows.

lowest 2 cm of the streak canal is especially important because of capacity of these tissues to act as a barrier to minimize milk leakage or entrance of environmental agents. Intuitively, the diameter of the streak canal is positively related to the rate of milk flow, but cows with the best balance of acceptable rates of milk flow and protection from bacterial invasion can expect greatest longevity in the herd. Teats vary in shape and size, from cylindrical to funnel-shaped. Teat ends also vary; some are flat, but others are round or pointed. Pointed teats are less common and are associated with slow milking times but resistance to mastitis. Round teats are common and occur on cows with faster milking times, but these cows exhibit some resistance to mastitis. Flat teat ends are less common, but these cows also tend to have faster milking times with less resistance to mastitis. Certainly the uniformity of milking machine teat cups means that cows with teats of large diameter or length are more likely to suffer milking machine–related trauma.

A lactation curve for a typical Holstein cow is illustrated in Figure 18.14A. However, it is important to realize that estimates of milk yield need to be evaluated in relationship to milk composition, state of maturity of the offspring, suckling patterns, diet, and behavior of the species. Practically, production curves are most reliable for dairy animals (cows, goats, and sheep) because these animals have been selected for ease of milking and handling, high yields of milk, and for their capacity to respond to machine or hand milking. Because of their usefulness as bioreactors to produce pharmaceutical proteins in their milk, renewed interest in milking of pigs has emerged in recent years. Garst et al. (1999a, b) reported results for animals that were milked four times per day as well as effects on litter weight gains. Milk yields peaked at about 19 days postpartum and declined to 45 days postpartum. As might be expected, sows that were milked four times per day had litters with substantially lower weights at the time of weaning. Average daily milk yield per sow was 1.1 liters per day or 43.1 ± 8.6 l for the entire lactation period. There were also substantial differences in milk yields between individual mammary glands. For example, anterior glands produced more than posterior glands (~40 vs. 15 ml per milking). Examples of pig milk yields are illustrated in Figure 18.14.

For other species, direct measurements of milk yield requires that the animals be sedated and/or injected with exogenous oxytocin. Under these circumstances the relevance of the data (other than comparison between treatments) can be questioned. Certainly it is unknown whether yields reflect "natural" levels of production or whether measures of composition are accurate. An alternate for estimating yields is the response to timed-suckling episodes. This typically involves removal of the suckling young for a period of time and then weighing the litter or offspring immediately before and after a set period when returned to the mother (Beal et al, 1990). For species in which the offspring are solely dependent on milk for nourishment, measurement of offspring weight gain is used as an indirect measure of milk production of the mother.

While there is likely some question of the accuracy of yield estimates for nondairy mammals, comparisons of peak milk yields between species give valuable insight toward physiological demands of lactation. In particular, scaling milk production relative to body weight or mammary gland weight suggests common relationships and illustrates the effect of genetic selection for milk production. Although the number of the known mammals evaluated is small, when data for 19 species–including mouse, hamster, rabbit, pig, human, goat, sheep, cow, and camel–are used, unselected species array in a regular pattern for relationships between milk yield and body weight, energy output in milk and body weight, and mammary weight versus body weight. Equations for these relationships include the following examples (Hanwell and Peaker, 1977).

$$\text{milk yield (kg/day)} = 0.084 \text{ body weight (kg)}^{0.77}$$

$$\text{energy output in milk (kcal/day)} = 127.2 \text{ body weight}^{0.69}$$

$$\text{mammary weight (kg)} = 0.045 \text{ body weight (kg)}^{0.82}$$

Per unit of body weight, smaller animals have higher milk yields, greater outputs of energy in their milk, and relatively larger mammary glands than other mammals. If data are averaged the relationship between mammary gland weight and milk yield can be expressed by the following equation:

$$\text{milk yield (kg/day)} = 1.67 \times \text{gland weight (kg)}^{0.95}$$

Because the exponent does not differ significantly from unity, on average, 1 g of mammary tissue from a lactating animal produces 1.67 ml of milk per day.

There must certainly be some variation in this ratio—i.e., variation in the degree of differentiation of the alveolar cells and contribution of accumulated secretions to weight measurements, stage of lactation, milking, or suckling patterns—but this value provides a reasonable rule of thumb for comparative purposes. It comes as no surprise to good dairy cattle managers that energy and metabolic demands on the high-producing dairy are very great. The energy and substrate demands to support increased milk production are met by a combination of increased feed intake and mobilization of body reserves. Indeed, the typical dairy cow is in a negative energy balance for much of early lactation. However, when compared with smaller mammals, these demands seem relatively less severe. This is a reflection of not only demands of the suckling young but also the fact that smaller mammals typically secrete a much more energy-dense milk than cows. As an extreme case it is estimated that the pygmy shrew (Sorex minutus), which weighs only 5 g, must more than double its food consumption during lactation and eat more than four times its body weight per day to meet the additional demands of lactation. Lactation in small animals generally involves a relatively short period of intense metabolic demand but in larger animals a longer period of lesser demand.

The relationship between milk yield and body weight is illustrated in Figure 18.15. The regression line for several species not selected for milk production is shown. Because certain species have been selected for high yields (dairy cows, dairy goats) values for some of these highly selected animals are also plotted as individual data points. Data points for these animals are above the calculated regression line for the nonselected species, i.e., well above 95% confidence intervals, reflecting greater than expected milk production. The success of genetic selection for milk yield in dairy cows, a trait with a heritability of only 0.2 to 0.3, is such that a typical Holstein cow has been converted to the metabolic size of a dog and exceptional cows to the metabolic size of rodents. Concern for good husbandry practices and health of dairy animals, particularly in the face of recent techniques (e.g., use of bovine somatotropin) to increase production and continuing genetic progress, is justified but it is equally important to view these physiological demands on the dairy cow within an appropriate frame of reference (Mepham, 1983).

Any discussion of milk synthesis also has to consider not only the nutrients necessary for milk synthesis but also the physiological adjustments necessary to supply these nutrients to the mammary gland. Requirements for high levels of milk production are staggering at first glance. For example, in the dairy cow the energy requirements for milk production can easily approach 80% of net energy of intake. Demands for

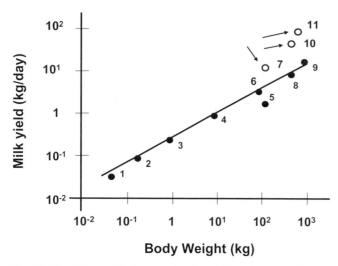

Fig. 18.15.   Relationship between body weight and milk yield. Comparisons between dairy (open circles) and nondairy animals are illustrated. 1 = mouse, 2 = hamster, 3= rat, 4 = fox, 5 = human, 6 = goat, 7 = dairy goat, 8 = sheep, 9 = beef cow, 10 = Holstein cow, 11 = Jersey cow. Adapted and redrawn from Hanwell and Peaker, 1977.

lactose production can require 85% of available glucose. It has been calculated that high-producing cows must mobilize adipose tissue and body nutrient reserves equal to approximately one-third of the milk produced during the first month or more of lactation. Clearly, finely tuned coordinated interactions between all the major physiological systems are necessary for success.

Galactopoiesis and bST

Administration of bST to lactating dairy cows increases the yield and efficiency of milk production. In response to injection of bST, milk secretion increases within a day and is maximized within a week. The increased milk yield is maintained as long as treatment is continued but quickly returns to control levels when bST is discontinued. The milk yield response is dose dependent and the response curve hyperbolic. At approximately 40 mg of bST/day, nearly maximal response is obtained. Milk yield achieved with near maximal doses of bST is impressive, with increases reported as high as 30–40%. Typically bST increases milk production by 4–6 kg/day, approximately a 10–15% increase in yield. The magnitude of response to a particular dose of bST depends upon biological variation, stage of lactation, and management parameters. The bST formulation currently approved for use in the United States is a prolonged-release n-methionyl-bST (Posilac, Monsanto Co.) that was approved by the United States Food and Drug Administration in

November 1993. It is administered at a dose of 500 mg per cow every 2 weeks. Package instructions are that treatment should be initiated after peak lactation at >60 days postcalving, when cows are at or near positive energy balance.

The first year after approval, average milk yield increased 3 kg, and this level of increase for bST-adopting herds has been maintained. Since not all cows in the bST herds are treated, i.e., some cows are not eligible <60 days postpartum, this is a conservative estimate of the effect of bST treatment on milk production (Bauman et al., 1999).

Given the voluminous literature and now widespread commercial use of bST in dairy cows in the U.S. and other countries, testing and evaluation of this technology has likely been the most intensely scrutinized new animal technology in history. Public debate about bST use was also extensive. Special interest groups and public individuals predicted dire consequences from adoption of bST for use in dairy cows. Among concerns that had little, if any, scientific basis, were that bST approval would cause a massive reduction in milk consumption, milk price would decline, and farmers would go bankrupt. Others predicted dire animal consequences. Media coverage was extensive near the time of approval by the Center of Veterinary Medicine of the Food and Drug Administration in 1994, with more than 800 reports in the first quarter of the year. At the current time the regulatory agencies of more than 50 countries have reviewed safety concerns and approved bST for use. It is estimated that more than 3 million cows currently receive bST supplementation. In the U.S. this includes animals in herds of all sizes, located in every region of the country. Scientific and anecdotal information support the view that bST is a safe, effective and profitable management tool for the dairy farmer. Although U.S. food laws do not mandate labeling of milk from bST-treated cows because the composition of the milk from the bST cows is equivalent to that of controls, a relatively small niche market has developed for milk obtained from herds not using bST. However, since there is no chemical test to distinguish the milk from bST and non-bST–treated cows, validation of milk from non-bST–treated cows simply depends on the fact that these producers sign a certification declaring that bST is not used on their farms. This is analogous to niche markets for other organic farmed products. A recent estimate is that milk from these farms constitutes less that 1% of fluid milk sales in the U.S. This suggests that the vast majority of consumers are interested in wholesome food products obtained at competitive prices. In fact, during the first year after approval milk consumption in the U.S. increased about 1%.

Reasons for some of the rancorous debate on the approval of bST for use in dairy cows were varied, but logic suggests that several elements were important. This was the first proposition for widespread treatment of animals with a recombinant DNA–derived product that impacted not animal health but animal production. Second, the wholesomeness of milk and milk products seems to occupy a special position when compared with many other food materials. Third, the now roundly refuted dire predictions of consequences on animal health (Collier et al., 2001) coincided with a growing affluence and associated "greening" of attitudes among many segments of the population. Finally, popular concerns that the adoption of the technology might hasten the disappearance of family farms and change the sociology of rural farm areas was seemingly carried along on a wave of nostalgia at the time. Certainly it was an interesting process to observe.

Mammary involution

Mammary involution can be stimulated at any stage of lactation by removal of suckling young or in dairy animals by suspending milking. Most of the detailed cellular and molecular research on mammary involution has focused on effects of acute induction of involution. However, after the peak of lactation a gradual involution occurs as the young are progressively weaned. In dairy cows there is also a gradual decline in milk production with time, even with regular milking. This decline is greater for cows that become pregnant soon after calving.

Cellular details of mammary involution have been most studied in rodents. Regardless of the differences in timing of events between species, i.e., days to hours in rodents versus days to weeks in ruminants, involution involves apoptosis (or programmed cell death) of the alveolar epithelial cells and tissue remodeling. Apoptosis of mammary epithelial cells occurs in several phases of mammary development, not just mammary involution. These include canalization of major mammary ducts in fetal development, rapid elongation of mammary ducts via the terminal end bud, and the waxing and waning of ductular growth during estrus or menstrual cycles. Apoptotic destruction of abnormal cells at early phases of carcinogenesis is also a likely mechanism for protection against breast cancer.

In rodents, removal of the suckling young and accumulation of milk at midlactation rapidly initiates involution of the mammary gland. Marked changes in gene expression are evident within 24 hours and evidence of widespread apoptosis observed by 48 hours. For example in rats, expression of mRNA for the caseins is reduced 95% and that of acetyl-CoA carboxylase, a key lipogenic enzyme, 98% within 24 hours.

Translational activity is also reduced. A second stage of involution is initiated between 72 to 96 hours with the activation of a series of tissue proteinases, including stromelysin 1 and 2, gelatinase A, and plasminogen activator. By this time remodeling of the mammary gland to prepare for a new reproductive cycle is well under way. Given the rapidity and magnitude of these tissue changes, it is not surprising that involution in the mouse is only partially reversible if suckling young are returned within 48 hours. Although much of the involution process is initiated by milk stasis, the continued secretion of lactogenic hormones associated with milking or suckling can delay the process. This is shown by experiments in which suckling is allowed in only selected glands. For example, in lactating sheep when both glands were nonsuckled for the first 15 days postpartum, the mammary prolactin receptor was reduced 84%; but in the nonsuckled gland of ewes with the opposite gland having continuing suckling stimulation, the prolactin receptor was reduced only 36%. Parenchymal DNA concentration was not affected by suckling treatments. However, RNA concentration followed a pattern similar to prolactin receptor: lowest when neither gland was suckled (2.1 mg/g), highest in suckled glands (7.4 mg/g), and intermediate in a nonsuckled gland companion to a suckled gland (3.8 mg/g). Alveolar structure was maintained in all treatments but the cytological appearance of the epithelial cells reflected changes in RNA concentration. Epithelial cells from ewes with neither gland suckled were poorly maintained, with many cells engorged with secretory vesicles and lipid droplets.

Involution in the ruminant mammary gland is decidedly slower, with less loss of alveolar structure. After 3 days of nonmilking casein and α-lactalbumin mRNA was reduced but β-lactoglobulin mRNA was unchanged. After a week, mRNA for the two milk proteins α_{-s1}casein and α-lactalbumin was dramatically lower (85 and 99%, respectively). After 4 days of nonsuckling alveolar structure was degenerated in the rodent and apoptosis, based on the degree of DNA laddering, is near maximal. However, even in nonpregnant, lactating beef cows, alveolar structure was largely intact in the absence of suckling, with only isolated areas of tissue degeneration evident even after several weeks. Nonetheless, based on quantitative histology, well-differentiated cells, common in suckled glands, were rare in nonsuckled glands. Interestingly, regression of the gland in the absence of suckling was not uniform. Structure of parenchymal tissue distant from the teat was better maintained. Even 42 days after cessation of suckling, areas of alveolar structure were present. Overall, alveoli from lactating glands had more cells per cross-section (30.4 ± 0.9) compared with 21.4 ± 0.8 in glands not suckled for 42 days. In total, these data illustrate that even a prolonged period of nonsuckling (42 days) does not result in complete destruction of the mammary alveoli. However, since total gland DNA was reduced (50 to 64% after 21 and 42 days of nonsuckling, respectively) cells are lost with prolonged milk stasis in the beef cow. Regardless, survival of de-differentiated alveolar cells should allow milk secretion to be reinitiated if milking is resumed. In dairy cows, resumption of milking after 12 days of nonmilking in selected glands caused a rapid recovery in milk production to near pretreatment values for those glands. When none of the glands were milked, recovery was impaired, i.e., only 28% of pretreatment yields were obtained. In contrast, return of suckling calves to their dams after a 28-day hiatus in beef cows was recently shown to restore milk production to about 50% of control. After 1 week of renewed suckling, milk yield had increased elevenfold (2.2 kg/d) and composition was near normal except for reduced lactose (3.7 versus 4.7%). These data do not mean that mammary involution does not occur in cattle; however, the extent and timing of events are more prolonged than for rodents (Akers et al., 1990; Lamb et al., 1999).

When extrapolated to the dairy cow with a dry period between lactations occurring 40–60 days prior to the birth of the calf, it is reasonable to suggest that tissue degeneration is certainly less than in rodents and likely less than in nonpregnant cows. Just as suckling or milking of contralateral glands acts to slow involution in companion nonmilked or nonsuckled glands, the involution process is also likely minimized during the typical dry period of dairy cows. During the later stages of the dry period, the mammary gland is growing and alveolar cells are preparing for lactogenesis. This overlap of lactation and pregnancy when cows are "dried off" in preparation for calving means those stimuli associated with mammary involution and milk stasis conflict with mammogenic and lactogenic stimuli of pregnancy. Cows are usually well into the last trimester of pregnancy, i.e., 40 to 60 days before calving at drying off; goats may be in early stages to the second trimester of pregnancy; and ewes are typically nonpregnant at the end of lactation. Differences in the management of the reproductive/lactation of these dairy animals are due to the seasonal nature of reproduction in goats and sheep, gestational length, and usual lactation periods. Among dairy animals the dairy cow is unique in this abrupt interface between successive lactations.

Dairy managers have developed methods to maximize profitability and milk production. Empirical evidence shows that the inclusion of a nonlactating or dry period between lactations is needed to maximize milk production in the dairy cow. Without a dry period, milk production in the subsequent lactation is reduced about 20%. Thus, the dry period is not essential but is beneficial. In fact, a dry period of 40–60 days seems optimal, since a dry period that is too short (less than 40 days) also impairs subsequent milk production. The dry period seems to be important because of effects on the mammary gland rather than effects on the nutritional status of the dam, as was once commonly believed. However, this is an area of intensive research activity, given the fact that better management, use of bST, and genetic improvement means that many dairy cows are producing rather large amounts of milk at the time when a dry-off period would normally occur.

Because of the typical breeding pattern, little attention has been given to determining an optimal dry period for goats or sheep. However, when lactating goats were hormonally induced to ovulate and mated during the usual seasonal anestrus period, they entered the next lactation without a dry period and they produced 12% less milk than controls. The data were confounded with possible effects of season. Consequently, in a second study these researchers used a within-animal experimental design to determine the effect of drying off on lactation in goats. One gland was milked continuously and the other dried off 24 weeks before parturition. There was no difference in subsequent milk production between udder halves. In contrast with the first study, this suggests a dry period is of no benefit. However, the dry period was relatively very long (i.e., three times the optimal length for the cow). Finally, the udder-half experimental design may be less than ideal for this evaluation. Interactions of glands of differing lactational states within the udder on cell turnover and lactogenesis have not been investigated. Since prepartum milking advances lactogenesis and milk production, milking one gland may conceivably advance lactogenesis and milk production in other glands. In nonpregnant ruminants milking delays mammary involution in other nonsuckled glands. Thus, it is possible that milking one gland during the prepartum period inhibits the ability of the opposite gland to produce maximally during the subsequent lactation, or that milk production was increased in glands milked continuously when the opposite gland was dried off. The importance of a dry period to maximize milk production in dairy goats and sheep is unsettled. Studies to determine the effects of pregnancy status, length of the dry period and other implications of the udder-half experimental design are warranted (Wilde et al., 1999).

References

Akers, R.M. 1985. Lactogenic hormones: Binding sites, mammary growth, secretory cell differentiation, and milk biosynthesis in ruminants. J. Dairy Sci. 68: 501–519.

Akers, R.M. 2002. Lactation and the Mammary Gland. Iowa State Press, Ames, Iowa.

Akers, R.M. 2006. Major advances associated with hormone and growth factor regulation of mammary growth and lactation in dairy cows. J. Dairy Sci. 89: 1222–1234.

Akers, R.M., D.E. Bauman, A.V. Capuco, G.T. Goodman, and H.A. Tucker. 1981. Prolactin regulation of milk secretion and biochemical differentiation of mammary epithelial cells in periparturient cows. Endocrinol. 109: 23–30.

Akers, R.M., D.E. Bauman, G.T. Goodman, A.V. Capuco, and H.A. Tucker. 1981. Prolactin regulation of cytological differentiation of mammary epithelial cells in periparturient cows. Endocrinol. 109: 31–40.

Akers, R.M., W.E. Beal, T.B. McFadden, and A.V. Capuco. 1990. Morphometric analysis of involuting bovine mammary tissue after 21 or 42 days of non-suckling. J. Anim. Sci. 68: 3604–3613.

Akers, R.M., A.V. Capuco, and J.E. Keys. 2006. Mammary histology and alveolar cell differentiation during late gestation and early lactation in mammary tissue of beef and dairy heifers. Livestock Sci. 105: 44–49.

Asimov, G.J. and N.K. Krouze. 1937. The lactogenic preparations from the anterior pituitary and the increase of milk yield in cows. J. Dairy Sci. 20: 289–306.

Bar-Peled, U., E. Maltz, I. Bruckental, Y. Folman, Y. Kali, H. Gacitua, A.R. Lehrer, C.H. Knight, B. Robinzon, H. Voet, and H. Tagari. 1995. Relationship between frequent milking or sucking in early lactation and milk production of high producing dairy cows. J. Dairy Sci. 78: 2726–2736.

Bauman, D.E. 1999. Bovine somatotropin and lactation: From basic science to commercial application. Domestic Anim. Endo. 17: 101–116.

Bauman, D.E., R.W. Everett, W.L. Weiland, and R.J Collier. 1999. Production responses to bovine somatotropin in northeast dairy herds. J. Dairy Sci. 82: 2564–2573.

Beal, W.E., D.R. Notter, and R.M. Akers. 1990. Techniques for estimation of milk yield in beef cows and relationships to calf weight gain and postpartum reproduction. J. Anim. Sci. 68: 937–943.

Capuco, A.V. and R.M. Akers. 1999. Mammary involution in dairy animals. J. Mammary Gland Biol. Neoplasia 4: 137–144.

Capuco, A.V., S. Ellis, D.L. Wood, R.M. Akers, and W. Garrett. 2002. Postnatal mammary ductal growth: Three-dimensional imaging of cell proliferation, effects of estrogen treatment and expression of steroid receptors in prepubertal calves. Tissue Cell 34: 143–154.

Capuco, A.V., P.A. Feldhoff, R.M. Akers, J.L. Wittliff, and H.A. Tucker. 1982. Progestin binding in mammary tissue of prepartum, nonlactating and postpartum, lactating cows. Steroids 40: 503–517.

Collier, R.J., J.C. Byatt, S.C. Denham, P.J. Eppard, A.C. Fabellar, R.L. Hintz, M.F. McGrath, C.L. McLaughlin, J.K. Shearer, J.J. Veenhuizen, and J.L. Vicini. 2001. Effects of sustained release bovine somatotropin (Sometribove) on animal health in commercial dairy herds. J. Dairy Sci. 84: 1098–1108.

Cowie, A.T. 1969. Lactogenesis. In The Initiation of Milk Secretion at Parturition, pp. 157–169. Edited by M. Reynolds and S.J. Folley. University of Pennsylvania Press, Philadelphia.

Cowie, A.T., I.A. Forsyth, and I.C. Hart. 1980. Hormonal Control of Lactation. Springer-Verlag Berlin, Heidelberg.

Garst, A.S., S.F. Ball, B.L. Williams, C.M. Wood, J.W. Knight, H.D. Moll, C.H. Aardema, and F.C. Gwazdauskas. 1999a. Technical note: Machine milking of sows—Lactational milk yield and litter weights. J. Anim. Sci. 77: 1620–1623.

Garst, A.S., S.F. Ball, B.L. Williams, C.M. Wood, J.W. Knight, H.D. Moll, C.H. Aardema, and F.C. Gwazdauskas. 1999b. Influence of pig substitution on milk yield, litter weights, and milk composition of machine milked sows. J. Anim. Sci. 77: 1624–1630.

Goodman, G.T., R.M. Akers, K.H. Friderici, and H.A. Tucker. 1983. Hormonal regulation of α-lactalbumin secretion from bovine mammary tissue cultured in vitro. Endocrinol. 112: 1324–1330.

Hanwell, A. and M. Peaker. 1977. Physiological effects of lactation on the mother. Symp. Zool. Soc. Lond. 41: 297–312.

Jenness, R. 1974. The composition of milk. In Lactation a Comprehensive Treatise, Vol III, pp. 3–96. Edited by B.L. Larson and V.R. Smith. Academic Press, New York and London.

Jenness, R. 1985. Biochemical and nutritional aspects of milk and colostrums. In Lactation. Edited by B.L. Larson, Iowa State Press, Ames, Iowa.

Keys, J.E., A.V. Capuco, R.M. Akers, and J. Djiane. 1989. Comparative study of mammary gland development and differentiation between beef and dairy heifers. Domestic Anim. Endocrinol. 6: 311–319.

Lamb, G.C., B.L. Miller, J.M. Lynch, D.M. Grieger, J.S. Stevenson, and M.C. Lucy. 1999. Suckling reinitiated milk secretion in beef cows after an early postpartum hiatus of milking or suckling. J. Dairy Sci. 82: 1489–1496.

Larson, B.L. 1985. Biosynthesis and cellular secretion of milk. In Lactation. Edited by B.L. Larson. Iowa State University Press, Ames, Iowa.

Lyons, W.R., C.H. Li, and R.E. Johnson. 1958. The hormonal control of mammary growth. Recent Progr. in Hormone Res. 14: 219–254.

McFadden, T.B., R.M. Akers, and A.V. Capuco. 1988. Relationships of milk proteins in blood with somatic cell counts in milk of dairy cows. J. Dairy Sci. 71: 826–834.

Mepham, T.B. 1983. Physiological aspects of lactation. In Biochemistry of Lactation, edited by T.B. Mepham, pp. 4–28. Elsevier Science Publishers, B. V. Amsterdam.

Nandi, S. 1958. Endocrine control of mammary gland development and function in the C3H/He Crgl mouse. J. Ntl. Cancer Inst. 21: 1039–1360.

Nickerson, S.C. and R.M. Akers. 1984. Biochemical and ultrastructural aspects of milk synthesis and secretion. Int. J. Biochem. 16: 855–865.

Nickerson, S.C. and J.W. Pankey. 1983. Cytological observations of the bovine teat end. Amer. J. Vet. Res. 44: 1433–1441.

Oftendal, O.T. 1984. Milk composition, milk yield and energy output at peak lactation: A comparative review. Symp. Zool. Soc. Lond. 51: 33–85.

Oftendal, O.T. 1997. Lactation in whales and dolphins: Evidence of divergence between baleen- and toothed-species. J. Mammary Gland Biol. Neoplasia 2: 205–230.

Purup, S., K. Sejrsen, and R.M. Akers. 1995. Effect of bovine GH and ovariectomy on mammary sensitivity to IGF-I in prepubertal heifers. J. Endocrinol. 144: 153–158.

Purup, S., K. Sejrsen, J. Foldager, and R.M. Akers. 1993. Effect of exogenous bovine growth hormone and ovariectomy on prepubertal mammary growth, serum hormones and acute in-vitro proliferative response of mammary explants from Holstein heifers. J. Endocrinol. 139: 19–26.

Purup, S., M. Vestergaard, M.S. Weber, K. Plaut, R.M. Akers, and K. Sejrsen. 2000. Local regulation of pubertal mammary growth in heifers. J. Anim. Sci. 78(Suppl. 3): 36–47.

Riddle, O., R.W. Bates, and S.W. Dykshorn. 1933. The preparation, identification and assay of prolactin—Hormone of the anterior pituitary. Am. J. Physiol. 105: 191–216.

Rosen, J.M., S.L. Wyszomierski, and D. Hadsell. 1999. Regulation of milk protein gene expression. Annu. Rev. Nutr. 19: 407–436.

Sejrsen, K. and S. Purup. 1997. Influence of prepubertal feeding level on milk yield potential of dairy heifers: A review. J. Anim. Sci. 75: 828–835.

Sejrsen, K., J. Foldager, M.T. Sorensen, R.M. Akers, and D.E. Bauman. 1986. Effect of exogenous bovine somatotropin on pubertal mammary development in heifers. J. Dairy Sci. 69: 1528–1535.

Sejrsen, K., J.T. Huber, H.A. Tucker, and R.M. Akers. 1982. Influence of plane of nutrition on mammary development in pre-and post-pubertal heifers. J. Dairy Sci. 65: 793–800.

Sejrsen, K., S. Purup, M. Vestergard, and J. Foldager. 2000. High body weight gain and reduced bovine mammary growth: Physiological basis and implications for milk yield potential. Domestic Anim. Endocrinol. 19: 93–104.

Sheffield, L.G. 1988. Organization and growth of mammary epithelia in the mammary fat pad. J. Dairy Sci. 71:2855–2874.

Sinha, Y.N. and H.A. Tucker. 1969. Mammary development and pituitary prolactin level of heifers from birth through puberty and during estrus cycle. J. Dairy Sci. 52: 507–512.

Smith, J.J., A.V. Capuco, and R.M. Akers. 1987. Quantification of progesterone binding in mammary tissue of pregnant ewes. J. Dairy Sci. 70: 1178–1185.

Smith, J.J., A.V. Capuco, W.E. Beal, and R.M. Akers. 1989. Association of prolactin and insulin receptors with mammogenesis and lobulo-alveolar formation in pregnant ewes. Int. J. Biochem. 21: 73–81.

Smith, K.L. and F.L. Schanbacher. 1973. Hormone induced lactation in the bovine. I. Lactational performance following injections of 17β-estradiol and progesterone. J. Dairy Sci. 56: 738–745.

Stelwagen, K. 2001. Effect of milking frequency on mammary functioning and shape of the lactation curve. J. Dairy Sci. 84: E204–E211.

Stricker, P. and R. Grueter. 1928. Action du lobe anterieur de l'hypophyse sur la montée laiteuse. CR Soc. Biol. (Paris) 99: 1978–1980.

Swett, W.W., P.C. Underwood, C.A. Matthews, and R.R. Graves. 1942. Arrangement of the tissues by which the cow's udder is suspended. J. Agric. Res. 65: 19–42.

Topper, Y.J. and C.S. Freeman. 1980. Multiple hormone interactions in the development of the mammary gland. Physiol. Rev. 60: 1049–1106.

Tucker, H.A. 1981. Physiological control of mammary growth, lactogenesis, and lactation. J. Dairy Sci. 64:1403–1421.

Tucker, H.A. 1987. Quantitative estimates of mammary growth during various physiological states: A review. J. Dairy Sci. 70: 1958–1966.

Tucker, H.A. 1994. Lactation and its hormonal control. In The Physiology of Reproduction, pp. 1065–1098. Edited by E. Knobil and J.D. Neill, 2nd ed., Raven Press, New York.

Tucker, H.A. 2000. Hormones, mammary growth, and lactation: A 41-year perspective. J. Dairy Sci. 83: 874–884.

Wilde, C.J., C.H. Knight, and D.J. Flint. 1999. Control of milk secretion and apoptosis during mammary involution. J. Mammary Gland Biol. 4: 129–136.

19 Reproduction

Contents

Introduction

What could be more fundamental to success of a species than reproduction? Understanding homeostasis and physiological controls are of limited use unless we can maintain our animals. Natural selection has produced an astounding variety of successful reproductive strategies. From an evolutionary viewpoint, the most favored pattern is one that results in the largest number of offspring reaching sexual maturity. Most population biologists have recognized two general patterns, namely, r-selection or K-selection. These terms were coined from logistic equations that were used to model growth of populations of animals in the wild.

For r-selection animals, the investment in each individual is small both in a physical and energetic sense.

Examples of this pattern of reproduction include fishes or amphibians that can produce extremely large numbers of eggs. The trade-off in producing so many small offspring is that there is little if any care of the offspring. They are produced and released into the environment to fend for themselves. It is estimated that only six out of a million mackerel fry survive to also reproduce. On the other hand, K-selection species produce fewer but larger offspring. Because these offspring are cared for—at least to some degree—during development, the chance that they will successfully reach reproductive age is far greater. Compared with the mackerel, individual K-selection animals may have a 50% chance of success. Clearly, for most agricultural operations the K-selection pattern predominates.

Energetic costs of parental care occur in two categories. First there is the cost that relates to transfer of nutrients to the developing neonate. For mammals the demands of lactation can be very large. The lactating mother can expend 40% of her energy producing milk. This can be even greater in high-producing dairy cows that have been selected for copious milk production. In other animals, for example, crop milk produced by pigeons and doves also represents a direct energetic expenditure cost. In addition, there are costs of behavioral responses to protect and nurture neonates.

As with most of the chapter topics, entire courses are devoted to these physiological specialties. Many animal science majors will take courses devoted to nutrition, lactation, and reproduction. Our goal for this chapter is not to substitute for a specialized course in reproduction but rather to provide some basics and stimulate your interest in more detailed study.

Overview of the female reproductive tract

The structures of the female reproductive tract include the ovaries, oviducts, uterus, cervix, vagina, and external genitalia. In farm animal species, the reproductive tract is positioned below the rectum. For cows and mares, this relationship is especially helpful because it allows the producer or veterinarian an opportunity to manually evaluate the reproductive tract by manipulation per rectum. This provides a practical means to determine the functional status of the ovary, diagnosis of pregnancy by determining presence or absence of a fetus within the uterus, or manipulation of the tract for purposes of artificial insemination (AI). As we have noted for other mucosal structures, the female tract is essentially a series of interconnected tubes with distinct layers of varying thickness. The outermost serosa is a thin layer of simple squamous epithelial cells. The next layer, the muscularis, is typically composed of an outer layer of smooth muscle cells arranged longitudinally and an inner layer of smooth muscle cells that form a continuous circular layer of cells. This arrangement allows for the generation of muscle contractions to aid transport of fluids and secretions, movement of ova and spermatozoa, passage of the early embryo, and ultimately expulsion of the fetus and fetal membranes at the time of parturition. Just under the muscularis, the submucosa provides connective tissue space to house blood and lymphatic vessels as well as nerves, and glands to support and nourish the internal lining of the reproductive tract mucosa. The lumen of all of the regions of the mucosa is lined by epithelial cells, but the structural and functional attributes of these cells vary from region to region to reflect different activities and variation in the reproductive cycle. To illustrate, a simple layer of columnar epithelial cells lines the oviduct, but some of the cells are also ciliated. Fluids that coat the surface allow for the beating of the cilia to propel ovulated eggs from the ovary into the oviducts and into the uterus for possible implantation if fertilization occurs. In contrast, a layer of stratified squamous epithelial cells provides for increased protection and lines the lumen of the reproductive tract in the posterior region of the vagina. Figure 19.1 illustrates the general histology of a cross section through the oviduct of a cow as well as specialization of the epithelial cells, i.e., presence of cilia.

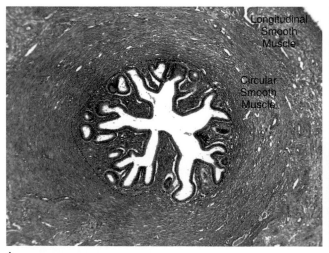
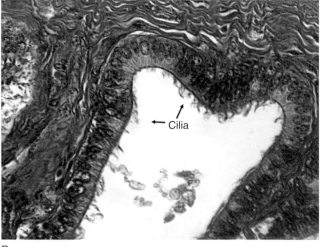

A   B

Fig. 19.1. Histology of the bovine female reproductive tract. Panel A shows a low-power (4×) view of a cross section of the oviduct. The region outlined with the dashed line contains the mucosa and submucosa. Most evident in this view is the highly folded mucosal surface surrounding the opening in the center of the oviduct. The surrounding muscularis occurs as circular and longitudinal layers, and it is evident as a band that surrounds the mucosa. A small edge of the serosa appears in the extreme upper-right corner. The mucosa is enlarged (40×) in Panel B. Here, the epithelial cells appear as columnar epithelial cells with evident cilia (arrows).

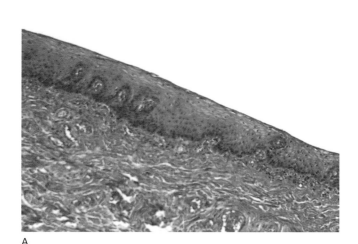

A

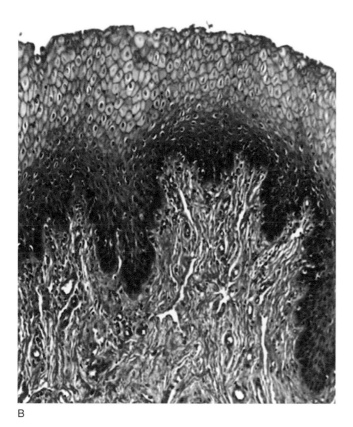

B

Fig. 19.2. Posterior vaginal epithelium of bovine. During the luteal phase (A), the epithelial cell layer is thinner than during the follicular phase (B) of the estrous cycle.

As you might suspect, there is substantial deviation in the surface epithelium at different locations of the reproductive tract. In addition, there are also marked variations associated with the stage of the estrous cycle. For example, Figure 19.2 illustrates the vaginal epithelium along the surface of the posterior vagina as well as differences associated with the stage of the estrus cycle. Unlike the oviduct, here the epithelial lining is composed of stratified squamous epithelial

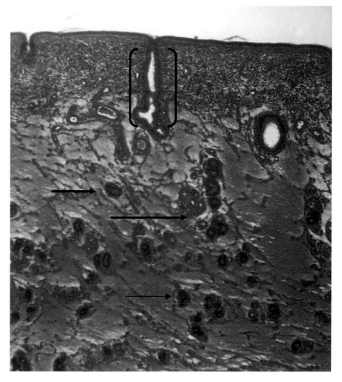

Fig. 19.3. Section of bovine uterus from a cow during the follicular phase of the estrus cycle (4×). A section through a uterine gland is evident (brackets) as well as older glands deeper within the muscularis (arrows).

cells. During the follicular phase of the estrus cycle, the layer of cells is thicker compared with the luteal phase.

For primates who express menses, variation in the uterine epithelium and in uterine glands is especially pronounced. Figure 19.3 shows the histological appearance of the uterus. Compared with other regions of the reproductive tract, the muscularis is extensive and the submucosa area has abundant glands that supply secretions that are especially important during pregnancy.

The entire reproductive tract develops in a retroperitoneal position. The tract is positioned against the peritoneum so that with continued growth the tract becomes completely surrounded. This new connective tissue sheath forms a continuous drape around the reproductive tract. This functions to suspend and maintain the ovaries, oviduct, uterus, and the anterior vagina. In this mature state this supporting tissue is called the broad ligament.

The ovaries, analogous to the testes in the male, are the primary reproductive organs since they produce the female gametes (sing. = ovum, pl. = ova). However, the ovaries produce not only gametes; they are also critical endocrine organs. Release of mature ova occurs with the rupture of follicles on the surface of the ovary. The ovum or ova enter the open end of the oviducts

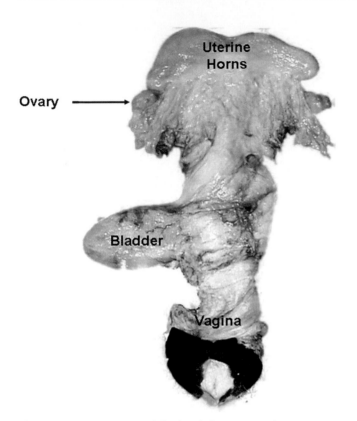

Fig. 19.4.   Gross anatomy of the female bovine reproductive tract.

to be directed to the uterus. Fertilization typically occurs within the oviduct during transit to the uterus. Figures 19.4 and 19.6 illustrate the gross anatomy of the primary structures of the reproductive tract of a cow and Figure 19.5 shows a dissected view of the vagina and cervix.

The paired ovaries are located in the lumbar region in close proximity to the kidneys. In sexually mature animals, the ovary undergoes dramatic but predictable cyclic development. For example, within a window of about 3 weeks in cows, pigs, or horses, ovulation occurs and the selected ovarian follicles are transformed into corpus luteum (sing.) or corpora lutea (pl.), which produce large quantities of progesterone. If fertilization does not occur, the corpus luteum regresses and a new crop of follicles mature. These follicles produce estrogen and selected follicle(s) proceed to undergo ovulation. This pattern constitutes an estrus cycle. The ovary is generally oval to rounded in shape with distinct regional differences and blisterlike structures— the follicles—near the outer surface. A connective tissue layer called the tunica albuginea covers and protects the ovary. This connective tissue band serves as support of a surface layer of epithelial unfortunately called the germinal epithelium. This is unfortunate because despite the promising name, these epithelial cells do not produce the gametes. Instead, beneath the tunica albuginea, within the ovarian cortex there are

populations of oocytes, which are recruited to develop into the mature follicles. The ovarian cortex also houses the corpus luteum as well as older degenerated corpora lutea called corpora albicantia. The center of the ovary is called the ovarian medulla, and it contains the blood, nerves, and lymphatic vessels that supply the ovary. The structure of the bovine ovary is illustrated in Figure 19.6.

In domestic species, the uterus consists of a body, a cervix (or neck) and two uterine horns. However, there are substantial variations in the shape and arrangement of the horns. For example, the body of the bovine uterus appears larger because the intercornual ligament, which acts to obscure the individual nature of the two uterine horns, covers the caudal region of the uterus. Among mammals there are three distinct types of uteri. The duplex uterus has two cervical canals, which acts to separate each uterine horn into distinct compartments. However, there are two types of duplex uteri. In the first case, there is a single vaginal canal opening to the outside. On the interior it divides to produce two vaginas and two cervices. This occurs in marsupials. In the North American opossum, for example, the male accommodates this circumstance by having a forked penis. The rabbit has a less complex arrangement; there are two uterine horns and two cervical canals but a single vaginal canal. The bicornuate uterus is characterized by the presence of two uterine horns and a small uterine body. In all of these cases, the uterus opens into the vagina via a single cervical opening. Cows, mares, and pigs all have this type of uterine structure. Primates on the other hand have a simplex uterus. There is a large uterine body but essentially no apparent uterine horns.

The appearance of the internal lining of the uterus, the endometrium, varies markedly during the estrous or menstrual cycles and during pregnancy. However, the tissue is highly glandular with a rich blood supply. The epithelial surface is a simple columnar epithelium in the mare but is composed of stratified columnar epithelial cells in ruminants. In addition, simple branched tubular glands provide secretions—called uterine milk—that are especially important during estrus and pregnancy. In many animals these uterine glands are scattered throughout the endometrium. But in ruminants, the internal uterine surface is punctuated by caruncles that are not glandular. These mushroomlike caruncles provide sites for attachment of fetal membranes in these animals. The smooth muscle of the uterus (the muscularis) is frequently called the myometrium.

The most caudal region of the uterus leads to the cervix. The cervix is a tough, connective tissue and smooth muscle sphincter that is tightly closed except during estrus and parturition. During estrus, the slight

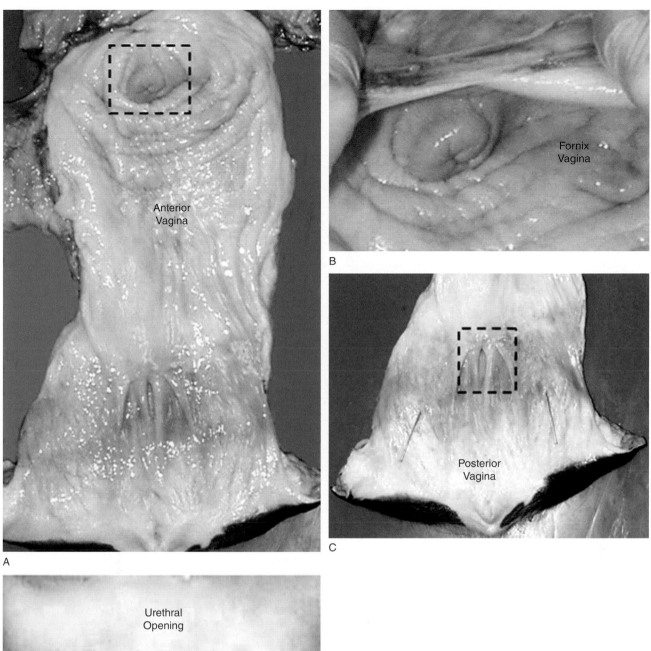

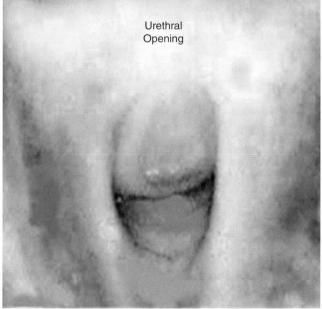

Fig. 19.5. Dissected view of the portions of the bovine vagina and cervix. The anterior vagina ends at the opening of the cervix (indicated by the dashed box, the external cervical os). The pocket on either side of the cervix (Panel B) (fornix vagina) can be a nemesis for those learning the art of artificial insemination. Toward the rear or posterior end of the vagina (Panel C) the opening to the urethra (Panel D) is recessed in the suburethral diverticulum, an area that has to be successfully navigated for placement of urine cannulas used for experiments requiring collection and monitoring of urine production in cows.

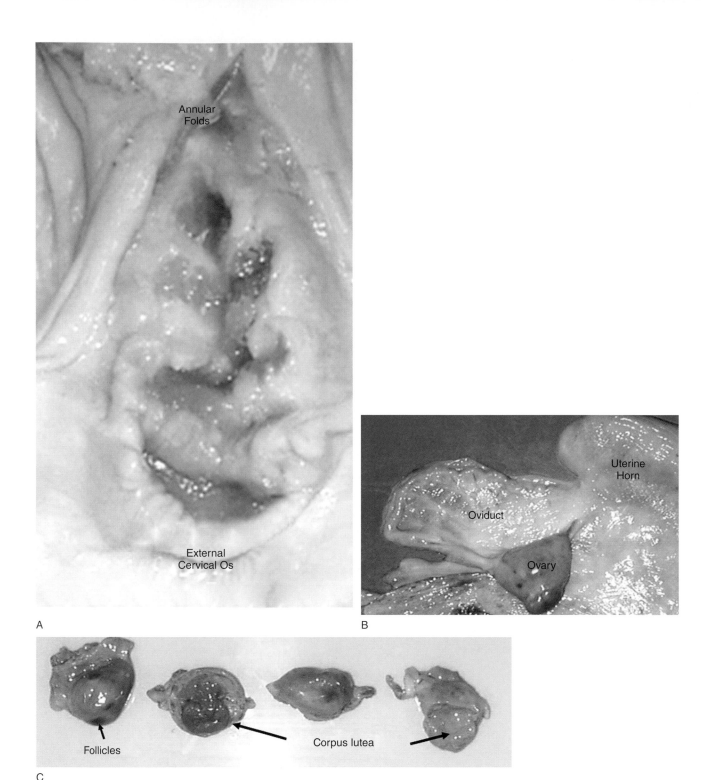

A

B

C

Fig. 19.6. Reproductive tract anatomy, continued. The upper panel (A) shows a bisected view of the cervix. The circular pattern of the annular folds is evident. The middle panel (B) shows the relationship between the uterine horns, oviduct, and ovary. The lower panel (C) illustrates variation in follicles and corpus lutea. The follicle to the left is nearing ovulation as indicated by the red points in the surface. The third follicle is relatively mature (evidenced by the fluid-filled cavity (center, reddish-brown area). The left corpus luteum is older than the more yellow body in the right of the panel.

Table 19.1. Comparative anatomy of female reproductive tracts, domestic farm animals.

Organ	Mare	Sow	Cow	Ewe
Oviduct	20–30 cm	15–30 cm	25 cm	15–19 cm
Uterus				
Type	Bipartite	Bicornuate	Bipartite	Bipartite
Horn	15–25 cm	40–65 cm	35–40 cm	10–12 cm
Body	15–20 cm	5 cm	2–4 cm	1–2 cm
Endometrium	Prominent longitudinal folds	Slight longitudinal folds	40–120 caruncles	88–96 caruncles
Cervix				
Lumen	Conspicuous folds	Corkscrewlike	2–5 annular rings	Annular rings
Opening to uterus	Clearly defined	Ill-defined	small and protruding	Small and protruding
Vagina	20–35 cm	10–15 cm	25–30 cm	10–14 cm
Vestibule	10–12 cm	6–8 cm	10–12 cm	2.5–3 cm

Modified from Frandson et al., 2003.

loosening of the cervix allows spermatozoa to enter the uterus. In ruminants the inner surface of the uterus is oriented in a series of circular folds or ridges called annular folds. Learning to traverse these folds can be a challenge to beginning artificial breeding technicians.

The vagina is the region of the reproductive tract within the pelvis positioned between the cervix on the cranial end and the vulva on the caudal end. The vulva or external genitalia is comprised of the right and left labia, which join at the midline to produce a commissure or union. The ventral commissure of the vestibule (the posterior vagina) houses the clitoris, the female homologue of the glans penis in males. It is composed of erectile tissue and is covered by stratified squamous epithelium. It is well supplied with sensory nerve endings. The functional significance is not well established in domestic animals, but clitoral stimulation at the time of insemination has been shown to increase conception rates in beef cows. Some comparative features of the female reproductive tract of various nonpregnant farm animals are given in Table 19.1.

Puberty in females

On the surface the definition of puberty seems simple enough; it is the age at which reproductive competence is achieved. However, in farm animals several criteria have been used to define puberty in females. For example, age at first estrus or heat can be a defining moment in cattle. However, this may or may not be associated with ovulation. Thus, this may not necessarily reflect reproductive competence. Ovulation can be evaluated by palpation of the ovary or ultrasound imaging in larger animals. However, in practical management terms the age at which a female can support pregnancy without harm to herself is probably an excellent definition. Although the physiological demands on the female to complete follicular development, ovulation, and transport of the fertilized ova to the uterus for implantation are relatively minor, the metabolic requirements to maintain the pregnancy and initiate lactation to support a rapidly growing neonate can be daunting. Thus, from a husbandry standpoint it is rarely an advantage for females to become pregnant at the earliest possible time.

Endocrinology of female puberty

In females the neurons of the hypothalamus that secrete GnRH must acquire the ability to secrete enough GnRH in response to feedback from ovarian estrogen to stimulate ovulation. This process is influenced by body mass, management, social cues, and genetics. For example, the range in months for the onset of puberty in cattle can be marked, i.e., as low as 8.5 months in Holsteins to 19.0 months in Brahman cattle. We begin by recalling the relationship between the hypothalamic hormones, the anterior pituitary hormones, and specifically the impact of the gonadotropin-releasing hormone or GnRH on secretion of Follicle Stimulating Hormone (FSH) and Luteinizing Hormone (LH). It is known that even in prepubertal animals exogenous GnRH is capable of stimulating secretion of FSH and LH from the anterior pituitary and that FSH and LH can stimulate follicular development in the ovary. However, sustained follicular development and maturation of selected follicles to undergo ovulation requires sustained secretion of these gonadotropic hormones. This suggests that the primary delay is a failure of the hypothalamus to produce enough GnRH in young animals.

Table 19.2.   Average age or time for selected reproductive attributes in some species.

Animal	Onset of Puberty	Age of First Breeding	Estrous Cycle	Estrus	Gestation
Bovine	9 to 24 mo	21 to 25 mo	21 d	18 hr	282 d
Ovine	4 to 14 mo	12 to 18 mo	17 d	1 to 2 d	150 d
Porcine	5 to 7 mo	8 to 10 mo	21 d	2 d	114 d
Equine	12 to 19 mo	24 to 36 mo	21 d	6 d	336 d

Senger (2003) has likened this gradual process to a rheostat in control of a light. As the rheostat is gradually turned higher, the lights in the room become more and more intense until maximal brightness is reached. You may recall that the hypothalamus has a number of specific nuclei. In functional terms, the secretion of GnRH is controlled by a tonically acting center located in the area of the dorsomedial nucleus. Before puberty, secretion of GnRH occurs at a relatively slow frequency and the amplitude of each of the secretory events is also rather low. This means that corresponding effects on secretion of FSH and LH from the anterior pituitary are also reduced. However, as ovarian development progresses secretion of estradiol from waves of growing follicles increases. Over time the estradiol (along with effects of environment, nutrients, and social interactions) has an escalating impact to increase the frequency and amplitude of bursts of GnRH secretion from this tonic center in the hypothalamus. This produces more FSH and LH and, in a positive cascade, more follicular activity.

However, ovulation requires not just low-level secretion of LH but rather a marked surge in the concentration. This is called the preovulatory LH surge. This depends on the activation of a second population of hypothalamic nuclei called the surge center. These nuclei are located more anterior in the hypothalamus in the area of the preoptic and anterior hypothalamic nuclei. Essentially, the prepubertal female is characterized by having insufficient ovarian-derived estradiol to stimulate the surge center as well as the absence of sensitivity to estradiol. As she matures, her hypothalamus becomes progressively more sensitive to estradiol.

Estrous cycles, estrus, and ovulation

The ovaries are, of course, the source of the female gametes (ova) and estrous cycles; in postpubertal animals, these cycles delineate periodic development or maturing of follicles, which results in release of eggs or ova that have the possibility of being fertilized. In a developmental sense, the sequence of cellular events required to create eggs is called oogenesis. The period when the female is receptive to sexual activity is called estrus or more commonly heat. An estrous cycle is simply the time from the beginning of one estrus period to another. It is worth taking a moment to clarify some of this confusing terminology. Estrus is a noun. (A cow displays estrus). Estrous is an adjective. (The average length of an estrous cycle in the Holstein dairy cow is 21 days.) A review of British and European scientific literature shows that oestrus and oestrous are the equivalent terms for estrus and estrous, respectively.

Animals that exhibit only one estrous cycle per year are monoestrous. In these animals it is usual for the estrus period to last several days. Examples are dogs, wolves, foxes, and bears. As a successful reproductive strategy, having the extended period of estrus increases the chance of a successful mating. In contrast, polyestrous species exhibit multiple cycles each year. However, these cycles are not necessarily uniformly distributed throughout the year. There are windows of inactivity when the animals are said to be anestrous. These animals are seasonal polyestrous. Even among animals that are not seasonal breeders, there can be interruptions in the usual regular pattern. For example, in cattle, which breed year-round, there is typically an anestrous period for several weeks or months after calving. This can be especially pronounced in beef cows that are suckling their calves. Table 19.2 provides a summary of selected reproductive measures in some common farm animals.

It is important to appreciate that there can be substantial differences between breeds. For example, onset of puberty in cattle can vary from a low of about 9 months in Holsteins to 19 months in Brahman cows. Similarly, Meishan pigs can show estrus as early as 3 months, but Yorkshire gilts average about 7 months. In the case of onset of puberty, several external factors are also important. In sheep and goats, season of birth or photoperiod can act to hasten or delay onset of puberty. Presence or absence of the opposite sex during the peripubertal period impacts cattle and swine, as does the density of housing in swine. In a large grouping of gilts normal puberty is 28 weeks, but in a smaller group (~3) puberty is typically delayed until 32 weeks. Age at onset of puberty is also greatly influenced by body size and condition. Onset of puberty is a particularly important aspect of farm animal management. In dairy cattle it is an advantage to breed females as soon as practical so that the animals enter the milking herd earlier. This has to be coupled with the animals also having the necessary body size and condition to avoid calving difficulties and successfully compete with older, stronger cows at the feed bunk. From a genetic viewpoint, minimizing the age at puberty in males likely has the greatest benefit. In other words, like many aspects of animal production—growth, lactation—reproduction is also markedly impacted by management of the animals.

We will use the dairy cow as our model species to describe the estrous cycle and process of ovulation. The general development of follicles is similar in most mammals. The ovary contains thousands of primary or dormant follicles. Essentially these are the ova, each of which is surrounded by a thin layer of cuboidal follicular or granulosa cells. In response to tonic secretion of FSH and LH some of these primary follicles commence enlargement to become small antral follicles. Antral follicles are those which exhibit the appearance of a fluid-filled space between the oocyte in the center and the surrounding granulosa cells. This population of antral follicles provides the source of follicles that are eligible for activation during sequential estrous cycles.

Based on tradition, the estrous cycle is divided into two phases, named after the dominant structures that are present on the ovary. The follicular phase in most animals is relatively short (~20% of the estrous period) but the preovulatory follicles that produce estradiol are in control. The follicular phase encompasses the time from the regression of the corpora lutea to the time of ovulation. This is not to say that there is no follicular activity at other stages of the estrous cycle. Indeed, there are populations of follicles that sequentially develop throughout the estrous cycle. However, as in many things, timing is everything. As described below, it is only the dominant follicle(s) that are part of a wave of development occurring near the time when the regression of the corpus luteum occurs that has the opportunity to be qualified for ovulation.

It is now known that several waves (typically three) of follicular development occur during the estrous cycle in cattle. Beginning after ovulation, groups or clusters of small or medium antral follicles become especially sensitive to gonadotropins. These follicles are described as recruited follicles. Among this group of recruited follicles, several are selected and begin to mature. However, typically only one of these selected follicles will win the maturity race so that it becomes the dominant follicle. Other selected follicles in this class begin to undergo regression or atresia. Even the dominant follicle is destined to undergo atresia if it is so unlucky to have been recruited in the first or second wave of follicular development during the estrous cycle. This developmental process is illustrated in Figure 19.7. Figure 19.8 illustrates changes in major

reproductive hormones during a bovine estrous cycle.

For a moment let's consider development of the ovary and specifically the relationship between the follicle and the oocytes. In the fetus, primordial germ cells migrate from the yolk sac to the immature ovary. These germ cells (now called an oogonium) become surrounded by a single layer of follicular cells. As the ovary matures, it is usual to find clusters or nests of these germ cells in the cortex of ovary (Fig. 19.7A). It is worth remembering that these cells undergo meiosis but they stop in the first prophase before the first division. In most animals the first of the two meiotic divisions is completed, producing the first polar body, at about the time of ovulation. The essential point is that unlike spermatogenesis, where each primary germ cell produces four spermatozoa, the maturation of the oocyte creates only one mature ovum and three polar bodies. Thereafter, some of these primary or primordial follicles are stimulated to growth, progressing first to a secondary follicle stage. This is characterized by an increase in the number of granulosa cells surrounding the oocyte (Fig. 19.7B). A tertiary follicle or antral follicle is characterized by the coalescence of fluid that appears between the granulosa cells so that a prominent space is evident (Fig. 19.7C). With progressive development, the stroma cells surrounding the follicle segregate into two distinct layers—the theca interna (closest to the layer of granulosa cells) and an outer theca externa. These layers give additional structural substance to the rapidly developing follicle. Moreover, the theca interna, if the follicle is a dominating ovulatory follicle, is destined to be a major source of steroid hormones. The granulosa cells are separated from the theca cells by the basement membrane. At this time the oocyte is typically displaced to one side of the follicle and antrum where it is surrounded by a cluster or cloud of granulosa cells called the cumulus oophorus (Fig. 19.8). Other granulosa cells remain in layers surrounding the oocyte adjacent to the theca interna. These cells are referred to as the membrana granulosa. The granulosa cells adjacent to the ovum secrete glycoproteins that form a protective layer called the zona pellucida. Figure 19.9 shows examples of developing follicles.

We have used the cow as our primary model, but it is clear that there are dramatic differences between farm species. The LH surge and ovulation in most farm animals (cow, sow, ewe, and mare) take place regularly independent of copulation (Fig. 19.10). These animals are spontaneous ovulators. In contrast, in rabbits, mink, camels, llamas, and alpacas ovulation requires copulation. Such animals are induced ovulators. In these animals, appearance of the preovulatory LH surge depends on neural reflexes produced by vaginal simulation. These animals (often depending

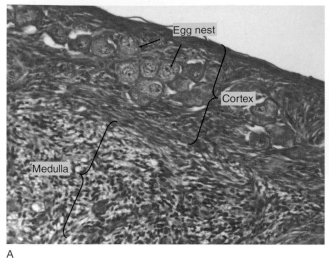

A

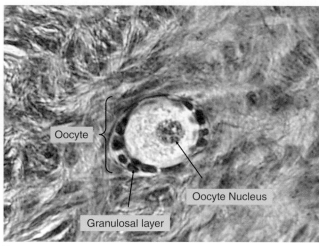

B

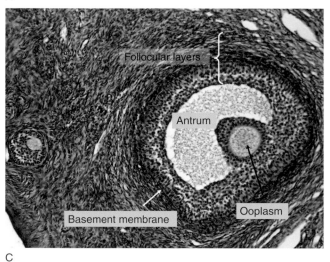

C

Fig. 19.7. Examples of follicular development in the bovine. The upper panel (A) shows a low-power view of the ovary. In the outer cortex larger clusters of cells (egg nest with arrows) are primordial oocytes. The center is called the medulla. The middle panel (B) illustrates the appearance of a secondary follicle. The oocyte with its evident nucleus and large area of cytoplasm is surrounded by multiple layers of granulosa cells (layer). The lower panel (C) illustrates a tertiary follicle. The antral space or antrum and surrounding layers of follicular cells are evident. In this particular case the nucleus of the oocyte is not apparent but the ooplasm can be seen. The basement membrane demarcates the boundary between the follicular and theca cells.

on season) have typical estrous cycles and associated follicular development, but the mature follicles undergo atresia if copulation does not occur.

Once ovulation occurs, the granulosa cells lining the now empty follicular cavity begin to divide, fill the space, begin a process called luteinization in response to high levels of LH, and create a structure called the corpus luteum (yellow body or CL). The CL is a powerful endocrine tissue that produces large amounts of progesterone. Secretion of progesterone prepares the uterus to receive the ovulated ovum or ova. If fertilization and implantation of the ova is successful, this produces maternal recognition of pregnancy and the usual regress of the CL does not take place. Progesterone concentrations in the blood are maintained throughout pregnancy. Some species are dependent on the CL for all of the progesterone needs, but in others the CL can actually be removed and pregnancy maintained because of progesterone produced by the placenta. Progesterone, especially in the later states of pregnancy, is critical for mammary development

needed to support lactation after the birth of the young.

If pregnancy is not established, the CL must regress for the animal to continue estrous cycles. In most domestic species, the signal to induce CL regression is prostaglandin F2α (PGF$_2$α). Secretion of PGF$_2$α begins to increase after ovulation with timing that corresponds with estrous cycle length in the species. Essentially, when PGF$_2$α secretion is sufficient, this stimulates a series of biochemical and cellular changes in the CL so that it regresses or undergoes luteolysis. This then allows for another estrous cycle to begin.

Certainly successful breeding depends on the ability to detect candidate animals in estrus. In situations where cattle breed naturally, herd bulls handle these demands very well. However, in dairy operations, it is not usual to maintain bulls for breeding. There are several practical reasons for this approach. First, dairy bulls are very large and potentially deadly animals. Thus, the physical needs for adequate handling and housing facilities can be substantial. Perhaps more

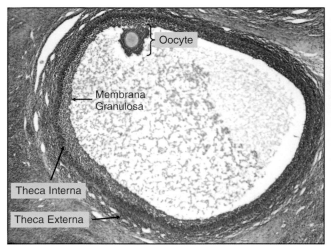

A

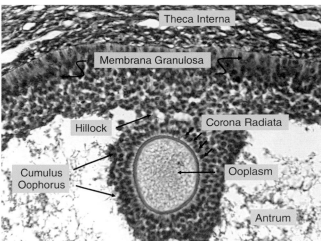

B

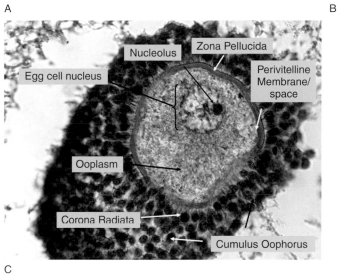

C

Fig. 19.8. Details of tertiary follicle development. In the upper panel (A) the antrum occupies most of the area. The ovum (without evident nucleus) appears to the upper left. The membrana granulosa (the edge of the layer of follicular cells) borders the antrum. To the outside theca interna and theca externa are evident as distinct layers. In the middle panel (B) regions of the cumulus oophorus and corona radiata (layer of granulosa cells that immediately surround the ovum) and hillock (group of granulosa that anchor the oocyte within the antral space) are illustrated. In the lower panel (C) some of the detail of the ooplasm can be seen as well as the oocyte nucleus, the nucleolus, and the zona pellucida and perivitelline space.

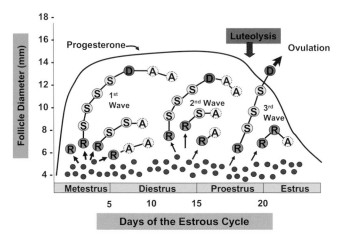

Fig. 19.9. Several follicular waves occur during the estrous cycle. The small filled circles represent gonadotropin-sensitive follicles. During each wave some follicles are recruited (R), some of these are selected (S), and some become dominant (D). Most eventually become regressed or become atretic (A). Only follicles recruited during the third wave or after luteolysis of the corpus luteum produced in the previous cycle will become eligible for ovulation.

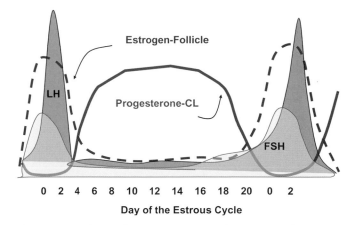

Fig. 19.10. Relative changes in secretion of major reproductive hormones during a bovine estrous cycle. During the follicular phase [proestrus + estrus] from about day 17 to 1, progesterone declines rapidly due to luteolysis and there is a correspondingly rapid increase in estrogen coming from recruited and selected follicles. This promotes increases in FSH with further stimulation of estrogen secretion and finally the dramatic LH surge that leads to ovulation.

importantly, genetic progress in dairy has depended on the ability to breed many cows to genetically superior bulls. This is only possible by use of AI. Without bulls to detect females in heat, this means that producers had to learn other methods of heat detection. Fortunately, behavioral cues in cattle are dramatic, and if animals are housed so that interactions between females are possible, i.e., appropriate pastures or lots with good footing, and there is sufficient time for observation, heat can be detected. Specifically, as the cow enters estrus she gradually begins to display activity that signals approaching sexual receptivity. These include increased physical activity (locomotion), bellowing, nervousness, and attempts to mount other females. As the period progresses, the female's willingness to accept a male increases. During this time the cow will display mating posture called lordosis. Such animals stand still so that herdmates will periodically engage in mounting behavior. The animal ready for breeding is said to be in standing heat. Observation of standing heat is the major cue for managers to breed these animals. To be most efficient—because spermatozoa deposited in the body of the uterus after AI have a limited viability period—it is important to have the inseminate deposited very near the time of ovulation. This means that most operations need to observe candidate animals at least twice daily and likely 30–45 min per session. Since labor is an important part of farm costs, it is not surprising that multiple techniques to better automate heat detection have been devised. As examples, patches placed on the rump of candidate animals, which contain packets of dye that rupture when the animal is mounted; mounted pressure sensors that send radio signals to a base station on the farm; or monitoring of activity via daily reading of pedometers are methods used to decrease the costs and increase the efficiency of heat detection. One of the more interesting experimental approaches was to train dogs to identify cows in heat.

In recent years, control of estrous cycles to more efficiently manage the breeding of cattle has become a reality through the use of estrus-synchronization schemes. This has become possible because of the availability of commercial formulations of $PGF_2\alpha$, GNRH, and progesterone. Indeed there are now effective schemes to allow the timed breeding of cows and heifers without the need for heat detection. As a recent example, Peeler et al. (2004) reported results from a trial in which heifers were synchronized using intravaginal progesterone inserts also called controlled internal drug release devices (CIDR), along with GNRH treatment and timed AI. Briefly, heifers were assigned to the protocol irrespective of stage of the estrous cycle. At this time they received a CIDR containing 1.38 g of progesterone and a 1 mg injection of ECP (estradiol cypionate). After 7 days the CIDR was removed and the heifers were given a 25 mg injection of $PGF_2\alpha$. On day 9 the heifers were given an injection containing 100 µg GNRH. The heifers were bred 48, 56, or 72 hr after the CIDR was removed. The first service pregnancy rates averaged 57.6%. There was no estrus detection in the study, but more importantly the success rate was similar to that obtained with laborious heat detection systems.

Fertilization and pregnancy

Assuming a successful ovulation and insemination has occurred, the reproductive story is just beginning. As spermatozoa ascend through the cervix, uterine body, and ultimately the oviduct, many are lost. However, those that remain must undergo a process called capacitation. These are biochemical changes to the sperm cells that are induced by secretions of the female reproductive tract. Capacitation is essential for fertilization. It is generally accepted that exposure of spermatozoa to seminal fluid during maturation in the testes or at the time of ejaculation leads to the coating of the cell surface with a complex layer of proteins and carbohydrates. Removal of these materials via the capacitation process in the female tract is essential for the spermatozoa to bind the oocyte. Fertilization typically occurs when the oocyte and spermatozoa meet in the ampulla region of the oviduct.

Interestingly, when the spermatozoa reach this area, swimming patterns change from very regular linear movements to a more erratic, even frenzied, motion. This change is induced by molecules secreted in this region of the oviduct and is thought to increase the opportunity of contact between sperm and oocyte. Fertilization depends on a complex series of steps (outlined in Fig. 19.11).

Sperm cells have very specific proteins associated with the acrosome portion of the head of the spermatozoa, which have an affinity for the zona pellucida of the oocyte. This outer layer of the oocyte is composed of three glycoproteins called zona protein 1, 2, and 3 (ZP1, ZP2, and ZP3, respectively). ZP1 and ZP2 are primarily structural proteins that maintain the space and organization of the zona pellucida. ZP3, in contrast, acts as an anchor or receptor for proteins found in the membrane of the sperm cell. Two binding sites are present. The primary zona binding region allows for the close adherence of the oocyte and sperm cell. A second site induces the acrosome reaction when ZP3 from the zona pellucida binds.

The acrosome is a lysosome-like membrane-bound structure that is oriented around the outer portion of the spermatozoa where it partially encapsulates the condensed nucleus of the spermatozoa. It contains

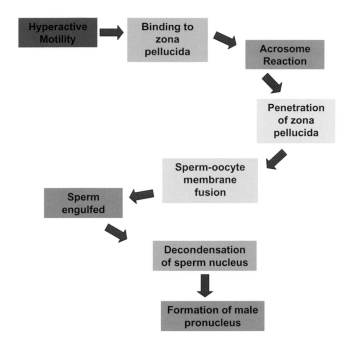

Fig. 19.11. Events following capacitation and fertilization.

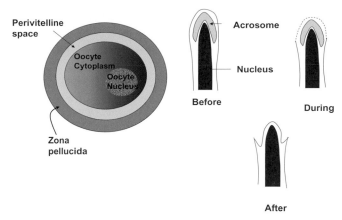

Fig. 19.12. The oocyte and fertilization. The upper left panel illustrates the structures of the oocyte. Before fertilization can take place the spermatozoon must penetrate the zona pellucida, enter the perivitelline space and ultimately fuse with the oocyte plasma membrane and be engulfed. The right illustrates events of the acrosomal reaction. During the reaction, the outer plasma membrane surrounding the sperm head fuses with the other membrane of the acrosome. This leads to release of the acrosomal contents. The end result is that the inner membrane of the acrosome encompasses the nucleus and continues in a continuous fashion with the remaining plasma membrane of the spermatozoon.

enzymes that are important for events associated with fertilization. The acrosome reaction is essential because it allows the spermatozoa to penetrate the zona pellucida and because it exposes the nucleus of the sperm cell, i.e., now surrounded by former inner membrane of the acrosome. After binding, the acrosomal reaction begins as the plasma membrane surrounding the sperm head forms fusion points with the acrosomal membrane. As small vesicles appear, this produces a morphological cellular landmark called vesiculation, which is used to identify cells that have undergone the acrosome reaction. Among the enzymes released, proacrosin has a very high affinity for the zona pellucida. This supports the close adherence of the oocyte and spermatozoa undergoing the acrosome reaction. When activated to acrosin, its hydrolytic action degrades the zona pellucida in the very local region where the sperm cell is attached. This is important because the continued presence of the zona pellucida is necessary for subsequent development. The continued beating of the tail of the spermatozoa supplies the mechanical force needed for the activated spermatozoa to penetrate through the zona pellucida to the perivitelline space, which surrounds the plasma membrane of the oocyte. When the spermatozoon gets to the perivitelline space, it binds to microvilli on the surface of the oocyte. The plasma membrane of the oocyte then fuses with the membrane surrounding the spermatozoon and engulfment occurs. After this event, dense vesicles—the cortical granules—previously produced inside the oocyte, migrate to the cell surface and release their contents by exocytosis. The proteases,

mucopolysaccharides, plasminogen activator, acid phosphatases, and peroxidases contained in the granules alter the biochemical properties of the zona pellucida so that additional sperm cannot enter; this is called the zona block. In some species, these substances also reduce the capacity of the oocyte plasma membrane to fuse with additional spermatozoa, the vitelline block. This gives another mechanism to prevent polyspermy (fertilization by more than one spermatozoon), which results in embryonic death. After the sperm nucleus is freed into the cytoplasm of the oocyte, it becomes the male pronucleus. However, this requires a major decondensation of the sperm nucleus. During the maturation of the spermatozoa in the testis, the nucleus becomes very highly compacted and ordered due to the creation of many disulfide cross links. In this state the chromosomes are essentially inert. Fortunately, the oocyte cytoplasm is rich in glutathione, which allows for the loosening of the chromosomes so that interaction can take place. The last step in fertilization is the fusion of male and female pronuclei. This is called syngamy. After this point, the zygote enters the first stages of embryo genesis. Structures of the oocyte and spermatozoa are illustrated in Figure 19.12.

Implantation and placentation

After a successful fertilization the embryo has to develop into a blastocyst, hatch from the surrounding zona pellucida, develop a functional trophoblast, and secrete signals that ultimately allow maintenance of the corpus luteum. After fusion of the male and female pronuclei, the single-celled egg is called a zygote. It can also be referred to as an embryo, which is defined as an organism in the early stages of development. Embryos typically have not acquired features that allow for recognition of a particular species. By contrast, a fetus—a potential offspring still within the uterus—can generally be recognized as a member of the species. *Conceptus* is defined as the product of conception, but it is poorly described. It is really a catchall term since it includes early and late embryos, the embryo plus extraembyronic membranes during preimplantation, and the fetus and placenta.

Soon after syngamy, the zygote initiates a series of mitotic divisions or cleavages. The first cleavage produces a two-celled embryo. Each of the cells at this time is called a blastomere. Subsequent divisions produce 4, 8, and 16 identical daughter cells. At these early stages the blastomeres are totipotent. In other words, each of the individual cells is capable of giving rise to a fully formed offspring. For example, identical twins can be produced in experimental situations by separating individual blastomeres, placing them into surrogate zona pellucida and allowing development in the uterus of a recipient female. It was long thought that adult or differentiated cells were not capable of this process. However, the production of Dolly the sheep from adult mammary gland fibroblast cells shows that it is possible, with just the correct conditions, to dedifferentiate cells so that they can become totipotent once again. Once beyond the 16-cell stage it becomes impossible to accurately count the growing ball of cells, so the structure is called a morula. With further divisions a blastocyst develops. It is characterized by the presence of inner cell mass (ICM), a fluid-filled cavity called a blastocoele, and a layer of cells around the periphery called the trophoblast. Figure 19.13 illustrates some of these stages of development.

During the morula stage the cells begin to segregate into two distinct populations, inner and outer cells. Cells in the ICM develop gap junctions, which allows for coordinated communication between the cells. The outer cells by contrast become linked by tight junctions. This allows for the creation of a unique environment with respect to ions inside the developing blastocoele. Specifically, increasing concentrations of Na^+ produce osmotic drive for water to enter the structure and expand the volume of the blastocoele. The ICM develops into the embryo while the trophoblast gives rise to the chorion, which eventually becomes the fetal component of the placenta. With continuing expansion of the blastocyst via fluid and cell proliferation, pressure increases, the trophoblast cells begin to

secrete enzymes, and an area of the zona pellucida degrades and ruptures. The blastocyst escapes or hatches and becomes a free-floating embryo within the lumen of the uterus. This development cycle is illustrated in Figure 19.14.

After hatching of the blastocyst, cell division occurs very rapidly. For example, in the cow on day 13 the blastocyst is about 3 mm in diameter. Over the next few days, the blastocyst increases in length to 250 mm and appears as a string or thread. By day 18 of gestation, the blastocyst occupies areas of both uterine horns. Much of this growth involves appearance of extraembyronic membranes, which is essential for the embryo to attach to the uterus of the dam for subsequent development. The outer trophoblast combined with the newly developed endoderm gives rise to the chorion and amnion. The yolk sac develops from the endoderm (see Figure 19.15).

Implantation is the attachment of the free-floating blastocyst to the uterine epithelium and corresponding growth or penetration of the epithelium by embryonic tissues. Just how dramatic and extensive this interaction is varies between species. In most farm animals, the degree of penetration is much less than in rodents and humans, for example. Implantation in most farm animals is considered noninvasive and primarily associated with cell-to-cell junctions between embryonic and uterine tissues. After fertilization, attachment occurs in the cow at about 35 days, in the sow at about 11 days, and in the mare at about 55 days.

Placentation refers to the development of the extraembyronic membranes or the placenta. The placenta and its layers allow for exchanges between the maternal and fetal circulations so that nutrients can be supplied and wastes removed. The chorion is the outermost membrane and therefore is in contact with the maternal uterine wall. The next layer toward the fetus is the allantois, which forms a continuous layer that creates a fluid-filled sac—the allantoic cavity—around the fetus. The amnion is the closest membrane to the fetus. It also forms a fluid-filled cavity in direct contact with the fetus. The amnion is fused to the inner layer of the allantois. When parturition occurs, the allantoic sac is expelled followed by the amniotic sac. Branches from the umbilical arteries and veins pass through the connective tissue between the allantois and chorion. The physical attachment of the conceptus to the uterus offers major reproductive advantages. Modification of the intrauterine environment as the fetus develops ensures that the developing fetus will be provided with nutrients and physiological support to maximize the chance for a successful birth. This was a major evolutionary step for eutherian mammals compared with lower animals that laid their eggs.

Connections between the chorion and the uterus are varied between species. By convention, the histologi-

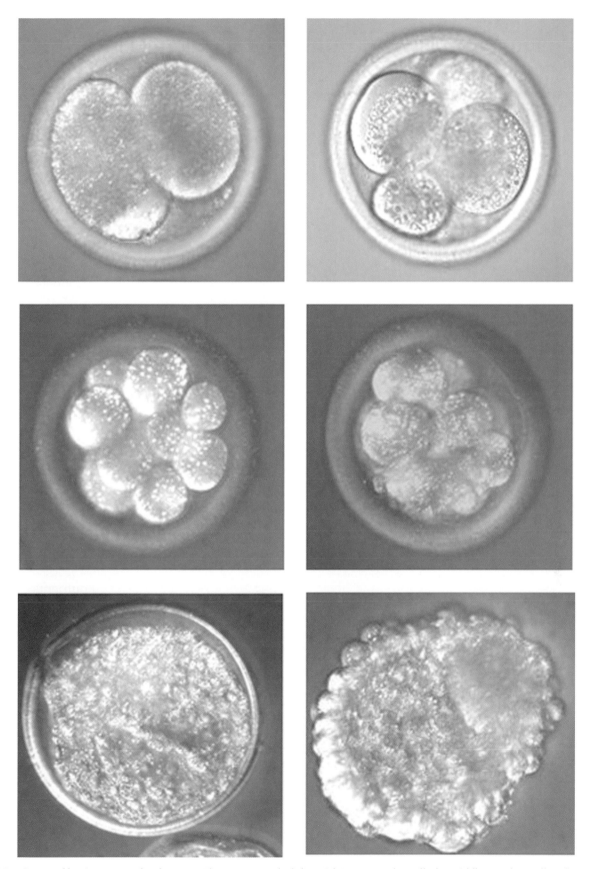

Fig. 19.13. Stages of bovine oocyte development. The upper panels (left to right) are 2- and 4-cell, the middle panels 8-cell and morula, and the lower panels expanded blastocyst and hatched blastocyst, respectively.

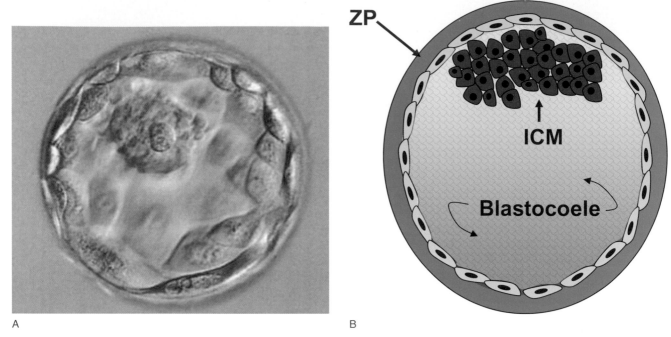

Fig. 19.14. Photograph and representation of preimplantation embryo just before hatching. The inner cell mass (ICM) (A) develops into the embryo and the trophoblast cells (lower arrows) that surround the expanding space or blastocoele give rise to the chorion. After expansion, hatching occurs so that the blastocyst escapes to become a free-floating embryo within the uterus prior to implantation (B).

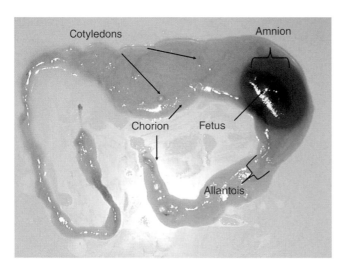

Fig. 19.15. Developing bovine fetus and associated membranes.

cal relationship between the fetal membranes and uterine epithelium is named beginning with the maternal side. For example, placenta of most farm animals is classified as epitheliochorial. This means that the chorion of the fetus is in direct contact with the uterine surface. This is the least intimate arrangement of the types of placentas. In hemochorial placentation fetal vessels and chorion are invaginated so that there is direct contact between a single layer of chorion epithelial cells and maternal blood. In hemoendothelial placentation, maternal blood can directly bathe the

outer surface of chorionic capillaries. The number of layers separating fetal and maternal circulations is important in part because this markedly affects transfer of immunoglobulins in utero. Since most farm animals have an epitheliochorial connection, calves, for example, are born without protective antibodies from the dam. Consequently, absorption of antibodies from the colostrum is very important. Primates, rabbits, rodents, and other species with the hemochorial or hemoendothelial arrangement are born with some antibodies that transfer in utero from the mother.

Placentation patterns also vary at a gross anatomy level based on the location or distribution of sites for exchange between the placenta and the uterus. In the horse and pig, extensions from the chorion (chorionic villi) project into crypts scattered over the entire surface of the endometrium. This is called a diffuse type of placenta. Ruminants have scattered attachments, which depend on a cotyledonary type of connection. In this situation, exchange takes place at distinct structures called placentomes. The placentomes are formed by the combined invagination of specific regions of the chorionic membrane, the cotyledons, into the buttonlike projections from the surface of the endometrium, the caruncles. Caruncles project from the surface of the uterus about 2 cm and vary from 1 to 10 cm in diameter. The caruncles also increase in size as pregnancy advances and are larger in the gravid horn than in the nongravid horn of the uterus.

Zonary placentas, found in dogs and cats, for example, are characterized by a major region of exchange that forms in a region near the center of the developing conceptus essentially in a band. In primates and rodents the discoid placenta type occurs. It is characterized by the presence of one of two distinct discs on a region of the chorion. The discs house the chorionic villi, which interconnect with the endometrium.

Exchanges that occur across the placenta involve typical mechanisms, i.e., diffusion, facilitated diffusion, and active transport. Glucose is the major energy source for the fetus. Since lipids do not readily cross the placenta, triglycerides are hydrolyzed and the fatty acids reesterified. With the exception of antibodies—depending on the placentation type—large proteins do not pass the placenta. Unfortunately, many toxic substances are readily absorbed. Appearance of alcohol fetal syndrome in humans is evidence of the ability of ethanol to pass the placenta and adversely affect fetal development. Substances that cause abnormal fetal development or birth defects are teratogenic.

The placenta is also a major endocrine organ during pregnancy. For example, mares produce a gonadotropin, equine chorionic gonadotropins (ECG), sometimes called pregnant mare serum gonadotropin (PMSG). The hormone acts like LH and serves to stimulate the maintenance of the primary CL on the ovary. Concentrations are especially high during the period from 40–100 days of gestation. In fact, this "extra" stimulus can promote additional luteinization of ovarian follicles to ensure that an adequate level of progesterone is maintained. When used in other species, PMSG has a very strong FSH-like action, so it is useful to induce follicular development, i.e., in superovulation and embryo transfer schemes.

In addition to the ovaries, in many species the placenta is a major source of estrogen and progesterone. For example, in sows or rabbits, lutectomy (surgical removal of the CL) will terminate the pregnancy any time during gestation. But in other species, the placenta can take over the necessary production of progesterone. The time when the placenta can take over and maintain the pregnancy in the cow, ewe, mare, and human is 7 months, 50 days, 70 days, and 50 days, respectively.

The placenta also produces a polypeptide in many species that has properties similar to Prl and GH, most commonly referred to as placental lactogen. Whether the GH- or Prl-like activity predominates varies markedly, as does the amount of placental lactogen that appears in the material circulation. In sheep and goats, concentrations of several hundred ng/ml are common near the time of parturition but concentrations are only 1–2 ng/ml in cattle.

Parturition

Parturition is divided into three phases: 1) initiation of uterine contractions, 2) expulsion of the fetus, and 3) expulsion of the fetal membranes. However, events leading to birth are really the result of a cascade of actions. During most of gestation, maintenance of high progesterone concentrations produce a quiet uterus. As birth approaches, luteolysis of the dominant CL and/or decreasing placental production of progesterone couples with increasing estrogen concentrations to prepare for parturition. Increasing estrogen also stimulates expression of oxytocin receptors in the myometrium. Activation of the fetal pituitary-adrenal axis is essential for the initiation of parturition. It is generally accepted that the fetus essentially becomes "stressed" so that it begins to secrete ACTH. This leads to fetal secretion of glucocorticoids. Its elevation acts to remove the progesterone block by stimulation of three enzymes in the placenta that increases the conversion of progesterone to estradiol. These enzymes are 17α hydrolyase (conversion of progesterone to 17α hydroxyprogesterone), 17, 20 lyase (conversion of 17α hydroxyprogesterone to androstenedione), and aromatase (conversion of androstenedione to estradiol). Fetal corticoids also promote synthesis of $PGF_2\alpha$, which acts to remove the progesterone block. Increasing estradiol and $PGF_2\alpha$ synergize to make the uterus more sensitive to actions that promote contractions. In some species (mares, humans, rabbits, and pigs), the hormone relaxin, which is produced by the ovary and/or placenta, acts to soften cervical tissues and allow pelvic ligament stretch to aid parturition.

As estradiol and glucocorticoids increase, the contracting uterus pushes the fetus toward the cervix. Neural signals originating in the cervix promote oxytocin release that produces more contractions, more pressure on the cervix, and then more oxytocin in a positive cascade. As the fetus enters the cervical canal the first stage of parturition is complete. Although estradiol and other hormones increase mucus secretion and general lubrication of the cervical canal and vagina, progressively stronger contractions are critical. With the fetus properly positioned, the feet and head put increasing pressure on the fetal membranes so that the membranes rupture, releasing amniotic fluid. This also acts as lubrication. As the fetus passes the birth canal it becomes hypoxic. This promotes fetal movement, which stimulates more uterine contraction. Along with active abdominal contractions of the dam, expulsion of the fetus is accomplished.

In most cases, the fetal membranes are expelled just after the fetus. The degree of disruption varies depending on the type of placentation, but it requires that the chorionic villi are removed from the crypts on the maternal side of the placenta. This is believed to be caused by active vasoconstriction of the arteries of the villi. This is important to minimize hemorrhage. Clearly, this is also much more likely in animals with hemochorial or hemoendothelial types of placentation.

The duration of parturition varies substantially between species. For example, in cows initial stages of parturition (start of contractions and cervical dilation) typically lasts 2 to 6 h, fetal expulsion 30 to 60 min, and expulsion of fetal membranes 6 to 12 h. Prolonged parturition is called dystocia. One cause of problems is excessive size of the fetus. Consequently care must be taken in breeding programs, especially when cross-breeding occurs. Another problem occurs when there is a failure of the fetus to become properly positioned for birth. For example, in cattle the calf is normally positioned as if it is diving head first with the front legs extended underneath the lower jaw. In about 5% of births, the calf is abnormally positioned. In some cases, normal birth becomes impossible so that a cesarean section is required. A third issue arises in normally monotocous species when there are multiple births. This can be the result of twins presenting simultaneously, one abnormally positioned fetus blocking birth of another, or uterine fatigue from prolonged parturition.

Overview of male reproductive tract

The reproductive tract of the male is made up of testis, epididymis, spermatic cord, accessory sex glands, and the penis. The testis is critical for production of spermatozoa and testosterone. The epididymis provides the environment needed for both the spermatozoa to mature and for storage. The accessory sex glands produce seminal plasma and fluids and the penis is the structure needed for copulation.

The testes lie outside the abdominal cavity within the scrotum, essentially a purselike structure that is derived from the skin and connective tissue of the abdominal wall. The testes develop in the abdomen, in a position medial to the embryonic kidney. A grouping of ducts within the testis develops so that they connect to the mesonephric tubules to eventually give rise to the epididymis, ductus deferens, and vesicular gland. The prostrate and bulbourethral glands develop from the embryonic sinus and the penis forms by tabulation and elongation of a tubercle that appears at the orifice of the urogenital sinus. This pattern of development depends on secretions from the fetal testis. Specifically, androgen production stimulates secretion of a glycoprotein called Mullerian-inhibiting substance, which prevents the female developmental pattern from proceeding. In other words, in the absence of blockage, the female development pattern is normal.

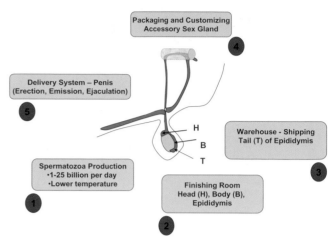

Fig. 19.16. Male reproductive function viewed as a manufacturing process: 1) Production of spermatozoa occurs in the seminiferous tubules of the testes; 2) spermatozoa are transported to the body and head of the epididymis; 3) in the tail of the epididymis, spermatozoa become functionally fertile; 4) addition of secretions from the accessory sex gland (seminal vesicles, prostate, etc.) provides seminal plasma; 5) sexual arousal and intromission provide the delivery system to the female reproduction tract.

The testes normally migrate in a caudal directly within the abdominal cavity to the inguinal ring. They pass through the enlarged foramen of the genitofemoral nerve (Lumbar; L3 and L4). This process requires the formation of a peritoneal sac that extends through the abdominal wall so that the testis is enclosed by an inguinal ligament of the testis called the gubernaculum testis. The migration is complete once the testes are in the scrotum. If this process fails the condition is called cryptorchidism. If both testes fail to descend, the male is sterile. This is because the lower temperature of the testes within the scrotum is required for spermatogenesis. As diagrammed in Figure 19.16, the various parts of the male reproduction system have been likened to a manufacturing operation. If successful, the end products are fully functional spermatozoa. Hormones (testosterone, FSH, and LH) and secretory products (fluids of the epididymis and seminal plasma) allow for appropriate movement, transport, and maturation of the spermatozoa.

The testes are responsible for the creation of the spermatozoa and they are very efficient. Depending on the species, 1 to 25 billion spermatozoa are produced per day. Once the cells are produced over a period of several days they pass thorough the rete tubules and enter the head (caput) and body (corpus) of the epididymis. In these locations, the cells are modified so that they become fertile. Cells that enter the tail (cauda) of the epididymis are capable of fertilization if removed and incubated in an appropriate buffer solution. This region of the epididymis serves as a reservoir for spermatozoa prior to ejaculation. With

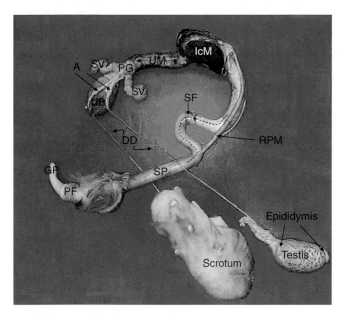

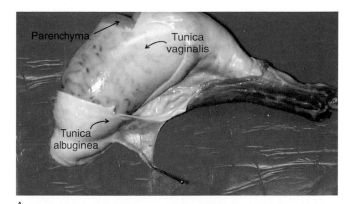

A

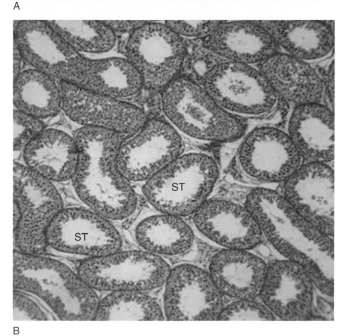

B

Fig. 19.17. Gross anatomy of the dissected reproductive tract of a bull. A = ampulla of ductus deferens, GP = glans penis, DD = ductus deferens, IcM = ischiocabernosus muscle, RPM = retractor penis muscle, PG = prostrate gland, PF = preputial fold, SF = sigmoid flexure, SP = shaft of penis, SV = seminal vesicles, UB = urinary bladder, UM = urethralis muscle.

Fig. 19.18. Gross anatomy of the bull testis and corresponding histological appearance of the testicular parenchymal tissue. The capsule surrounding the testis (tunica vaginalis and (tunica albuginea) supports the parenchymal tissue (A). The striking feature of the testis is the abundance of seminiferous tubules (ST), responsible for the production of the spermatozoa (B).

sexual arousal, the spermatozoa in the tail of the epididymis are transported via contractions of the smooth muscle of the epididymal duct and the ductus deferens to the pelvic urethra. The final packaging involves the addition of fluids produced by the accessory sex glands (ampulla of the ductus deferens, seminal vesicles, prostrate gland, and bulbourethral glands). The noncellular component of the semen is called seminal plasma. Some of these basic structural elements are illustrated in Figure 19.17.

Spermatogenesis

The functional tissue of an organ is called the parenchyma of the organ. Testicular parenchyma is comprised of the seminiferous tubules and the interstitial cells of Leydig. However, the support of these cells requires a rich supply of capillaries, lymphatic vessels, and connective tissues. The testis is surrounded by a tough capsule composed of two elements. The tunica vaginalis (visceral tunic) is closest to the testicular parenchyma and the tunica albuginea, a tougher outer connective tissue layer. Tissue projections from the capsule penetrate into the testicular tissue to create supporting septa for the seminiferous tubules where they join a central connective tissue band called the mediastinum. When the testis is cut longitudinally, it appears that there are elongated islands of parenchymal tissue separated by faint bands of connective

tissue. Examples of the gross and microscopic anatomy of the testis are shown in Figure 19.18.

The seminiferous tubules are the key to spermatogenesis. As the images in Figures 19.17 and 19.18 suggest, they are very highly convoluted structures with a complex array of developing cells (germinal epithelium) that make up the wall of the tubule. The end of each seminiferous tubule joins with the rete tubules that are continuous with the epididymis. The tubule is surrounded by peritubular cells, connective tissue elements, capillaries, and the Leydig cells. Within the basement membrane the basal compartment contains the Sertoli cells and the developing population of germ cells, the spermatogonia. Essentially, the cycle of differentiation involves sequential

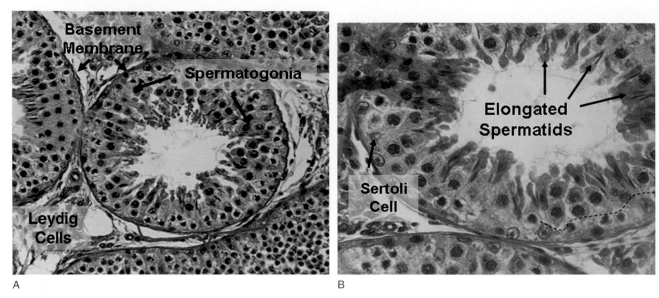

Fig. 19.19. Histology of seminiferous tubules is illustrated. The left panel (A) provides an overview of the seminiferous tubules with their distinct basement membranes. In the regions between the tubules islands of cells, Leydig cells (lower-left corner), are responsive to gonadotropin (FSH and LH) secretion and in turn produce locally high concentrations of testosterone. Testosterone, in addition to its affect on secondary sex characteristics, is also important in the differential of the germ cells. The right panel (B) provides higher magnification to illustrate the presence of Sertoli cells and spermatogonia of the basal compartment as well as presence of spermatids and elongated spermatids in the adluminal compartment. The thin dashed line shows the approximate boundary between the basal and adluminal compartments.

development of the germ cells until the mature spermatozoa are released into the luminal space of the seminiferous tubule. The Sertoli cells are the only somatic cells that are part of the internal structure (inside the basement membrane) of the seminiferous tubules. As the spermatogonia develop, their destiny is largely controlled by the Sertoli cells. Specifically, each of the Sertoli cells tends or anchors a maximum number of germ cells. This means that the absolute number of spermatozoa produced per day is directly linked with the density of Sertoli cells within the seminiferous tubules. In many ways the Sertoli cells are analogous to the granulosal cells of the ovarian follicles. The layer of Sertoli cells near the basement membrane are linked to one another by tight junctions. This produces a barrier that allows different local environments within the basal region compared with the area near the lumen of the tubule (the adluminal compartment). The basal region houses the spermatogonia and the early spermatocytes. The adluminal region has all the other germ cells, i.e., primary and secondary spermatocytes, spermatids, elongated spermatids, and mature spermatozoa. Cells of the seminiferous tubules are illustrated in more detail in Figure 19.19. Because not all the cells in regions of the tubules mature simultaneously, a survey of sections shows varying stages of maturity. Figure 19.20 shows a section of seminiferous tubule with fully formed spermatozoa nearing the point of being released into the lumen; this would be Stage VIII of the development.

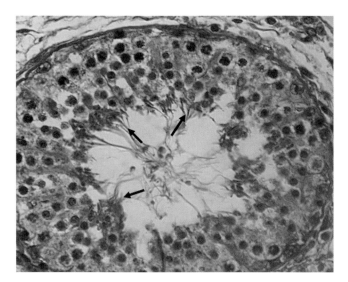

Fig. 19.20. Stage VIII development of bull spermatogenesis. Several clusters of mature spermatozoa (arrows) are nearing release into the lumen of the seminiferous tubule.

This developmental process can be characterized in several ways. A *cycle* is described as a series of changes in a given region of the tubular epithelium between appearances of the same developmental stage. A *stage* is a well-characterized histological-cellular profile of the epithelium that defines a particular period of spermatogenesis. A *wave of development* defines the sequential order of stages of spermatogenesis that occur along the length of the tubule. As an example, if you begin at the time when a "crop" of new spermatozoa have been released into the lumen of the tubule, this region of the germinal epithelium is described as being in Stage I of spermatogenesis. The appearance is characterized by the complete absence of spermatozoa, and the presence of primary spermatogonia and Sertoli cells (near the basement membrane), and some round spermatids in the adluminal area but little else. By Stage II some elongation of some of the spermatids begins. In Stage III the elongating spermatids begin to clump or bunch in close association with the apical regions of the Sertoli cells. In Stage IV secondary spermatocytes appear. Stages V–VIII are characterized by continued expansion of the epithelium until the new crop of mature spermatozoa "back out" of their docking stations with the Sertoli cells and are released so the cycle in that region of the tubule can begin once more.

The peritubular cells, basement membrane, and junctional complexes of the Sertoli cells combine to create a so-called blood testis barrier that prevents large molecular weight materials and immune cells from entering the adluminal area of the seminiferous tubules. This is important because it prevents autoimmune reactions from impacting the developing spermatozoa as they undergo meiosis.

Sperm storage, maturation, and delivery

Once spermatozoa are shed into the luminal space of the seminiferous tubules, the efferent ducts converge into the rete tubules and then a single epididymal duct. Here, the cells and fluids (rete fluid) combine. The head of the epididymis is the initial segment. The head and body of the epididymis provide an environment, governed at least in part by the effects of testosterone, for maturation of the spermatozoa. Like the seminiferous tubules, the epididymis is also highly convoluted. In many species, if extended it would reach 60 m. It is surrounded by smooth muscle so that rhythmic contractions progressively propel the spermatozoa to the tail of the epididymis. Transit times vary, but in bulls, for example, it takes 9–14 days for the trip from the head through the tail. Once in the tail, smooth muscle activity is reduced unless there is sexual stimulation. Sexual stimulation induces smooth muscle contractions in the tail so that spermatozoa are propelled into the ductus deferens. However, transit through the body and head of the epididymis are not affected. This means that the tail region of the epididymis, especially the distal region, serves as a reservoir. Thus, sperm number per ejaculate is dramatically impacted by ejaculation frequency. In a practical sense, this explains the need for not overstocking breeding

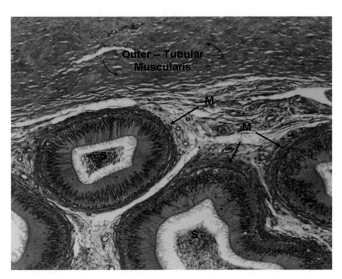

Fig. 19.21. Image of the body region of the bovine epididymis. Part of the thick muscular tunic (outer tubular muscularis) that surrounds the entire structure is shown, as well as smooth muscle (M and arrows) surrounding the highly convoluted epididymal tubular elements.

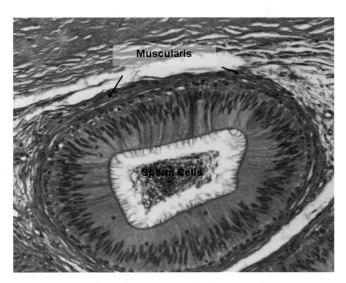

Fig. 19.22. Histological appearance of tail region of the epididymis. Note the distinct layer of smooth muscle (muscularis) surrounding the tubule, the cluster of spermatozoa in the luminal area, and the pseudostratified epithelial cells with cilia that line the internal surface.

males so that maximum fertility is maintained. In short, the breeding capacity depends primarily on the epididymal tail reserves rather than the rate of sperm production.

Given the continuous production of several billion spermatozoa daily, there is also a continuous loss of spermatozoa irrespective of sexual activity. Since there is no reabsorption of spermatozoa, periodic contraction of the epididymis and ductus deferens produces a flow of cells into the pelvic urethra where they are flushed with urination. Figures 19.21 and 19.22

illustrate histological features of the epididymis. Notice the accumulation of spermatozoa in the lumen of the caudal regions, presence of a distinct muscularis (contrast with the seminiferous tubules), and distinct presence of the stratified, ciliated epithelium that lines the internal surface of the epididymis.

Reproduction in birds

It is apparent even to the casual observer that there are dramatic reproductive differences between mammals and birds. Chickens (gallus domesticus) are familiar as domesticated birds in the poultry industry. These birds are believed to be descended from Red Jungle fowl found in southeastern Asia. We take advantage of the prodigious egg production of these animals to provide a breakfast staple around the world and meat for our tables. Indeed, the world population of chickens is approximately 24 billion.

Before World War II, most egg production came from farm flocks of only a few hundred hens. Beginning in the 1950s and 1960s, changing technology and creation of specialized equipment shifted production from these small farm flocks to larger, vertically integrated (direct association between growers and producers and egg or meat wholesalers) large enterprises. In the major egg-producing states, flocks of 100,000 laying hens are not unusual, and some flocks number more than 1 million. Each of the 235 million laying birds in the U.S. produces from 250 to 300 eggs a year. Our purpose is to provide some highlights and comparative aspects with a focus on the domestic chicken.

Mature male chickens are called roosters and cocks or cockerels if immature. Castrated roosters are called capons. Young females are called pullets and mature females are called hens. Roosters are usually differentiated from hens by their striking plumage and often bright feathers on their necks.

Given the opportunity, flocks of chickens are gregarious and maintain a distinct social or pecking order. A mature rooster that finds food may call the other chickens by making a clucking sound and by picking up and dropping the food. This behavior also occurs in hens when they call their chicks. As a part of a courting ritual, the rooster may drag the wing opposite the hen and turn in a circle around the hen. When she becomes acclimated to responding to his vocalization, the rooster may mount the hen and proceed with the fertilization. Similar behaviors can be observed during the spring-summer mating season with various songbirds.

Most wild birds usually lay one or more eggs in a group called a clutch and then stop laying additional eggs to incubate eggs in the nest. These birds display yearly breeding cycles. On the other hand, domestic chickens are continuous breeders and under the best conditions are reproductively active throughout the year. Seasonal disruption of reproduction in birds is an adaptive response to ensure that newly hatched chicks can be cared for under conditions most suitable for survival. A common mechanism for ending the breeding season of wild birds in northern latitudes depends on hypothalamic signaling and subsequent hormonal response of the birds to an increasing photoperiod. In other words, the birds become refractory to normally stimulating long days. This results in regression of the gonads. Recovery or the ability to respond positively to long-day photoperiods is reestablished only after birds are exposed to short photoperiods for 40 to 60 days.

Avian reproduction is best understood in domestic chicken and turkeys. In fact, the modern poultry industry depends on a well-developed understanding of the reproductive cycle and how best to manipulate and control it for maximum egg production. Birds lay eggs in groups or clutches of one or more eggs. This is followed by a rest period and then another cycle. Clutch size, as well as the numbers of clutches laid in a breeding season, varies with species, but the principle is the same. Domestic hens usually lay five or more eggs in a clutch, with a day's break between clutches.

Hens ovulate in the morning and almost never after 3:00 p.m. under a normal photoperiod. The final stages to prepare the terminal egg for laying takes from 25 to 26 h. This period includes approximately 3.5 h to add the layers of albumen (egg white) around the yolk, 1.5 h for shell membranes, and 20 h needed for shell formation. Ovulation of the next egg in sequence (part of the clutch) begins within an hour of laying the previous egg. This means that the hen starts to slowly get behind as each day passes. After several days she gets so far behind that she would have to ovulate after 3:00 p.m. Since this does not happen, the next ovulation is delayed and the clutch cycle is broken. After a couple of days the sequence begins again with a new clutch of eggs.

Sometimes a hen will stop laying additional eggs and begin to focus on the incubation of eggs. This is called "broodiness" or "going broody." A broody chicken will doggedly sit on her nest and protest or peck if disturbed. While brooding, the hen maintains constant temperature and humidity, and also turns the eggs regularly. At the end of the 21-day incubation period, if the eggs are fertilized they will hatch and the broody hen will take care of her chicks. Since individual eggs do not all hatch at the same time (the hen lays only one egg approximately every 25 h), the hen will usually stay on the nest for about 2 days after the first egg hatches. During this time, the newly hatched

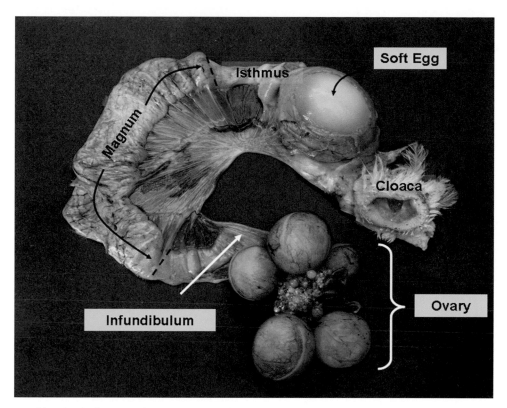

Fig. 19.23. Structures of female chicken reproductive tract. The ovary with multiple oocytes in various stages of development is apparent. After ovulation, the egg progresses through segments of the oviduct, infundibulum, magnum, and isthmus. In this illustration, a mature egg after albumin deposition (soft egg), but before shell formation, is shown. The mature egg is subsequently laid after passage into the cloaca. Original photograph provided courtesy of Dr. Frank Robinson, University of Alberta.

chicks live off the egg yolk they absorb just before hatching. The hen can sense the chicks peeping inside the eggs and will gently cluck to stimulate them to break out of their shells. If the eggs are not fertilized and do not hatch, the hen will eventually lose interest and leave the nest.

Avian female reproductive system

The right ovary and oviduct are present during early embryonic development in birds, but asymmetrical migration of precursor germ cells to the left ovary ultimately results in regression of the right ovary in most species. Thus, the mature reproductive system consists of a single left ovary and its oviduct. The ovary of a chick embryo contains ~500,000 oocytes at time of hatching when oogenesis ends. The ovary in immature birds exhibits a mass of small ova, many of which are visible to the unaided eye. It is typical that 250 to 500 ova are ovulated during the life of most domesticated birds. Figure 19.23 gives the parts of an avian reproductive tract.

Follicle growth is characterized into three phases: 1) slowly growing, small (60 to 100 µm) follicles that

occurs over periods of months or years; 2) growth over a period of months with rapid deposition of yolk protein; and 3) very rapid growth during the typical 6–11 days prior to ovulation when the majority of yolk proteins and lipids are deposited in the egg. During phase 3 in the chicken, the follicle adds 2 g of protein per day and increases in diameter from 8 to 37 mm. Yolk proteins are made in the liver. The ovary enlarges greatly during the breeding season. The chicken ovary is divided into two lobes, each with follicles. The ovary in a hen exhibits a clear hierarchy of progressively developing follicles (Fig. 19.24). This explains the cycle of egg laying to create the clutch of eggs.

The follicles in birds bear little resemblance to those in mammals. There is no antrum or follicular fluid, but the follicle is filled with yolk. The mass of yolk grows rapidly, which is important because it provides all of the nourishment for the developing embryo. This mass progressively decreases as the embryo grows. In chickens, posthatching nutrition is also mostly from the yolk for a short time since it is not completely absorbed when the chick hatches.

Ovulation causes release of a mature egg. The egg, with its extensive nutrient reserves is picked up by the infundibulum and carried into the magnum, which is

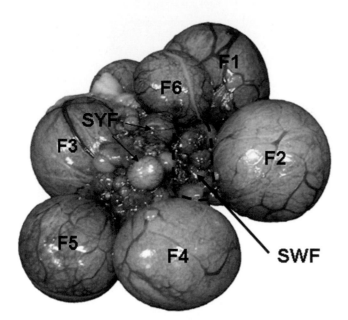

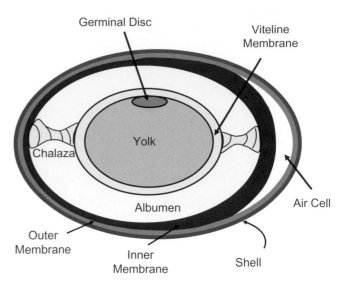

Fig. 19.25. Parts of a chicken egg.

Fig. 19.24. Progressively developing follicles of a laying hen ovary. F1–F6 illustrate sequential development of follicles and thus eggs destined for ovulation. Small yellow follicles (SYF) are those that are beginning to sequester yolk proteins. Small white follicles (SWF), some of which appear in the area bounded by the dashed box, are follicles in still earlier stages of development. Original photograph provided courtesy of Dr. Frank Robinson, University of Alberta.

An average hen egg weighs about 60 g. Of this weight, the shell constitutes 11%; the white, 58%; and the yolk, 31%. These proportions are generally consistent for small or large eggs. Figure 19.25 illustrates the structures of a chicken egg.

the largest segment of the oviduct. Over about 3 h the egg receives a coating of albumen. The egg then passes into the isthmus, where the shell membranes are deposited. This takes about 1 h. The egg then moves to the uterus, or shell gland, where the shell is added, and in some birds, pigment is added in characteristic patterns. The egg then passes into the vagina and cloaca for laying.

The shells of newly deposited eggs are completely filled. The air cell forms by contraction of the contents during cooling and by the loss of moisture. A high-quality egg has only a small air cell. The yolk is positioned in the center of the albumen and is surrounded by the colorless vitelline membrane. The germinal disc is the site of fertilization and is attached to the yolk. On either side of the yolk there are two, twisted, whitish cordlike structures called chalazae. These structures support the yolk in the center of the albumen. Most of the albumen is thick. Surrounding the albumen there are two shell membranes and the shell itself. The shell contains several thousand pores that permit gas exchange.

By the way, the yellow of your breakfast egg is the true oocyte. The yellow of the egg is a single cell and the yolk represents a massive lipid inclusion in its cytoplasm. The largest single cell in existence is the yolk of an ostrich egg, which can have a diameter of 6 in.

Avian male reproductive system

Fundamentals are similar to male mammals in that male birds have two testes that produce sperm. A bird's testes (or ovary for that matter) greatly increase in size during the breeding season. Their small size during the rest of the year lightens the load for flight. The cloaca is the outlet for eggs and sperm.

Male birds have paired abdominal testes located anterior to the cranial lobe of each kidney. The vas deferens emerges medially and passes caudally alongside the ureters to the cloaca where it has a common opening with the ureter in the urodeum. The distal portion of the vas deferens becomes straightened and then abruptly widens at the point where it joins the cloaca. This enlarged structure has a bean-shaped appearance when it is filled with stored semen during the breeding season.

Sperm production occurs in the seminiferous tubules of the testes. Like mammals, sperm formation is temperature sensitive. Thus, maturation is improved with reduced temperatures typical of evening and nighttime hours and in some cases by the development of scrotallike external thermoregulatory swellings, which house the seminal glomera. Accessory organs include the paracloacal vascular bodies, dorsal proctodeal gland, and lymphatic folds. These structures are either directly adjacent to the cloaca or a part of its structure.

Few male birds have a penislike structure. Thus, most achieve fertilization via a cloacal kiss. This involves positioning the male on the back of the female with a twisting of his tail under hers and the touching of the cloaca of each. During copulation or in response to massage, a phallic-like swelling occurs in the accessory lymphatic folds of the cloaca. The paracloacal bodies are essential to this event because they act to store lymph fluid, which promotes swelling.

In chickens after copulation or insemination (turkeys), spermatozoa are stored in specialized storage tubules located in the uterovaginal region of the female. These cells remain viable for up to 2 weeks in chickens and 3 weeks or more in turkeys. Most evidence suggests that spermatozoa fill these glands sequentially and that there is no mixing between successive copulations or inseminations. However, sperm cells from the most recent copulation are most likely to fertilize an ovum. After each egg is laid, spermatozoa are released from these glands where they migrate to the infundibulum of the oviduct where fertilization occurs.

Reproductive technologies

A variety of techniques often called assisted reproductive technologies (ART)—e.g., in vitro fertilization (IVF), superovulation, embryo transfer (ET), and freezing, etc.—are popularized because they are used to assist couples incapable of conceiving naturally. However, these tools have their origins in reproductive physiology of laboratory and farm animals. For example, scientists worked for many years to perfect IVF before it was recognized that sperm cells have to undergo capacitation in the female reproductive tract before fertilization. This ultimately led to methods to induce capacitation and therefore routinely successful IVF. Advances in one aspect of reproduction thus allow progress in other areas. For example, ET would not be practical without endocrine tools to induce superovulation and methods to routinely collect, fertilize, and freeze eggs. Cloning and development of transgenic animals depended on development of techniques to visualize, micromanipulate, and culture eggs and embryos. Several of these key techniques are outlined in subsequent sections.

Artificial insemination

The AI industry is an excellent example of a practical link between scientific understanding, rapid adoption of practical procedures, and creation of an entirely new agricultural industry. The foundations to understanding semen preservation and storage did not occur overnight. However, it was clear especially to dairy producers that techniques to select and preserve semen from genetically superior bulls would rapidly increase genetic progress. Specifically, a highly selected sire could potentially be mated with thousands of females. The first commercial AI using fresh semen dates back to 1937, but this was built on a long history of discoveries.

For example, in 1677 Leeuwenhoek was the first to see spermatozoa with his newly created microscope. The Italian Spallanzani discovered in 1780 that a dog could be impregnated with the cellular portion of semen and that semen could be cooled and used at a later time. The Russian professor Ivanov developed techniques for collection of semen and insemination of cattle, horses, sheep, and pigs by the early 1930s. A Danish scientist, Sorenson, who had connections with Ivanov, established the first AI cooperative for dairy producers in 1933.

The extension dairy specialist E. J. Perry from Rutgers University was visiting Denmark at this time and returned to establish the first AI cooperative in the United States in 1937. This exploded with the creation of seven AI cooperatives by 1939. This pace of development continued as more AI organizations appeared and the number of cows inseminated increased dramatically. To control costs, many small cooperatives ultimately consolidated.

It is estimated that 60% of U.S. dairy cows are artificially inseminated. In contrast, more than 90% of dairy cows in Europe are bred using AI. The two largest AI organizations are privately owned companies with national and worldwide semen distribution efforts. The largest of these, American Breeders Service Global, sells approximately 3.5 million breeding services per year. The second largest is Select Sires.

Although methods for collecting semen and insemination have been available for many years, it is likely that the commercial industry would not have developed as rapidly without several critical research discoveries: 1) the development of semen extenders that would protect sperm cells against temperature shock and thereby allow cold storage, 2) the realization that bull semen could be extended (diluted) to breed large numbers of cows from each ejaculate, and 3) the discovery of methods for frozen storage of bull spermatozoa. In 1939, Drs. Phillips and Lardy at the University of Wisconsin discovered that egg yolk would protect sperm cells from temperature shock upon cooling. The protection was due to phospholipids and lipoproteins in the egg yolk. Extenders combining egg yolk with phosphate, citrate, and bicarbonate buffers were soon developed, and they form the basis for extenders in use today. Heated milk was also found to be a satisfactory semen extender and to provide temperature shock protection.

Spermatozoa were some of the first cells frozen, i.e., by English scientists in 1949. Dr. Polge and co-workers discovered that glycerol in the extender media would protect fowl and bull spermatozoa from damage during freezing. Early freezing and storage was accomplished with dry ice and alcohol at a temperature of –79°C. Afterward, liquid nitrogen became the coolant of choice because its –196°C temperature provided longer and safer storage conditions. The first U.S. calf (named Frosty) from frozen semen was born in 1953.

Dairy producers use AI in their herds because of the following advantages: 1) ready access to genetically superior sires, 2) added disease protection by maintaining a herd closed to new animals, 3) absence of need to keep a dangerous bull on the farm and 4) organized breeding management and record services. In swine operations, AI is often used to decrease the cost of maintaining males at the production unit. In turkeys, AI is used because mating cannot occur naturally because of development of very large-breasted birds.

The techniques are generally available for use of AI in other species, but use is limited for economic reasons—or in horses because the registry of offspring is restricted. Changes in industry structure, however, often drive changes in the use of AI. For example, in the swine industry the growth of large farm units in the 1990s led to the adaptation of AI to reduce expenses of maintaining males. In the horse industry a change in the Quarter Horse Association regulations to allow the registration of foals from AI with cooled and shipped semen has increased the use of AI.

In vitro fertilization (IVF)

The relevance of in vitro fertilization as a research tool has been recognized for many years. The first report of offspring (rabbits) produced this way was in 1959. The first "test-tube" human infant was born in 1978. In cattle, successful fertilization occurs more readily with oocytes that are ovulated compared with those collected from ovarian follicles. Regardless, this in part explains the importance of collecting eggs from animals that are superovulated (hormonally treated so that a greater than normal number of eggs are produced and ovulated) for both embryo transfers and cloning (i.e., genetically superior donors) as well as donors of eggs to be used in transgenic trials.

Methods to improve techniques for oocyte collection and culture conditions to produce a greater percentage of successful oocytes collected from ovaries are under active development. These in vitro maturation (IVM) efforts are closely tied with ultrasound-guided follicular aspiration, also called transvaginal ovum recovery. In this method, an aspiration needle inserted through a guide within a transvaginal ultrasound probe is passed through the vaginal wall and into each follicle while applying a vacuum. Typically, 6 to 8 oocytes can be collected per ovary or more following superovulation. In theory, regardless of superovulation, it is possible to recover 10 to 20 oocytes every 10 to 14 days. Current IVM and IVF methods would be expected to produce 3–5 embryos suitable for implantation.

The advantage of this system is the ability to collect oocytes from cows of known genetic merit, at least twice weekly for extended periods of time, as source material for IVF and microinjection of DNA (see below). This procedure has been shown to yield about 10% greater development of microinjected zygotes to the blastocyst stage and a greater percentage of transferred blastocysts developing to term compared to use of slaughterhouse-derived oocytes.

Embryo transfer (ET)

Although embryo transfer (ET) has been in the popular press recently, because of implications to human reproduction, the basic techniques have been known for many years. The first recorded successful case in 1890 by the physiologist Walter Heap was done with rabbits. By the 1930s, transfers with sheep and goats were reported, and in the 1950s, the first successful embryo transfers in cattle occurred in Cambridge, England. The first successful ET in cattle in the U.S. was in 1951 and commercial ET work began in the 1970s. The first Holstein ET calf was registered in 1974. The popularity of ET in the dairy industry increased dramatically with development of nonsurgical methods for recovery of embryos and subsequent implantation of either freshly collected or frozen embryos. The first successful nonsurgical embryo collection was reported in 1964 and the first North American calf from a frozen embryo was in 1977. Further development of the ultrasound transvaginal collection method combined with improvements in IVM will likely further increase use of ET to expand populations of genetically superior cattle or to allow for cloning of transgenic animals. At the current time, approximately 80% of young AI sires are produced by ET; approximately 12,000 ET heifers are registered each year.

Finally, it also is possible to determine the sex of embryos using PCR techniques designed to amplify male specific sequences on the Y chromosome. Briefly, only a small sampling of cells from the blastocyst (perhaps only one cell) can be utilized. The detection of these sequences in the amplified DNA from these cells would indicate a male, and the absence of the sequences would indicate a female. Biopsied cells are quickly reproduced. In France, where this technology has been rapidly adopted, many dairy producers will no longer transfer embryos without having them sexed.

Sexed semen

Since the initiation of AI, countless numbers of techniques have been investigated with the goal of separating spermatozoa into X- and Y-bearing cells as a means to control sex of offspring. Most of these methods were only marginally better than chance and suffered from poor repeatablity.

However, in the 1980s a breakthrough in semen sexing technology was made by USDA researchers. The patents for this technology were subsequently licensed to a company named XY Inc. of Fort Collins, Colorado. Commercialization of sexed semen in the U.S. was initiated with a 2003 license granted to Sexing Technologies (ST) in Navasota, Texas. Sexed bovine semen is now commercially available.

Briefly, the method utilizes a flow cytometer and associated nontoxic DNA dyes to sort sperm and simultaneously detect the 3 to 4% difference in DNA content between male and female sperm. The first step in this procedure is to dilute sperm to a very low concentration and stain them with a fluorescent dye. The sample is passed under pressure through the flow cytometer. As single sperm cells pass through an internal laser beam, the fluorescent dye is excited. Because of the larger X chromosome, female sperm emit less fluorescence than the Y chromosome–bearing male spermatozoa. Detectors measure the amount of fluorescence and assign positive or negative charges to each droplet containing a single sperm. Charged deflector plates then split the single stream into three streams: positively charged particles containing one sex go one way and negatively charged droplets containing the other sex are deflected in the opposite direction; uncharged droplets containing multiple sperm or unidentified sperm pass through the machine without being deflected. Based on multiple research trials, the procedure separates sperm of the two sexes with approximately 90% accuracy.

There are, however, several major limitations that have hampered widespread implementation of AI using sex-sorted semen. Reduced conception rate is an issue. Given the necessary manipulation, the sorting process negatively impacts sperm viability and longevity compared to normally cryopreserved semen.

In addition, the procedure is extremely slow and relatively inefficient. To properly sort, sperm must be precisely oriented as they pass through the laser and fluorescence detectors in the flow cytometer. Due to the flat shape of bovine sperm heads, only about 30%

are correctly oriented and half of these are female. This means only 15% of the sperm entering the procedure are recovered as a marketable product. Although 3,000 to 5,000 sperm of each sex can be sorted per second; it still takes approximately 1.3 hr of sorting to produce enough semen for a standard 20 million sperm/straw dosage. This resulted in commercialization of a product with about tenfold fewer spermatozoa per insemination. Because of the low sperm numbers per dose and compromised sperm viability, sex-sorted semen is recommended only for use in well-managed, highly fertile virgin heifers. Data summarized to this time indicates that herds that typically achieve a 60 to 65% conception rate in virgin heifers with normal semen can expect a 45 to 55% conception rate with sexed semen. Sex-sorted semen is not currently recommended for use in lactating cows (because of inherently reduced conception rates, compared with heifers).

Cloning

Cloning is the creation of a new individual that is genetically identical to the source individual. Identical (monozygotic) twins come from an embryo that spontaneously splits, resulting in natural cloning. Cloning animals is a technique that may well assist animal industries in maintaining high-quality livestock to supply future food and fiber needs. Identifying and reproducing superior livestock genetics ensures that herds are maintained at the highest quality possible. Animal cloning offers potential benefits to consumers, farmers, and endangered species—for example, allowing farmers and ranchers to accelerate the reproduction of their most productive and healthiest livestock. Cloning can be used to protect endangered species. For example, in China, panda cells are being kept on reserve should this species' numbers be threatened by extinction.

In 1997, cloning was revolutionized when Dr. Ian Wilmut and his colleagues at the Roslin Institute in Edinburgh, Scotland, successfully cloned a sheep named Dolly. Dolly was the first mammal cloned using nonembryonic cells. Wilmut and his colleagues transplanted a nucleus from a mammary gland fibroblast of a Finn Dorsett sheep into the enucleated egg of a Scottish blackface ewe. The nucleus-egg combination was stimulated with electricity to fuse the two and to stimulate cell division. The new cell divided and was placed in the uterus of a blackface ewe to develop. Dolly was subsequently born. Dolly was shown to be genetically identical to the Finn Dorsett mammary cells and not to the blackface ewe. This clearly demonstrated that she was a successful clone (it took 276 attempts before the experiment was

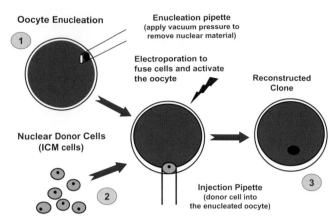

Fig. 19.26. Overview of micromanipulation and cloning. Step 1 indicates the removal or enucleation of the existing nucleus of a fertilized oocyte. This is accomplished by micromanipulating the egg under differential contrast or phase contrast microscope. The egg is held with slight vacuum with a microscopic blunted holding pipette (not shown) while a fine dissection pipette is used to aspirate the nucleus of the egg. Step 2 indicates the collection of the nucleus of a donor cell, in this case cells from the interstitial cell mass (ICM) from the embryo of an animal scheduled for cloning. In step (3) the donor cell nucleus is injected and a slight electrical charge is used to induce fusion of the donor nucleus and egg. The newly generated egg is allowed to develop and then frozen or implanted in a surrogate dam.

successful). Dolly has since grown and reproduced several offspring of her own through normal sexual means. Therefore, Dolly is a viable, healthy clone.

Nuclear transfer in livestock using cells of the interstitial cell mass (ICM) of a donor blastocyst is relatively routine. Nuclear transfer is accomplished by the fusion of a donor cell to the unfertilized ova, which has been enucleated. Before the success of somatic cell nuclear transfer, it was possible to obtain cells from transgenic early bovine embryos as a source of nuclear material for donation to an enucleated oocyte.

The most common cloning method, known as "somatic cell nuclear transfer" or simply "nuclear transfer," requires two kinds of cells. One is a somatic cell, which is collected from the animal scheduled to be cloned (known as the "genetic donor"). A somatic cell is any cell other than a sperm cell or egg cell. The other kind of cell required for cloning is an egg cell, which is collected from a female of the same species. In the lab, the nucleus of the egg cell is removed. The nucleus from the donor somatic is then inserted into the enucleated egg. A charge is applied resulting in the fused egg.

The activated egg is then placed in a culture medium. Over the course of several days, a blastocyst forms. The blastocyst is subsequently implanted in the uterus of a recipient female (sometimes referred to as "surrogate mother") where it continues to develop. After a full-term pregnancy, the recipient gives birth to an

animal that is essentially the identical twin of the genetic donor. Since Dolly, several university laboratories and companies have used various modifications of the nuclear transfer technique to produce cloned mammals, including cows, pigs, monkeys, and mice. This technique is outlined in Figure 19.26.

Transgenic animals

Farmers began manipulating genome of animals soon after domestication of livestock began. Certainly most of this genetic gain arose from the selection of individuals considered superior to be retained as breeding stock. Production of transgenic animals is in many ways an extension of this effort. This became possible as a consequence of the ability of scientists to develop recombinant DNA and thereby isolate individual genes for the transfer of copies into the genome of other animals. A "transgenic" animal is one that integrates recombinant DNA into its own genetic material.

The primary method for the production of transgenic animals is through the introduction of foreign genes by microinjection of DNA into one pronucleus of fertilized ova. This procedure was described in 1980 for mice and has been used mostly for the production of transgenic animals. Fertilized ova can be collected prior to the time of cell division after superovulation or following IVF of oocytes collected from slaughterhouse ovaries. The apparent potential viability of in vivo collected zygotes is higher than for the superovulated zygotes, but the number of potential cells available for gene insertion makes the slaughterhouse-provided oocytes more practical for transgenic work in cattle. Review summaries indicate that for DNA microinjected into over 11,500 IVF slaughterhouse-derived ova, only 9% developed to the morula/blastocyst stage. Of 478 embryos transferred to recipients, 90 (19%) produced calves. Ten percent of the calves were transgenic, and a heifer from the study was induced to lactate and shown to secrete human α-lactalbumin in her milk. The rate of transgenesis, based on microinjected zygotes, was .08% (Ayares, 2000). This technique is illustrated in Figure 19.27.

Indeed, a variety of proteins used in human medicine (human growth hormone, insulin, erythropoietin, etc.) are recombinant proteins derived from the transferring genes coding for the production of these proteins into bacterial cells. Bacterial cells containing these choice proteins are subsequently grown in large incubators and the proteins harvested and purified. The recombinant bovine somatotropin used to enhance lactation performance in dairy cows or the rennet used in cheese making is derived in a similar process.

In recent years, scientists have utilized these technologies to link genes of interest with gene promoters that would drive the production of specific proteins in selected tissues and especially the mammary gland. It has been possible to utilize promoter regions of

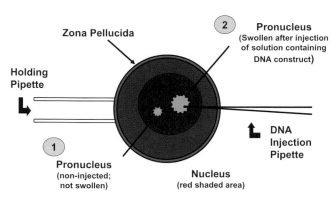

Fig. 19.27. Microinjection and transgenic animals. Step 1 indicates the normal appearance of the pronucleus of a fertilized egg. For insertion of the gene constructs, the egg is positioned with a holding pipette and the injection pipette containing a solution with multiple copies of the DNA construct (Step 2) is used to inject a small volume (~1 pl) into the pronucleus. In response, the organelle swells.

specific milk protein genes (caseins, α-lactalbumin, β-lactoglobulin) to direct secretion of a variety of proteins into milk. These transgenic animals are then bred and the lactating animals used as living bioreactors, e.g., the milk used as a source to purify and isolate the desire protein products (Table 19.3).

The production of pharmaceutical proteins (assuming investment and support continues) likely holds a more immediate application than transgenic tools to improve livestock performance. Safe and effective proteins produced from transgenic animals can be produced with current technologies, and products can be available in unlimited quantities and at reasonable costs to consumers. Many of these products will be the result of using the mammary gland of sheep and goats and possibly cows and pigs as bioreactors for the production of human recombinant proteins.

Despite the potential benefits, there are limitations in technology because of availability of appropriate genes for DNA insertion and the inefficiencies of production of transgenic livestock. More genes are likely to become available as more basic genome projects identify candidates. But low efficiencies for transgene integration and low embryonic survival rates because of embryo manipulation are large impediments.

Table 19.3. Selected listing of milk protein gene promoters and expression of recombinant proteins in milk.

Promoter and Expressed Protein	Animal	Concentration per Milliliter
Bovine α-lactalbumin	Rat	2.4 mg
Bovine α-lactalbumin	Mouse	1.5 mg
Human α-lactalbumin	Cow	2.4 mg
Bovine α$_{s1}$-casein		
hEPO[a]	Mouse	0.2 mg
hIGF-I[b]	Rabbit	1 mg
hlactoferrin	Cow	Not reported
Goat β-casein	Mouse	22 mg
hLAtPA[c]	Goat	
hAnti-thrombin III	Goat	
Ovine β-lactoglobulin		
hAAT[d]	Mouse	5 µg to 21 mg
hAAT	Sheep	5 µg to 35 mg
hFactor IX	Sheep	25 ng
hInterferon γ	Mouse	20 ng
hFibrinogen	Sheep	5 mg
Mouse whey acidic protein		
hGH[e]	Mouse	3.5 mg
Protein C	Mouse	3 µg
Protein C	Pig	1 mg
hFactor VIII	Pig	2.7 mg

[a] hEPO-recombinant human erythropoeitin.
[b] hIGF-I-recombinant human insulinlike growth factor-I.
[c] hLAtPA-recombinant human long acting tissue plasminogen activator.
[d] hAAT-recombinant human α-1-antitrypsin.
[e] hGH-recombinant human growth hormone.
Adapted from Gwazdauskas, 2002.

Integration efficiencies are less than 30% in laboratory mice, and lower in livestock species. The low integration and reproductive efficiencies are acceptable for laboratory species, but these costs become less acceptable for use in livestock species.

Choice of gene construct is probably the most important decision for attempting to design livestock to have a significant impact on the agricultural and consuming community. The construct usually contains a regulatory element (promoter, enhancer) from one gene ligated to a structural gene sequence. This combination allows for theoretical direction of the expression of the structural gene to specific areas of production, at specific times, and allows for regulation of the amount of product produced.

Transgenic technology for the improvement of animal production or performance has been touted for nearly 2 decades since the first publication of the "super" mouse with an added growth hormone (GH) construct. The prospect for improvement of dairy, beef, swine, and sheep production and health through transgenesis is still rudimentary. Part of the delay in real progress with transgenic animal production has been the fact that DNA injected into the egg insertion (with current techniques for livestock species) is incorporated at random sites in the genome. This can produce negative effects. For example, addition of a GH gene in swine led to overproduction of GH and insulinlike growth factor I (IGF-I) and subsequent physiological conditions similar to excessive GH production in acromegaly. Additionally, the high cost of animals and their care, the lack of inbred lines, long generation intervals, and production of small numbers (one or two) of offspring per female in sheep and cattle have lowered the chances for meaningful progress in livestock species with this approach. However, as indicated previously, utilization of the mammary gland as a bioreactor offers interesting possibilities for large-scale production of recombinant proteins that cannot be done with bacterial cell cultures.

References

Ayares, D.L. 2000. Transgenic protein production: Achievements using microinjection technology and the promise of nuclear transfer. J. Anim. Sci. 78 (Suppl. 3): 8–18.

Bearden, H.J., J.W. Fuquay, and S.T. Willard. 2004. Applied Animal Reproduction, Pearson Prentice Hall, London.

Frandson, R.D., W.L. Wilke, and A.D. Fails. 2003. Anatomy and Physiology of Farm Animals 6th Edition. Lippincott Williams and Wilkins, Ambler, Pennsylvania.

Gwazdauskas, F.C. 2002. Gamete and embryo technology-transgenic animals. Encyclopedia of Dairy Science. Edited by H. Roginski, J.W. Fuquay, and P.F. Fox. Academic Press, New York and London.

Krisher, R.L., J.R. Gibbons, and F.C. Gwazdauskas. 1995. Nuclear transfer in the bovine using microinjected donor embryos: Assessment of development and deoxyribonucleic acid detection frequency. J. Dairy Sci. 78: 1282–1288.

Peeler, I.D., R.L. Nebel, R.E. Pearson, W.S. Swecker, and A. Garcia. 2004. Pregnancy rates after timed AI of heifers following removal of intravaginal progesterone inserts. J. Dairy Sci. 87: 2868–2873.

Randall, D., W. Burggen, and K. French. 2002. Eckert Animal Physiology. W.H. Freeman and Company, New York.

Senger, P.L. 2003. Pathways to Pregnancy and Parturition. Current Concepts, Inc. Pullman, WA.

Weigel, K.A. 2004. Exploring the role of sexed semen in dairy production systems. J. Dairy Sci. 87: E120–E130.

Whittow, G.C., Editor. 2000. Sturkie's Avian Physiology, 5th Edition. Academic Press, San Diego, California.

Glossary

11-cis-retinal: A carotenoid constituent of visual pigments. It is the oxidized form of retinol, which functions as the active component of the visual cycle. It is bound to the protein opsin forming the complex rhodopsin. When stimulated by visible light, the retinal component of the rhodopsin complex undergoes isomerization at the 11-position of the double bond to the *cis* form; this is reversed in "dark" reactions to return to the native *trans* configuration.

2, 3-bis-phosphoglycerate (BPG): A three-carbon isomer of the metabolic intermediate 1,3-bisphosphoglycerate. It is notable because it binds to deoxygenated hemoglobin in the red blood cell. In so doing, it indirectly regulates the ability of red blood cells to release oxygen near tissues that need it most.

5-hydroxytryptamine: A monoamine neurotransmitter synthesized in serotonergic neurons in the central nervous system (CNS) and enterochromaffin cells in the gastrointestinal tract.

A

Abdominal cavity: The space bounded by the abdominal walls, diaphragm, and pelvis, it contains most of the organs of digestion, the spleen, the kidneys, and the adrenal glands.

Abdominopelvic cavity: The portion of the ventral body cavity that contains abdominal and pelvic subdivisions. It also contains the peritoneal cavity.

Abduction: To move away from the midline of the body or from an adjacent part or limb.

Abomasum: The fourth and final stomach compartment of the stomach in ruminants. It serves primarily in the acid hydrolysis of microbial and dietary protein, preparing these protein sources for further digestion and absorption in the small intestine.

Absolute refractory period: The period following stimulation during which no additional action potential can be evoked.

Absorption: The active or passive uptake of gases, fluids, or solutes.

Accessory organs: Organs that assist with the functioning of other organs within a system.

Accessory pancreatic duct: An additional duct called duct of Santorini, which connects directly to the duodenum.

Accommodation reflex: A reflex action of the eye, in response to focusing on a near object, and then looking at a distant object (and vice versa), comprising coordinated changes in convergence, lens shape, and pupil size. It is dependent on cranial nerve II (afferent limb of reflex), higher centers, and cranial nerve III.

Acetylcholine: A white crystalline derivative of choline that is released at the ends of nerve fibers in the somatic and parasympathetic nervous systems and is involved in the transmission of nerve impulses in the body.

Acetylcholinesterase: Any of various enzymes in the blood and in certain tissues that catalyze the hydrolysis of acetylcholine.

Acetyl CoA: A small molecule that carries acetyl groups in cells. It is a critical part of energy production by cells.

Acquired reflex: An acquired response that is under the control of (conditional on the occurrence of) a stimulus.

Acromion: Bone comprising the tip of the shoulder.

Acrosome: A saclike organelle positioned on the anterior end of the sperm head. It contains enzymes that are necessary for sperm penetration of the egg at fertilization.

Actin: A protein found in muscle that, together with myosin, functions in muscle contraction.

Active transport: The mediated transport of biochemicals and other atomic/molecular substances across membranes.

Active zone: The region on the surface of functional (globular) proteins that fit and interact chemically with other molecules of complementary shape and charge.

Adduction: To move inward toward the median axis of the body or toward an adjacent part or limb.

Adenine: A purine, i.e., one of the types of nitrogenous bases found in nucleic acids such as DNA and RNA.

Adenohypophysis: The anterior lobe of the pituitary gland.

Adenosine diphosphate (ADP): A molecule of adenine with two phosphate groups attached. It is an important precursor for generation of adenosine triphosphate (ATP).

Adenosine triphosphate (ATP): A critical cellular molecule composed of adenine with three phosphate groups attached. The third phosphate depends on a high energy bond, which, when broken, can be used by the cell to produce energy.

Adenylate cyclase: An essential cellular enzyme localized in the cytoplasmic side of the plasma membrane. When activated it converts ATP to cyclic AMP (cAMP). cAMP serves as an intracellular regulator for hormone action.

Adrenal gland: Paired endocrine glands located at the superior pole of each kidney. The adrenal has a cortex and medulla. The cortex is responsible for production of two major classes of steroid hormones: glucocorticoids and mineralocorticoids. The adrenal medulla produces the catecholamines epinephrine and norepinephrine.

Adrenaline: *See* epinephrine.

Adrenergic fibers: Nerve fibers that release norepinephrine.

Adrenergic receptors: Cellular proteins that bind norepinephrine and epinephrine and similar molecules. They mediate neural signaling in the CNS and hormonal signaling via epinephrine in some peripheral tissues. The name was derived because epinephrine and norepinephrine were originally called adrenalin and noradrenalin.

Adrenocorticotropic hormone (ACTH): A glycoprotein hormone made in the anterior lobe of the pituitary. It controls secretion of glucocorticoids (cortisol, corticosterone, etc.) from the adrenal cortex.

Adventitia: The superficial layer of connective tissue surrounding an internal organ; fibers are continuous with those of surrounding tissues, providing support and stabilization.

Aerobic respiration: Respiration in which molecular oxygen is consumed and carbon dioxide and water are produced.

Afferent: Carrying to or toward a center.

Afferent nerve: A nerve conveying impulses from the periphery to the central nervous system; also called the centripetal nerves.

Afferent neuron: A nerve cell that carries impulses toward the central nervous system. These neurons are initiate nerve impulses following receptor stimulation.

Afterload: The arrangement of a muscle so that it lifts a weight from an adjustable support or works against a constant opposing force to which it is not exposed when at rest.

Agonist: A substance that can combine with a cell receptor to produce a reaction typical for that substance.

Agranulocytes: Nongranular leukocytes (monocytes or lymphocytes).

Air sacs: One of innumerable spherical outcroppings of the respiratory bronchioles in the mammalian lung, the primary sites of gas exchange with the blood.

Albumin: A common liver-produced protein found in many tissues, including plasma. It is soluble in water and a principle component in egg white.

Alimentary tract: The tubular portion of the digestive tract. *See also* gastrointestinal tract (GI tract).

Alkaline tide: A period of urinary neutrality or alkalinity after meals.

All *trans*-retinal: Retinol and derivatives of retinol that play an essential role in metabolic functioning of the retina, the growth of and differentiation of epithelial tissue, the growth of bone, reproduction, and the immune response. Dietary vitamin A is derived from a variety of carotenoids found in plants. It is enriched in the liver, egg yolks, and the fat component of dairy products.

Allantois: A sac connected to the embryo that makes respiration by the embryo possible. It also stores excretions.

Allometric growth: A growth rate of an organ or tissue that is faster than the rate of general body growth.

Allosteric protein: A protein (most often in reference to an enzyme) that changes conformation (and thereby functional capacity) when it binds to another molecule or when covalent changes alter its shape.

α-lactalbumin: A specific milk protein synthesized and secreted by the alveolar epithelial cells. The protein is also part of the lactose synthetase enzyme. It appears in the whey fraction of milk.

Alveolar ducts: Part of the respiratory passages beyond a respiratory bronchiole; from it arise alveolar sacs and alveoli.

Alveolar macrophages: The cells within the lungs that phagocytose microbes and particulate matter, e.g., inhaled dust. They are mainly sited within the alveoli where they arrive via the capillaries after production within bone marrow from monocytes.

Alveolar sac: An air-filled chamber that supplies air to several alveoli; also, terminology used to describe the glandular structures in the mature mammary gland.

Alveolar ventilation rate: An index of respiratory efficiency; it measures volume of air wasted and flow of fresh gases in and out of alveoli.

Alveoli: Blind pockets at the end of the respiratory tree, lined by a simple squamous epithelium and surrounded by a capillary network; sites of gas exchange with the blood; a bony socket that holds the root of a tooth.

Alveoli (mammary): Multicellular, spherical, hollow units of the mammary gland that are responsible for synthesis and secretion of milk. Milk is secreted into and stored in the internal lumenal space of the alveoli between milking or suckling episodes.

Amacrine cells: Interneurons in the retina that operate at the Inner Plexiform Layer, the second synaptic retinal layer where bipolar cells and ganglion cells synapse.

Aminopeptidase: An enzyme that is used as a biomarker to detect damage to the kidneys, and that may be used to help diagnose certain kidney disorders.

Amnion: The innermost of the fetal membranes, it forms the fluid-filled sac that surrounds and protects the developing fetus. The amnion and amniotic fluid protect the developing embryo from shock and permit movement.

Amoeboid action: The flowing movement of the cytoplasm of a phagocyte.

AMPA (α-amino-3-hydroxy 5-methylisoaxzole-4-propionic acid) receptors: A non–NMDA-type ionotropic transmembrane receptor for glutamate that mediates fast synaptic transmission in the central nervous system (CNS). Its name is derived from its ability to be activated by the artificial glutamate analog, AMPA. AMPARs are found in many parts of the brain and are the most commonly found receptor in the nervous system.

Amygdaloid body: Almond-shaped groups of neurons located deep in the medial temporal lobes of the brain in complex vertebrates. Shown in research to perform a primary role in the processing and memory of emotional reactions, the amygdalae are considered part of the limbic system.

Anaerobic glycolyis: The anaerobic metabolic breakdown of a nutrient molecule, such as glucose, without net oxidation. Fermentation does not directly produce energy in cells; it merely allows glycolysis (a process that yields two ATP per glucose) to continue.

Anal canal: The distal portion of the rectum that contains the anal columns and ends at the anus.

Anaphase: A stage of mitosis during which the chromosomes separate and move away from each other.

Anastomosis: The joining of two tubes, usually referring to a connection between two peripheral vessels without an intervening capillary bed.

Anatomical dead space: The volume of the conducting airways from the external environment down to the terminal bronchioles.

Anatomical position: An anatomical reference position; the body viewed from the anterior surface with the palms facing forward. For domestic species, this would be four legs on the ground and head facing forward.

Anatomy: The study of the structure of the body.

Anencephaly: Congenital absence of most of the brain and spinal cord.

Anestrus: Term that can refer to the absence of estrus without ovulation, the period of sexual quiescence between two estrous cycles, or prolonged failure of estrus in mature animals.

Anisotropic: Having physical properties that differ according to the direction of measurement.

Annular cartilage: The lowermost of the laryngeal cartilages, it may be palpated just below the thyroid prominence adjacent the cricoid cartilage and the first tracheal ring is the cricothyroid membrane, a site used for rapid emergency airway access (cricothyroidotomy).

Antagonist: Something, such as a muscle, disease, or physiological process that neutralizes or impedes the action or effect of another.

Anterior: On or near the front, or ventral surface, of the body.

Anterior chamber: The fluid-filled space inside the eye between the iris and the cornea's innermost surface, the endothelium.

Anterior horn: The front section of the lateral ventricle of the brain, extending forward from Monro's foramen; also called the ventral horn.

Anterior median fissure: The longitudinal groove in the midline of the anterior aspect of the medulla oblongata, continuous with the anterior median fissure of the spinal cord and ending at the foramen cecum medullae oblongatae.

Anterior neuropore: The anterior opening leading from the central canal of the embryonic neural tube to the exterior.

Anterior segment: The front third of the eye that includes the structures in front of the vitreous humour: the cornea, iris, ciliary body, and lens.

Anterior vagal trunks: A nerve trunk (or trunks) formed by fibers from both left and right vagus nerves.

Antibody: Proteins produced by B lymphocytes (plasma cells) that are produced in response to exposure to a specific antigen. Antibodies are members of the immunoglobulin family of proteins.

Anticodon: The sequence of three nucleotides in the transfer RNA that is complementary to the three nucleotide sequence of the messenger RNA. The anticodon corresponds to a specific amino acid also attached to the tRNA during active protein synthesis.

Antidiuretic hormone (ADH): A hormone produced in the hypothalamus but stored and released from the posterior lobe of the pituitary. Its secretion promotes reabsorption of water by the distal convoluted tubules and collecting ducts of the kidney nephrons.

Antigen: Usually a foreign substance that, when it enters the body, elicits an immune response (antibody production or cell-mediated response).

Antiport: A form of membrane carrier protein that transports two different ions or molecules across a membrane in opposite directions. The transfer can occur with both ions simultaneously or sequentially .

Antithrombin: Any substance that inhibits or prevents the effects of thrombin so that blood does not coagulate.

Anus: The external opening of the anal canal.

Aorta: The large, elastic artery that carries blood away from the left ventricle and into the systemic circuit.

Aortic arch: The curve between the ascending and descending portions of the aorta.

Aortic body: A receptor in the aortic arch sensitive to changing oxygen, carbon dioxide, and pH levels of the blood.

Aortic valve: A one-way valve that permits the flow of blood from the left ventricle into the aorta during ventricular emptying but prevents the backflow of blood from the aorta into the left ventricle during ventricular relaxation.

Apex: Extremity of a conical or pyramidal structure. The apex of the heart is the rounded tip directed anteriorly and slightly inferiorly.

Apical: The tip of a cell or a structure. For example, in activity secreting epithelial cells, products are packaged and ultimately released from the cell at the apical end of the cell.

Apneustic area: A respiratory center whose chronic activation would lead to apnea at full inhalation.

Aponeurosis: A sheetlike fibrous membrane resembling a flattened tendon that serves as a fascia to bind muscles together or to connect muscle to bone.

Aponeurotic attachments: Fibrous or membranous sheets connecting a muscle and the part it moves.

Apoptosis: One of the main types of programmed cell death (PCD). As such, it is a process of deliberate life relinquishment by a cell in a multicellular organism.

Apositional growth: The enlargement of a bone by the addition of cartilage or bony matrix at its surface.

Appendicular: Pertaining to the upper or lower limbs.

Aqueous humor: The clear, watery fluid in the eye that fills the space between the back surface of the cornea and the front surface of the vitreous humour.

Arachnoid granulations: Any of numerous villuslike projections of the cranial arachnoid through the dura into the superior sagittal sinus or into its lateral venous lacunae; also called the arachnoid villus or pacchionian body.

Arachnoid mater: One of the three meninges, the membranes that cover the brain and spinal cord. It is interposed between the two other meninges, the more superficial dura mater and the deeper pia mater, and is separated from the pia mater by the subarachnoid space.

Arbor vitae: White matter of the cerebellum.

Arytenoid cartilages: A pair of small cartilages in the larynx.

Ascending aorta: Part of the aorta from which the coronary arteries arise.

Ascending segment: A part of the large intestine.

Ascites: The overproduction and accumulation of peritoneal fluid.

Aspartate: A salt or ester of aspartic acid.

Association area: An area of the cerebral cortex where motor and sensory functions are integrated.

Astigmatism: A refractive error of the eye in which there is a difference in degree of refraction in different meridians. It is typically characterized by an aspherical, nonfigure of revolution cornea in which the corneal profile slope and refractive power in one meridian are greater than that of the perpendicular axis.

ATP: *See* adenosine triphosphate (ATP).

ATP synthase: Enzyme complex located in the inner membrane of the mitochondria that catalyzes the formation of ATP from ADP and inorganic phosphate as a consequence of oxidative phosphorylation.

ATPase: General name for a large class of enzymes that catalyze reactions that hydrolyze ATP, thereby liberating energy for biochemical processes.

Atria: Thin walled chambers of the heart that receive venous blood from the pulmonary or systemic circuit atrial natriuretic peptide.

Atrioventricular (AV) node: Specialized cardiocytes that relay the contractile stimulus to the bundle of His, the bundle branches, the Purkinje fibers, and the ventricular myocardium; located at the boundary between the atria and ventricles.

Auditory ossicles: The three smallest bones in the body. They are positioned within the middle ear space and serve to transmit sounds from the air to the fluid-filled labyrinth (cochlea). The absence of the auditory ossicles would cause a moderate to severe hearing loss.

Auditory tube: A passageway that connects the nasopharynx with the middle ear cavity; also called the eustachian tube or pharyngotympanic tube.

Auricle: A broad, flattened process that resembles the external ear; in the ear, the expanded, projecting portion that surrounds the external auditory canal; also called the pinna. In the heart it is the externally visible flap formed by the collapse of the outer wall of a relaxed atrium.

Auscultation: The technical term for listening to the internal sounds of the body, usually using a stethoscope.

Autocrine: Mechanism whereby ligands (growth factors, hormones) produced by a particular cell act to modify the action of that cell.

Autonomic nervous system: Efferent division of the peripheral nervous system that innervates cardiac and smooth muscles and glands; also called the involuntary or visceral motor system.

Autoregulation: Changes in activity that maintain homeostasis in direct response to changes in the local environment; does not require neural or endocrine control.

Autorhythmic: Spontaneous and periodic; for example, in smooth muscle it implies spontaneous (without nervous or hormonal stimulation) and periodic contractions.

Autorhythmic fibers: Self-excitable and repeatedly generated action potentials that trigger heart contractions. They continue to stimulate a heart to beat even after it is removed from the body!

Axial skeleton: The bones constituting the head and trunk of a vertebrate body.

Axon: The elongate extension of a neuron that conducts an action potential.

Axon hillock: In a multipolar neuron, the portion of the cell body adjacent to the initial segment.

Axon terminals: The branched endings of a neuronal axon, which release a neurotransmitter that influences target cells in close association with the axon terminals.

B

Baroreceptor reflex: A reflexive change in cardiac activity in response to changes in blood pressure.

Baroreceptors: The receptors responsible for baroreception.

Basal cells: The innermost layer of the epidermis; also called the Stratum Germinativum or Stratum Basale. Cells produced here in the germinal layer form the prickle cells in the above layer (the Stratum Spinosum).

Basal lamina: The thin layer of extracellular matrix that creates a boundary between the epithelial cells and the surrounding stromal tissue and between other cell types; also called the basement membrane.

Basophils: Circulating granulocytes (white blood cells) similar in size and function to tissue mast cells.

Bicarbonate ions: HCO_3^-; anion components of the carbonic acid-bicarbonate buffer system.

Bicuspid valve: The left atrioventricular (AV) valve; also called the mitral valve.

Bile duct: Any of a number of long tubelike structures that carry bile.

Bilirubin: A pigment that is the by-product of hemoglobin catabolism.

Biliverdin: Green bile pigment formed from the oxidation of bilirubin.

Biogenic amines: Class of neurotransmitters, including catecholamines and indolamines.

Biopsy: To remove a small piece of tissue or cells (biopsy of embryo) from a living animal for analysis or study.

Bipolar cell: As a part of the retina, the bipolar cell exists between photoreceptors (rod cells and cone cells) and ganglion cells.

Bipolar neuron: Neuron with an axon and a dendrite extending from opposite sides of the cell body.

Blastocoele: The cavity in the center of the blastocyst.

Blastocyst: An early embryo composed of an inner cell mass, the blastocoele, and trophoblast.

Blastomere: A cell created by the cleavage divisions of the early embryo.

Blind spot: The specific region of the retina where the optic nerve and blood vessels pass through to connect to the back of the eye.

Blood-brain barrier: The isolation of the central nervous system from the general circulation;

primarily the result of astrocyte regulation of capillary permeability.

Blood pressure: A force exerted against vessel walls by the blood in the vessels, due to the push exerted by cardiac contraction and the elasticity of the vessel walls; usually measured along one of the muscular arteries, with systolic pressure measured during ventricular systole and diastolic pressure during ventricular diastole.

Bohr effect: The increased oxygen release by hemoglobin in the presence of elevated carbon dioxide levels.

Bolus: Any kind of ball-shaped organic structure of an organism or of its discharged substances.

Bone remodeling: The continuous turnover of bone matrix and mineral that involves first, an increase in resorption (osteoclastic activity), and later, reactive bone formation (osteoblastic activity).

Bony collar: A bone collar that forms concurrently with the primary ossification center. Cells of the perichondrium begin to form bone. The bone collar holds together the shaft, which has been weakened by the disintegration of the cartilage. The connective tissue about the bone collar, previously a perichondrium, is now called periosteum.

Boyle's law: The principle that, in a gas, pressure and volume are inversely related.

Brachiocephalic: Relating to the arm and the head.

Brachiocephalic trunk: An artery that arises from the arch of the aorta and divides into the right subclavian and right carotid arteries.

Brain stem: The portion of the brain—consisting of the medulla oblongata, pons Varolii, and midbrain—that connects the spinal cord to the forebrain and cerebrum.

Bronchi: A branch of the bronchial tree between the trachea and bronchioles.

Bronchial tree: The trachea, bronchi, and bronchioles.

Bronchioles: The branching air passageways inside the lungs.

Brush-border: The epithelial surface consisting of microvilli.

bST or bovine somatotropin: A protein hormone, also called the growth hormone (GH), that is produced in the anterior pituitary gland. A common terminology is to use a lowercase letter to indicate the species of origin (e.g., pST for porcine somatotropin) and a lowercase *r* to indicate that the protein is derived by recombinant DNA technology. For example, rbST stands for recombinant bovine somatotropin or growth hormone.

Buccal: Pertaining to the cheeks.

Bulk flow: The movement of large particles and macromolecules across a plasma membrane.

C

Calcification: Impregnation with calcium or calcium salts; also called calcareous infiltration.

Calcitonin: A 32–amino acid polypeptide hormone that is produced primarily by the C cells of the thyroid and, in many other animals, in the ultimobranchial body.

Calmodulin: A ubiquitous, eukaryotic calcium-binding protein that regulates cellular processes by modifying the activity of specific calcium-sensitive enzymes.

Calsequestrin: The principal calcium-binding protein present in the sarcoplasmic reticulum of cardiac and skeletal muscle.

Calvaria: The skullcap, consisting of the superior portions of the frontal, parietal, and occipital bones.

Canaliculi: Microscopic passageways between cells; bile canaliculi carry bile to bile ducts in the liver; in bone, canaliculi permit the diffusion of nutrients and wastes to and from osteocytes.

Cancellous bone: Structure composed of a network of bony struts or spikes; also called spongy bone.

Canine: Referring to the cuspid tooth.

Capacitance vessels: The capacitance of a vessel is a measure of how easily it stretches.

Capacitation: Activation of spermatozoa that occurs after deposition into the female reproductive tract. It involves release of enzymes from the acrosome of the sperm cells and is necessary for fertilization.

Capillary: A small blood vessel, located between an arteriole and a venule, whose thin wall permits the diffusion of gases, nutrients, and wastes between plasma and interstitial fluids.

Capillary bed: The network of capillaries supplying an organ.

Capillary exchange: A dynamic process that has the role of supplying extravascular cells with the substances essential for survival.

Capillary hydrostatic pressure (HP$_c$): In capillaries, hydrostatic pressure is exerted by blood. Thus, capillary hydrostatic pressure (HP$_c$) is equivalent to the blood pressure in the capillaries.

Carbamino compounds: The combination of CO_2 with terminal amine groups in blood protein of which the most important is the globin of hemoglobin.

Carbaminohemoglobin: Hemoglobin bound to carbon dioxide molecules.

Carbohydrate: Organic compound composed of carbon, hydrogen, and oxygen in a 1 : 2 : 1 ration. Examples include glucose, lactose, starch, and cellulose. Many are critical for ATP production in cells.

Carboxyl group: A carbon atom linked to an oxygen atom by a double bond and to a hydroxyl group.

This combination is common in fatty acids and amino acids.

Carboxyl terminal (C terminal): The end of a protein chain that has a free carbonyl group.

Carcinoma: Refers to a cancer of the epithelial cells or the epithelium. It is the most common type of cancer.

Cardia: The area of the stomach surrounding its connection with the esophagus.

Cardiac accelerator nerves: Sympathetic nerves responsible for increasing cardiac rate.

Cardiac center: Part of the medulla oblongata responsible for controlling the heart rate.

Cardiac cycle: One complete heartbeat, including atrial and ventricular systole and diastole.

Cardiac muscle: The muscle of the heart, consisting of anastomosing transversely striated muscle fibers formed of cells united at intercalated discs; also called the myocardium or, simply, heart muscle.

Cardiac notch: The lateral deflection of the anterior border of the left lung. It is produced to accommodate the space taken up by the heart.

Cardiac output: The amount of blood ejected by the left ventricle each minute; normally about 5 l.

Cardiac reserve: The potential percentage increase in cardiac output above resting levels.

Cardiocytes or cardiac myocytes: A type of involuntary mononucleated striated muscle found exclusively within the heart. Its function is to "pump" blood through the circulatory system by contracting.

Cardiogenic shock: Essentially the failure to pump, it is a condition wherein the heart is so inefficient that it cannot sustain adequate circulation.

Cardiovascular center: Poorly localized centers in the reticular formation of the medulla oblongata of the brain. It includes cardioacceleratory, cardioinhibitory, and vasomotor centers.

Carotid bodies: A small cluster of chemoreceptors and supporting cells located near the bifurcation of the carotid artery. It measures changes in blood pressure and the composition of arterial blood flowing past it, including the partial pressures of oxygen and carbon dioxide, and is also sensitive to changes in pH and temperature.

Carotid sinus: A dilated segment at the base of the internal carotid artery whose walls contain baroreceptors sensitive to changes in blood pressure.

Caruncle: In ungulates, this is the buttonlike area of the uterine endometrium that creates the maternal side of the cotyledonary placenta.

Caseins: Proteins that constitute the largest group of specific proteins found in milk. They are empirically defined by their precipitation from milk at pH 4.6 and their capacity to produce micelles containing calcium. Major subtypes include α, β, and γ caseins.

Catecholamines: Epinephrine, norepinephrine, dopamine, and related compounds.

Caudate nucleus: An elongated, curved mass of gray matter consisting of three portions: an anterior, thick portion that projects into the anterior horn of the lateral ventricle; a portion extending along the floor of the body of the lateral ventricle; and an elongated, thin portion that curves downward and backward in the temporal lobes to the wall of the lateral ventricle; also called the caudatum.

Caudodorsal blind sac: A region of the rumen.

Caveoli: A small vesicle or recess, especially one communicating with the outside of a cell and extending inward, indenting the cytoplasm and the cell membrane.

Cecum: An expanded pouch at the start of the large intestine.

Cell body: The body of a neuron; also called the soma.

Cellular immunity: That part of the immune system that depends on the actions of specialized cells to provide protection. Protection is most closely associated with activation of a class of lymphocytes, the T cells.

Cellular physiology: The study of how cells work.

Cementum: Bony material that covers the root of a tooth and is not shielded by a layer of enamel.

Central chemoreceptors: Receptors located in the medulla near the respiratory center that respond to changes in extracellular fluid H^+ concentration resulting from changes in arterial P_{CO_2} and adjust respiration accordingly.

Central nervous system: Brain and spinal cord.

Centriole: A small organelle located near the nucleus of the cell. It is involved in synthesis of microtubules and in cell division.

Cephalic: Pertaining to the head.

Cephalization: An evolutionary trend in the animal kingdom toward centralization of neural and sensory organs in the head or anterior region of the body.

Cerebral aquaduct: The slender cavity of the midbrain that connects the third and fourth ventricles; also called the aqueduct of Sylvius.

Cerebral peduncles: The massive bundle of corticofugal nerve fibers passing longitudinally over the ventral surface of the midbrain on each side of the midline.

Cerebroventricles: Fluid-filled spaces in the brain.

Cerebrum: The largest portion of the brain, including practically all the parts within the skull except the medulla, pons, and cerebellum, and now usually referring only to the parts derived from the telencephalon and including mainly the cerebral hemispheres that are joined at the bottom by the corpus callosum. It controls and integrates motor, sensory, and higher mental functions, such as thought, reason, emotion, and memory.

Cervical thoracic air sacs: A pair of air sacs located on each side in the neck region of birds; one sac usually extends from each lung, but sometimes a series of cervical sacs are located along the neck, as in geese.

Cervix: The proximal portion of the uterus, it forms the boundary between the vagina and uterus.

Chaperone: An intracellular protein that allows other proteins to avoid alterations in folding or conformation so that the supported protein maintains its function.

Chemical synapses: Specialized junctions through which cells of the nervous system signal to one another and to nonneuronal cells such as muscles or glands.

Chemically gated channels: Channels in the plasma membrane that open or close in response to the binding of a specific chemical messenger with a membrane receptor site that is in close association with the channel.

Chemoreceptor: A cell or group of cells that transduce a chemical signal into an action potential.

Chemoreceptor reflex: Chemoreceptors that detect decrease in blood oxygen, increase in carbon dioxide, or decrease in pH and produce an increased rate and depth of respiration, and, by means of the vasomotor center, vasoconstriction.

Chemotaxis: The attraction of phagocytic cells to the source of abnormal chemicals in tissue fluids.

Chloride shift: The movement of plasma chloride ions into red blood cells in exchange for bicarbonate ions generated by the intracellular dissociation of carbonic acid.

Choanae: Openings from the nasal cavity into the nasopharynx. They are also known as internal nares.

Cholecystokinin (CCK): A duodenal hormone that stimulates the contraction of the gallbladder and the secretion of enzymes by the exocrine pancreas; also called pancreozymin.

Cholesterol: A common lipid with a characteristic four-ring structure; it is important for membrane fluidity and as the precursor for a myriad of steroids.

Cholinergic neurons: Nerve endings that, upon stimulation, release acetylcholine.

Chondroblasts: Cells of growing cartilage tissue responsible for increasing tissue mass.

Chondrocyte: The primary cell type found in developed cartilage.

Chondroitin sulfate: A major proteoglycan found in cartilage.

Chordae tendineae: Fibrous cords that stabilize the position of the AV valves in the heart, preventing backflow during ventricular systole.

Chordamesoderm: The middle germ layer that develops into muscle, bone, cartilage, blood, and connective tissue.

Chorion: The outer extraembyronic membrane that is derived from the trophoblastic ectoderm. It develops villi that make the fetal sites of placental attachment.

Choroid plexus: A vascular proliferation of the cerebral ventricles that serves to regulate intraventricular pressure by secretion or absorption of cerebrospinal fluid.

Choroids: The vascular layer of the eye lying between the retina and the sclera. The choroid provides oxygen and nourishment to the outer layers of the retina.

Chylomicrons: Relatively large droplets that may contain triglycerides, phospholipids, and cholesterol in association with proteins. They are synthesized and released by intestinal cells and transported to the venous blood by the lymphatic system.

Chyme: A semifluid, acidic mixture of ingested food and digestive secretions that forms in the stomach during the early phases of digestion.

Cilia: Extensions of the plasma membrane containing doublets of parallel microtubules. They are approximately 5 to 10 micrometers in length. There are two types of cilia: 1) motile cilium, which constantly beats in one direction, and 2) nonmotile cilium, which cannot beat and usually serves as a sensor.

Ciliary body: The part of the eye containing the ciliary muscle and ciliary processes.

Ciliary muscles: A smooth muscle that affects zonules in the eye (fibers that suspend the lens in position during accommodation), enabling changes in lens shape for light focusing.

Ciliary processes: Processes formed by the inward folding of the various layers of the choroid, i.e., the choroid proper and the lamina basalis, and are received between corresponding folds of the suspensory ligament of the lens.

Cingulate: A gyrus in the medial part of the brain. It partially wraps around the corpus callosum and is limited above by the cingulate sulcus.

Circulatory shock: When mean arterial blood pressure falls so low that adequate blood flow to the tissues can no longer be maintained.

Circumduction: The circular movement of a limb such that the distal end of the limb delineates an arc.

Circumvallate papilla: one of the large, dome-shaped papillae on the superior surface of the tongue that form a V, separating the body of the tongue from the root.

Circumventricular organs: Sites in the neuroendocrine system that allow factors to "circumvent" the

Brain Blood Barrier. These organs secrete or are sites of action of different hormones, neurotransmitters, and cytokines.

Citric acid cycle: This fundamental biochemical pathway (also called the TCA, tricarboxylic acid cycle, or Krebs cycle) is central to aerobic respiration. Acetyl groups derived from nutrient sources are area oxidized to CO_2 and H_2O. In the process, the coenzymes NAD and FAD become oxidized and are ultimately utilized in the electron transport chain of the mitochondria to produce ATP.

Clavicular air sac: A single, median air sac between the clavicles and surrounding the bifurcation of the trachea of birds.

Cloaca: The common opening in birds through which the intestinal, urinary, and reproductive tracts empty.

Clostridium botulinum: A bacterium that occurs widely in nature and is a cause of botulism; its six main types, A to F, are characterized by distinct but pharmacologically similar, very potent neurotoxins.

Clot: A network of fibrin fibers and trapped blood cells; also called a thrombus if it occurs within the circulatory system.

Clot retraction: Condensation of the clot into a denser, compact structure; caused by the elastic nature of fibrin.

Cochlea: A coiled, tapered tube containing the auditory branch of the mammalian inner ear. Its core component is the Organ of Corti, the sensory organ of hearing.

Cochlear duct: An endolymph-filled cavity inside the cochlea, located between the scala tympani and the scala vestibuli, separated by the basilar membrane and Reissner's membrane (the vestibular membrane), respectively.

Codon: Sequence of three bases in a DNA or strand of mRNA that corresponds with the instructions for incorporating a specific amino acid into a growing protein chain.

Coenzymes: Organic molecules that serve as cofactors required for the action of certain enzymes. Most coenzymes are derived from vitamins.

Cofactor: A companion molecule necessary for function of many enzymes. Most often this is either a metal ion or organic molecule.

Collagen: The most abundant class of proteins in the body, collagens are predominating in the extracellular matrix surrounding cells and in connective tissues.

Collaterals: A branch of a nerve axon or blood vessel.

Colloid osmotic pressure (OP$_c$): Pressure created in a fluid.

Colon: The large intestine.

Colostrum: Mammary gland secretion that accumulates prior to the onset of normal milk production. It is rich in antibodies.

Common hepatic duct: The duct formed by the junction of the right hepatic duct (which drains bile from the right functional lobe of the liver) and the left hepatic duct (which drains bile from the left functional lobe of the liver).

Compact bone: Dense bone that contains parallel osteons.

Complementarity of structure and function: An essential concept to understanding of how an animal works and its limitations. In short, the principle that function and structure are interdependent.

Complete fracture: Break involving the entire width of the bone.

Complete tetanus: An acute, often fatal disease that is characterized by spasmodic contraction of voluntary muscles, especially one occurring in the neck and jaw, and that is caused by the bacterium *Clostridium tetani*, which usually enters the body through an infected wound and produces a neurotoxin; also called lockjaw.

Compound fracture: A fracture in which broken bone fragments lacerate soft tissue and protrude through an open wound in the skin.

Concentration gradient: The difference in concentration of a material between tissue regions or locations within cells. For example, the concentration of sodium is typically higher in the extracellular fluid than the cytoplasm. Movement of molecules down their concentration gradients is often utilized to "drive" various transport functions.

Concentric: Having a common center or center point, as of circles.

Concentric lamellae: One of the tubular layers of bone surrounding the central canal in an osteon; also called Haversian lamellae.

Conchae: Three pairs of thin, scroll-like bones that project into the nasal cavities; the superior and medial conchae are part of the ethmoid, and the inferior conchae are separate bones.

Cones: Cells in the retina of the eye that function only in relatively bright light. They gradually become less concentrated toward the periphery of the retina.

Conjunctiva: A membrane that covers the sclera (white part of the eye) and lines the inside of the eyelids. It helps lubricate the eye by producing mucus and tears, although a smaller volume of tears than the lacrimal gland.

Connexon: Hollow cylinders made of transmembrane proteins that connect adjacent cells at gap junctions, allowing chemical substances to pass through.

Continuous capillary: A capillary in which pores are absent; it is less permeable to large molecules than other types of capillaries.

Contractility: The ability to contract; possessed by skeletal, smooth, and cardiac muscle cells.

Control center: One of three interdependent components of homeostatic control mechanisms; it determines the set point.

Conus medullaris: The terminal end of the spinal cord. It occurs near lumbar nerves 1 (L1) and 2 (L2). After the spinal cord terminates, the spinal nerves continue as dangling nerves called the cauda equina.

Convergence: The converging of many presynaptic terminals from thousands of other neurons on a single neuronal cell body and its dendrites so that activity in the single neuron is influenced by the activity in many other neurons.

Convergent: The coordinated turning of the eyes inward to focus on an object at close range.

Coracoid process: A long curved projection from the neck of the scapula, overhanging the glenoid cavity and giving attachment to the short head of the biceps, the coracobrachial muscle, the smaller pectoral muscle, and the coracoacromial ligament.

Cori cycle: A metabolic pathway that allows lactic acid produced by muscle action to be to be converted to glucose by the liver. This action typically occurs during muscle rest.

Cornea: The transparent front part of the eye that covers the iris, pupil, and anterior chamber, providing most of an eye's optical power.

Corpora quadrigemina: The four colliculi—two inferior, two superior—located on the posterior aspect of the midbrain.

Corpus callosum: The commissural plate of nerve fibers connecting the two cerebral hemispheres except for most of the temporal lobes; also called the commissure of cerebral hemispheres.

Corpus luteum (CL): Yellow-to-orange structures formed on the surface of the ovary after ovulation from granulosal and thecal cells from the ruptured follicle. The CL produces progesterone and oxytocin.

Corpus striatum: Either of two gray and white, striated bodies of nerve fibers located in the lower lateral wall of each cerebral hemisphere.

Corticoids: General name for the class of steroid hormones secreted by the adrenal gland.

Costal cartilages: The cartilage forming the anterior continuation of a rib.

Cotransport: A membrane carrier system in which the transfer of one molecule depends on the simultaneous transfer of another molecule.

Cotyledons: In ruminants, the points of attachment between the fetal and maternal placenta. It is composed of the maternal cotyledon (the caruncle of the uterus + the fetal cotyledon from the chorion of the conceptus).

Covalent bond: A common chemical bond in which electrons are shared between atoms.

Cranial: Pertaining to the head.

Cranial base: The structure that forms the inferior aspect of the cranium and is divided by bony ridges into three distinct fossae.

Cranial nerves: Nerves that emerge from the brain stem instead of the spinal cord.

Cranial vault: Eight skull bones that surround and protect the brain; braincase.

Cranium: The braincase; the skull bones that surround and protect the brain.

Creatine kinase: The enzyme that catalyzes the transfer of phosphate from phosphocreatine to ADP, forming creatine and ATP; important in muscle contraction.

Creatine phosphate: An organic compound found in muscle tissue and capable of storing and providing energy for muscular contraction; also called phosphocreatine.

Cricoid cartilage: A ring-shaped cartilage that forms the inferior margin of the larynx.

Crop: A thin-walled expanded portion of the alimentary tract that is found in many animals and is used for the storage of food prior to digestion.

Crossed-extensor reflex: A withdrawal reflex. When the reflex occurs, the flexors in the withdrawing limb contract and the extensors relax, while in the other limb the opposite occurs.

Crossmatching: Matching blood types.

Cryptorchidism: Failure of the testicles to descend into the scrotum during fetal development. The undescended testis remains in the abdominal cavity.

Crystallins: A water-soluble structural protein found in the lens of the eye accounting for the transparency of the structure. Crystallins from a vertebrate eye lens are classified into three types: alpha, beta, and gamma.

Curare: A purified preparation or alkaloid obtained from the Chondrodendron tomentosum, it is used to relax skeletal muscles.

Cyclic AMP: An important intracellular signaling molecule, it is formed by the action of the enzyme adenylate cyclase on ATP. Its appearance is typically induced by binding of a particular hormone to its surface receptor.

Cyclicity: The condition during which the female displays estrus cycles with predictable duration.

Cystic duct: A duct that carries bile between the gallbladder and the common bile duct.

Cytokines: Small growth factor–like proteins that serve to regulate the activity of the various immune system cells.

Cytokinesis: The dividing of cytoplasm between two cells at the time of mitosis.

Cytology: The study of the structure, organelles, and function of cells.

Cytoplasm: The portion of the cell interior not occupied by the nucleus.

Cytosine: A pyrimidine which is one of the two classes of nitrogenous bases found in nucleic acids such as DNA and RNA.

Cytoskeleton: The network of microtubules and microfilaments found in the cytoplasm of the cell.

Cytosol: The fluid portion of a cytoplasm, it is effectively prepared by breaking the cells apart and saving the supernatant from a $100,000 \times g$ centrifugation minus any lipid.

Cytoxic T cell: An activated lymphocyte, part of cellular immunity, also called a killer T cell, it acts to destroy cells that have been infected by viruses by releasing enzymes.

D

Dale's Principle: A principle postulated by the English neuroscientist Henry Hallett Dale, which states that, although different neurotransmitters can be produced at different synapses within the brain, individual neurons are capable of releasing only one neurotransmitter from its axonal terminal. Dale's Principle has been shown to be false because many nerve terminals release neuropeptides as well as amino acids or amines.

Dalton's Law: Named for the English chemist John Dalton (1766–1844). In a mixture of gases, the portion of the total pressure resulting from each type of gas is determined by the percentage of the total volume represented by each gas type.

Dark adaptation: The ability of the eye to adjust to various levels of darkness and light.

Dark cells: Cells that line the endolymphatic space of the ear.

De novo: Refers to a synthesis process occurring within a tissue or cell.

Deamination: The removal of an amine group from a molecule often in relation to the metabolism of the amino acids from proteins.

Deciduous: An adjective meaning "temporary" or "tending to fall off" (derived from the Latin word *decidere*, to fall off).

Decomposition reaction: Description of a chemical reaction that results in the breaking down of a larger molecule into its component parts, i.e., a protein into amino acids or starch into glucose monomers.

Defensins: Locally produced tissue proteins that can protect cells from infection by bacteria.

Deglutition: Swallowing.

Dehydration synthesis: A chemical reaction wherein a larger molecule is created by covalently bonding smaller molecules together. In the process water is often produced.

Deltoid tuberosity: A bump or raised area on the outside of the humerus where the deltoid muscle attaches.

Denaturation: Dramatic change in the tertiary structure of a protein or other macromolecule that leaves it nonfunctional. This can be caused by heating (egg albumin after frying or poaching) or exposure to chemicals.

Dendrite: A branching process of a neuron that receives stimuli and conducts potentials toward the nerve cell body.

Dentate gyrus: One of the two interlocking gyri composing the hippocampus.

Dentin: The bonelike material that forms the body of a tooth; it differs from bone in that it lacks osteocytes and osteons.

Deoxygenated blood: Blood whose red blood cells carry very little oxygen, as found in all veins except the pulmonary vein; also called oxygen-poor blood.

Deoxyhemoglobin: Hemoglobin without oxygen bound to it.

Depolarization: A reduction in membrane potential from resting potential; movement of the potential from resting toward 0 mV.

Depression: An inward displacement of a body part.

Dermis: A deep layer of the skin, it is primarily composed of dense irregular connective tissue. A hypodermic injection, for example, would be placement of the material just under the skin into the adjacent tissue.

Descending segment: The portion of the large intestine that leads to the rectum.

Desmin: A component of the cytoskeleton—important structural components of living cells. Their size is intermediate between that of microfilaments and microtubules.

Desmosomes: A structure that forms the site of adhesion between two cells, consisting of a dense plate in each adjacent cell separated by a thin layer of extracellular material; also called the macula adherens.

Diabetes insipidus: A disease characterized by the production of large amounts of dilute urine and intense thirst. It is named because the symptoms are similar to those common in diabetes mellitus, but the cause is insufficient production of antidiuretic hormone (ADH) rather than insulin insufficiency or failure of insulin action.

Diabetes mellitus: A disease caused by either failure of the endocrine pancreas to produce sufficient amounts of insulin or failure of insulin function.

Diacylglycerol: A lipid produced in the plasma membrane after the cleavage of inositol phospholipids. This usually occurs following hormone signaling. It is two fatty acid chains linked to glycerol.

Diapedesis: The movement of white blood cells through the walls of blood vessels by migration between adjacent endothelial cells.

Diaphysis: The shaft of a long bone.

Diastole: Period of the cardiac cycle when either the ventricles or the atria are relaxing.

Diastolic blood pressure: Pressure measured in the walls of a muscular artery when the left ventricle is in diastole.

Diencephalon: The posterior part of the prosencephalon, composed of the epithalamus, the dorsal thalamus, the subthalamus, and the hypothalamus.

Diestrus: The stage of the estrus cycle characterized by major secretion of progesterone from the corpus luteum and periods of minimal or no reproductive behavior.

Differential blood count: A common laboratory procedure often using a stained blood smear to tabulate the relative proportions of classes of white blood cells in a sample. Variations from normal proportions for a given species or stage of development is used diagnostically.

Diffuse placenta: The placental type characterized by the distribution of chorionic villi across the surface of the chorion (e.g., pigs, mares).

Diffusion: Passive molecular movement from an area of higher concentration to an area of lower concentration.

Digestion: The chemical breakdown of ingested materials into simple molecules that can be absorbed by the cells of the digestive tract.

Digestive tract: An internal passageway that begins at the mouth, ends at the anus, and is lined by a mucous membrane; also called the gastrointestinal tract.

Dipeptidase: An enzyme that catalyzes the hydrolysis of dipeptides into their constituent amino acids.

Diploë: The diploic veins are found in the skull and drain the diploic space. This is found in the bones of the vault of the skull, and is the marrow-containing area of cancellous bone between the inner and outer layers of compact bone. The diploic veins drain this area to the outside of the skull and are usually four in number: one frontal, two parietal, and one occipital.

Directly gated: Also called a transmitter or ligand-gated channel, in which the ligand receptor and ion channel are one and the same.

Disaccharide: A sugar molecule composed of two simpler sugars, e.g., glucose + galactose, to yield milk sugar or lactose.

Displaced fractures: A break or fracture in which the two ends of the broken bone are separated from one another.

Distal: Away from the origin. For example, the wrist is distal from the elbow, or the distal convoluted tubules of the kidney nephrons are distant from the proximal (near the site of filtration) convoluted tubules.

Distributing arteries: Medium-sized artery with a tunica media composed principally of smooth muscle; regulates blood flow to different regions of the body.

Divergence: The diverging, or branching, of a neuron's axon terminals so that activity in this single neuron influences the many other cells with which its terminals synapse.

Diverticulum: A sac or pouch in the wall of the colon or other organ.

DNA (deoxyribonucleic acid): The critical polynucleotide created by covalent bonding of nucleotides, phosphate groups, and deoxyribose in repeating chains. It is the basis for transference of genetic information.

Dolichephalic: Having a disproportionately long head.

Dominant follicle: The final maturation stage of follicle development in cattle, i.e., the follicle likely destined to ovulate.

Dopamine: An important neurotransmitter in the central nervous system.

Dorsal: Toward the back, posterior.

Dorsal root: The afferent sensory root of a spinal nerve. At the distal end of the dorsal root is the dorsal root ganglion, which contains the neuron cell bodies of the nerve fibers conveyed by the root.

Dorsal root ganglion: A nodule on a dorsal root that contains cell bodies of neurons in afferent spinal nerves. All of the axons in the dorsal root convey somatosensory information, bringing sensory information into the brain and spinal cord.

Dorsal sac: Toward the back, posterior.

Down-regulation: A term frequently used to describe a reduced response to hormone stimulation over time. It often reflects a decrease in the number of available hormone receptors.

Downstroke or falling phase: The repolarization phase of an action potential in which the cell or neuron membrane potential moves toward a more negative value.

Duct: A tubular canal or passageway most often associated with secretion of products from a glandular organ.

Ductus arteriosus: A vascular connection between the pulmonary trunk and the aorta that functions throughout fetal life; it normally closes at birth or shortly thereafter and persists as the ligamentum arteriosum.

Duodenal gland: Small gland that opens into the base of intestinal glands. It secretes a mucuslike alkaline substance.

Duodenal papilla: A conical projection from the inner surface of the duodenum that contains the opening of the duodenal ampulla.

Duodenum: The proximal region of the small intestine that contains short villi and submucosal glands.

Dura mater: The tough fibrous membrane covering the brain and the spinal cord and lining the inner surface of the skull; also called the dura pachymeninx.

Dural sinuses: Venous channels found between layers of dura mater in the brain. They receive blood from internal and external veins of the brain and ultimately empty into the internal jugular vein. Damage to the walls of the dural sinuses may result in dural sinus thrombosis.

Dystocia: Difficult birth, a term often used in animal management–recording schemes to indicate that an animal required assistance with giving birth.

Dystophin: A structural protein found in small amounts in normal muscle but absent or present in abnormal amounts in individuals with muscular dystrophy.

E

Eccentric: Departing from a recognized, conventional, or established norm or pattern.

Eccrine glands: A common type of sweat gland that produces primarily a watery secretion containing dissolved salts.

Ectoderm: One of three germinal cell layers (ectoderm, mesoderm, and endoderm) in the developing embryo. The mammary gland, for example, is derived from the ectoderm.

Edema: Abnormal accumulation of fluid in body parts or tissues; causes swelling. It is common surrounding the udder of first-calf heifers.

Effector: A peripheral gland or muscle cell innervated by a motor neuron.

Effector organ: The muscles or glands that are innervated by the nervous system and that carry out the nervous system's orders to bring about a desired effect, such as a particular movement or secretion.

Efferent: Away from.

Efferent nerve: A nerve conveying impulses from the central nervous system to the periphery; also called a centrifugal nerve.

Elastic cartilage: A yellowish flexible cartilage in which the matrix is infiltrated by a network of elastic fibers; it occurs primarily in the external ear, eustachian tube, and some cartilages of the larynx and epiglottis; also called yellow cartilage.

Elastin: A relatively common extracellular matrix protein, which gives strength and flexibility to tissues. For example it allows the expansion and recovery of the aorta or the spring in the fibroelastic cartilage of the external ear.

Electrical synapses: A mechanical and electrically conductive link between two abutting neurons that is formed at a narrow gap between the pre- and postsynaptic cells known as a gap junction.

Electrocardiogram (ECG or EKG): A graphic record of the electrical activities of the heart, as monitored at specific locations on the body surface.

Electrochemical gradient: The simultaneous existence of an electrical gradient and concentration (chemical) gradient for a particular ion.

Electron acceptor: An atom or molecule that easily takes up an electron, thereby becoming reduced in the process.

Electron carrier: A molecule that transfers an electron from a donor molecule to an acceptor molecule, e. g., cytochrome c in the mitochondria in conversion of NADH to NAD.

Electron transport: The movement of electrons from a higher to lower energy via movement along a series of carrier molecules—for example, the oxidative phosphorylation process inside mitochondria.

Elevation: Movement in a superior, or upward, direction.

Embryology: The study of embryonic development, focusing on the first 2 months after fertilization.

Emesis: Vomiting.

Enamel: Crystalline material similar in mineral composition to bone, but harder and without osteocytes, which covers the exposed surfaces of the teeth.

End buds: The swollen terminal ends of mammary ducts in the gland of peripubertal rodents. These structures are responsible for the rapid growth and elongation of the ductular tree. Although alveolar budlike structures in the mammary glands of peripubertal ruminants serve as sites of focus for rapid growth of mammary ducts, ruminants apparently do not have morphologically similar end buds.

End diastolic volume (EDV): The volume of blood in the ventricle at the end of diastole, when filling is complete.

End systolic volume (ESV): The volume of blood in the ventricle at the end of systole, when emptying is complete.

Endocardium: The simple squamous epithelium that lines the heart and is continuous with the endothelium of the great vessels.

Endochondral ossification: The conversion of a cartilaginous model to bone; the characteristic mode of formation for skeletal elements other than the bones of the cranium, the clavicles, and sesamoid bones.

Endocrine: A control system of ductless glands that secrete chemical "instant messengers" called hormones, which circulate within the body via the bloodstream to affect distant cells within specific organs.

Endocrinology: Study of the endocrine system.

Endocytosis: The uptake of material into a cell by the invagination of the plasma membrane followed by internalization of membrane-surrounded vesicles.

Endolymph: The fluid contained in the membranous labyrinth of the inner ear. The main cation of this unique extracellular fluid is potassium.

Endoneurium: The innermost layer of connective tissue in a peripheral nerve, forming an interstitial layer around each individual fiber outside the neurolemma. In some circumstances; also called the epilemma, sheath of Henle, or sheath of Key and Retzius.

Endoplasmic Reticulum (ER): A cellular organelle composed of a network of membranous sacs or tubules whose intercompartment is continuous with the Golgi apparatus. The outer surface is frequently studded with ribosomes. In this situation newly made proteins are often vectored into the cisteral space of the ER to transport to the Golgi. Without ribosomes it is called smooth endoplasmic reticulum (SER); with ribosomes it is called rough endoplasmic reticulum or RER.

Endosteum: An incomplete cellular lining on the inner (medullary) surfaces of bones.

Endothelium: A single layer of simple squamous cells that line the walls of the heart, blood vessels, and lymphatic vessels.

End-product inhibition: A process whereby the accumulation of the last product in a biochemical pathway acts to inhibit further production of the product.

Enterendocrine cells: Endocrine cells scattered among the epithelial cells that line the digestive tract.

Enteric nervous system: An interdependent part of the autonomic nervous system. Despite its many interactions with other parts of the ANS, it can be regarded as a nerve body of its own.

Enterogastric reflex: The reflexive inhibition of gastric secretion; it is initiated by the arrival of chyme in the small intestine.

Enterokinase: An enzyme in the lumen of the small intestine that activates the proenzymes secreted by the pancreas.

Eosinophil: A microphage (white blood cell) with a lobed nucleus and red-staining granules; it participates in the immune response and is especially important during allergic reactions.

Ependymal cells: A type of neuroglia cell lining the central canal of the spinal cord or the brain.

Epicardium: A serous membrane covering the outer surface of the heart; also called the visceral pericardium.

Epidermal growth factor (EFG): A protein, which along with its related receptors (EGFR or ERBB1), makes up a family of related growth factors and receptors that are believed to be involved in regulation of mammary growth and mammary cancer and other tissue development in many species. Receptors for this family include EGRR as several ligands such as amphriegulin, TGF-α, and ERBB2 (called HER in humans and Neu in rodents).

Epidermis: The outer or superficial layer of the skin. It is composed of stratified squamous epithelial cells with selected specialized immune cells and associated sensory elements.

Epidural space: The space between the walls and the dura mater of the vertebral canal.

Epiglottic: Pertaining to, or connected with, the epiglottis.

Epinephrine: A catecholamine hormone secreted by the adrenal medulla and a neurotransmitter, released by certain neurons and active in the central nervous system. It is stored in the chromaffin granules and is released in response to hypoglycemia, stress, and other stimuli. It is a potent stimulator of the adrenergic receptors of the sympathetic nervous system and a powerful cardiac stimulant that accelerates the heart rate and increases cardiac output. It also promotes glycogenolysis and exerts other metabolic effects.

Epineurium: The outermost layer of connective tissue of a peripheral nerve, surrounding the entire nerve and containing its supplying blood vessels and lymphatics.

Epiphyseal line: The line of junction of the epiphysis and diaphysis of a long bone where growth in length occurs.

Epiphyseal plate: The plate of cartilage between the shaft and the epiphysis of a long bone during its growth; also called the epiphyseal cartilage.

Epiphysis: The head of a long bone.

Epiploic appendages: One of a number of small processes of peritoneum projecting from the serous coat of the large intestine except the rectum; it is generally distended with fat.

Epithelium: A tissue composed of a layer of cells. It is one of four primary body tissues. Epithelium lines both the outside (skin) and the inside cavities and lumen of bodies. Epithelial cells are also the primary functional (parenchymal) parts of organs and glands.

Equilibrium: The sense of balance, which maintains physical balance in animals.

Equilibrium potential: The potential that exists when the concentration gradient and opposing electrical gradient for a given ion exactly counterbalance each other so there is no net movement of the ion.

Eructation sequence: The coordinated neural and mechanical steps that occur when a ruminate animal regurgitates material to "chew its cud."

Erythrocytes: A red blood cell; it has no nucleus and contains large quantities of hemoglobin.

Erythropoiesis: The process of erythrocyte formation.

Erythropoietin (EPO): A hormone released by tissues, especially the kidneys, exposed to low oxygen concentrations; stimulates erythropoiesis (red blood cell formation) in bone marrow.

Esophageal hiatus: The defect in the diaphragm through which the esophagus passes from the thorax into the abdomen.

Esophagus: A muscular tube that connects the pharynx to the stomach.

Estrogen: A steroid hormone produced predominately in female reproductive tissues (ovary, placenta) associated with development of sexual receptivity and secondary sex characteristics (mammary development, characteristic female body development).

Estrous cycle: The reproductive cycle of nonprimate females defined as the period from one estrus (heat) to the next. Consecutive ovulations can also be used to signal cycles. Each cycle consists of a follicular and luteal phase.

Estrus: Period during which the female is sexually receptive to the male.

Ethmoid bone: A light spongy bone located between the eye sockets, forming part of the walls and septum of the superior nasal cavity, and containing perforations for the passage of olfactory nerve fibers.

Ethmoidal: Of, relating to, or being a light spongy bone located between the orbits, forming part of the walls and septum of the superior nasal cavity and containing numerous perforations for the passage of the fibers of the olfactory nerves.

Eutherian mammal: Those that produce a placenta.

Eversion: A turning outward, as of the eyelid.

Ewe: An adult female sheep.

Excitable membrane: Membranes that propagate action potentials, a characteristic of muscle cells and nerve cells.

Excitation-contraction coupling: The process whereby the spreading depolarization is converted into force production by muscle fibers.

Excitatory postsynaptic potential (EPSP): A small depolarization of the postsynaptic membrane in response to neurotransmitter binding, bringing the membrane closer to threshold.

Excretion: A removal from body fluids.

Excretory lacrimal ducts: Tear ducts.

Exocrine: Glands that secrete their products and temporarily store their secretions in a duct.

Exocytosis: Fusion of a membrane-enclosed intracellular vesicle with the plasma membrane, followed by the opening of the vesicle and the emptying of its contents to the outside.

Expiratory reserve volume: The amount of additional air that can be voluntarily moved out of the respiratory tract after one normal exhalation.

Extension: A pulling or dragging force exerted on a limb in a distal direction.

External nares: The entrance from the exterior to the nasal cavity.

External respiration: The diffusion of gases between the alveolar air and the alveolar capillaries and between the systemic capillaries and peripheral tissues.

Exteroceptor: A sense organ, such as the ear, that receives and responds to stimuli originating from outside the body.

Extracellular matrix: A complex network or mesh of proteins (collagen, elastin, etc.) and polysaccharides (glycosaminoglycans, etc.) secreted by cells. It serves as a structure scaffold for tissue and organ development and tissue function.

Extrafusal muscle fibers: A class of muscle fiber innervated by alpha motor neurons. Contraction of these fibers allows for movement. Extrafusal muscle fibers and associated alpha motor neurons are called a motor unit. The connection between alpha motor neurons and extrafusal muscle fiber is a neuromuscular junction.

Extraocular muscles: The six muscles that control the movements of the eye. The actions of the extraocular muscles depend on the position of the eye at the time of muscle contraction.

Extrapyramidal system: A neural network located in the brain that is part of the motor system involved in the coordination of movement. Extrapyramidal neurons, like related gamma system neurons, excite or inhibit anterior horn cells.

Extrinsic muscles: The six skeletal muscles that attach to and move each eye.

Eyebrows: A bony ridge above the eye that protects the eye and bears a tuft of facial hair in most mammals. The main function of the eyebrows is to prevent moisture (mostly sweat and rain) from dripping into the eye.

Eyelashes: The hairs that grow at the edge of the eyelid. Eyelashes protect the eye from debris and perform some of the same function as whiskers do on a cat or a mouse, in the sense that they are sensitive to being touched, thus providing a warning that an object (such as an insect or dust mote) is near the eye (which is then closed reflexively).

Eyelids: A thin fold of skin and muscle that covers and protects an eye.

F

F actin: One of the major protein components found in muscle, existing as F actin or G actin.

Facial: Pertaining to the face.

Facilitated diffusion: The passive movement of a substance across a cell membrane by means of a protein carrier.

Falciform ligament: A sheet of mesentery that contains the ligamentum teres, the fibrous remains of the umbilical vein of the fetus.

Far point of vision: Distance from the eye where accommodation is not needed to have the image focused on the retina.

Fascia: A sheet or band of fibrous connective tissue enveloping, separating, or binding together muscles, organs, and other soft structures of the body.

Fast glycolytic fibers: Muscle fibers with low myoglobin content, few mitochondria, few blood capillaries, and a large amount of glycogen. Also called fast twitch B or fatigable fibers, they hydrolyze ATP very quickly, fatigue easily, and are needed for sports such as sprinting.

Fast oxidative fibers: Muscle fibers that contain large amounts of myoglobin, many mitochondria, and many blood capillaries. Also called fast twitch A or fatigue-resistant fibers, they generate ATP by the aerobic system, split ATP at a slow rate, have slow contraction velocity, are resistant to fatigue, are found in large numbers in postural muscles, and are needed for aerobic activities such as long distance running.

Fatty acid: A common lipid composed of a carboxylic acid typically attached to a long hydrocarbon chain. Examples are palmitic or oleic acid.

Fenestrated: Pierced with one or more small openings.

Fenestrated capillaries: Capillaries with openings that allow larger molecules to diffuse.

Ferritin: A protein that stores iron in the body. The serum ferritin level—the amount of ferritin in your blood—is directly proportional to the amount of iron stored in your body.

Fibrinolysis: The breakdown of the fibrin strands of a blood clot by a proteolytic enzyme.

Fibroblast growth factor (FGF): One of a number of ~18,000 dalton proteins from a family with at least 23 members. FGFs were first isolated from bovine pituitary, but they are known to be widely distributed and are involved in tissue growth and development, including embryonic development.

Fibroblasts: Connective tissue cells responsible for the production of extracellular fibers and the secretion of the organic compounds of the extracellular matrix.

Fibrocartilage: Cartilage containing an abundance of collagen fibers; it is located around the edges of joints, in the intervertebral discs, the menisci of the knee, and so on.

Fibrous tunic: Outer layer of the eye; composed of the sclera and the cornea.

Filiform papillae: Thin, longer papillae that don't contain taste buds but which are the most numerous. These papillae are mechanical and not involved in gustation.

Filtration: The movement of a fluid across a membrane whose pores restrict the passage of solutes on the basis of size.

Filum terminale: A fibrous extension of the spinal cord, from the conus medullaris of the neural tube.

First-class lever: An anatomical structure that acts as a hinge or point of support.

Fissures: A normal groove or furrow, as in the liver or brain, that divides an organ into lobes or parts.

Fixed macrophages: Macrophages that are resident cells in a particular tissue or organ as opposed to circulating monocytes that are recruited to a tissue because of chemotaxis.

Flat bones: A bone having a thin, flattened shape, as the scapula.

Flexion: The act of bending a joint or limb in the body by the action of flexors.

Flexor reflex: Reflex initiated by a painful stimulus (actual or perceived); causes automatic withdrawal of the threatened body part from the stimulus.

Folia: A broad, thin, leaflike structure, as of the cerebellar cortex.

Foliate papillae: The leaf-shaped ridges on the lateral borders of the tongue.

Follicle Stimulating Hormone (FSH): A glycoprotein hormone produced in the anterior pituitary gland in response to secretion of gonadotropic releasing hormone (GnRH) from the hypothalamus. FSH promotes follicular development in females and Sertoli cell function in males.

Follicular phase: The period of the estrous cycle when the dominate follicle produces estradiol. Females display behavioral estrus and ovulation during this time.

Foramen of Magendie: An opening in the hollow nerve tube connecting the fourth ventricle of the brain with the subarachnoid space.

Foramen ovale: Hole or opening in a bone or between body cavities.

Foramina of Luschka: Along with the median aperture, they comprise the three openings in the roof of the fourth ventricle. They are found at the extremities of the lateral recesses.

Fornix: An archlike anatomical structure or fold, such as the arched band of white matter located beneath the corpus callosum of the brain.

Fornix vagina: The cranial region of the vagina that creates a crypt extending to the cervix.

Fourth ventricle: A cerebrospinal fluid-filled space within the hindbrain bordered dorsally by the cerebellum and ventrally by the tegmentum.

Fovea: A part of the eye, a spot located in the center of the macula. The fovea is responsible for sharp central vision.

Frank-Starling law of the heart: Intrinsic control of the heart such that increasing the end diastolic volume, i.e., increased venous return, results in a greater stroke volume.

Freemartin: A sterile heifer born twin to a bull. It has incomplete development of the reproduction tract and malelike behavior.

Frontal lobe: The largest portion of each cerebral hemisphere, anterior to the central sulcus.

Frontal plane: A sectional plane that divides the body into an anterior portion and a posterior portion; also called the coronal plane.

Frontonasal suture: Separates the frontal bones from the nasal bones.

Frontoparietal suture: A suture extending across the skull between the parietal and frontal bones.

Fulcrum: An anatomical structure that acts as a hinge or point of support.

Fully saturated: A fatty acid molecule with no double bonds between any of its carbon atoms.

Functional syncytium: A group of smooth or cardiac muscle cells that are interconnected by gap junctions and function electrically and mechanically as a single unit.

Fundus: The base of an organ.

Fungiform papillae: Mushroom-shaped papillae (projections) on the tongue. They are located on the top surface of the tongue, toward the back. They have taste buds on their surface that can distinguish the four tastes: sweet, sour, bitter, and salty.

Funiculi: One of three major divisions of white matter in the spinal cord, consisting of fasciculi.

G

G actin: Globular protein molecules that, when bound together, form fibrous actin (F actin).

G protein: A generic term for a member of a large family of guanine triphosphate (GTP)-binding proteins that are important elements in cell signaling. The binding of a hormone or other signaling ligand in this family activates these cellular proteins, many of which act as kinases.

Galactopoiesis: This term refers to the maintenance of continuation of an established lactation. For example, secretion of growth hormone and prolactin are believed to be essential for maintaining lactation in most species, so these hormones would be classified as galactopoietic hormones.

Gamma Amino Butryic acid (GABA): A neurotransmitter of the central nervous system whose effects are generally inhibitory.

Gamma motor neurons: Regulates the gain of the stretch reflex by adjusting the level of tension in the intrafusal muscle fibers of the muscle spindle. This mechanism sets the baseline level of activity in α motor neurons and helps to regulate muscle length and tone.

Ganglia: A tissue mass that contains the dendrites and cell bodies (or "somata") of nerve cells—in most cases, ones belonging to the peripheral nervous system. Within the central nervous system such a mass is often called a nucleus. An interconnected group of ganglia is called a plexus.

Ganglion cell: A type of neuron located in the retina of the eye that receives visual information from photoreceptors via various intermediate cells such as bipolar cells, amacrine cells, and horizontal cells.

Gap junction: A gap between adjacent cell membranes containing very fine latticelike connections that allows physiologic components to pass directly from cell to cell; also called a nexus.

Gastric glands: The tubular glands of the stomach whose cells produce acid, enzymes, intrinsic factor, and hormones.

Gastric inhibitory peptide (GIP): A duodenal hormone released when the arriving chyme contains large quantities of carbohydrates; triggers the secretion of insulin and a slowdown in gastric activity.

Gastric pits: Small pit in the mucous membrane of the stomach at the bottom of which are the mouths of the gastric glands that secrete mucus, hydrochloric acid, intrinsic factor, pepsinogen, and hormones.

Gastrin: A hormone produced by enteroendocrine cells of the stomach, after exposure to mechanical stimuli or stimulation of the vagus nerve, and of the duodenum, after exposure to chyme that contains undigested proteins.

Gastroileal reflex: Peristaltic movements that shift materials from the ileum to the colon; triggered by the arrival of food in the stomach.

Gastrointestinal tract: Also referred to as the GI tract, the alimentary canal, (nourishment canal) or the gut, it is the system of organs within multicellular animals. It takes in food, digests it to extract energy and nutrients, and expels the remaining waste.

Generator potential: A small depolarization produced by neurotransmitter binding or activation of a sensory receptor in the nervous system.

Germ layers: The ectoderm, mesoderm, and endoderm, which are the earliest recognizable tissues in the developing embryo.

Gestation: The act or faculty of tasting.

Gingivae: The gums.

Gizzard: An adapted stomach that is found in birds, earthworms, and other animals. It has a thick, muscular wall, enabling powerful grinding action.

Gland of the third eyelid: A gland also known as a nictitating membrane, which can move across the eyeball to give the sensitive eye structures additional protection in particular circumstances.

Glaucoma: A group of diseases of the optic nerve involving loss of retinal ganglion cells in a characteristic pattern of optic neuropathy.

Glenoid cavity: The hollow in the head of the scapula into which the head of the humerus sits to make the shoulder joint; also called the glenoid fossa.

Globus pallidus: The inner and lighter gray portion of the lentiform nucleus of the brain; also called the pallidum.

Glottis: The passageway from the pharynx to the larynx.

Glucose: A six-carbon (hexose) sugar that is fundamental to the metabolism of cells. It is stored as a polymer in animal cells as glycogen.

Glucuronic acid: A carboxylic acid that has the structure of a glucose molecule that has had its sixth carbon atom (of six total) oxidized. Its formula is $C_6H_{10}O_7$.

Glutamate: A salt of glutamic acid.

Glycerol: A simple three-carbon polyalcohol that is often derived from the catabolism of glucose. Among other functions, it serves as a precursor in the formation of mono-, di-, or triglycerides.

Glycine: A nonessential amino acid derived from the alkaline hydrolysis of gelatin and used as a nutrient and dietary supplement; also used in biochemical research and in the treatment of certain myopathies.

Glycogen: A storage form of glucose; a polysaccharide composed of repeating glucose units. Granules of glycogen are found in liver and muscle cells.

Glycolytic: The metabolic breakdown of glucose and other sugars that releases energy in the form of ATP.

Glycoprotein: A protein that has one or more covalently linked oligosaccharide chains. These proteins are common as integral proteins of the outer surface of the plasma membrane of cells.

Goblet cell: A goblet-shaped, mucus-producing, unicellular gland in certain epithelia of the digestive and respiratory tracts.

Golgi or Golgi apparatus: The cellular organelle linked with packaging and processing (phosphorylation, glycosylation, etc.) of proteins destined to be secreted from the cell. Stacks of Golgi membranes and associated secretory vesicles are abundant in the apical cytoplasm of fully differentiated secretory epithelial cells, e.g., mammary, pancreatic, etc.

Golgi tendon receptors: Proprioceptors located in tendons, close to the point of skeletal muscle insertion; important to smooth onset and termination of muscle contraction.

Golgi type I neurons: A nerve cell having a long axon that leaves the gray matter of the central nervous system, of which it forms a part.

Golgi type II neurons: A nerve cell having a short axon that ramifies in the gray matter of the central nervous system.

Gonadotropin releasing hormone (GnRH): A decapeptide hormone produced by hypothalamic neurons. Release into the portal blood supplying the anterior pituitary causes secretion of gonatotropins (Follicle Stimulating Hormone, FSH, and luteinizing hormone, LH).

Granulocytes: White blood cells containing granules that are visible with the light microscope; includes eosinophils, basophils, and neutrophils; also called granular leukocytes.

Gray matter: Brownish-gray nerve tissue, especially of the brain and spinal cord, composed of nerve cell bodies and their dendrites and some supportive tissue; also called gray substance or substantia grisea.

Gray ramus: A bundle of postganglionic sympathetic nerve fibers that are distributed to effectors in the body wall, skin, and limbs by way of a spinal nerve.

Greater curvature: The larger, longer outside dimension of the stomach.

Greater omentum: A large fold of the dorsal mesentery of the stomach; hangs anterior to the intestines.

Growth factors: Small peptides that act by an autocrine, a paracrine, or a classic endocrine loop to stimulate or inhibit growth and development of tissues or cells.

GTP (guanosine triphosphate): A critical nucleoside involved in reactions for synthesis of RNA, protein synthesis, and cell signaling.

Gyri: Any of the prominent, rounded, elevated convolutions on the surfaces of the cerebral hemispheres (singular = gyrus).

H

H zone: Area in the center of the A band in which there are no actin myofilaments; contains only myosin.

Habenula: A circumscriptive cell mass embedded in the posterior end of the medullary stria of the thalamus, from which it receives most of its afferent fibers; also called the habena, pedunculus of pineal body (or gland).

Hard palate: The bony roof of the oral cavity, formed by the maxillary and palatine bones.

Haustra: Saclike pouches along the length of the large intestine that result from tension in the taenia coli.

Haversian system: A central canal and the concentric osseous lamellae encircling it, occurring in compact bone.

Hearing: The sense by which sound is perceived.

Heat shock proteins: Also called stress-response proteins, these are produced by cells in response to elevated temperatures or other stressors and are believed to help the cell survive.

Helicotrema: The part of the cochlear labyrinth where the scala tympani and the scala vestibuli meet. It is also known as the cochlear apex.

Hematocrit: The percentage of the volume of whole blood contributed by cells; also called the volume of packed red cells (VPRC) or packed cell volume (PCV).

Hematoma: A tumor or swelling filled with blood.

Hematopoiesis: Blood cell formation; hemopoiesis.

Hematopoietic stem cells: Undifferentiated cells, usually located in the bone marrow, that are capable of dividing and producing daughter cells, which become various blood system components.

Hemopoiesis: Blood cell formation and differentiation.

Henry's Law: Named for the English chemist William Henry (1775–1836). The concentration of a gas dissolved in a liquid is equal to the partial pressure of the gas over the liquid times the solubility coefficient of the gas.

Hepatic artery: An artery that distributes blood to the liver, pancreas, and gallbladder as well as to the stomach and duodenal portion of the small intestine.

Hepatic growth factor (HGF): A heparin-binding protein that has also been referred to as hematopoietin or scatter factor. It has proliferation and differentiation on multiple cell types, including liver, muscle, and mammary cells.

Hepatic portal vein: The vessel that carries blood between the intestinal capillaries and the sinusoids of the liver.

Hepatocyte: A liver cell.

Hepatoduodenal ligament: The portion of the lesser omentum extending between the liver and duodenum.

Hepatopancreatic ampulla: Commonly called the Ampulla of Vater, it is formed by the union of the pancreatic duct and the bile duct.

Hepatopancreatic sphincter: Controls secretions from the liver, pancreas, and gallbladder into the duodenum of the small intestine. It is a sphincter muscle located at the surface of the duodenum.

Heterotopic: Ectopic, positioned outside the normal location.

Hiatal hernia: The protrusion (or hernia) of the upper part of the stomach into the thorax through a tear or weakness in the diaphragm.

Hilum/hilus: A localized region where blood vessels, lymphatic vessels, nerves, and/or other anatomical structures are attached to an organ.

Hippocampus: The complex, internally convoluted structure that forms the medial margin of the cortical mantle of the cerebral hemisphere, borders the choroid fissure of the lateral ventricle, is composed of two gyri with their white matter, and forms part of the limbic system.

Histamine: The chemical released by stimulated mast cells or basophils to initiate or enhance an inflammatory response.

Histology: The study of tissues.

Histone(s): A group of proteins, high in arginine and lysine, they are closely associated with DNA in the chromosomes.

Holocrine glands: Glands that contain secretory cells that accumulate their products; then the cells are sloughed and disrupted to create the secretion from the glands—for example, the crop sac glands of some birds.

Homeorrhesis: This indicates a state of adjusted or altered physiology to support a particular activity or function (e.g., lactation or reproduction).

Homeostasis: The maintenance of a relatively constant internal environment.

Horizontal cells: The laterally interconnecting neurons in the outer plexiform layer of the retina. There are three basic types—HI, HII, and HIII—and all three are multipolar cells.

Hyaline cartilage: Semitransparent opalescent cartilage that forms most of the fetal skeleton and that consists of cells that synthesize a surrounding matrix of hyaluronic acid, collagen, and protein; in the adult, it is found in the trachea, larynx, and joint surfaces.

Hyaline cartilage rings: C-shaped bands of cartilage that provide the rigid structure apparent in the trachea.

Hyaloid canal: A branch of the ophthalmic artery, which is itself a branch of the carotid artery. It is contained within the optic stalk of the eye and extends through the vitreous humor to the lens.

Hydrocephalus: A usually congenital condition in which an abnormal accumulation of fluid in the cerebral ventricles causes enlargement of the skull and compression of the brain, destroying much of the neural tissue.

Hydrochloric acid (HCl): The aqueous (water-based) solution of hydrogen chloride (HCl) gas. It is a strong acid, the major component of gastric acid, and of wide industrial use.

Hydrophilic: Refers to molecules that readily associate or dissolve in water—for example, ethanol.

Hydrophobic: Refers to molecules that do not readily dissolve in water—for example, oil and water.

Hyperalgesia: An extreme sensitivity to pain, which in one form is caused by damage to nociceptors in the body's soft tissues.

Hypercapnia: High plasma carbon dioxide concentrations, commonly as a result of hypoventilation or inadequate tissue perfusion.

Hyperopia: Also known as hypermetropia or colloquially as farsightedness or longsightedness, it is a defect of vision caused by an imperfection in the eye (often when the eyeball is too short or when the lens cannot become round enough), causing inability to focus on near objects, and in extreme cases causing a sufferer to be unable to focus on objects at any distance.

Hyperpolarization: An increase in membrane potential from resting potential; potential becomes even more negative than at resting potential.

Hypertonia: Extreme tension of the muscles or arteries.

Hypertonic: Refers to any fluid with a high enough concentration of solutes to cause water to move out of the cell (cell shrinkage) because of osmosis.

Hypocapnia: A low plasma P_{CO2} concentration commonly as a result of hyperventilation.

Hypothalamo-hypophyseal portal system: A unique circulatory arrangement that allows small quantities of hypothalamic releasing hormones to flow directly down the pituitary stalk to the anterior pituitary without being diluted in the general circulation, thus making these hormones much more potent.

Hypotonic: Refers to any fluid with a low enough concentration of solutes to cause water to move into the cell (cell swelling and possible rupture) because of osmosis.

Hypovolemic shock: The most common form of shock; results from extreme blood loss.

I

I band: A pale band of actin on each side of the Z line of a striated muscle fiber.

Ileocecal valve: A fold of mucous membrana that guards the connection between the ileum and the cecum.

Ileum: The distal 2.5 m of the small intestine.

Immunity: Resistance to injuries and diseases caused by foreign compounds, toxins, or pathogens.

Incisive: Having the power to cut.

Incisors: The first kind of tooth in heterodont mammals.

Incomplete break: The break goes only partway through the bone. An incomplete fracture is also known as a greenstick fracture.

Incomplete tetanus: Myograph recording, or situation in which individual muscle twitches are apparent.

Incus: The anvil-shaped small bone or ossicle in the middle ear. It connects the malleus to the stapes. The incus exists only in mammals, and is derived from a reptilian upper jawbone, the quadrate bone.

Inferior colliculus: The structure in the brain that lies caudal to its counterpart, the superior colliculus, above the trochlear nerve and at the base of the projection of the medial geniculate nucleus (MGN) and the lateral geniculate nucleus (LGN).

Inferior oblique muscle: A thin, narrow muscle, placed near the anterior margin of the floor of the orbit.

Inferior rectus muscles: A muscle in the orbit that depresses, adducts, and rotates the eye laterally.

Inferior sagittal sinus: An unpaired dural sinus in the lower margin of the falx cerebri.

Inferior vena cava: The vein that carries blood from the parts of the body inferior to the heart to the right atrium.

Infraspinous fossa: The hollow on the dorsal aspect of the scapula inferior to the spine, giving attachment chiefly to the infraspinatus muscle.

Infundibulum: The funnel-shaped, unpaired prominence of the base of the hypothalamus behind the optic chiasm, continuous below the stalk of the pituitary gland. The funnellike opening of the oviduct is also called the infundibulum.

Ingestion: The introduction of materials into the digestive tract by way of the mouth.

Inhibin: A hormone, produced by Sertoli cells in the male and granulosa cells in the female, that acts to inhibit secretion of FSH.

Inhibitory postsynaptic potential (IPSP): Hyperpolarization in the postsynaptic membrane that causes the membrane potential to move away from the threshold.

Innate reflexes: An automatic instinctive unlearned reaction to a stimulus.

Inner ear: Structure comprising both the organ of hearing (the cochlea) and the labyrinth or vestibular apparatus, which is the organ of balance located in the inner ear consisting of three semicircular canals and the vestibule.

Inner hair cells: Bulbous cells that are medially placed in one row in the organ of Corti. In contrast to the outer hair cells, the inner hair cells are fewer in number, have fewer sensory hairs, and are less differentiated.

Inner synaptic layers: Where inner nuclear layer cells contact ganglion cells.

Insertion: The point or mode of attachment of a skeletal muscle to the bone or other body part that it moves.

Inspiratory areas: Nuclei located in the respiratory center of the brain stem that are involved in control of inspiration.

Inspiratory reserve volume: The maximum amount of air that can be drawn into the lungs over and above the normal tidal volume.

Insula: An oval region of the cerebral cortex, lateral to the lentiform nucleus, and buried in the fissure of Sylvius.

Insulin: The protein hormone produced by the β cells of the endocrine pancreas (Islets of Langerhans). When blood glucose is elevated it is secreted, which (in normal circumstances) stimulates the uptake of glucose to maintain normal blood glucose concentration.

Insulin receptor substrate (IRS): These proteins are intracellular mediators of IGF-I and insulin action. Binding insulin or IGF-I to their cell surface receptors causes autophosphorylation or the receptor and creation of docking sites for IRS family members. When IRS docks, this allows further interactions, a cascade of other signaling molecules, including the p85 substrate of PI3K.

Insulinlike growth factor I (IGF-I): A small growth factor (~7.4 kD) that appears in circulation largely in response to growth hormone stimulation of the liver. However, it is also locally produced in the stromal tissue of a number of organs. It is a potent stimulator of cell proliferation and is involved in prevention of apoptosis.

Insulinlike growth factor binding proteins (IGFBPs): These proteins comprise a family of at least six well-characterized members and several relatives that can bind IGF-I. They are believed to modulate the biological effectiveness of IGF-I. IGFBP-2, 3, and 4 are evident in serum, but IGFBPs are also produced within various tissues.

Integration: The process by which the nervous system processes and interprets sensory input and makes decisions about what should be done at each moment.

Integrins: Family of transmembrane proteins that are important in adhesion of cells to the extracellular matrix and in cell signaling.

Interatrial septum: Wall between the atria of the heart.

Intercalated discs: Regions where adjacent cardiocytes interlock and where gap junctions permit electrical coupling between the cells.

Interleukins: Group of growth factorlike proteins produced primarily by immune tissues that regulate growth and activation of various immune cells.

Intermediate mass: A type of mesoderm that is located between the paraxial mesoderm and the lateral plate.

Internal capsule: A layer of white matter separating the caudate nucleus and thalamus from the lentiform nucleus and serving as the major route by which the cerebral cortex is connected with the brain stem and the spinal cord.

Internal nares: The entrance from the nasal cavity to the nasopharynx.

Internal respiration: The diffusion of gases between interstitial fluid and cytoplasm.

Internasal suture: The line of union between the two nasal bones.

Interneurons: Association neurons; central nervous system neurons that are between sensory and motor neurons.

Interoceptors: A specialized sensory nerve receptor that receives and responds to stimuli originating from within the body.

Interphase: The usually prolonged period of a cell cycle between the end of one mitosis and the next; this includes G_1, S, and G_2 phases.

Interstitial growth: A form of cartilage growth through the growth, mitosis, and secretion of chondrocytes in the matrix.

Interventricular foramen of Monroe: Channels that connect the paired lateral ventricles with the third ventricle at the midline of the brain. As channels, they allow cerebrospinal fluid (CSF) produced in the lateral ventricles to reach the third ventricle and then the rest of the brain's ventricular system.

Interventricular septum: The wall between the ventricles of the heart.

Intervertebral foramen: Any of the openings into the vertebral canal bounded by the pedicles of adjacent vertebrae above and below, the vertebral bodies in front, and the articular processes behind.

Intestinal glands or crypts of Lieberkühn: Glands found in the epithelial lining of the small intestine. Named for the 18th-century German anatomist Johann Nathanael Lieberkühn, the crypts secrete various enzymes, including sucrase and maltase.

Intestinal villi: Multicellular projections from the wall of the small intestine that protrude into the lumen of the intestine. They are covered with absorptive epithelial cells.

Intrafusal muscle fibers: Muscle fibers that comprise the muscle spindle. They are fibers walled off from the rest of the muscle by a collagen sheath. This sheath has a spindle or fusiform. Although the intrafusal fibers are wrapped with sensor receptors, their counterparts, extrafusal muscle fibers, are responsible for the power-generating component of muscle and are innervated by motor neurons.

Intramembranous ossification: The formation of bone within a connective tissue without the prior development of a cartilaginous model.

Intraocular pressure: The fluid pressure inside the eye. It may become elevated due to anatomical problems, inflammation of the eye, genetic factors, or as a side effect from medication.

Intrapulmonary primary bronchus: The section between the pulmonary hilus and the ostium of the abdominal air sac.

Intrinsic factor: A glycoprotein, secreted by the parietal cells of the stomach, that facilitates the intestinal absorption of vitamin B_{12}.

Intrinsic muscles: Muscles located within the structure being moved.

Intron: The noncoding segments of DNA that are transcribed in the production of mRNA but then excised by RNA splicing enzymes before the mature mRNA exits the nucleus for protein synthesis.

Inversion: A chromosomal defect in which a segment of the chromosome breaks off and reattaches in the reverse direction.

Involuntary striated muscle: Also called cardiac muscle.

Ionotropic receptors: A group of intrinsic transmembrane ion channels that are opened in response to binding of a chemical messenger, as opposed to voltage-gated ion channels or stretch-activated ion channels.

IP_3: Inositol trisphosphate, a small molecule produced by the breakdown of the inositol phospholipid PIP_2 following stimulation by hormone binding. IP_3 acts as a second messenger by releasing Ca^{++} from storage in RER.

Iris: The most visible part of the eye of vertebrates.

Irregular bones: Any of a group of bones having peculiar or complex forms, such as the vertebrae.

Isometric: Of or involving muscular contraction against resistance in which the length of the muscle remains the same.

Isotonic: Of or involving muscular contraction in which the muscle remains under relatively constant tension while its length changes.

Isotropic: Identical in all directions; invariant with respect to direction.

Isovolumetric contraction phase: The period of cardiac contraction before the pressure inside the heart chamber is sufficiently elevated to open the heart valves and induce blood flow.

J

Janus protein tyrosine kinases (JAKS): Cellular kinases that become activated when certain cytokine family members (e.g., prolactin and growth hormone) bind to their surface receptors on target cells. They are involved in signal transduction.

Jejunum: The middle part of the small intestine.

K

K-complexes: An EEG waveform that occurs during stage 2 sleep. It consists of a brief high-voltage peak, usually greater than 100 μV, and lasts for longer than 0.5 sec. K-complexes occur randomly throughout stage 2 sleep, but may also occur in response to auditory stimuli.

Kinocilium: A special structure connected to the hair cells of the inner ear's cochlea of amphibia.

Kupffer cells: Stellate reticular cells of the liver; phagocytic cells of the liver sinusoids.

L

Labyrinth: A system of fluid passages in the inner ear.

Lacrimal canals: The small channels in each eyelid that commence at minute orifices, puncta lacrimalia, on the summits of the papillæ lacrimales, seen on the margins of the lids at the lateral extremity of the lacus lacrimalis.

Lacrimal glands: Paired glands, one for each eye, that secrete lacrimal fluid. Each gland is about the size of an almond (2 cm) and sits alongside the eyeball within the orbit, nestled in the lacrimal fossa of the frontal bone.

Lacrimal sac: The upper dilated end of the nasolacrimal duct, lodged in a deep groove formed by the lacrimal bone and frontal process of the maxilla.

Lactase: A member of the β-galactosidase family of enzymes, it is involved in the hydrolysis of the disaccharide lactose into constituent galactose and glucose monomers.

Lacteal: A terminal lymphatic within an intestinal villus.

Lactogenesis: The onset of lactation that occurs near the time of parturition. It occurs in two phases, with limited structural and functional differentiation of the mammary alveolar cells after lobulo-alveolar development during gestation, followed by dramatic differentiation and copious milk secretion within hours or days of parturition. Hormones (e.g., prolactin or glucocorticoids) that promote this process are called lactogenic hormones.

Lacuna: A small pit or cavity.

Lamina propria: The reticular tissue that underlies a mucous epithelium and forms part of a mucous membrane.

Laryngopharynx: The division of the pharynx that is inferior to the epiglottis and superior to the esophagus.

Lateral geniculate: A part of the brain, which is the primary processor of visual information, received from the retina, in the central nervous system.

Lateral geniculate body of the thalamus: A part of the brain that is the primary processor of visual information, received from the retina, in the central nervous system.

Lateral rectus muscle: A muscle in the orbit. It is one of six extraocular muscles that control the movements of the eye and the only muscle innervated by the abducens nerve, cranial nerve VI.

Lateral sulcus (lateral fissure, Sylvian fissure): The deepest and most prominent of the cortical fissures of the brain, extending between frontal and temporal lobes and then back and slightly upward over the lateral aspect of the cerebral hemisphere.

Leak channels: Resting channels allow ions to cross the membrane down their electrochemical gradient, whether or not the cell is depolarized.

Left colic flexure: A bend in the colon, known as the "splenic flexure," that is near the spleen.

Lens fiber: Epithelial cell that makes up the lens of the eye.

Lentiform nucleus: The large, cone-shaped mass of gray matter that forms the central core of the cerebral hemisphere, whose convex base is formed by the putamen and whose apical part consists of the globus pallidus; also called the lenticular nucleus.

Lesser curvature: The inside curve of the stomach, found opposite the greater curve located on the outer edge.

Lesser omentum: A small pocket in the mesentery that connects the lesser curvature of the stomach to the liver.

Leukocyte: A white blood cell.

Leukopoiesis (or leucopoiesis): The production of white blood cells.

Leydig cells: Cells in the interstitial tissue of the testis that secrete testosterone.

Ligamentum arteriosum: The fibrous strand in adults that is the remnant of the ductus arteriosus of the fetal stage.

Ligand: Any molecule that binds to a specific site on a protein; term often used in reference to hormones or growth factors binding to their receptors.

Ligand-gated ion channel: Also referred to as LGICs, or ionotropic receptors, a group of intrinsic transmembrane ion channels that are opened in response to binding of a chemical messenger, as opposed to voltage-gated ion channels or stretch-activated ion channels.

Light adaptation: Ability of the eye to adjust to various levels of darkness and light.

Linear fracture: A fracture that runs parallel to the long axis of a bone; also called a fissured fracture.

Lingual frenulum: An epithelial fold that attaches the inferior surface of the tongue to the floor of the mouth.

Lobar arteries: Arteries that pass between lobes of the kidney.

Lobar (secondary) bronchi: Branch from a primary bronchus that conducts air to each lobe of the lungs. There are two branches in the left lung and three branches from the primary bronchus in the right lung.

Lobulo-alveolar: A developmental term that indicates a structural grouping of several alveoli, their terminal ducts and related common ducts, and surrounding supporting connective tissue.

Long bone: One of the elongated bones of the extremities, consisting of a tubular shaft, which is composed of compact bone surrounding a central marrow-filled cavity, and two expanded portions that usually serve as articulation points.

Longitudinal pillars: Supporting layers in the rumen. They provide some compartmentalization as well as mixing.

Long-term potentiation: The long-lasting enhancement in efficacy of the synapse between two neurons.

Lower respiratory system: A system composed of the larynx, trachea, and lungs.

Lung compliance: A static measure of lung and chest recoil, expressed as a change in lung volume per unit change in airway pressure, e.g., $l/cm\ H_2O$.

Luteal phase: The phase of the estrus cycle characterized by major production of progesterone and the presence of a functional corpus luteum.

Luteinization: The process by which granulosal and thecal cells are transformed into luteal cells following ovulation.

Luteinizing hormone (LH): A hormone produced in the anterior pituitary gland. It causes ovulation and development of the CL in females and stimulates Leydig cells to secrete testosterone in males.

Lymphocyte: A cell of the lymphatic system that participates in the immune response.

Lysosome: A membrane-bound organelle that contains hydrolytic enzymes. These organelles are activated to destroy damaged cells (apoptotic actions) and are important in the action of neutrophils.

M

M line: A fine dark band in the center of the H band in the myofibrils of striated muscle fibers; also called the M band.

M phase: Period of the cell cycle during which the nucleus and cytoplasm of the cell divide.

Macrophage: A protective cell type common in connective tissue, lymphatic tissue, and certain body organs that phagocytizes tissue cells, bacteria, and other foreign debris. It is important as an antigen presenter to T cells and B cells in the immune response.

Macula lutea: An oval yellow spot near the center of the retina. It has a diameter of about 1.5 mm and is often histologically defined as having two or more layers of ganglion cells.

Magnocellular: Cells in the brain concerned primarily with visual perception. In particular, these cells are responsible for resolving motion and coarse outlines.

Malleus: A hammer-shaped small bone or ossicle of the middle ear that connects with the incus and is attached to the inner surface of the eardrum.

Maltase: An enzyme produced by the cells lining the small intestine to break down disaccharides.

Mammillary bodies: A pair of small round bodies, resembling two breasts, located in the brain and forming part of the limbic system. They are located at the ends of the anterior arches of the fornix.

Mammogenic: Substances that stimulate mammary growth and development. For example, the ovarian hormone estrogen is a classic example of a mammogenic hormone.

Manubrium: The upper segment of the sternum with which the clavicle and the first two pairs of ribs articulate.

Margination: The arrangement of neutrophils along an endothelial cell border prior to diapedesis into a tissue area.

Mass peristalsis: A powerful peristaltic contraction that moves fecal materials along the colon and into the rectum.

Maxillary: Of or relating to a jaw or jawbone, especially the upper one.

Maxillary sinus: One of the paranasal sinuses. It is an air-filled chamber lined by a respiratory epithelium that is located in a maxillary bone and opens into the nasal cavity.

Mean arterial pressure (MAP): The average pressure responsible for driving blood forward through the arteries into the tissues throughout the cardiac cycle; it equals cardiac output times total peripheral resistance.

Meatus: An opening or entrance into a passageway.

Mechanical nociceptors: Receptors that respond to excess pressure or mechanical deformation.

Mechanoreceptors: A specialized sensory end organ that responds to mechanical stimuli such as tension or pressure.

Medial forebrain bundle: A fiber system running longitudinally through the lateral zone of the hypothalamus, connecting it with the midbrain tegmentum and various components of the limbic system.

Medial geniculate: A nucleus of the thalamus that acts as a relay for auditory information. It receives its input from the inferior colliculus and sends information out to the auditory cortex.

Medial rectus muscle: A muscle in the orbit. As with most of the muscles of the orbit, it is innervated by the inferior division of the oculomotor nerve (cranial nerve III).

Median: Of, relating to, or situated in or near the plane that divides a bilaterally symmetrical animal into right and left halves; mesial.

Mediastinum: The central tissue mass that divides the thoracic cavity into two pleural cavities; it includes the aorta and other great vessels, the esophagus, trachea, thymus, the pericardial cavity and heart, and a host of nerves, small vessels, and lymphatic vessels. In males, the area of connective tissue attaching a testis to the epididymis, proximal portion of ductus deferens, and associated vessels.

Medullary cavity: The space within a bone that contains the marrow.

Medullary rhythmicity area: The center in the medulla oblongata that sets the background pace of respiration; it includes inspiratory and expiratory centers.

Meibomian glands: A special kind of sebaceous glands at the rim of the eyelids, responsible for the supply of sebum, an oily substance that prevents evaporation of the eye's tear film; also called the tarsal glands.

Meissner's corpuscles: A type of mechanoreceptor and, more specifically, a tactile corpuscle (corpusculum tactus). They are distributed throughout the skin, but concentrated in areas especially sensitive to light touch, such as the fingertips, palms, soles, lips, tongue, face, nipples, and the external skin of the male and female genitals. They are primarily located just beneath the epidermis within the dermal papillae.

Meissner's plexus (submucosal): A sensory network formed by nerve branches, which have perforated circular muscular fibers of the small intestine. This plexus lies in the submucosal of the intestine. It also contains ganglia from which nerve fibers pass to the muscularis mucosae and to the mucous membrane.

Melatonin: A hormone derived from serotonin and produced by the pineal gland that stimulates color change in the epidermis of amphibians and reptiles and that is believed to influence estrus in mammals.

Membranous labyrinth: A system of fluid passages in the inner ear, comprising the vestibular system and the auditory system, which provides the sense of balance.

Meningeal layers: The layers of protective tissue surrounding the central nervous system.

Meninges: A membrane, especially one of the three membranes enclosing the brain and spinal cord.

Merkel's discs: Mechanoreceptors found in the skin and mucosa of vertebrates that provide touch information to the brain. Each ending consists of a Merkel cell in close apposition with an enlarged nerve terminal.

Mesaticephalic: The ratio of the maximum width of the head to its maximum length, multiplied by 100.

Mesencephalon: The portion of the vertebrate brain that develops from the middle section of the embryonic brain; also called the midbrain.

Mesenchyme: Refers to the tissue or cells derived from the embryonic mesoderm. In developing glands—mammary, for example—the stromal tissue that surrounds the developing epithelial ducts contains precursor cells capable of being induced to differentiate into one of several different stromal tissue cell types (i.e., endothelial, fibroblast, adipocyte).

Mesentery: A double layer of serous membrane that supports and stabilizes the position of an organ in the abdominopelvic cavity and provides a route for the associated blood vessels, nerves, and lymphatic vessels.

Mesothelium: A simple squamous epithelium that lines one of the divisions of the ventral body cavity.

Metabotropic receptors: Receptors indirectly linked with ion channels on the plasma membrane of the cell through signal transduction mechanisms.

Metaphysis: The zone of growth between the epiphysis and diaphysis during development of a bone.

Metarteriole: A vessel that connects an arteriole to a venule and that provides blood to a capillary plexus.

Metestrus: A stage of the estrous cycle between ovulation and formation of the corpus luteum.

Microtubules: Hollow tubes composed of tubulin, measuring approximately 25 nm in diameter and usually several micrometers long. It helps provide support to the cytoplasm of the cell and is a component of certain cell organelles, such as centrioles, spindle fibers, cilia, and flagella.

Middle ear: The portion of the ear internal to the eardrum and external to the oval window of the cochlea. The middle ear contains three ossicles, which amplify vibration of the eardrum into pressure waves in the fluid in the inner ear.

Midsagittal plane: A plane passing through the midline of the body that divides it into left and right halves.

Minor duodenal papilla: Site of the opening of the accessory pancreatic duct into the duodenum.

Mitogen-activated protein kinase (MAPK): A protein kinase that performs an essential step in relaying signals for the plasma membrane to the cell nucleus. It is activated by a variety of proliferation or differentiation signals from outside target cells.

Mitral valve: *See* bicuspid valve.

Mixed nerve: A nerve that contains both sensory and motor fibers.

Modiolus: The central bony pillar of the cochlea, but also the muscle of facial expression found near the risorus muscle, between the lateral edge of the orbicularis oris, and the insertion of the zygomatic major muscle.

Molars: The rearmost and most complicated kind of tooth in most mammals. In many mammals they grind food, hence the name, which means "millstone."

Monoamine oxidase (MAO): An enzyme in the cells of most tissues that catalyzes the oxidative deamination of monoamines such as serotonin.

Monocytes: Phagocytic agranulocytes (white blood cells) in the circulating blood.

Monoglyceride: A lipid molecule consisting of a single fatty acid bound to a molecule of glycerol.

Monosaccharide: A simple sugar with the general formula $(CH_2O)_x$, where $x = 3$ to 7; examples are glucose and ribose.

Monosynaptic reflex: A reflex that provides automatic regulation of skeletal muscle length.

Monotocous: Animals that typically give birth to single offspring.

Morula: A stage of early embryonic development while the egg is still within the confines of the zona pellucida. It is characterized by the appearance of blastomeres from initial cleavage divisions.

Motor areas: The cortical area that influences motor movements.

Motor end plate: The flattened end of a motor neuron that transmits neural impulses to a muscle.

Motor nerve: A nerve that passes toward or to muscles or glands.

Motor neurons: Neurons that innervate skeletal, smooth, or cardiac muscle fibers.

Motor unit: A single somatic motor neuron and the group of muscle fibers innervated by it.

mRNA: Messenger ribonucleic acid (mRNA) specifies the amino acid sequence of a protein. In eukaryotes, it is derived from a larger precursor immature mRNA produced by RNA polymerase in the cell nucleus from a complementary strand of DNA. Processing of this immature RNA stand to remove sections corresponding with the noncoding introns yields the mRNA used for protein synthesis.

Mucosa: A mucous membrane; the epithelium plus the lamina propria.

Mucosa-associated lymphatic system (MALT): The extensive collection of lymphoid tissues linked with the digestive system.

Multiparous: A term indicating an animal that has had more than one pregnancy and birth.

Multipennate: A muscle whose internal fibers are organized around several tendons.

Multiple motor unit summation: Increased force of contraction of a muscle due to recruitment of motor units.

Multipolar neuron: One of three categories of neurons consisting of a neuron cell body, an axon, and two or more dendrites.

Multiunit smooth muscle: A smooth muscle mass that consists of multiple discrete units that function independently of one another and that must be separately stimulated by autonomic nerves to contract.

Muscarinic: A highly toxic alkaloid, $C_9H_{20}NO_2$, related to the cholines, derived from the red form of the mushroom *Amanita muscaria* and found in decaying animal tissue.

Muscle fatigue: The decline in the ability of a muscle to create force; it can be caused by barriers or interferences at many of the differing stages of muscle contraction, and it is primarily regulated by the reduction in the release of $Ca2+$ (calcium) ions from the sarcoplasmic reticulum, along with falling ATP levels.

Muscle fiber: A cylindrical multinucleate cell composed of myofibrils that contract when stimulated.

Muscle spindles: A stretch receptor in vertebrate muscle.

Muscle tone: The continuous and passive partial contraction of muscles. It helps maintain posture.

Muscularis externa: Concentric layers of smooth muscle responsible for peristalsis.

Muscularis mucosae: The layer of smooth muscle beneath the lamina propria; it is responsible for moving the mucosal surface.

Myelin: An insulating sheath around an axon; it consists of multiple layers of neuroglial membrane. It significantly increases the impulse propagation rate along the axon.

Myelocele: Protrusion of the spinal cord in cases of spina bifida.

Myelomeningocele: Protrusion of the spinal membranes and spinal cord through a defect in the vertebral column; also called the meningomyelocele.

Myenteric (or Auerbach's) plexus: Parasympathetic motor neurons and sympathetic postganglionic fibers located between the circular and longitudinal layers of the muscularis externa located in the esophagus, stomach, and intestines.

Myoblasts: A primitive muscle cell having the potential to develop into a muscle fiber; also called a sarcoblast.

Myocardium: The cardiac muscle tissue of the heart.

Myoepithelial cells: Specialized cells that form a network surrounding the mammary alveoli. In response to oxytocin, these cells contract to cause milk ejection.

Myofibrils: One of the threadlike longitudinal fibrils occurring in a skeletal or cardiac muscle fiber; also called a sarcostyle.

Myofilaments: Any of the ultramicroscopic filaments, made up of actin and myosin, that are the structural units of a myofibril.

Myoglobin: An oxygen-binding pigment that is especially common in slow skeletal muscle fibers and cardiac muscle cells.

Myogram: The tracing of muscular contractions made by a myograph.

Myomesin: A 185 kDa protein located in the M band of striated muscle where it interacts with myosin and titin, possibly connecting thick filaments with the third filament system.

Myoneural junction: The synaptic connection of the axon of a motor neuron with a muscle fiber.

Myopia: Sometimes called short-sightedness or near-sightedness, it is a refractive defect of the eye in which collimated light produces image focus in front of the retina when accommodation is relaxed.

Myosin: The most common protein in muscle cells, a globulin responsible for the elastic and contractile properties of muscle and combining with actin to form actomyosin.

Myosin light-chain kinase (MLCK): This protein is important in the mechanism of contraction in smooth muscle. Once there is an influx of calcium into the smooth muscle, either from the sarcoplasmic reticulum or, more importantly, from the extracellular space, contraction of smooth muscle fibers may begin. First, the calcium will bind to calmodulin. This binding will activate the MLCK, which will go on to phosphorylate the myosin light chains. This will enable the myosin light chains to bind to the actin filament so that contraction may start.

Myotatic reflex: Tonic contraction of the muscles in response to a stretching force, due to stimulation of muscle proprioceptors; also called the stretch reflex.

N

Nasal bones: Two small oblong bones, varying in size and form in different individuals; they are placed side by side at the middle and upper part of the face, and they form, by their junction, the bridge of the nose. Each has two surfaces and four borders.

Nasal cavity: A chamber in the skull that is bounded by the internal and external nares.

Nasolacrimal duct: A duct that carries tears from the lacrimal sac into the nasal cavity.

Nasomaxillary suture: The suture uniting the nasal bone and the maxilla.

Nasopharynx: A region that is posterior to the internal nares and superior to the soft palate and ends at the oropharynx.

Near point of vision: Closest point from the eye at which an object can be held without appearing blurred.

Nebulin: An actin-binding molecule, which is localized to the I band in skeletal muscle.

Necrosis: Death of cells or tissues through injury or disease, especially in a localized area of the body.

Negative chronotropic factors: Factors that act to slow normal heart rhythm, and therefore heart rate.

Negative feedback: A corrective mechanism that opposes or negates a variation from normal limits.

Neostigmine: A drug that inhibits acetylcholinesterase, used in its bromide form orally and its methylsulfate form parenterally to treat myasthenia gravis.

Nerve: Any of the cordlike bundles of nervous tissue made up of myelinated or unmyelinated nerve fibers and held together by a connective tissue sheath through which sensory stimuli and motor impulses pass between the brain or other parts of the central nervous system and the eyes, glands, muscles, and other parts of the body.

Nerve growth factor (NGF): First identified because of effects on the salivary gland, there are multiple members: NGF, neurotropin 1–6, etc. These peptides are needed for development of the sympathetic nervous system and play a role in follicular development in the ovary.

Nervous system: Fast-acting control system that triggers muscle contraction or gland secretion.

Net filtration pressure (NFP): The net difference in the hydrostatic and osmotic forces acting across the glomerular membrane that favors the filtration of protein-free plasma into Bowman's capsule.

Neural crest: A component of the ectoderm, this is one of several ridgelike clusters of cells found on either side of the neural tube in vertebrate embryos. It has been referred to as the fourth germ layer, due to its great importance.

Neural tube: A dorsal tubular structure in the vertebrate embryo formed by longitudinal folding of the neural plate and differentiating into the brain and spinal cord.

Neurocoel: The central canal and ventricles of the spinal cord and brain; the myelencephalic cavity.

Neuroglia: Cells in the nervous system other than the neurons; it includes astrocytes, ependymal cells, microglia, oligodendrocytes, satellite cells, and Schwann cells.

Neuromuscular junction: The junction between a nerve fiber and the muscle it supplies.

Neurons: A cell in neural tissue that is specialized for intercellular communication through 1) changes in membrane potential, and 2) synaptic connections.

Neurotransmitter: A chemical compound released by one neuron to affect the transmembrane potential of another.

Neurotransmitter-gated channels: Cell membrane channels of neurons that are activated by the binding of neurotransmitters.

Neurotrophic factors: Secreted by cells in a neuron's target field, these act by prohibiting the neuron from apoptosis.

Neutrophil: A microphage that is very numerous and normally the first of the mobile phagocytic cells to arrive at an area of injury or infection.

Nicotinamide adenine dinucleotide (NAD): A molecule that serves as a coenzyme for oxidative pathways (glycolysis, Krebs cycle, electron transport chain). It serves to transfer electrons in oxidative-reduction reactions and is derived from niacin.

Nicotinic: Of or relating to nicotine.

Nicotinic receptor: Ionotropic receptors that form ion channels in plasma membranes.

Nictitating membrane: A membrane that can move across the eyeball to give the sensitive eye structures additional protection. It is often called a third eyelid or haw and may be referred to as the plica semilunaris.

Nitric oxide (NO): A recently identified local chemical mediator released from endothelial cells and other tissues. It exerts multiple effects, ranging from local vasodilation to acting as a toxic agent against foreign invaders or as a neurotransmitter.

NMDA receptor: A brain receptor activated by the amino acid glutamate, which, when excessively stimulated, may cause cognitive defects in Alzheimer's disease; also called the N-methyl-D-aspartate receptor.

Nociceptor: A sensory receptor that responds to pain.

Node of Ranvier: The area between adjacent neuroglia where the myelin covering of an axon is incomplete.

Noggin: A slang term that means "head."

Nondisplaced fracture: A simple crack in the bone that has not caused the bone to move from its normal anatomic position; also called a hairline fracture.

Nonstriated involuntary muscle: Another name for smooth muscle.

Noradrenaline: *See* norepinephrine.

Norepinephrine: A catecholamine neurotransmitter in the peripheral nervous system and central nervous system, it is released at most sympathetic neuromuscular and neuroglandular junctions, and a hormone secreted by the adrenal medulla; also called noradrenaline.

Nuclear bag fibers: Fibers that lie in the center of each intrafusal muscle fiber of a muscle spindle. Each has a large number of nuclei concentrated in bags, which cause excitation of both the primary and secondary nerve fibers.

Nuclear chain fibers: Fibers numbering 3–9 per muscle spindle, which are half the size of the nuclear bag fibers. Their nuclei are aligned in a chain and they excite the secondary nerve. Nuclear chain fibers are static; nuclear bag fibers are dynamic.

Nucleosidases: Hydrolytic enzymes that catalyze the hydrolysis of a nucleotide into a nucleoside and a phosphate.

Nucleus cuneatus: A wedge-shaped nucleus in the closed part of the medulla oblongata. It contains cells that give rise to the cuneate tubercle, visible on the posterior aspect of the medulla.

Nucleus gracilis: The medial of the three nuclei of the dorsal spinal column, receiving dorsal root fibers conveying sensory innervation of the leg.

Nulliparous: A female that has not become pregnant.

O

Occipital bone: A bone at the lower and posterior part of the skull, consisting of basilar, condylar, and squamous sections. It encloses the foramen magnum.

Occipital lobe: The posterior lobe of each cerebral hemisphere, having the shape of a three-sided pyramid and containing the visual center of the brain.

Oestrous: British spelling of estrous.

Oestrus: British spelling of estrus (sexual receptivity or heat in the female).

Olfaction: The sense of smell.

Olfactory: Of, relating to, or connected with the sense of smell.

Olfactory (Bowman's) glands: Any of the tubular and often branched glands occurring beneath the olfactory epithelium of the nose.

Olfactory bulb: A structure of the vertebrate forebrain involved in olfaction, the perception of odors.

Olfactory cortex: The sensory system used for olfaction.

Olfactory receptors: A type of G protein–coupled receptor in olfactory receptor neurons. In vertebrates, the olfactory receptors are located in the olfactory epithelium.

Oligodendrocyte: Central nervous system neuroglia cell type that maintains cellular organization within the gray matter and provides a myelin sheath in areas of white matter.

Olivary nuclei: A smooth oval prominence of the ventrolateral surface of the medulla oblongata lateral to the pyramidal tract, corresponding to the olivary nucleus; also called the oliva or olive.

Omasoabomasal orifice: The opening between the omasum and abomasum of the ruminant stomach compartments.

Omasum: Also known as the "manyplies" because of its appearance like pages of a wet book, it is the third compartment of the stomach in ruminants. Though its functions have not been well studied, it appears to primarily aid in the absorption of water, magnesium, and fermentation acids.

Oncotic pressure: Pressure exerted by the vitreous humor of the eye.

Oocyte: The developing egg.

Opsin: A group of light-sensitive 35–55 kDa membrane-bound G protein–coupled receptors found in photoreceptor cells of the retina. They are involved in vision, mediating the conversion of a photon of light into an electrochemical signal, the first step in the visual transduction cascade.

Optic chiasm: A flattened quadrangular body that is the point of crossing of the fibers of the optic nerves; also called the optic decussation.

Optic chiasma: The part of the brain where the optic nerves partially cross. Specifically, the nerves connected to the right eye that associate the right visual field of the left eye and vice versa for the left eye.

Optic disc: The point in the eye where the optic nerve fibres leave the retina.

Optic radiation: A collection of axons from relay neurons in the lateral geniculate nucleus of the thalamus carrying visual information to the visual cortex (also called the striate cortex) along the calcarine fissure.

Optic vesicles: An evagination on either side of the embryonic forebrain from which the optic nerve and retina develop.

Ora serrata: The serrated junction between the retina and the ciliary body. This junction marks the transition from the simple nonphotosensitive area of the retina to the complex, multilayered photosensitive region.

Oral: Pertaining to the mouth.

Organ physiology: The study of specific organs, e.g., cardiac or ovarian.

Origin: The point of attachment of a muscle that remains relatively fixed during contraction of the muscle.

Oropharynx: The middle portion of the pharynx, bounded superiorly by the nasopharynx, anteriorly by the oral cavity, and inferiorly by the laryngopharynx.

Osmosis: The movement of water across a selectively permeable membrane from one solution to another solution that contains a higher solute concentration.

Ossification: The formation of bone.

Ossification center: The site where bone begins to form in a specific bone or part of bone as a result of the accumulation of osteoblasts in the connective tissue.

Osteoblast: A cell that produces the fibers and matrix of bone.

Osteocyte: A bone cell responsible for the maintenance and turnover of the mineral content of the surrounding bone.

Osteogenesis: Formation and development of bony tissue; also called osteogeny.

Osteoid: The bone matrix, especially before calcification.

Osteomalacia: A disease occurring primarily in adults that results from a deficiency in vitamin D or calcium and is characterized by a softening of the bones with accompanying pain and weakness; also called adult rickets or late rickets.

Osteon: The basic histological unit of compact bone, consisting of osteocytes organized around a central canal and separated by concentric lamellae.

Osteonal canal: Located at the center of osteons, this canal contains blood vessels, a nerve, and bone fluid.

Osteoprogenitor cells: A mesenchymal cell that differentiates into an osteoblast; also called a preosteoblast.

Otolithic membrane: A gelatinous membrane located in the vestibular apparatus of the inner ear, which plays an essential role in the brain's interpretation of equilibrium. Both the saccular macula and utricular macula are covered by an otolithic membrane.

Outer ear: The external portion of the ear, which includes the eardrum.

Outer hair cells: Acoustical preamplifiers.

Outer synaptic layers: The location within the retina where connections are made between photoreceptors and cells of the inner nuclear layer, and the nuclear layer cells contact ganglion cells.

Oxidative: A reaction in which the atoms in an element lose electrons and the valence of the element is correspondingly increased.

Oxidative phosphorylation: The process of ATP synthesis during which an inorganic phosphate group becomes attached to ADP. It occurs via the electron transport chain in the mitochondria and to a lesser extent as a result of substrate level phosphorylation.

Oxygen debt: The amount of extra oxygen required by muscle tissue to oxidize lactic acid and replenish depleted ATP and phosphocreatine following vigorous exercise.

Oxygen-hemoglobin dissociation curve: A graph describing the relationship between the percentages of hemoglobin saturated with oxygen and a range of oxygen partial pressures.

Oxyhemoglobin: An oxygen-bound form of hemoglobin.

Oxytocin: A hormone produced by neurons in the hypothalamus and released by nerve terminals in the posterior pituitary gland. Primary systemic effects are to elicit milk ejection and uterine contractions. However, oxytocin is also produced locally by the corpus luteum.

P

P wave: A deflection of the ECG corresponding to atrial depolarization.

Pacemaker cells: A device by which the contractions of the heart are controlled by electrical impulses; these impulses occur at a rate that controls the beat of the heart. The cells that create these rhythmical impulses are called pacemaker cells.

Pacinian corpuscle: An encapsulated receptor found in deep layers of the skin that senses vibratory pressure and touch.

Palate: The horizontal partition separating the oral cavity from the nasal cavity and nasopharynx; it is divided into an anterior bony (hard) palate and a posterior fleshy (soft) palate.

Palatine bones: Pertaining to the palate.

Palatopharyngeal arches: Either of two ridges or folds of mucous membrane passing from the soft palate to the wall of the pharynx and enclosing the palatopharyngeal muscle.

Palpebral fissure: A fissure that separates the upper and lower eyelids.

Pancreatic duct: A tubular duct that carries pancreatic juice from the pancreas to the duodenum.

Pancreatic islets: Aggregations of endocrine cells embedded within the exocrine tissue of the pancreas; also called the islets of Langerhans.

Paneth cells: Cells that provide host defense against microbes in the small intestine. They are functionally similar to neutrophils. When exposed to bacteria or bacterial antigens, these cells secrete antimicrobial molecules into the lumen of the crypt, thereby contributing to maintenance of the gastrointestinal barrier.

Papillae: Any of the small projections on the top of the tongue, in particular vallate and fungiform papillae, that contain taste buds.

Papillary muscle: A nipplelike conical projection of myocardium within the ventricle; the chordae tendineae are attached to the apex of the papillary muscle.

Parahippocampal gyrus: A long convolution located on the medial surface of the temporal lobe of the brain and forming the lower part of the gyrus fornicatus; also called the hippocampal gyrus.

Paranasal sinuses: Bony chambers, lined by respiratory epithelium, that open into the nasal cavity; the frontal, ethmoidal, sphenoidal, and maxillary sinuses.

Parasympathetic divisions: One of the two divisions of the autonomic nervous system; also called the craniosacral division; generally responsible for activities that conserve energy and lower the metabolic rate.

Parasympathetic subdivision: One of three divisions of the autonomic nervous system. Sometimes called the "rest and digest" system, the parasympathetic system conserves energy as it slows the heart rate, increases intestinal and gland activity, and relaxes sphincter muscles in the gastrointestinal tract.

Parenchyma: The functional portion of a tissue or organ. For example, in the exocrine pancreas the acini that produce and secrete enzymes are parenchyma.

Parietal cells: Cells of the gastric gland that secrete hydrochloric acid and intrinsic factor.

Parietal lobe: The middle portion of each cerebral hemisphere, separated from the frontal lobe by the central sulcus, from the temporal lobe by the lateral sulcus, and from the occipital lobe only partially by the parieto-occipital sulcus on its medial aspect.

Parietal serosa: The part of the double-layered membrane that lines the walls of the ventral body cavity.

Parieto-occipital sulcus: A deep fissure on the medial surface of the cerebral cortex marking the border between the parietal lobe and the cuneus of the occipital lobe; also called the parieto-occipital fissure.

Parotid salivary gland: Large salivary glands that secrete saliva that contain high concentrations of salivary (alpha) amylase.

Partial pressure: The pressure exerted by a single component of a mixture of gases.

Parvocellular (P cells): Slow-conducting neurons that transmit information about color vision, texture, pattern, and visual acuity. The cells transmit the information to the lateral geniculate nucleus.

Passive immunity: Immunity that is derived from transfer rather than activation of an animal's own immune system. Examples include antibodies passed to the fetus in utero or across the gut of the newborn via colostrum ingestion.

Pelvic cavity: The inferior subdivision of the abdominopelvic cavity, it encloses the urinary bladder, the sigmoid colon and rectum, and male or female reproductive organs.

Pelvic symphysis: The midline cartilaginous joint uniting the superior rami of the left and right pubic bones.

Perception: Recognition and interpretation of sensory stimuli based chiefly on memory.

Pericardial cavity: The space between the parietal pericardium and the epicardium (visceral pericardium) at the outer surface of the heart.

Pericarditis: An inflammation of the pericardium.

Pericardium: The fibrous sac that surrounds the heart; its inner, serous lining is continuous with the epicardium.

Perichondrium: The dense irregular fibrous membrane of connective tissue covering the surface of cartilage except at the endings of joints.

Perikaryon: The cytoplasm that surrounds the nucleus in the cell body of a neuron.

Perilymph: Extracellular fluid located within the cochlea (part of the ear) in two of its three compartments; the scala tympani and scala vestibuli.

Perineurium: The sheath of connective tissue enclosing a bundle of nerve fibers.

Periosteum: The thick fibrous membrane covering the entire surface of a bone, except its articular cartilage, and serving as an attachment for muscles and tendons.

Peripheral nervous system: The portion of the nervous system consisting of nerves and ganglia that lies outside the brain and spinal cord.

Peristalsis: A wave of smooth muscle contractions that propels materials along the axis of a tube such as the digestive tract, the ureters, or the ductus deferens.

Peritoneal cavity: *See* abdominopelvic cavity.

Peritoneum: The serous membrane that lines the peritoneal cavity.

Phagocytosis: The amoebalike engulfment of extracellular material by one of the immune cells, most often neutrophils or macrophages.

Pharyngotympanic: *See* auditory tube.

Pharynx: The throat; a muscular passageway shared by the digestive and respiratory tracts.

Philtrum: The midline groove in the upper lip that runs from the top of the lip to the nose.

Phosphatase: An enzyme that hydrolyses phosphoric acid monoesters into a phosphate ion and a molecule with a free hydroxyl group.

Phosphatidyinositol-3-kinase (PI3K): An enzyme involved in the synthesis of the phosphoinositide family of lipid second messengers. Members of this family of intracellular signaling molecules are thought to be critical to suppress signals that can cause apoptosis or programmed cell death.

Phosphodiesterease: Enzymes that split phosphodiester bonds—for example, in the conversion of cyclic AMP to AMP.

Phospholipid: A class of essential lipids needed for creation of cellular membranes. They are usually composed of two fatty acids attached to glycerol and an additional polar group, e.g., choline.

Phosphorylation: The addition of a phosphate group to a protein, most often by the action of an enzyme called a kinase.

Photopigments: Located in photoreceptor outer segment disc membranes, they change their conformation on the perception of photons. The conformational change allows the photopigment to interact with transducin and to start the visual cascade.

Photoreceptor: A specialized type of neuron found in the eye's retina that is capable of phototransduction. More specifically, the photoreceptor sends signals to other neurons by a change in its membrane potential when it absorbs photons.

Physiology: The study of function, which deals with the ways organisms perform vital activities.

Pia mater: The fine vascular membrane that closely envelops the brain and spinal cord under the arachnoid and the dura mater.

Pigmented layer: The layer of the retina that consists of a single stratum of cells. In the eyes of albinos, the cells of this layer contain no pigment.

Pineal body: A small, unpaired, flattened glandular structure lying in the depression between the two superior colliculi of the brain and secreting the hormone melatonin; also called the conarium, epiphysis, or pineal gland.

Pitch: The tone of a sound, determined by the frequency of vibrations (that is, whether a sound is a C or G note).

Placenta: The reproduction structure that allows metabolic exchanges between fetus and mother. It is composed of a embryonic tissue (the chorion) and maternal tissue (endometrium). The placenta also functions as an endocrine organ during gestation.

Plasmin: A proteolytic enzyme important in dissolution of blood clots. It converts fibrin to soluble components.

Plasminogen: An inactive form of plasmin found in blood and tissue fluids.

Pleura: The serous membrane that lines the pleural cavities.

Pleural cavities: Subdivisions of the thoracic cavity that contain the lungs.

Pleural membrane: The membrane lining the lung and the chest cavity.

Pleurisy: An inflammation of the pleura; also called pleuritis.

Plica: A permanent transverse fold in the wall of the small intestine.

Pluripotent stem cells: Precursor cells—for example, those that reside in the bone marrow and continuously divide and differentiate to give rise to each of the types of blood cells.

Pneumotaxic area: A center in the reticular formation of the pons that regulates the activities of the apneustic and respiratory rhythmicity centers to adjust the pace of respiration; also called pneumotaxic center.

Pneumothorax: The introduction of air into the pleural cavity.

Polycythemia: An excessive or abnormal increase in the number of erythrocytes.

Polyestrous: Exhibiting multiple estrous cycles distributed throughout the year, i.e., no seasonal anestrous.

Polyestrus: Exhibiting multiple episodes of estrus distributed throughout the year.

Polymorphonuclear leukocytes: Another name for a neutrophil, the name describes the fact that the cell has a lobed nucleus, which makes it appear as if it has multiple (*poly*) nuclei.

Polysynaptic reflex: A reflex in which interneurons are interposed between the sensory fiber and the motor neuron(s).

Polytocous: Mammals that give birth to multiple offspring (litters).

Pontine reticulospinal tract: Any of several fiber tracts descending to the spinal cord from the reticular formation of the pons and medulla oblongata. Some fibers conduct impulses from the neural mechanisms regulating cardiovascular and respiratory functions to the spinal cord; others form links in extrapyramidal motor mechanisms affecting muscle tonus and somatic movement.

Portal triad: Branches of the portal vein, hepatic artery, and hepatic duct bound together in the connective tissue that divides the liver into lobules.

Positive chronotropic factors: Agents that increase heart rate.

Postcentral gyrus: The anterior convolution of the parietal lobe, bounded in front by the central sulcus and in back by the interparietal sulcus.

Posterior chamber: A narrow chink behind the peripheral part of the iris of the eye and in front of the suspensory ligament of the lens and the ciliary processes.

Posterior cranial fossa: Part of the intracranial cavity, located between the Foramen magnum and Tentorium cerebelli. It contains the brain stem and cerebellum.

Posterior (dorsal) horns: The occipital division of the lateral ventricle of the brain, extending backward into the occipital lobe; also called the dorsal horn.

Posterior median sulcus: The longitudinal groove marking the posterior midline of the medulla oblongata and continuous below with the posterior median sulcus of the spinal cord; also called the posterior median fissure.

Posterior neuropore: The posterior opening leading from the central canal of the embryonic neural tube to the exterior.

Posterior segment: The back two-thirds of the eye, which includes the anterior hyaloid membrane and all structures behind it: the vitreous humor, retina, choroid, and optic nerve.

Postganglionic: Located posterior or distal to a ganglion.

Postsynaptic membrane: The portion of the cell membrane of a postsynaptic cell that is part of a synapse.

Postsynaptic potential: Changes in the membrane potential of the neuron that receives information at a synapse.

Posttranslational modification: Enzyme-mediated changes to proteins made after initial synthesis. This most often occurs in the Golgi apparatus and can include phosphorylation, glycosylation, or methylation.

Potential difference: The separation of opposite charges; requires a barrier that prevents ion migration.

P–Q interval: Time elapsing between the beginning of the P wave and the beginning of the QRS complex in the electrocardiogram; also called the PR interval.

Precapillary sphincter: A smooth muscle sphincter that regulates blood flow through a capillary.

Precentral gyrus: The posterior convolution of the frontal lobe, bounded in back by the central sulcus and in front by the precentral sulcus.

Preganglionic: Situated proximal to or preceding a ganglion, especially a ganglion of the autonomic nervous system.

Premolars: Transitional teeth located between the canine and molar teeth.

Presbyopia: The eye's diminished power of accommodation, which occurs with aging.

Presynaptic inhibition: A reduction in the release of a neurotransmitter from a presynaptic axon terminal as a result of excitation of another neuron that terminates on the axon terminal.

Presynaptic membrane: The synaptic surface where neurotransmitter release occurs.

Pretectal nuclei: A structure located in the midbrain. It receives binocular input from the eyes and is involved with the pupillary light reflex.

Prevertebral ganglia: Any of the sympathetic ganglia lying in front of the vertebral column, including the celiac and the superior and inferior mesenteric ganglions.

Primary fissure: The trilobed structure of the brain, lying posterior to the pons and medulla oblongata and inferior to the occipital lobes of the cerebral hemispheres, responsible for the regulation and coordination of complex voluntary muscular movement and the maintenance of posture and balance.

Primary hyperalgesia: Pain sensitivity that occurs directly in the damaged tissues.

Primary motor area: A group of networked cells in mammalian brains that controls movements of specific body parts associated with cell groups in that area of the brain. The area is closely linked by neural networks to corresponding areas in the primary somatosensory cortex.

Primary visual cortex: The part of the cerebral cortex that is responsible for processing visual stimuli. It is the simplest, earliest cortical visual area. It is highly specialized for processing information about static and moving objects and is excellent in pattern recognition.

Primiparous: A term indicating a mammal that is experiencing its first pregnancy or that is in the period following the birth of its first offspring.

Proerythroblasts: The precursor of the erythroblast, which in turn produces red blood cells or erythrocytes.

Proestrus: The stage of the estrus cycle between luteolysis and onset of estrus (heat).

Progenitor cells: A less mature cell in a developmental pathway. For example, in the immune system B lymphocytes are the precursors of plasma cells.

Progesterone: A steroid hormone primarily produced by the ovary (corpus luteum) and placenta. It is necessary for maintenance of pregnancy as well as normal mammary development.

Prohormone: A precursor of a hormone, it usually refers to a larger protein structure, which is cleaved to produce the active agent.

Prolactin (Prl): A protein produced in the anterior pituitary gland, it is a critical regulator of mammary gland function and other physiological processes, including regulation of fluid balances and some aspects of behavior.

Pronation: To turn or rotate (the foot) by abduction and eversion so that the inner edge of the sole bears the body's weight.

Proprioceptors: A sensory receptor, commonly found in muscles, tendons, joints, and the inner ear, that detects the motion or position of the body or a limb by responding to stimuli within the organism.

Prosencephalon: The most anterior of the three primary regions of the embryonic brain, from which the telencephalon and diencephalon develop.

Prostacyclin: A prostaglandin produced in the walls of blood vessels that acts as a vasodilator and inhibits platelet aggregation.

Prostaglandin (PG): A large group of structurally related hormone or growth factor–like regulators (including PGE, PGF, PGA, and PGB) found in tissues throughout the body. They are derived from arachidonic acid and exhibit multiple actions.

Proteoglycan: An example of a common extracellular matrix molecule, it consists of a glycoaminoglycans (GAG) chains attached to a protein core. These molecules are important in maintenance of intercellular spaces.

Protraction: The extension of teeth or other maxillary or mandibular structures into a position anterior to the normal position.

Proventriculus: A section of the avian digestive tract, located before the gizzard.

Pseudo-unipolar neuron: Another term for unipolar neuron.

Pulmonary arteries: Vessels that deliver blood to the lungs to be oxygenated.

Pulmonary circuit: Blood vessels between the pulmonary semilunar valve of the right ventricle and the entrance to the left atrium of the heart. It describes the blood flow to and from the lungs.

Pulmonary circulation: The closed loop of blood vessels carrying blood between the heart and lungs.

Pulmonary trunk: The large elastic artery that carries blood from the right ventricle of the heart to the right and left pulmonary arteries.

Pulmonary valve: A one-way valve that permits the flow of blood from the right ventricle into the pulmonary artery during ventricular emptying but prevents the backflow of blood from the pulmonary artery into the right ventricle during ventricular relaxation.

Pulmonary veins: Vessels that deliver freshly oxygenated blood from the respiratory zones of the lungs to the heart.

Pulmonary ventilation: The movement of air into and out of the lungs.

Pulp cavity: The internal chamber in a tooth, containing blood vessels, lymphatic vessels, nerves, and the cells that maintain the dentin.

Pulse pressure: Difference between systolic and diastolic pressure.

Pupil: The opening in the middle of the iris. It appears black because most of the light entering is absorbed by the tissues inside the eye.

Purine: One of two categories of nitrogenous ringed compounds found in RNA and DNA (the others are the pyrimidines); examples are adenine and guanine.

Purkinje cells: Any of numerous neurons of the cerebral cortex having large flask-shaped cell bodies with massive dendrites and one slender axon; also called the Purkinje corpuscles.

Putamen: The outer, larger, and darker gray of the three portions into which the lentiform nucleus of the brain is divided.

Pyloric region: The region of the stomach that connects to the duodenum.

Pyloric sphincter: A sphincter of smooth muscle that regulates the passage of chyme from the stomach to the duodenum.

Pylorus: The gastric region between the body of the stomach and the duodenum; it includes the pyloric sphincter.

Pyramidal system: a massive collection of axons that travel between the cerebral cortex of the brain and the spinal cord.

Pyrimidine: One of two classes of nitrogenous bases found in DNA and RNA examples; a sample is cytosine. The other class is purine.

Q

QRS complex: The principal deflection in the electrocardiogram, representing ventricular depolarization.

Quiescent period: The time interval of no activity occurring between each pulse during transmission.

R

Radioimmunoassay (RIA): A sensitive assay method to measure the concentration of hormones and other factors in biological fluids. The technique depends on the ability to produce antibodies against the substance under study and to label it with a radioisotope.

Ramp retina: The human retina has a smooth concave surface, but the horse has a ramp retina, which is irregular and inconsistent in its concave appearance.

Ras protein: An example of a large family of GTP-binding proteins that serve to relay signals from cell surface receptors to the cell nucleus. It was named for the ras gene, first identified in viruses that cause sarcoma in rats.

Reabsorption: The net movement of interstitial fluid into the capillary.

Receptive fields: A sensory neuron is a region of space in which the presence of a stimulus will alter the firing of that neuron. Receptive fields have been identified for neurons of the auditory system, the somatosensory system, and the visual system.

Receptor: A specialized cell or group of nerve endings that responds to sensory stimuli.

Receptor potential: The transmembrane potential difference of a sensory cell.

Rectum: The inferior 15 cm (6 in) of the digestive tract.

Red bone marrow: Bone marrow characterized by meshes of the reticular network that contain the developmental stages of red blood cells, white blood cells, and megakaryocytes.

Red muscle fibers: Those fibers that have a red appearance; they contain high levels of myoglobin and oxygen-storing proteins and tend to have more mitochondria and blood vessels than the white ones.

Red nucleus: A large, well-defined, somewhat elongated cell mass of reddish-gray hue that is located in the mesencephalic tegmentum, receives a massive projection from the contralateral half of the cerebellum, receives an additional projection from the ipsilateral motor cortex, and whose efferent connections are with the contralateral half of the rhombencephalic reticular formation and spinal cord.

Reduced hemoglobin: Hemoglobin that is not combined with O_2.

Referred pain: Pain that is felt in a part of the body at a distance from its area of origin.

Reflex arch: The receptor, sensory neuron, motor neuron, and effector involved in a particular reflex; interneurons may be present, depending on the reflex considered.

Refracted: The ability of the eye to bend light so that an image is focused on the retina.

Relative refractory period: The period that follows the absolute refractory period; the interval during which a threshold stimulus is unable to trigger an action potential unless the stimulus is particularly strong.

Releasing hormones: The general name given a number of small peptides synthesized by hypothalamic neurons whose release into the hypothalamic-hypophyseal portal blood system control secretion of anterior pituitary hormones.

Renin: The enzyme released by cells of the juxtaglomerular apparatus when renal blood flow declines; it converts angiotensinogen to angiotensin I.

Residual volume: The amount of air remaining in the lungs after maximum forced exhalation.

Resistance: Hindrance of flow of blood or air through a passageway (blood vessel or respiratory airway, respectively).

Resorption: The act or the process of resorbing.

Respiratory bronchiole: The smallest bronchiole (0.5 mm in diameter) that connects the terminal bronchiole to the alveolar duct.

Respiratory burst: The rapid release of reactive oxygen species (superoxide radical and hydrogen peroxide) from different types of cells.

Respiratory capacities: The amount of air that can be forcibly expelled from the lungs following breathing in as deeply as possible.

Respiratory membrane: The membrane that consists of the epithelial cells of the alveolus, the endothelial cells of the capillary, and the two fused basement membranes of these layers. Gas exchange occurs across this respiratory membrane.

Respiratory pump: A mechanism by which changes in the intrapleural pressures during the respiratory cycle assist the venous return to the heart; also called the thoracoabdominal pump.

Respiratory rhythmicity center: An area of the brain stem that is involved in the control of respiration.

Resting membrane potential: The voltage that exists across the plasma membrane during the resting state of an excitable cell. Values range from −50 to −200 millivolts, depending on cell type.

Reticular activating system (RAS): The name given to part of the brain (the reticular formation and its connections) believed to be the center of arousal and motivation in animals. It is situated at the core of the brain stem between the myelencephalon (medulla oblongata) and metencephalon (midbrain).

Reticulocyte: An immature erythrocyte.

Reticulorumen: The first chamber in the alimentary canal of ruminant animals, it is composed of the rumen and reticulum.

Retina: A thin layer of neural cells that lines the back of the eyeball of vertebrates and some cephalopods.

Retinal: A carotenoid constituent of visual pigments. It is the oxidized form of retinol, which functions as the active component of the visual cycle. It is bound to the protein opsin forming the complex rhodopsin. When stimulated by visible light, the retinal component of the rhodopsin complex undergoes isomerization at the 11-position of the double bond to the cis-form. This is reversed in "dark" reactions to return to the native *trans* configuration.

Retinal isomerase: An enzyme that catalyzes the conversion of the *trans* form of retinaldehyde to 11-cis-retinal, a reaction needed in the regeneration of the visual pigments.

Retraction: The act of pulling apart, usually as part of a surgical procedure.

Retroperitoneal: Located behind or outside the peritoneal cavity. For example, both male and female reproductive tracts and kidney are retroperitoneal.

Rhinencephalon areas: A part of the brain involved with olfaction.

Rhodopsin: Also known as visual purple, it is expressed in vertebrate photoreceptor cells. It is a pigment of the retina that is responsible for both the formation of the photoreceptor cells and the first events in the perception of light.

Rhombencephalon: The portion of the embryonic brain from which the metencephalon and myelencephalon develop, including the pons, cerebellum, and medulla oblongata; also called the hindbrain.

Rib: One of a series of long, curved bones occurring in pairs and extending from the spine to or toward the sternum.

Right colic (hepatic) flexure: A bend in the colon that is adjacent to the liver, and is therefore also known as the hepatic colic flexure.

Rigor mortis: Muscular stiffening following death; also called postmortem rigidity.

Rods: Photoreceptor cells in the retina of the eye that can function in less intense light than can the other type of photoreceptor, cone cells.

Root canals: The narrow extension of the pulp cavity that projects into the roots.

Rotation: Regular and uniform variation in a sequence or series, as in the recurrence of symptoms of a disease.

Rough endoplasmic reticulum (RER): The cellular organelle involved in translation of mRNA for synthesis of proteins for secretion from cells. It appears in transmission electron micrographs as parallel arrays of intracellular membranes studded with ribosomes.

Round ligament: The fibromuscular band that is attached to the uterus on either side in front of and below the opening of the uterine tube; it passes through the inguinal canal to the labium majus.

Ruffini ending: One of the four main cutaneous mechanoreceptors. Named after Angelo Ruffini, they are slowly adapting receptors found in the dermis and subcutaneous tissue of the skin. These thin cigar-shaped encapsulated sensory endings measure pressure when the skin is stretched. Their main function is thermoreception.

Rugae: Mucosal folds in the lining of the empty stomach that disappear as gastric distension occurs.

Rumen: The larger part of the reticulorumen, which is the first chamber in the alimentary canal of ruminant animals.

Ruminant: Any hoofed animal that digests its food in two steps, first by eating the raw material and regurgitating a semidigested form known as cud, and then eating the cud, a process called ruminating.

Rumination: An eating disorder characterized by having the contents of the stomach drawn back up into the mouth, chewed for a second time, and swallowed again. In some animals, known as ruminants, this is a natural and healthy part of digestion and is not considered an eating disorder.

S

Sacroiliac joint: The joint between the sacrum, at the base of the spine, and the ilium of the pelvis, which are joined by ligaments. Inflammation of this joint is known as *sacroiliitis*, one cause of disabling low back pain.

Sagittal plane: A sectional plane that divides the body into left and right portions.

Saltatory conduction: Transmission of an action potential along a myelinated fiber in which the nerve impulse appears to leap from node to node.

Sarcolemma: A thin membrane enclosing a striated muscle fiber.

Sarcomere: One of the segments into which a fibril of striated muscle is divided.

Sarcoplasm: The cytoplasm of a striated muscle fiber.

Sarcoplasmic reticulum: The endoplasmic reticulum found in striated muscle fibers.

Satellite cells: Any of the cells that encapsulate the bodies of nerve cells in many ganglia.

Scala media: An endolymph-filled cavity inside the cochlea, located between the scala tympani and the scala vestibuli, separated by the basilar membrane and Reissner's membrane (the vestibular membrane), respectively.

Scala tympani: The name of one of the perilymph-filled cavities in the cochlear labyrinth. It is separated from the scala media by the basilar membrane, and it extends from the round window to the helicotrema, where it continues as scala vestibuli.

Scala vestibuli: A perilymph-filled cavity inside the cochlea of the inner ear. It is separated from the scala media by Reissner's membrane and extends from the oval window to the helicotrema where it joins the scala tympani.

Scapula: Either of two large, flat, triangular bones forming the back part of the shoulder. More commonly called the shoulder blade.

Schwann cells: Neuroglia responsible for the neurilemma that surrounds axons in the peripheral nervous system.

Sclera: The (usually) white outer coating of the eye made of tough fibrin connective tissue, which gives the eye its shape and helps protect the delicate inner parts.

Scleral venous sinus (canal of Schlemm): A circular channel in the eye that collects aqueous humor from the anterior chamber and delivers it into the bloodstream.

Seasonal anestrus: A period of anestrous produced by exposure of either short (mare) or long (ewe) photoperiods.

Seasonal polyestrus: The term for exhibiting multiple estrous cycles during certain times of the year.

Sebaceous ciliary gland: Holocrine glands found in the skin of mammals. They secrete an oily substance called sebum (Latin, meaning "fat" or "tallow") that is made of fat (lipids) and the debris of dead fat-producing cells.

Second messenger: An intracellular molecule whose concentration changes as a consequence of a hormone binding to a cell surface receptor. The released molecule serves to carry the signal of the hormone (first messenger) into the target cell to elicit a reaction. The first second messenger identified in conjunction with the effects of glucagon was cyclic AMP.

Secondary hyperalgesia: Pain sensitivity that occurs in surrounding undamaged tissues.

Secondary ossification center: About the time of birth, a secondary ossification center appears in each end (epiphysis) of long bones. Periosteal buds carry mesenchyme and blood vessels in and the process is similar to that occurring in a primary ossification center.

Secretin: A hormone secreted by the duodenum that stimulates the production of buffers by the pancreas and inhibits gastric activity.

Secretion: The process of segregating, elaborating, and releasing chemicals from a cell, or a secreted chemical substance or amount of substance.

Segmentation: A morphogenesis process that divides a metazoan body into a series of semirepetitive segments.

Selectins: A family of transmembrane molecules expressed on the surface of leukocytes and activated endothelial cells.

Self-propagating: Propagating by one's self or by itself.

Semicircular canals: A group of three half-circular, interconnected tubes located inside each ear that are the equivalent of three gyroscopes located in three planes perpendicular.

Semicircular ducts: Consists of three oval ducts arranged at right angles to one another; an integral part of the equilibrium mechanism.

Seminiferous tubules: The highly convoluted tubules, located in the testes, that produce spermatozoa.

Sensations: A perception associated with stimulation of a sense organ or with a specific body condition.

Sensory areas: The main cerebral areas that receive sensory information from thalamic nerve projections.

Sensory input: Input that includes somatic sensation and special senses.

Sensory nerve: An afferent nerve conveying impulses that are processed by the central nervous system to become part of the organism's perception of itself and of its environment.

Sensory neurons: Nerve cells within the nervous system responsible for converting external stimuli from the organism's environment into internal electrical motor reflex loops and several forms of involuntary behavior, including pain avoidance.

Septum pellucidum: A thin membrane of nervous tissue that forms the medial wall of the lateral ventricles in the brain. It is also called the septum lucidum.

Serosa: *See* serous membrane.

Serosal fluid: Clear, watery fluid secreted by cells of a serous membrane.

Serotonin: A neurotransmitter in the central nervous system; a compound that enhances inflammation and is released by activated mast cells and basophils.

Serous cell: A cell that produces a serous secretion.

Serous membrane: A squamous epithelium and the underlying loose connective tissue; the lining of the pericardial, pleural, and peritoneal cavities.

Serous pericardium: The lining of the pericardial sac composed of a serous membrane.

Sertoli cells: Cells located in the seminiferous tubules of the testes that are thought to control spermatogenesis. They contain FSH receptors and were named for the Italian reproductive physiologist Enrico Sertoli.

Serum: The ground substance of blood plasma from which clotting agents have been removed.

Sesamoid bone: A bone that forms within a tendon.

Sharpey's fibers: A matrix of connective tissue consisting of bundles of strong collagenous fibers connecting periosteum to bone. They are part of the outer fibrous layer of periosteum, entering into the outer circumferential and interstitial lamellae of bone tissue.

Short bone: A bone whose dimensions are approximately equal, consisting of a layer of cortical substance enclosing the spongy substance and marrow.

Short day breeders: Sexually mature females that begin to initiate estrous cycles during periods with reduced photoperiods, i.e., short days.

Sigmoid colon: The S-shaped portion of the colon, 18 cm long, between the descending colon and the rectum.

Signal peptide: A small sequence of amino acids in the structure of a newly synthesized protein if the protein will be transported to the Golgi apparatus for packaging and secretion from the cell.

Signal transduction: The relaying of a signal from one form to another. In physiological processes, this is the process whereby extracellular signals are converted into intracellular responses.

Signaling transducers and activators of transcription (STATs): Regulators that make a group of transcription factors (seven are recognized) that are sequestered in the cytoplasm until activated by the binding of a cytokine or growth factor receptor. Ligand binding causes aggregation of receptor (cytokine) subunits and initiation of a cascade of tyrosine phosphorylation events, during which receptor-linked JAKs become activated to cause phosphorylation of the receptor. This creates a docking or binding site for a STAT that is, in turn, phosphorylated by the receptor. Phosphorylated STAT dissociates from the receptor, dimerizes, and translocates to the cell nucleus to interact with the promoters of specific genes. For example, STAT-5 is known to be essential for the hormone prolactin to induce production of mRNA for milk proteins.

Simple fracture: A bone fracture that causes little or no damage to the surrounding soft tissues; also called a closed fracture.

Single-unit smooth muscle: The most abundant type of smooth muscle. It is made up of muscle fibers that are interconnected by gap junctions so that they become excited and contract as a unit; also known as visceral smooth muscle.

Sinoatrial (SA) node: The natural pacemaker of the heart. It is located in the wall of the right atrium.

Sinusoidal capillary: A capillary with a caliber of from 10–20 μm or more; it is lined with a fenestrated type of endothelium.

Sinusoids: An exchange vessel that is similar in general structure to a fenestrated capillary. The two differ in size (sinusoids are larger and more irregular in cross section), continuity (sinusoids have gaps between endothelial cells), and support (sinusoids have thin basal laminae, if they have them at all).

Skeletal muscle: Muscle composed of cylindrical multinucleate cells with obvious striations; the muscle(s) attached to the body's skeleton; voluntary muscle.

Sleep spindles: A burst of brain activity, visible on an EEG, that occurs during stage 2 sleep. It consists of 12–16 Hz waves that occur for 0.5 to 1.5 sec.

Sliding filament theory: The concept that a sarcomere shortens as the thick and thin filaments slide past one another in the muscle cell.

Slow oxidative fibers: Fibers that generate energy for ATP resynthesis by means of a long-term system of aerobic energy transfer. They tend to have a low activity level of ATPase, a slower speed of contraction with a less-developed glycolytic capacity. They contain large and numerous mitochondria, and, coupled with the high levels of myoglobin, that gives them a red pigmentation. They have been demonstrated to have a high concentration of mitochondrial enzymes, and thus they are fatigue resistant.

Slow-wave sleep: A term used to describe stages 3 and 4 sleep.

Smell: The ability to perceive odors; also called olfaction.

Smooth muscle: Spindle-shaped cells with one centrally located nucleus and no externally visible striations (bands). It is found mainly in the walls of hollow organs.

Soft palate: The fleshy posterior extension of the hard palate, separating the nasopharynx from the oral cavity.

Solitary nucleus: A slender compact bundle of primary sensory fibers that accompany the vagus, glossopharyngeal, and facial nerves and convey information from stretch receptors and chemoreceptors in the walls of the cardiovascular, respiratory, and intestinal tracts and impulses generated by the receptor cells of the taste buds in the tongue.

Somatic afferent: Fibers that receive information from external sources.

Somatic efferent: Nerve fibers that are responsible for muscle contraction.

Somatic nervous system: That part of the peripheral nervous system associated with the voluntary control of body movements through the action of skeletal muscles, and also the reception of external stimuli.

Somatic reflexes: Reflexes that activate skeletal muscle.

Somatomedin hypothesis: An older idea stating that nearly all of the effects attributed to growth hormone were mediated by GH induction of IGF-I in the liver. When first isolated, IGF-I and IGF-II were known as somatomedin A and B, respectively.

Somatostatin: A 14—amino-acid peptide produced in the hypothalamus and other brain areas as well as the pancreas and gut. It is primarily known for its role in inhibiting the secretion of growth hormone, but it is also likely important in GI tract—nervous system interactions.

Somites: A segmental mass of mesoderm in the vertebrate embryo, occurring in pairs along the notochord and developing into muscles and vertebrae.

Spatial summation: A summation of the local potentials in which two or more action potentials arrive simultaneously at two or more presynaptic terminals that synapse with a single neuron.

Special senses: Any of the five senses related to the organs of sight, hearing, smell, taste, and touch.

Spermatogenesis: The process of creating spermatozoa. It depends on proliferation, meiosis, and differentiation of precursor cells (primary spermatocytes).

Sphenoid bone: A compound bone with winglike processes, situated at the base of the skull.

Sphincter of the hepatopancreatic ampulla (sphincter of Oddi): Controls secretions from the liver, pancreas, and gallbladder into the duodenum of the small intestine.

Spicules: A needlelike structure or part.

Spina bifida: A congenital defect in which the spinal column is imperfectly closed so that part of the meninges or spinal cord may protrude, often resulting in neurological disorders; also called hydrocele spinalis.

Spinal nerves: Any of 31 pairs of nerves emerging from the spinal cord, each attached to the cord by two roots, anterior or ventral and posterior or dorsal (the latter provided with a spinal ganglion). The two roots unite in the intervertebral foramen but divide again into ventral and dorsal rami, or anterior and posterior primary divisions (the former supplying the foreparts of the body and limbs and the latter the muscles and skin of the back).

Spinal reflex: A reflex arc involving the spinal cord.

Spinothalamic tract: A large ascending bundle of fibers in the ventral half of the lateral funiculus of the spinal cord, arising in the posterior horn at all levels of the cord and continuing into the brain stem. It is composed in the spinal cord of a lateral part that conveys impulses associated with pain and temperature sensation and of an anterior part that is involved in tactile sensation.

Spiral ganglion: Cell bodies of sensory neurons that innervate hair cells of the organ of Corti are located in the spiral ganglion.

Spiral organ or organ of Corti: The organ in the inner ear of mammals that contains auditory sensory cells, or "hair cells."

Splanchnic circulation: The blood vessels serving the digestive system.

Splanchnic nerves: Part of the sympathetic nervous system, which is part of the autonomic nervous system. Most sympathetic preganglionic nerves synapse in the sympathetic trunk lying beside the spinal cord, but splanchnic nerves pass through the trunk, travel near their target organ, and synapse in prevertebral ganglia.

S–T segment: The part of an electrocardiogram immediately following the QRS complex and merging into the T wave.

Stapedius muscle: The smallest striated muscle in the body. At just over 1 mm in length, its purpose is to stabilize the smallest bone in the body, the stapes.

Stem cells: Primal undifferentiated cells that retain the ability to produce an identical copy of when they divide (self-renew) and differentiate into other cell types.

Stercobilin: A tetrapyrrole chemical compound created by bacterial action on bilirubin and subsequent oxidation.

Stereocilia: Mechanosensing organelles of hair cells, which respond to fluid motion or fluid pressure changes in numerous types of animals for various functions, primarily hearing.

Sternebrae: One of the four segments of the primordial sternum of the embryo, the fusion of which forms the body of the adult sternum.

Sternum: A long flat bone, articulating with the cartilages of the first seven ribs and with the clavicle, forming the middle part of the anterior wall of the thorax, and consisting of the corpus, manubrium, and xiphoid process; also called the breastbone.

Stimulus transduction: The conversion of a stimulus from one form to another.

Streptokinase: An extracellular metallo-enzyme produced by beta-hemolytic streptococcus and used as an effective and cheap clot-dissolving medication—in some cases, of myocardial infarction (heart attack) and pulmonary embolism.

Stretch reflex: *See* myotatic reflex.

Striated muscles: Muscles that are marked by stripes or bands.

Stroke volume (SV): The amount of blood pumped out of a ventricle during one contraction.

Stroma: The supporting elements in a tissue or organ. For example, in the mammary gland this would be the connective tissue elements that surround and support the ducts and alveoli.

Sty: An inflammation of the sebaceous glands at the base of the eyelashes.

Subarachnoid space: The space between the arachnoid membrane and pia mater that is filled with cerebrospinal fluid and contains the large blood vessels that supply the brain and spinal cord.

Submucosa: The region between the muscularis mucosae and the muscularis externa.

Submucosal glands: Glands that are situated below (*sub*) or underneath the mucosal tissue.

Submucosal (or Meissner's) plexus: A plexus of unmyelinated nerve fibers, derived chiefly from the superior mesenteric plexus and ramifying in the intestinal submucosa.

Subscapular fossa: A depression in either of two large, flat, triangular bones forming the back part of the shoulder or scapula.

Substance P: A short-chain polypeptide that functions as a neurotransmitter, especially in the transmission of pain impulses from peripheral receptors to the central nervous system.

Substantia gelatinosa: The apical part of the posterior horn of the gray matter of the spinal cord composed largely of very small nerve cells and whose gelatinous appearance is due to its very low content of myelinated nerve fibers. It functions in the integration of sensory stimuli that gives rise to the sensations of heat and pain; also called Rolando's gelatinous substance.

Substantia nigra: A layer of large pigmented nerve cells in the mesencephalon that produce dopamine and whose destruction is associated with Parkinson's disease; also called nigra.

Subthalamic nucleus: A circumscript nucleus that is located in the ventral part of the subthalamus, receives a massive projection from the lateral segment of the globus pallidus, and projects to both pallidal segments and to the mesencephalon.

Sucrase: The enzyme involved in the hydrolysis of sucrose to fructose and glucose. It is secreted by the tips of the villi of the epithelium in the small intestines.

Sulci (sing. = sulcus): A depression or fissure in the surface of an organ, most especially the brain.

Summation: An accumulation of effects, especially those of muscular, sensory, or mental stimuli.

Superior cervical ganglion: The largest of the cervical ganglia, it is placed opposite the second and third cervical vertebrae. It is reddish-gray, usually fusiform in shape, sometimes broad and flattened, and occasionally constricted at intervals. It is believed to be formed by the coalescence of four ganglia, corresponding to the upper four cervical nerves.

Superior colliculi: The part of the brain that sits below the thalamus and surrounds the pineal gland in the mesencephalon of vertebrate brains. This structure comprises the rostral aspect of the midbrain, anterior to the periaqueductal gray and adjacent to the inferior colliculus. The inferior and superior colliculi are known collectively as the *corpora quadrigemina*, or four twins.

Superior oblique muscle: A fusiform muscle in the upper, medial side of the orbit whose primary action is intorsion and whose secondary actions are to abduct (laterally rotate) and depress the eyeball (i.e., make the eye move outward and downward).

Superior rectus muscle: A muscle in the orbit. It is one of the extraocular muscles.

Superior sagittal sinus: An unpaired dural sinus in the sagittal groove.

Superior vena cava: The vein that carries blood to the right atrium from parts of the body that are superior to the heart.

Superovulation: The ovulation of an abnormally large number of ova for a given species. This is usually a result of exogenous hormonal treatment. It is often used to produce ova for embryo transfer, cloning, or transgenic manipulation of animals.

Supination: The rotation of the forearm such that the palm faces anteriorly.

Supporting cells: Cells that serve to provide support and protection and perhaps contribute to the nutrition of principal or other cells of certain organs; such cells are found in the labyrinth of the inner ear, organ of Corti, olfactory epithelium, taste buds, and seminiferous tubules.

Suppressors of cytokine signaling (SOCS): Intracellular proteins that regulate the activity of signaling pathways, especially STAT-associated pathways.

Suprachiasmatic nucleus: A nucleus in the hypothalamus, so named because it resides immediately above the optic chiasm (OX). It consists of two nuclei, each of which lies on either side of the hemisphere separated by the third ventricle (3V). Its principal function is to create the circadian rhythm, which regulates the body functions over the 24-hr period.

Supraglenoid tubercle: A projection of bone located superior to the glenoid cavity. It is the attachment site for the tendon of the long head of the biceps brachii m.

Supraspinous fossa: Smaller than the infraspinatus fossa, it is concave, smooth, and broader at its vertebral than at its humeral end; its medial two-thirds gives origin to the supraspinatus.

Surface tension: The force at the liquid surface of an air-water interface resulting from the greater attraction of water molecules to the surrounding water molecules than to the air above the surface; it is a force that tends to decrease the area of a liquid surface and resists stretching of the surface.

Sympathetic chains: Chains that extend from the base of the skull to the coccyx.

Sympathetic division: The division of the autonomic nervous system that is responsible for "fight or flight" reactions; it is primarily concerned with the elevation of metabolic rate and increased alertness.

Sympathetic subdivision: The subdivision that activates what is often termed the "fight or flight" response. This response is also known as Sympathetico-adrenal response of the body; the preganglionic sympathetic fibers that end in the adrenal medulla (but also all other sympathetic fibers) secrete acetylcholine, which activates the secretion of adrenaline (epinephrine) and to a lesser extent noradrenaline (norepinephrine) from it.

Symporter: Also known as a cotransporter, it is an integral membrane protein that is involved in secondary active transport. It works by binding to two molecules at a time and using the gradient of one solute's concentration to force the other molecule against its gradient.

Synapse: The junction across which a nerve impulse passes from an axon terminal to a neuron, a muscle cell, or a gland cell.

Synaptic bouton: Axonal terminals; the bulbous distal endings of the terminal branches of an axon; also called synaptic knob.

Synaptic cleft: The fluid-filled space at a synapse.

Synaptic delay: The period between the arrival of an impulse at the presynaptic membrane and the initiation of an action potential in the postsynaptic membrane.

Synaptic plasticity: The ability of the connection, or synapse, between two neurons to change in strength.

Synaptic vesicles: Small membranous sacs containing a neurotransmitter.

Syndesmochorial placenta: A type of epitheliochorial placenta in which endothelial epithelium becomes eroded so that material capillaries are exposed to the chorionic epithelial tissue.

Synergist: Muscle that aids the action of a prime mover by effecting the same movement or by stabilizing joints across which the prime mover acts to prevent undesirable movements.

Syrinx: The name for the vocal organ of birds. Located at the base of a bird's trachea, it produces sounds without the vocal cords that mammals have.

Systemic circuit: The vessels between the aortic valve and the entrance to the right atrium; the system other than the vessels of the pulmonary circuit.

Systemic circulation: The closed loop of blood vessels carrying blood between the heart and body systems.

Systems physiology: The study of the function of specific systems such as the cardiovascular, respiratory, or reproductive systems.

Systole: A period of contraction in a chamber of the heart, as part of the cardiac cycle.

Systolic blood pressure: The peak arterial pressure measured during ventricular systole.

T

T tubule (transverse tubule): The extension of the muscle cell plasma membrane (sarcolemma) that protrudes deeply into the muscle cell.

T wave: A deflection of the ECG corresponding to ventricular depolarization.

Tapetum lucidum: A reflecting layer immediately behind, and sometimes within, the retina of the eye of many vertebrates (though not humans); it serves to reflect light back to the retina, increasing the quantity of light caught by the retina.

Tarsal plates: Two thin, elongated plates of dense connective tissue, about 2.5 cm in length; one is placed in each eyelid, and contributes to its form and support.

Taste: One of the most common and fundamental of the senses of animals. It is the direct detection of chemical composition, usually through contact with chemoreceptor cells.

Tectorial membrane: A gelatinous membrane, attached to the bony spiral lamina, which overlies the hair cells within the cochlea of the inner ear.

Tectum: A rooflike structure of the body, especially the dorsal part of the mesencephalon.

Tegmentum: A part of the midbrain consisting of white fibers running lengthwise through gray matter.

Telodendria: The terminal axonal branches that end in synaptic knobs.

Temporal lobe: The lowest of the major subdivisions of the cortical mantle of the brain, containing the sensory center for hearing and forming the rear two-thirds of the ventral surface of the cerebral hemisphere. It is separated from the frontal and parietal lobes above it by the fissure of Sylvius.

Temporal summation: The summation of the local potential that results when two or more action potentials arrive at a single synapse in rapid succession.

Tendon: A band of tough, inelastic fibrous tissue that connects a muscle with its bony attachment and consists of rows of elongated cells; minimal ground substance; and densely arranged, almost parallel, bundles of collageneous fibers.

Tendon reflex: A myotatic or deep reflex in which the muscle stretch receptors are stimulated by percussing the tendon of a muscle.

Tensor tympani muscle: A muscle that originates from the cartilagenous wall of the eustachian tube (also called the auditory tube) and the bony wall surrounding the tube.

Terminal bouton: An enlarged axon terminal or presynaptic terminal.

Testosterone: The major male sex steroid, it is produced in the interstitial tissue of the testes by Leydig cells.

Tetrodotoxin: A potent neurotoxin, found in many puffer fish and certain newts.

Thermoreceptors: A sensory receptor that responds to heat and cold.

Thick filament: A cytoskeletal filament in a skeletal or cardiac muscle cell, it is composed of myosin, with a core of titin.

Thin filament: A cytoskeletal filament in a skeletal or cardiac muscle cell, consists of actin, troponin, and tropomyosin.

Third ventricle: A narrow, vertically oriented cavity in the midplane below the corpus callosum that communicates with each of the lateral ventricles through the interventricular foramen.

Thoracic cavity: A cavity that is surrounded by the ribs and muscles of the chest.

Thoracic inlet: The superior thoracic aperture refers to the superior opening of the thoracic cavity. It is referred to anatomically as the thoracic inlet and clinically as the thoracic outlet.

Thorax: The chest.

Threshold: The transmembrane potential at which an action potential begins.

Thromboplastin: A protease that converts prothrombin to thrombin in the early stages of blood clotting; also called thrombokinase.

Thrombopoietin (TPO): A glycoprotein hormone, produced mainly by the liver and the kidney, that regulates the production of platelets by the bone marrow. It stimulates the production and differentiation of megakaryocytes, the bone marrow cells that fragment into large numbers of platelets.

Thyroid: An endocrine gland whose lobes are lateral to the thyroid cartilage of the larynx.

Thyroxin: Also called T4, it is a hormone produced by the thyroid gland; it is less potent than T3 triiodothyronine, which is also produced in lesser amounts by the thyroid gland.

Tidal volume (TV): The volume of air moved into and out of the lungs during a normal quiet respiratory cycle.

Tissue factor (TF): A protein present in subendothelial tissue, platelets, and leukocytes necessary for the initiation of thrombin formation from the zymogen prothrombin. Thrombin formation ultimately leads to the coagulation of blood.

Tissue plasminogen activator: A thrombolytic agent (clot-busting drug). It's approved for use in certain patients having a heart attack or stroke. This drug can dissolve blood clots, which cause most heart attacks and strokes.

Titin: A giant 3 MDa muscle protein and a major constituent of the sarcomere in vertebrate striated muscle. It is a multidomain protein, which forms filaments approximately 1 μm in length spanning half a sarcomere. Titin has a number of functions, including the control of assembly of muscle thick filaments, a role in muscle elasticity, and the generation of passive tension.

Trabecula: A connective tissue partition that subdivides an organ.

Trachea: The windpipe, an airway extending from the larynx to the primary bronchi.

Transducin: The name given to the heterotrimeric G protein that is naturally expressed in vertebrate retina rods and cones (a different transducin gene is expressed in each cell type).

Transferrin: A plasma protein that transports iron through the blood to the liver, spleen, and bone marrow.

Transforming growth factor β (TGF-β): One of a number of structurally related growth factors involved in the regulation of growth, differentiation, and development of the many organ systems.

Transverse: Lying across the long axis of the body or of a part.

Transverse colon: The part of the colon from the hepatic flexure (the turn of the colon by the liver) to the splenic flexure (the turn of the colon by the spleen). The transverse colon hangs off the stomach, attached to it by a wide band of tissue called the mesocolon. The transverse colon is mobile (unlike the parts of the colon immediately before and after it), and it is very mobile in the abdomen of some individuals.

Transverse fissure: A short but deep fissure, about 5 cm long, extending transversely across the undersurface of the left portion of the right lobe, nearer its posterior surface than its anterior border.

Transverse fracture: A fracture in which the line of break forms a right angle with the axis of the bone.

Triad: The transverse tubule, and the terminal cisternae on each side of it, in a skeletal muscle fiber.

Tricuspid valve: The right atrioventricular valve, which prevents the backflow of blood into the right atrium during ventricular systole.

Trigger zone: A specific area that, when stimulated by touch, pain, or pressure, excites an attack of neurologic pain.

Triglyceride: A lipid that is composed of a molecule of glycerol attached to three fatty acids.

Trypsin inhibitor: Chemicals that reduce the bioavailability of trypsin, an enzyme essential to nutrition of many animals.

Tuber cinereum: A prominence of the base of the hypothalamus, extending ventrally into the infundibulum and pituitary stalk.

Tunic: One of the enveloping layers of a part; one of the coats of a blood vessel; one of the coats of the eye; one of the coats of the digestive tract.

Tunica externa: The outermost layer of connective tissue fibers that stabilizes the position of a blood vessel.

Tunica interna: The innermost layer of connective tissue fibers in a blood vessel; it consists of the endothelium plus an underlying elastic membrana.

Tunica media: The middle layer of connective tissue fibers in a blood vessel; it contains collagen, elastin, and smooth muscle fibers in varying proportions.

Tympanic membrane: Colloquially known as "the eardrum," it is a thin membrane that separates the external ear from the middle ear. Its function is to transmit sound from the air to the ossicles inside the middle ear.

Type I alveolar cells: The single layer of flattened epithelial cells that forms the wall of the alveoli within the lungs.

Type II alveolar (or septal, cells): The cells within the alveolar walls that secrete pulmonary surfactant.

U

Ultradian rhythms: The regular recurrence in cycles of less than 24 hr from one stated point to another, as certain biologic activities which occur at such intervals, regardless of conditions of illumination.

Undershoot: A temporary decrease below the final steady-state value that may occur immediately following the removal of an influence that had been raising that value.

Unipennate: Of or being a muscle whose fibers are attached obliquely to one side of a lateral tendon.

Unipolar neuron: A neuron in which embryological fusion of the two processes leaves only one process extending from the cell body.

Unmyelinated axon: An axon whose neurilemma does not contain myelin and across which continuous propagation occurs.

Upper respiratory system: The nasal cavity, pharynx, and associated structures.

Upstroke: The rising or depolarization phase of the action potential.

Urobilin: A compound derived from urobilinogen and ultimately from the bilirubin excreted in bile.

Urobilinogen: A colorless product of bilirubin reduction. It is formed in the intestines by bacterial action. Part of it is resorbed and returned to the liver, while the rest is excreted in feces. Trace amounts can be detected in urine.

Uterus: A hollow, tubular organ with layers of smooth muscle and internal epithelial lining. It connects the cervix and the oviducts. It is responsible for sperm transport to the site of fertilization in the oviducts, accepts the early embryo, and houses the fetus during gestation.

Uvea: The middle of the three concentric layers that make up an eye.

V

Vagus nerve: Also called pneumogastric nerve or cranial nerve X, it is the tenth of twelve paired cranial nerves, and is the only nerve that starts in the brain stem (within the medulla oblongata) and extends, through the jugular foramen, down below the head, to the abdomen. The vagus nerve is arguably the single most important nerve in the body.

Variable: A quantity that is capable of assuming any of a set of values.

Varicosities: A varicose enlargement or swelling.

Vascular endothelial growth factor: A substance made by cells that stimulates new blood vessel formation, a mitogen for vascular endothelial (vessel lining) cells.

Vascular tunic: The middle of the three concentric layers that make up an eye; also called the uvea.

Vasoconstriction: A reduction in the diameter of arterioles due to the contraction of smooth muscles in the tunica media, it elevates peripheral resistance and may occur in response to local factors through the action of hormones, or from stimulation of the vasomotor center.

Vasodilation: An increase in the diameter of arterioles due to the relaxation of smooth muscles in the tunica media, it reduces peripheral resistance and may occur in response to local factors through the action of hormones, or after decreased stimulation of the vasomotor center.

Vasomotor center: The chief dominating or general center, which supplies all the unstriped muscles of the arterial system with motor nerves, situated in a part of the medulla oblongata; it is a center of reflex action, by the working of which afferent impulses are changed into efferent, vasomotor impulses leading either to dilation or constriction of the blood vessels.

Vasomotor nerve fibers: Sympathetic nerve fibers that cause the contraction of smooth muscle in the walls of blood vessels, thereby regulating blood vessel diameter.

Vasomotor tone: A relatively constant frequency of sympathetic impulses that keep blood vessels partially constricted in the periphery.

Venous return: The volume of blood returned to each atrium per minute from the veins.

Venous valves: A multicuspid structure located inside a vein. The valve cusps are attached to the vein wall and grow in a conjoined state.

Ventral: Pertaining to the anterior surface.

Ventral respiratory group: The area that controls expiration and acts to increase the force of inspiration.

Ventral root: The efferent motor root of a spinal nerve. At its distal end, the ventral root joins with the dorsal root to form a mixed spinal nerve.

Ventricles: A fluid-filled chamber; in the heart, one of the large chambers discharging blood into the pulmonary or systemic circuits; in the brain, one of four fluid-filled interior chambers.

Vermis: The narrow middle zone occurring between the two hemispheres of the cerebellum.

Vestibular apparatus: The sensory system that provides the dominant input about our movement and orientation in space.

Vestibular membrane: A membrane inside the cochlea of the inner ear. It separates scala media from scala vestibuli.

Vestibular nystagmus: Rapid involuntary rhythmic eye movement, with the eyes moving quickly in one direction (quick phase), and then slowly in the other (slow phase).

Vestibule: An enlarged area at the beginning of a canal, i.e., inner ear, nose, larynx.

Visceral afferent: A pathway coming into the central nervous system that carries subconscious information derived from the internal viscera.

Visceral pleura: Serous membrane investing the lungs and dipping into the fissures between the several lobes.

Visceral serosa: The part of the double-layered membrane that lines the outer surfaces of organs within the ventral body cavity.

Vision: Visual perception via the visual system; one of the senses.

Visual pigments: Chemicals functioning in the visual cycle in retinal rod cells. Through excitation by visible light, a series of complex molecular changes occur that serve to trigger, in the optical nerve endings, an impulse transmitted to the brain, resulting in the perception of vision.

Vocal ligament: The band that extends on either side from the thyroid cartilage to the vocal process of the arytenoid cartilage.

Voltage-gated channels: Channels in the plasma membrane that open or close in response to changes in membrane potential.

Voluntary striated: Also called skeletal muscle.

W

Wandering macrophages: The macrophages that migrate to a wound to effect cellular defenses against invading pathogens.

Wave summation: An increase in the frequency with which a muscle is stimulated, which increases the strength of contraction.

White blood cells (WBCs): Leukocytes; the granulocytes and agranulocytes of blood.

White matter: Whitish nerve tissue, especially of the brain and spinal cord, chiefly composed of myelinated nerve fibers and containing few or no neuronal cell bodies or dendrites; also called alba, substantia alba, or white substance.

White muscle fibers: Those fibers that contain low levels of myoglobin and oxygen-storing proteins and have a white appearance.

White rami: A bundle of nerve fibers that connect a sympathetic ganglion with a spinal nerve and are divided into two kinds, one consisting of myelinated preganglionic fibers.

Withdrawal reflex: A spinal reflex intended to protect the body from damaging stimuli. The classic example is when you touch something hot and withdraw your body part from the hot object.

Woven bone: Bony tissue characteristic of the embryonic skeleton in which the collagen fibers of the matrix are arranged irregularly in the form of interlacing networks; also called nonlamellar bone or reticulated bone.

X

Xiphoid cartilage: The posterior and smallest of the three divisions of the sternum, below the gladiolus and the manubrium; also called xiphoid or xiphoid process.

Xiphoid process: The cartilage at the lower end of the sternum; also called ensiform cartilage, ensiform process, xiphisternum, or xiphoid cartilage.

Y

Yellow bone marrow: Bone marrow in which the meshes of the reticular network are filled with fat.

Z

Z discs (or Z lines): Delicate membranelike structures found at either end of a sarcomere to which the actin myofilaments attach.

Zonular fibers: A ring of fibrous strands connecting the ciliary body with the crystalline lens of the eye.

Zygomatic arch: The arch formed by the temporal process of the zygomatic bone and the zygomatic process of the temporal bone; also called zygoma.

Index